Improving Quality of Life for People with Disabilities Through Smart Technologies

Ikram Ur Rehman
https://orcid.org/0000-0003-0115-9024
University of West London, UK

Moustafa Nasralla
Prince Sultan University, Saudi Arabia

Drishty Sobnath
https://orcid.org/0009-0001-9639-0079
Heriot Watt University, UAE

Muazzam Ali Khan Khattak
Quaid-i-Azam University, Pakistan

Sundus Ali
https://orcid.org/0000-0002-5496-8303
NED University of Engineering and Technology, Pakistan

IGI Global
Scientific Publishing
Publishing Tomorrow's Research Today

Vice President of Editorial	Melissa Wagner
Director of Acquisitions	Mikaela Felty
Director of Book Development	Jocelynn Hessler
Production Manager	Mike Brehm
Cover Design	Jose Rosado

Published in the United States of America by
IGI Global Scientific Publishing
701 East Chocolate Avenue
Hershey, PA, 17033, USA
Tel: 717-533-8845 | Fax: 717-533-7115
Website: https://www.igi-global.com E-mail: cust@igi-global.com

Library of Congress Cataloging-in-Publication Data

Names: Rehman, Ikram Ur, 1985- editor | Nasralla, Moustafa, 1987- editor | Sobnath, Drishty, 1990- editor | Khattak, Muazzam Ali Khan, 1981- editor | Ali, Sundus, 1986- editor
Title: Improving quality of life for people with disabilities through smart technologies / edited by Ikram Ur Rehman, Moustafa Nasralla, Drishty Sobnath, Muazzam Ali Khan Khattak, and Sundus Ali.
Description: Hershey, PA : IGI Global Scientific Publishing, [2026] | Includes bibliographical references and index. | Summary: "This book intends to provide a comprehensive understanding of how smart technologies can address the challenges faced by people with disabilities in navigating their environment, performing everyday tasks, and engaging in education and employment. It explores innovative solutions, such as intelligent transportation systems, smart healthcare, smart education and Ambient Assisted Living (AAL), that can improve accessibility and independence while ensuring inclusivity and sustainability"-- Provided by publisher.
Identifiers: LCCN 2025026764 (print) | LCCN 2025026765 (ebook) | ISBN 9798337320335 hardcover | ISBN 9798337320342 paperback | ISBN 9798337320359 ebook
Subjects: LCSH: Technology and people with disabilities | People with disabilities--Services for | Technological innovations--Social aspects
Classification: LCC HV1568 .I47 2026 (print) | LCC HV1568 (ebook) | DDC 362.4/048--dc23/eng/20250812
LC record available at https://lccn.loc.gov/2025026764
LC ebook record available at https://lccn.loc.gov/2025026765

British Cataloguing in Publication Data
A Cataloguing in Publication record for this book is available from the British Library.

Table of Contents

Preface xiii

Chapter 1
Digital Technology Improving the Quality of Life for People With Disabilities . 1
Yogita Lamba, Department of Political Sciences, International Relations, Indira Gandhi National Open University, India
S. Srinivasan, Department of Humanities and Social Sciences, Graphic Era University, Dehradun, India
Ajay Kumar Singh, Department of Humanities and Social Sciences, Graphic Era University, Dehradun, India

Chapter 2
Enhancing Quality of Life for Students With Disabilities Through Accessible Smart Technologies in Higher Education 45
Nthabiseng Istorina I. Mahetlana, University of South Africa, South Africa
Marubini Christinah Sadiki, University of South Africa, South Africa

Chapter 3
The Role of AI and ML in Telemedicine and Smart Healthcare 75
J. John Shiny, Velammal College of Engineering and Technology, India
S. Haranya, Velammal College of Engineering and Technology, India
T. Sathiyarupa, Velammal College of Engineering and Technology, India
Jaithun Shifaya B. S., Velammal College of Engineering and Technology, India
P. Y. Sivanithi, Velammal College of Engineering and Technology, India

Chapter 4
AI-Powered Intelligent Transportation Technologies to Improve Accessibility and Mobility for Individuals With Disabilities 119
Ghulam Fiza, NED University of Engineering and Technology, Karachi, Pakistan
Hira Mariam, NED University of Engineering and Technology, Karachi, Pakistan

Chapter 5
Machine Learning to Enhance Road and Traffic Safety for Senior and Disabled Citizens 167
Soorya Sathish, Heriot-Watt University, Dubai, UAE
Cristina Turcanu, Heriot-Watt University, Dubai, UAE

Chapter 6
Smartwatch-Based Semi-Supervised Fall Detection Using Anomaly Detection Techniques 203
Meshall Alshalaan, King Abdullah University of Science and Technology, Saudi Arabia
Fouzi Harrou, King Abdullah University of Science and Technology, Saudi Arabia
Ying Sun, King Abdullah University of Science and Technology, Saudi Arabia

Chapter 7
Evolving Approaches to Static American Sign Language Fingerspelling Recognition 237
Ajay Menon, School of Mathematical and Computer Sciences, Heriot Watt University, Dubai, UAE
Mahmoud A. A. Mousa, School of Mathematical and Computer Sciences, Heriot Watt University, Dubai, UAE

Chapter 8
Deep Learning-Based Pakistan Sign Language Interpretation for Enhancing Communication for Individuals With Hearing Disabilities 273
Mehwish Raza, NED University of Engineering and Technology, Pakistan
Majida Kazmi, NED University of Engineering and Technology, Pakistan
Fauzia Yasir, NED University of Engineering and Technology, Pakistan

Chapter 9
Security, Privacy, and Trust in Smart Systems for People With Visual Disabilities 315
Bülent Gürsel Emiroğlu, Kırıkkale University, Turkey

Chapter 10
Adaptive Materials for Transformative Rehabilitation 357
Rajni Verma, CGC University, Mohali, India
Mahapara Abbass, MMEC, Maharishi Markandeshwar University, Mullana, India
Amandeep Singh Wadhwa, University Institute of Engineering and Technology, Panjab University, Chandigarh, India
Shalom Akhai, MMEC, Maharishi Markandeshwar University, Mullana, India

Chapter 11
Advancing Skin Cancer Diagnosis Using Computer Vision to Aid the Visually Impaired 397
Ratish Palanisamy, Heriot-Watt University, UAE
Drishty Sobnath, Heriot-Watt University, UAE
Heba Elshimy, Heriot-Watt University, UAE

Chapter 12
Development of an IoT-Enabled Wearable Device for Monitoring Elbow Movements in Children With Cerebral Palsy Using MAS, AMS, and QUEST: Improving Quality of Life of Cerebral Palsy Children 443
S. Thangam, Amrita School of Computing, Amrita Vishwa Vidyapeetham, Bengaluru, India
Ananya Ganapathi, Amrita School of Computing, Amrita Vishwa Vidyapeetham, Bengaluru, India
Deivanai Saravanan, Amrita School of Computing, Amrita Vishwa Vidyapeetham, Bengaluru, India
Sneha Thejassu Raghavan, Amrita School of Computing, Amrita Vishwa Vidyapeetham, Bengaluru, India

Compilation of References 467

About the Contributors 539

Index 547

Detailed Table of Contents

Preface...xiii

Chapter 1
Digital Technology Improving the Quality of Life for People With Disabilities . 1
Yogita Lamba, Department of Political Sciences, International Relations, Indira Gandhi National Open University, India
S. Srinivasan, Department of Humanities and Social Sciences, Graphic Era University, Dehradun, India
Ajay Kumar Singh, Department of Humanities and Social Sciences, Graphic Era University, Dehradun, India

According to the WHO, 16% of the global population lives with a disability, with 200 million facing significant functional challenges. Rising chronic illnesses like diabetes, cancer, and mental disorders make disability a growing global health and human rights concern. The UN's SDGs for inclusive growth face setbacks as many individuals encounter physical, mental, social, and economic barriers. The UN Disability Inclusion Strategy highlights the indivisibility of human rights. This study examines smart technologies and digital strategies to improve accessibility and quality of life for persons with disabilities. Conducted in Dehradun District, it assesses 53 individuals with disabilities to evaluate how digital technology enhances their lives. Data analysis is carried out using SPSS. The study aims to identify obstacles, assess current solutions, and propose innovative, user-centric smart technologies to bridge the disability divide, ensuring better social and economic inclusion.

Chapter 2
Enhancing Quality of Life for Students With Disabilities Through Accessible Smart Technologies in Higher Education 45
Nthabiseng Istorina I. Mahetlana, University of South Africa, South Africa
Marubini Christinah Sadiki, University of South Africa, South Africa

The integration of smart technologies in higher education has the potential to significantly enhance the quality of life for students with disabilities by fostering greater accessibility, independence, and inclusion. This chapter explores how emerging digital tools such as assistive software, artificial intelligence, adaptive learning systems, and smart campus infrastructure can address the unique challenges faced by students with disabilities. The chapter highlights how institutions can implement these technologies to create an inclusive learning environment by examining case studies, best practices, and policy frameworks. Furthermore, it discusses the barriers to technology adoption, including financial constraints, lack of awareness, and infrastructural limitations, while proposing strategies for overcoming these challenges. This chapter underscores the transformative role of smart technologies in ensuring equitable educational opportunities and improving the overall well-being of students with disabilities in higher education.

Chapter 3
The Role of AI and ML in Telemedicine and Smart Healthcare 75
J. John Shiny, Velammal College of Engineering and Technology, India
S. Haranya, Velammal College of Engineering and Technology, India
T. Sathiyarupa, Velammal College of Engineering and Technology, India
Jaithun Shifaya B. S., Velammal College of Engineering and Technology, India
P. Y. Sivanithi, Velammal College of Engineering and Technology, India

The field of medicine is changing as a result of the new ways that artificial intelligence and machine learning are being used in telemedicine and smart healthcare to improve patient care and streamline the delivery of healthcare.AI and ML systems can detect the beginning of disease, optimize treatment regimens, and enhance clinical results by evaluating enormous volumes of health data. They delve into the development of intelligent healthcare systems through increased diagnostic precision, individualized treatment regimens, and wearable remote monitoring, it can improve healthcare. They can streamline administrative tasks, offer 24/7 virtual medical support, and boost patient engagement with tailored health education. Additionally, they can optimize clinical trials, improve resource management, and support evidence-based clinical decisions, leading to better patient outcomes. Overall, AI and ML helps in streamline the diagnostic process and contribute to better healthcare outcomes.

Chapter 4
AI-Powered Intelligent Transportation Technologies to Improve Accessibility and Mobility for Individuals With Disabilities 119
Ghulam Fiza, NED University of Engineering and Technology, Karachi, Pakistan
Hira Mariam, NED University of Engineering and Technology, Karachi, Pakistan

This chapter examines how artificial intelligence (AI) can revolutionize the development of intelligent and inclusive transportation solutions that improve accessibility for impaired people. The chapter begins by exploring the difficulties that these various groups of disabled people face when using public transit. It then highlights AI-based technologies that are redesigning transportation, from natural language processing (NLP) and machine learning (ML) to Internet of Things (IoT) enabled real-time monitoring and computer vision (CV). It then discusses the exceptional needs of several disabilities that are met by AI applications, such as communication assistance, adaptive urban design, smart navigation, and autonomous vehicles. The chapter finally explains the associated challenges for the implementation of such advanced technologies including regulatory, ethical, and technical concerns, while presenting insights into policy recommendations and future trends for creating inclusive, AI-powered transportation networks in smart cities.

Chapter 5
Machine Learning to Enhance Road and Traffic Safety for Senior and Disabled Citizens 167
Soorya Sathish, Heriot-Watt University, Dubai, UAE
Cristina Turcanu, Heriot-Watt University, Dubai, UAE

Machine learning (ML) models have the potential to improve road safety by predicting and preventing accidents. Building on this idea, this study examines how ML can enhance safe transportation for the elderly and people with disabilities, who often face significant mobility challenges. Traditional transport safety strategies tend to react to accidents rather than proactively address risks, further disadvantaging these vulnerable road users. This chapter explores how predictions based on specific ML models can analyse accident patterns and inform specific safety measures. By integrating AI-based accident prediction with intelligent traffic systems, adaptive signals, and accessibility-focused solutions, this research explores solutions and recommendations to guide urban planning and create safer and more inclusive transport networks tailored to those who need them most.

Chapter 6
Smartwatch-Based Semi-Supervised Fall Detection Using Anomaly Detection Techniques 203
Meshall Alshalaan, King Abdullah University of Science and Technology, Saudi Arabia
Fouzi Harrou, King Abdullah University of Science and Technology, Saudi Arabia
Ying Sun, King Abdullah University of Science and Technology, Saudi Arabia

Fall detection systems are crucial for seniors to mitigate significant health risks and severe fall-related injuries. Traditional supervised methods rely on extensive labeled datasets, which are challenging and time-consuming. Imbalanced datasets, where fall events are rare compared to daily activities, further complicate training. To bypass these challenges, we propose a semi-supervised fall detection approach using a One-Class Support Vector Machine (1SVM) with accelerometric data from smartwatches. 1SVM needs only fall-free data for training and effectively detects falls without labels. Specifically, we applied 1SVM to six features extracted from the accelerometric data, smoothed magnitude, moving window min-max difference, variance, maximum, and minimum. We evaluated this approach using publicly available smartwatch data named the SmartFall dataset, demonstrating 1SVM's superior performance with an accuracy of 87%, outperforming SVM, k-nearest neighbors (KNN), and Naive Bayes.

Chapter 7
Evolving Approaches to Static American Sign Language Fingerspelling Recognition 237
Ajay Menon, School of Mathematical and Computer Sciences, Heriot Watt University, Dubai, UAE
Mahmoud A. A. Mousa, School of Mathematical and Computer Sciences, Heriot Watt University, Dubai, UAE

This review synthesizes research on static American Sign Language (ASL) alphabet recognition from images, comparing traditional machine learning pipelines, convolutional neural network (CNN) transfer learning, and hybrid or transformer-based models. The analysis spans 2016 to 2025 studies that detail preprocessing, model design, and quantitative results on datasets such as the ASL Alphabet and Sign Language MNIST. Classical approaches using engineered features with classifiers such as Support Vector Machines (SVMs) or Random Forests perform well in controlled settings but rely on robust segmentation and handcrafted descriptors. Transfer learning on CNN backbones, including MobileNetV2, ResNet, EfficientNet, DenseNet, and the Visual Geometry Group (VGG) models, achieves near-perfect within-dataset accuracy; pure and modified Vision Transformers (ViTs) and CNN–transformer hybrids also reach ceiling-level performance with favorable speed-to-accuracy tradeoffs. Most evaluations remain closed set and seldom report signer-independent splits, cross-dataset transfer, or deployment metrics.

Chapter 8
Deep Learning-Based Pakistan Sign Language Interpretation for Enhancing Communication for Individuals With Hearing Disabilities 273
Mehwish Raza, NED University of Engineering and Technology, Pakistan
Majida Kazmi, NED University of Engineering and Technology, Pakistan
Fauzia Yasir, NED University of Engineering and Technology, Pakistan

Sign language recognition is a critical area within computer vision and assistive technology, promoting inclusive communication for individuals with hearing impairments. While various international sign languages have been widely studied, Pakistan Sign Language (PSL) remains underexplored. This chapter, per the authors, presents a real-time PSL recognition system using the YOLOv5 object detection framework. A custom dataset of 3,963 images, augmented to 9,522 using rotation, noise addition, and exposure adjustment, was developed using hand signs from students at the Ida Rieu School for the Blind and Deaf. The model achieved an accuracy of 94.67%, outperforming previous PSL systems in static sign classification. Comparative analysis shows improved generalization in real world conditions, particularly with complex backgrounds and partial occlusions. Unlike earlier approaches limited to controlled environments, this system demonstrates practical applicability in educational contexts. Future work includes optimizing for low-power edge deployment and dynamic sign recognition.

Chapter 9
Security, Privacy, and Trust in Smart Systems for People With Visual Disabilities 315
Bülent Gürsel Emiroğlu, Kırıkkale University, Turkey

As smart systems become increasingly prevalent, ensuring their accessibility, security, privacy, and trustworthiness is paramount for individuals with visual disabilities. These users face unique interaction barriers. This chapter explores the intersection of smart technologies and these challenges, focusing on the heightened importance of security and privacy and their implications for user trust. It outlines essential design considerations for creating inclusive technologies, emphasizing multimodal feedback and compatibility with assistive tools. By highlighting case studies, best practices, and emerging trends, the chapter aims to provide valuable insights for researchers, practitioners, and policymakers dedicated to enhancing the quality of life for people with visual disabilities.

Chapter 10
Adaptive Materials for Transformative Rehabilitation 357
Rajni Verma, CGC University, Mohali, India
Mahapara Abbass, MMEC, Maharishi Markandeshwar University, Mullana, India
Amandeep Singh Wadhwa, University Institute of Engineering and Technology, Panjab University, Chandigarh, India
Shalom Akhai, MMEC, Maharishi Markandeshwar University, Mullana, India

This chapter examines how smart materials are driving a paradigm shift in disability rehabilitation, offering groundbreaking solutions to restore mobility, independence, and dignity. By leveraging responsive technologies like shape-memory alloys, electroactive polymers, and piezoelectric sensors, smart materials enable adaptive, personalized therapies that address the unique challenges faced by individuals with physical, sensory, or neurological disabilities. The chapter highlights real-world applications—from AI-powered prosthetics to self-adjusting exoskeletons—while addressing barriers like cost and accessibility. It concludes with a vision for an inclusive future where smart materials erase limitations and redefine what's possible in rehabilitation.

Chapter 11
Advancing Skin Cancer Diagnosis Using Computer Vision to Aid the Visually Impaired 397
Ratish Palanisamy, Heriot-Watt University, UAE
Drishty Sobnath, Heriot-Watt University, UAE
Heba Elshimy, Heriot-Watt University, UAE

Skin cancer is one of the most common forms of cancer, with early detection being crucial for effective treatment. Individuals with visual impairment often struggle to monitor skin lesions independently, typically depending on caregivers or dermatologists for assistance. This study develops a skin cancer detection system using dermoscopic images from the HAM10000 dataset, evaluating four deep learning models to assist caregivers and dermatologists in providing faster analysis for the individuals who are visually impaired. The research employs segmentation masks to crop images during preprocessing, with data augmentation and transfer learning for optimizing performance. Among the models used, EfficientNetV2-L achieved the highest accuracy of 95.1% and a recall of 86.3% for malignant lesions in binary classification, showing reliable classification of cancerous lesions. This system helps caregivers and dermatologists with a tool to efficiently monitor skin health for visually impaired individuals, reducing diagnostic delays and supporting faster decision making.

Chapter 12
Development of an IoT-Enabled Wearable Device for Monitoring Elbow Movements in Children With Cerebral Palsy Using MAS, AMS, and QUEST: Improving Quality of Life of Cerebral Palsy Children 443
S. Thangam, Amrita School of Computing, Amrita Vishwa Vidyapeetham, Bengaluru, India
Ananya Ganapathi, Amrita School of Computing, Amrita Vishwa Vidyapeetham, Bengaluru, India
Deivanai Saravanan, Amrita School of Computing, Amrita Vishwa Vidyapeetham, Bengaluru, India
Sneha Thejassu Raghavan, Amrita School of Computing, Amrita Vishwa Vidyapeetham, Bengaluru, India

Cerebral palsy (CP) is a group of permanent movement disorders that significantly affect a child's ability to move and maintain balance and posture. Among the many challenges faced by children with CP, restricted joint movement, particularly in the elbows, severely impacts daily activities and motor development. The research proposes the design and development of an IoT-enabled wearable device aimed at assisting and monitoring elbow movements in children with cerebral palsy. The proposed solution integrates sensors such as accelerometers, muscle sensor, and flex sensors to capture real-time data on elbow flexion and extension. Tardieu, Modified Ashworth, Range of motion and Active movement scales are used for spasticity and movement assessment in order to provide thorough input. The sensor data is then transmitted to a cloud-based platform via WiFi. The proposed IoT solution provides real-time support for children with CP and offers a scalable platform for continuous improvement in therapeutic interventions.

Compilation of References 467

About the Contributors 539

Index 547

Preface

INTRODUCTION

Advancements in smart technologies are redefining what is possible for individuals living with disabilities. From intelligent assistive devices to AI-driven healthcare systems, these innovations are dismantling long-standing barriers and enabling greater independence, mobility, communication, and overall well-being. As global populations age and chronic illnesses rise, the need for inclusive, technology-driven solutions has never been more urgent. In this context, the integration of digital tools, advanced materials, and adaptive systems holds remarkable potential to transform lives across physical, sensory, and cognitive domains.

Despite this potential, the disability divide persists in many societies. Inequities in access, affordability, digital literacy, and policy support continue to limit the benefits of technological progress for millions who stand to gain the most. Effective solutions must therefore be designed with a deep understanding of diverse user needs, cultural contexts, and structural barriers. This requires multidisciplinary collaboration—bringing together researchers, technologists, medical professionals, policymakers, and disability communities themselves.

This volume, *Improving Quality of Life for People with Disabilities Through Smart Technologies*, seeks to bridge research and practice by highlighting innovative, evidence-based approaches shaping the future of accessibility. Each chapter contributes insights into cutting-edge systems, applications, and methodologies that support inclusion in healthcare, transportation, communication, education, and rehabilitation. As editors, our goal is to present a comprehensive and globally informed reference that underscores both the promise and the responsibility of using smart technologies to foster a more equitable world.

CHAPTER OVERVIEW

Chapter 1 investigates how digital technologies enhance daily living for individuals with disabilities through a focused study conducted in Dehradun District, India. The authors assess both the benefits and persistent challenges, offering data-driven insights into inclusive digital ecosystems.

Chapter 2 explores accessible smart technologies within higher education, emphasizing adaptive learning systems, assistive software, and AI-based tools that help students with disabilities navigate academic environments more independently and equitably.

Chapter 3 examines the transformative role of AI and machine learning in telemedicine and smart healthcare. The authors highlight advancements in diagnostics, patient monitoring, and personalized treatment that enhance clinical outcomes for diverse patient populations.

Chapter 4 turns to intelligent transportation systems, demonstrating how AI-powered tools—from computer vision to IoT-enabled accessibility support—can improve mobility for individuals with physical, sensory, and cognitive impairments.

Chapter 5 focuses on machine learning–based road-safety enhancements for elderly and disabled citizens. Predictive modeling and adaptive infrastructure solutions are presented as mechanisms to build safer, more inclusive urban landscapes.

Chapter 6 presents a semi-supervised smartwatch-based fall detection approach using anomaly-detection techniques. The proposed method addresses the challenges of imbalanced datasets and offers promising results for real-time safety monitoring.

Chapter 7 provides a comprehensive review of static American Sign Language (ASL) fingerspelling recognition, comparing classical machine learning, CNN-based transfer learning, and transformer-enabled approaches for improved communication accessibility.

Chapter 8 introduces a deep learning model for Pakistan Sign Language interpretation using YOLOv5. The system demonstrates high accuracy and real-world applicability, addressing a significant gap in assistive communication technologies for the deaf community in Pakistan.

Chapter 9 evaluates security, privacy, and trust considerations in smart systems for individuals with visual disabilities. The chapter underscores the importance of inclusive design principles, multimodal feedback, and robust protections for sensitive user data.

Chapter 10 examines how adaptive smart materials enhance rehabilitation through responsive prosthetics, exoskeletons, and therapeutic devices, envisioning a future where personalized, tech-enabled interventions redefine physical recovery.

Chapter 11 investigates the role of computer vision in assisting visually impaired individuals with early skin cancer detection. The study evaluates advanced deep learning models and demonstrates how AI tools can support caregivers and clinicians.

Chapter 12 presents an IoT-enabled wearable device for monitoring elbow movements in children with cerebral palsy. Integrating multiple sensors and clinical assessment scales, the proposed system offers a scalable approach to improving therapeutic outcomes.

CONCLUSION

As this collection demonstrates, smart technologies are reshaping the global landscape of disability inclusion. Across sectors and disciplines, researchers are developing tools that not only compensate for impairments but actively enhance autonomy, communication, safety, and participation. This shift marks a profound evolution: technologies are no longer peripheral aids, but integral enablers of human potential.

Yet the path forward requires careful attention to ethics, equity, and the lived experiences of people with disabilities. Innovation must be guided by principles of accessibility, affordability, security, and user-centered design. Technologies must be responsive to real-world contexts, adaptable to diverse needs, and grounded in collaborative dialogue with the communities they aim to serve. Without this grounding, even the most advanced tools risk reinforcing existing disparities.

We hope this book serves as both a reference and an inspiration for continued progress. By bringing together global research efforts, we aim to illuminate emerging opportunities while acknowledging the work still to be done. It is our conviction that through sustained collaboration and responsible innovation, smart technologies will continue to expand the boundaries of what is possible—building societies where every individual can participate fully and thrive with dignity.

Chapter 1
Digital Technology Improving the Quality of Life for People With Disabilities

Yogita Lamba
https://orcid.org/0009-0007-6196-1111
Department of Political Sciences, International Relations, Indira Gandhi National Open University, India

S. Srinivasan
https://orcid.org/0009-0002-0179-9849
Department of Humanities and Social Sciences, Graphic Era University, Dehradun, India

Ajay Kumar Singh
https://orcid.org/0000-0003-0429-0925
Department of Humanities and Social Sciences, Graphic Era University, Dehradun, India

ABSTRACT

According to the WHO, 16% of the global population lives with a disability, with 200 million facing significant functional challenges. Rising chronic illnesses like diabetes, cancer, and mental disorders make disability a growing global health and human rights concern. The UN's SDGs for inclusive growth face setbacks as many individuals encounter physical, mental, social, and economic barriers. The UN Disability Inclusion Strategy highlights the indivisibility of human rights. This study examines smart technologies and digital strategies to improve accessibility and quality of life for persons with disabilities. Conducted in Dehradun District, it assesses

DOI: 10.4018/979-8-3373-2033-5.ch001

53 individuals with disabilities to evaluate how digital technology enhances their lives. Data analysis is carried out using SPSS. The study aims to identify obstacles, assess current solutions, and propose innovative, user-centric smart technologies to bridge the disability divide, ensuring better social and economic inclusion.

INTRODUCTION

According to World Health Organization (WHO) 16% of the world's population (1 in 6 persons) live with some kind of disability, out of them approximately 200 million face considerable difficulties in functioning (WHO, 2022). With the rising global average ageing population, increasing chronic health related issues like diabetes, cancer, and mental health disorders, and the higher risk of disability in older people, in the years to come disability is going to become a greater concern in world health arena and a significant issue of human rights (Lang et al., 2011; Dev et al., 2025). United Nations' SDGs aiming to achieve inclusive growth faces setback as significant population faces barriers to inclusion due to disabilities (physical, mental, social and economic).

Digital inclusion can provide persons with disabilities access to education, financial services and skill development and further enabling them to get employment. Similarly, smart technologies can enable them to live an independent life. An inclusive digital economy for people with disabilities – creation of new jobs, inclusive workplaces, and production of smart devices for ease-of-living- is the way ahead to meet potential economic growth, utilizing its labor-force to the fullest. Since no single organization can resolve these issues on its own, cooperation and a public-private strategy are essential to achieving digital fairness (Yadav et al., 2021).

The UN Disability Inclusion Strategy reaffirms that complete realization of human rights is indivisible and integral part of fundamental of being. Smart technologies and associated digital strategies aimed at improving the quality of life for persons with disabilities through access to facilities and services using smart technologies (Bricout et al., 2021). The aim of the study is to improve accessibility of people with disabilities in social and economic spheres through user-centric and customized smart technology solutions (Vojinovic et al., 2024).

The United Nation presented its first ever report on Sustainable Development Goals and People with Disabilities in 2018 titled "Realization of Sustainable Development Goals by, for and with persons with disabilities" (Eberle et al., 2022). The report viewed the persons with disabilities as both agents and beneficiaries of development and thereby called for concrete actions to be adopted for inclusion of the worlds 15% population in developmental process as they remain at a significant disadvantage regarding most of the sustainable development goals (Leal Filho et al.,

2019). Analyzing the current status, UN 2018 Special Report on SDG and Persons with Disabilities highlighted –The need for inclusive policies to ensure equitable access to services and opportunities. The importance of accessibility in both physical and virtual environment, thus marking the significance of role of smart information and communication technologies in addressing these gaps and empowering the persons with disabilities (Jamwal et al., 2022). The smart technologies, software, devices & equipments that assist people with disabilities perform their day to day tasks with ease are called Assistive Technology, thereby improve their quality of life and empower them (Srinivasan & Rajavel, 2025).

Types of Persons With Disabilities and Their Special Needs for Smart Technologies

Cognitive Disability- A condition in which the person's ability to think, learn, remember and take decisions is compromised, it is known as cognitive disability. People with cognitive disability have difficulty remembering and completing tasks, and therefore requires assistance with processing information, memory and organization. Smart technology provides solutions through reminders, calendars, and software that convert Text –to -Speech or Speech –to –Text (Szabó et al., 2023).

Mobility Disability- A wide range of conditions can lead to mobility disability in a person- it could be balance and coordination disability or walking disability, which impacts the physical activities of the person (Mahmoudi-Dehaki et al., 2025). Mobility aids must not be seen limited to wheelchairs as they also include accessible transportation like self driving cars to powered wheelchairs and exo-skeletons. Some of these are discussed in detail in this chapter further. Physical limitations at larger level include inaccessibility to public spaces which can be resolved through curb -cuts at the point of street and side walk meeting, along with lifts and ramps in public infrastructure (Mann, 2005).

Visually Impaired- According to World Health Organization (WHO), globally 2.2 billion people have vision impairment and this account to a total cost of US $411 Billion, posing an enormous financial burden (Rizzo et al., 2023). Smart technologies offer immense potential for vision impairment with tools like smart eyewear, smart canes, screen readers, Optical Character Recognition (OCR) that converts to digital text for readers, etc. Smart technology used in eye-care and eye- treatments can also help avoid vision impairment from worsening.

Speech Disability- Speech impairments or speech disorders are difficulties that affect a person's ability to communicate effectively, the causes of it range from development delays or neurological conditions. AI-powered speech recognition and augmentative communication systems (Bhardwaj et al., 2024).

Disabilities Associated with Age – Aging is a natural process and so are the growing disabilities like physical and cognitive with age. Elderly people (65 years and above) develop mobility issues, vision disabilities and cognitive decline, and require special devices to make their old age easier. Smart technologies like mobility aids (smart scooters and wheelchairs), health monitoring systems (GPS enabled), and assistive communication devices help them accept their old age with ease (Klingbeil et al., 2004; Oladele et al., 2021) .

Hearing Disabilities- Hearing loss impacts communication ability negatively and also has an effect on person's security, this leads to isolation and depression. Low-tech assistive devices include vibrating alarm clocks and flashing doorbells. Smart tech assistive devices known as Assistive Listening Devices (ALDs) are specialized technologies devised for individuals with hearing loss – this includes Bluetooth systems, Infrared systems, induction loops etc (Rominger & Eiten, 2019; Ekpete, 2024) .

Children born with Disabilities- According to UNICEF data, nearly 240 Million children in the world suffer from some of disability in the world today. One of the major being learning disability (LD), which requires special assistive technology including computer programs and tablet applications that provide word prediction capabilities (WordQ), text – to – speech (example: Kurzweil 3000) etc. These smart technologies have the potential to make children with disabilities have access to education and open up opportunities to live and build a dignified life for themselves (Ekepete, 2024).

Social and Economic Disabilities- Individuals with disparities face deprivation and disparity in multiple social and economic sectors like education, employment, income and overall quality of life, often stemming from systemic discrimination. These disparities often remain overseen on framing and implementation of governmental policies and programs. Smart technologies play important tool for government and policy makers to address these socio-economic disabilities by implementing accessible digital services and providing subsidized assistive technologies to foster social inclusion and economic integration through financial inclusion (internet banking and mobile banking that allowing people with physical disabilities) (Santoso, 2023).

Smart Home for the People With Disabilities

The advent of smart technology based ecosystem for home called smart home has greatly enhanced the quality of life of disabled persons by ensuring safety and independence. These technologies include voice-activated assistants like the Amazon's Alexa which on command can control lights, thermostats, vacuum cleaners and multiple electronic devices linked to it. Smart homes ensure low dependence on others through adaptive equipment like automated door openers and adjustable counter tops specifically catering to the needs of persons with mobility impairments. Researchers found technology to have improved the participation, independence and quality of life among the people with disabilities and other complex needs (Jamwal et al., 2022).

AI equipped 'smart homes' include use of smart monitoring system and mental disabilities like Alzheimer or dementia (Srinivasan et al., 2025). The different forms of smart homes based on their distinctive purposes are as follows:

1. Smart Homes for people with disabilities due to old age (dementia, memory loss, mobility, vision loss etc.)
2. Smart Homes for people with speech related disabilities.
3. Smart Homes for people cognitive or other mental disabilities
4. Smart Homes for people with physical disabilities related to movement.
5. Smart Homes for people with low vision.

Studying the integration of smart homes for intellectually disabled persons, researchers analyzed that smart home technologies not just foster autonomy and enhance accessibility through voice or visual feedback system by alleviating caregiver's burden, but smart home technologies also have social and psychological benefits of enhancing self-esteem and social inclusion. The study further finds extremely positive attitude of intellectually disabled persons towards using safety technologies (Ojasalo et al., 2010).

Definition of Smart Environment: Smart environments improve the quality of life for persons with disabilities. Smart homes enhance accessibility, independence, and safety, while smart cities extend these benefits to public spaces through inclusive infrastructures that ensure mobility, communication, and participation. The shift from smart homes to smart cities moves from individual empowerment to collective inclusion, connecting personal well-being with community accessibility (Attar et al., 2024).

Smart Homes to Smart Cities

Digital technologies improve the quality of life for persons with disabilities by enhancing accessibility, independence, and safety in smart homes. Yet, their greater potential lies in extending to public spaces through smart cities, which ensure mobility, communication, and participation at a societal level. This shift marks a move from individual empowerment to collective inclusion, bridging personal well-being with community accessibility (Srinivasan et al., 2025).

Section Ending Recommendations

Smart Homes: "Smart homes enhance daily living and independence, but these benefits must expand to public spaces for wider inclusion."

Smart Cities: "Inclusive smart city frameworks complement personal technologies by enabling broader participation and equal opportunities."

Socio-Cultural Challenges

While smart homes and cities enhance accessibility and independence, socio-cultural challenges—such as attitudes toward disability, social stigma, and limited awareness—can hinder adoption and effective use. Addressing these barriers is essential to ensure that technological advancements translate into real inclusion and equal participation in both personal and public environments (AI-Homoud, 2025).

Smart Cities for the People With Disabilities

Currently, over half of the total population of persons with disabilities resides in urban areas and it is estimated that 15% of urban population will constitute people living with disabilities by 2050. The concept of developing smart cities provides an optimistic opportunity to create equitable urban landscapes for people of disabilities by accessible infrastructure and services.

Smart cities refer to urban areas that utilize digital technologies and data driven solutions for efficient resource management to improve quality of urban services and operations, thereby improve quality of life of the residents and address various challenges related to urbanization (Kitchen, 2019). Smart cities offer diverse tools to enhance accessibility and quality of life through IoT infused infrastructure and inclusive transportation systems benefitting not only individuals with disabilities but also whole community by promoting sustainability and socio-economic inclusion of all (Pearson & Shafik, 2024).

Table 1. Key Domain for Smart Cities for PWDs

Key Domains of Smart Cities for PWDs (Physical and Cognitive)
Technology integration: AI, IoT, sensors, automation etc. Data driven decision making: Traffic management Urban Mobility: Smart pedestrian pathways and PWDs friendly infrastructure Quality of life of vulnerable people: Smart parking and buildings Safety and Security: Smart CCTVs and Healthcare tracking Citizen engagement: e Governance & e-participation Connectivity: sustainable mobility to schools, colleges and public places

Robotics for the People With Disabilities

Robotics has high potential to benefit the lives of persons living with disabilities be it physical or mental. Apart from the obvious role as a manipulator in form of mounted on a desk, wheelchair or body born, it also aids in mobility, education and communication. Therefore, assistive robotics is the collection of connected technologies to serve the needs of people with various kinds of disabilities (Hillman, 2006). For hundreds of years, people with lower limb impairments have had to rely on crutches and wheelchairs to navigate the world. However, their mobility still remains limited, and long-term wheelchair use can have both negative physical and mental affect. South Korean researchers developed wearable robots– robotic exosuit or exoskeleton that helps paraplegics walk again fully upright without any need for crutches simply by wearing it. This reduced the dependence on wheelchair as the primary solution.

Generally, robots can offer companionship to older adults, helping them feel less alone. It is useful for assisting older people. Similarly, Assistive Mobile Manipulators (AMMs) display immense potential to one day help people with disabilities by serving as surrogates, therefore would give them the autonomy in performing small regular tasks like scratching, picking and socializing (Chen et al., 2013).

General Smart Technologies for the Persons With Disabilities

Smart technologies include smart devices like computers, laptops, phones etc. and a network of technologies that provide real-time information which helps people maker better informed decisions and provide smart solutions to their problems (Washburn et al., 2009). For the ultimate goal is to make disabled people to be accepted in society as 'normal' and to live an independent and life of dignity. To make them integrated in the society, people with disabilities must be integrated into smart technology (Troussas et al., 2020).

Virtual Assistance

Multiple intelligent devices installed into the home environment as part of smart-home, provide residents with both assistance in physical mobility and also, 24 Hours real-time health monitoring. The modern 'home-installed systems' are not only versatile in functioning but also tend to provide emotional support to the user, example – performing functions without causing any inconvenience to them (Stefanov et al., 2004).

Voice Assistance

Voice assistant technologies are software based smart technologies that have the ability to interpret human speech and respond to it via synthesized voices, the most famous in current times are the Apple's Siri, Google Assistant, and Amazon's Alexa. These are found as an inbuilt feature of your smart phones or smart speakers. From ordering food online to booking train tickets, from shopping clothes to buying medicines, the modern world functions are performed in online sphere and have become the very basic aspects of well being, however this is also creating a divide as people with disabilities falling behind in adapting to these technologies. For example: most of these functions require using a website or application, which is not easy for the visually impaired. The voice assistants have the ability to access application through voice command and thereby place orders. Similarly, voice assistants can perform basic functions like drawing the drapes, checking the lock on gate, turning lights ON/OFF, and operating other electronic appliances. These functions make lives of people living with disabilities like the visually impaired or mobility impaired to perform the very basic functions themselves, giving them independent and dignified quality of life (Doobransky & Hargittai, 2006; Humphry & Chesher, 2021; Tajadod, 2021).

Self Driving Cars

Autonomous Vehicles: (AVs) have long promised a greater opportunities and freedom for the people with disabilities. From no deny of service based on prejudice, to providing independent transportation options self-driving cars allow disabled community better access to employment and services. Wheelchair –accessible robotaxis with smart technologies like Smartphone control are being developed my private companies like Cruise.

BACKGROUND OF THE STUDY

Digital technology significantly improves the quality of life for people with disabilities by addressing challenges in mobility, communication, education, and employment. The integration of assistive technologies, AI, and IoT supports independence and participation (Srinivasan et al., 2025). With 1.3 billion people (16% of the global population) living with disabilities, inclusive digital solutions are essential. Assistive tools like screen readers, speech recognition, and adaptive devices support those with visual, hearing, and physical impairments. AI applications enhance communication through predictive text, voice-to-text, and translation.

Wearables such as smart prosthetics and exoskeletons improve mobility and daily functioning. In education, digital platforms and accessible LMS offer personalized learning using tools like text-to-speech, closed captions, and adaptive software. Employment opportunities have grown through remote work and digital accessibility. Global organizations like the UN and WHO promote digital inclusion through frameworks such as the CRPD. However, barriers like affordability, low digital literacy, and poor infrastructure, especially in low- and middle-income countries, still exist. Ethical concerns including privacy, bias, and lack of user-centered design also need attention. This study examines how digital technologies impact people with disabilities, identifies key enablers and obstacles, and offers policy suggestions to enhance digital inclusivity and create a more inclusive society.

SCOPE OF STUDY

This study aims to explore the smart technologies and associated strategies necessary to enhance quality of life of people with disabilities. The research will focus on: This study focuses on individuals with disabilities from diverse socioeconomic and technological backgrounds. It aims to understand the varying accessibility challenges experienced by specially-abled persons across urban, suburban, and rural settings. These technologies contribute to enhancing ease of living and social inclusion for individuals with disabilities. TIt emphasizes the need for digital tools that are not only functional but also user-friendly for specially-abled users. Such engagement ensures that solutions are inclusive, practical, and rooted in real-world experiences. The study also undertakes a comprehensive policy analysis to assess the effectiveness of current frameworks and regulations in promoting digital inclusivity. It seeks to identify gaps and suggest improvements for addressing the unique needs of specially-abled users.

A critical component of the research involves examining the issue of technology acceptance among specially-abled individuals, particularly in rural areas where infrastructure and digital literacy may be limited. In addition to these areas, the study investigates other persistent roadblocks to digital inclusivity, such as affordability, stigma, and lack of awareness or training. Furthermore, it assesses the potential of emerging technologies—including artificial intelligence and other cutting-edge tools—in enhancing accessibility and user experience. The research also includes an evaluation of international frameworks and user-centric initiatives aimed at promoting digital inclusion for persons with disabilities, providing a global perspective on best practices and scalable models. By leveraging surveys, interviews, and case studies, the study seeks to offer actionable and scalable solutions. Its overarching goal is to reduce the digital exclusion of specially-abled individuals and to ensure their full participation in socio-economic activities in the era of digital transformation.

RESEARCH OBJECTIVES

1. Identify Barriers: Investigate the specific problems that specially-abled persons have while accessing and using smart technologies including digital services.
2. Assess Digital Literacy: Determine the current level of digital literacy among specially-abled persons and how it affects their ability to navigate emerging technologies and digital world.
3. Evaluate Existing Solutions: Assess the efficacy of current digital strategies, methods, and technology in meeting the demands of specially-abled populations.
4. Propose innovative strategies: Create actionable and user-centered recommendations for improving the accessibility and inclusion of specially-abled persons.
5. Encourage Policy Advocacy: Propose policy frameworks that assure long-term digital inclusion while also addressing the special needs of the specially-abled persons.

RESEARCH QUESTIONS

◇ **Barriers to Access** – Main digital challenges faced by people with disabilities, including socioeconomic, regional, cultural, and linguistic factors.
◇ **Digital Literacy and Skills** – The role of training and awareness in enabling effective use of smart technologies.
◇ **Inclusive Design and Customization** – Importance of user-centric features and tailoring assistive technologies to diverse needs.
◇ **Perceptions and Community Support** – Trust, usefulness, and the role of community systems in bridging digital gaps.
◇ **Policies and Global Best Practices** – Regulatory frameworks and successful strategies from other regions to promote long-term digital inclusion.

RELEVANT REVIEW

Impact of Smart Technologies on the Life of PWDs

Inclusive Workplaces: SMARTDISABLE project was launched to provide persons with disabilities with adequate and accessible workplace environment, enabling them to access ICTs effectively, with the major component of this project is known as 'Smart Help' for persons with disability. Smart Help solution is applicable in all profession settings, from offices and manufacturing to hospitals etc. (Kbar et al., 2015). As per the study 'Smart Help' provides the following solutions:

a. Auto Emergency Response to assist persons with disabilities in emergency scenarios.
b. Intelligent intervention on the basis of behavior of individual with disability to guide and warn them.
c. Voice recognition along with keyboard and mouse.
d. Favorable opportunities for individuals with disabilities to participate at workplace.

Inclusive Education: According to UNICEF, globally nearly 240 Million children living with disabilities are being denied basic rights with 42% less likely to have foundational reading and numerical skills and 49% more likely to have never attended school. World Bank's study Disability Gaps in Educational Attainment and Literacy that studied 19 developing countries highlights that primary school completion for children with disabilities in these countries is only 48% accounting for three in ten children with disabilities have never been in school.

Software programs to teach sign language using Android in Kerala (India) for a school for the deaf which showed positive results as learners were able to use the same books for learning vocabulary in sign language (Joy & Balakrishnan, 2019). Multimedia resource developed and tested to teach arithmetic skills to 11 deaf students of Grade 1 after compared to conventional teaching approach in Grade 1 in two boarding schools for deaf learners (Techaraungrong et al., 2017). Similarly, assistive technology provides aid in multiple domains including communication, learning and mobility. Educational Technology commonly known as EdTech has played significant role in enabling learners with disabilities in accessing school and thereby educational and social exclusion, enabling them to enjoy the benefits of school curriculum and participate in various educational activities (Lynch et al., 2024).

Financial Inclusion: World Health Organization (WHO) has categorized the obstacles faced by people with disabilities (PWDs) to financial inclusion into 5:

1. Lower demand of formal financial services among people with disabilities compared to those without disabilities.
2. Banks have low expectations of people with disabilities and are not welcomed by the banks.

3. Need of more appropriate technologies to overcome communication barriers faced by people with disabilities. Information and Communication Technology (ICT) currently present lags behind in meeting the web accessibility needs.
4. Financial services not tailored to meet the needs of people with disabilities
5. Need of inclusive infrastructure to make formal financial systems more accessible to people with disabilities.

FinTech adoption doesn't directly impact the financial well-being and financial inclusion of people with disabilities. More than FinTech, financial well-being of people with disabilities can be explained based on mediating factors (financial knowledge, access and behavior), financial access being the most significant of these all (Gafoor & Amilan, 2024). To address financial barriers experienced by persons with disabilities there is need to include ICT, digital innovation and multi -stakeholder collaboration (Puli et al., 2024).

Women with Disabilities: According to UNFPA report, female with disabilities are ten times more likely to experience violence than their non-disabled counterparts. In India, 11.8 Million women and girls with disabilities face augmented vulnerabilities. UNFPA advice leveraging technology to empower women and girls with disabilities as digital solutions can bridge accessibility gaps. Digital innovations like AI-powered chatbots and emergency alert systems provide crucial support. UNICEF report by Alessandaro Di Rosa and Megan T. Tucker (2022) – Accessible and Inclusive Digital Solutions for Girls with Disabilities recommends

i. Engaging with the caregivers of girls with disabilities and other stakeholders.
ii. Investing in digital skills education for girls with disabilities
iii. Careful designing of digital tools to reach girls with disabilities

There is however a major research gap in this aspect, smart technologies for women with disabilities.

Elderly & Age Related Disabilities: Around 10% of people above the age of 65 years suffer from cognitive impairments that directly impact their ability to independently perform any daily task. One such common cognitive disability is Alzheimer that results in a decline in cognitive performance in the elderly population. A person with Alzheimer would be unable to take care of themselves, perform household chores etc. In general, people with cognitive disabilities are among the lowest in using assistive technologies and therefore there's a growing need to develop smart technologies that meet the specific demands of this group (Mann, 2005).

Current Status of Smart Technologies and Associated Issues

Digital Divide and Overcoming the Information Gap

People with disabilities are at a disadvantage in accessing information mainly due to physical and cognitive barriers that further limit their social interactions and participation and economic opportunities. The digital divide here refers to the disparities in access to use of and literacy about technology. According to US government reports, more than 1 in 3 disabled persons i.e. 38% in the United States do not own a computer. While 84% of people above the age of 15 years use internet for some work or another, the percentage of internet users among people with disabilities in the United States still remain low at 65% (Gell et al., 2015).

This existence of information divide faced by persons with disabilities, particularly in relation to access to and utilization of digital technologies can be solved through building smart environment which needs proper (Nam & Park, 2017). The largest groups affected are likely to be the elderly, the physically and mentally disabled and the chronically sick (Commission for Rural Communities, 2005; Social Exclusion Unit, 2001, p. 12). Thus it creates a vicious cycle of social and digital exclusion among the people with disabilities. Smart environment and smart society have the potential to further widen the information divide experienced by people with disabilities in the future. Thus a targeted ICT education program aimed to improve the skills of people with disabilities is the need of the hour (Nam & Park, 2017). Smart homes are a road to independent living for people with disabilities; however a major setback that lies ahead is the affordability challenge and implementation constraints. While smart homes are becoming more of a need than a luxury day by day, they however are still not economically accessible to the common people (Ahmed et al., 2016).

Table 2. Role of Smart Homes and overcoming the accessibility issues

MART HOME FEATURES	APPLIATIONS	BENEFITS WITH DISABILITIES	POTENTIAL
Monitoring Systems	1. Fire and smoke detection with alarm 2. Temperature, ventilation, lighting monitoring	1. Physical mobility 2. Hearing 3. Vision 4. Cognitive 5. Elderly	1. Help in emergency detection 2. Help in monitoring for disabled people
Special Assistive Technologies	1. Voice command controlled appliances 2. Hand free systems 3. Powered wheelchairs	1. Physical mobility 2. Vision 3. Hearing 4. Elderly	1. Decrease need of caregivers 2. Make daily activities easy
Security Systems	1. Security front door cameras 2. Intelligent door and window locks 3. Facial recognition systems	1. Physical mobility 2. Elderly 3. Vision 4. Speech 5. Cognition 6. Hearing	1. Provide secure home environment to people with disabilities living alone
Interactive Communication Systems	1. Medical systems for interaction with patients from home 2. Social interaction assistance systems	1. Physical mobility 2. Hearing 3. Elderly 4. Cognitive 5. Vision 6. Speech	1. Help in accessing medical care 2. Help in maintain social relations
Home Automation Systems	1. Remote controlled home appliances 2. Intelligent household devices	1. Physical Mobility 2. Elderly 3. Cognitive 4. Hearing 5. Vision 6. Speech	1. Ease of living 2. Improve quality of life 3. Less dependence on caregivers

Role of Smart Cities Around the Globe and Overcoming the Challenges

Smart cities showed positive impact on enhancing accessibility to public services, healthcare, and transportation etc. for people with disabilities in Saudi Arabia. The integration of smart traffic systems and intelligent public spaces and transportation made it easier for PWDs to interact with city environment (Attar et al., 2024). Smart technologies are used in public spaces in Smart cities to make it more inclusive, such as providing real –time information on accessibility features with better signage, ramps and tactile paths. However, despite advancements, not all smart technologies are accessible to PWDs, especially as they lack proper design considerations (for instance visual and auditory disabilities). Smart city planners are encouraged to prioritize universal design principles, ensuring that smart city technologies are usable by everyone, regardless of their disabilities (Zhou et al., 2024).

Developed V/s Developing

When it comes to smart technologies there is not debate that strong hold on research and finances, the forerunners are the developed states like USA, European nations, South Korea etc. According to reports by Statista, USA leads the way in smart home technologies and adaptation, with more than 25 Million of USA houses as smart homes. Similarly, reports suggest that implementation and adaptation of smart homes in other developed countries like UK, Germany, South Korea and China rose to 500% within the year 2020. The global smart home size is was valued at $80 Billion in 2022. Persons with disabilities in Africa face multifaceted challenges in accessing ICT and it highlights the intersection of disability with poverty, education, infrastructure and policy (Wanjiku Wang'ang'a, 2024). Total Communication with Animation Dictionary (TCAD) helped deaf learners in primary schools of Thailand improve retention skills using sign language, lip reading, finger spelling etc. (Wicha et al., 2012). An analytical study of 7 Low and Middle Income Countries conducted by GSMA 'The Digital Exclusion of Women with Disabilities' identified that the disability gap for internet widens progressively with each stage. As instance GSMA highlights in Kenya persons with disabilities are 11% less likely to own a mobile phone than those not disabled, and 85% less likely to use it. The gap varies majorly by country, for example- in Bangladesh 55% PWDs are less likely to own a mobile than those without disabilities.

In Egypt, a proposal of a new smart home wireless sensor network suitable for Alzheimer people and the elderly called E/D- WSH system which provides complete solution for whole home environment based on RFID system, proximity sensor, gas leakage detection system etc. (Katsivelis et al., 2017). Use of EdTech for people with disabilities in low and middle income countries needs further long term and robust research that includes learners, curriculum design to comprehensively understand the impact on improving education experiences for the children with disabilities (Lynch et al., 2024).

Existing Technologies Issues and How to Overcome Them

Majority of Information and Communications Technology (ICT) designs currently used are inaccessible which creates barriers, developing innovative technologies offer unprecedented support- millions have access to digital versions and new tools like GPS, imagine recognition, near-field communication and internet connectivity allow independent living.

Table 3. Relevant Recent Research Study

S. No.	Author and Year	Country	Objective	Methodology	Outcome of the study
1.	(Soar & Croll, 2007)	Australia	To examine how Assistant technologies (AT) can be effectively integrated in smart homes to improve quality of life of people with disabilities.	Case study approach. 1. Designing and development of a prototype of a smart home. 2. Testing and evaluation in real life settings. 3. Qualitative and quantitative data collection through interviews and observations.	1. AT reduce the reliance on medical staff and caregivers. 2. AT improved quality of life enabling PWDs to live more independently. 3. AT enable caregivers to receive real –time health data, this improves personalized care and response time. 4. Smart homes can integrate technologies to meet specific need of people with disabilities.
2.	(Nam & Park, 2017)	South Korea	Understanding the role of ICT particularly Smart Homes in bridging the gaps for disabilities.	Qualitative research methodology: 1. Case study analysis of existing smart homes. 2. Interviews and surveys for data collection. 3. Comparative analysis.	Positive impact in reducing information divide for people with disabilities by: 1. Improving access to information and overcoming barriers such as physical accessibility, sensory impairments etc. 2. Enhancing communications by allowing PWDs to interact with media and services, increasing the independence. Highlighted challenges and barriers like: 1. Lack of awareness 2. High cost 3. Technological literacy
3.	(Almufaresh et al., 2024)	Pakistan	To develop a conceptual model for integrating AI into inclusive technologies aimed at enhancing disability inclusion.	Conceptual and theoretical: 1. Literature review of existing literature on inclusive technology. 2. Conceptual model development based on interviews and surveys	1. Development of a conceptual model outlining strategies and approaches for designing inclusive AI. 2. Highlighted the role of AI in disability inclusion, underscoring the potential of AI in reducing barriers and create equitable opportunities for disabled persons. 3. Importance of ethical considerations, privacy and policy frameworks.

continued on following page

Table 3. Continued

S. No.	Author and Year	Country	Objective	Methodology	Outcome of the study
4.	(Liu et al., 2016)	Egypt	The aim is to develop and assess smart home systems that have the potential to solve common challenges, such as mobility, safety and health monitoring.	Designing and implementation: 1. Researchers designed a smart home system with various technologies like sensors, automation etc. 2. Smart Technologies implemented: sensor networks, automation household tasks, health monitoring systems, etc. 3. Testing and evaluation	1. Participants reported higher satisfaction with their living conditions. 2. Sensor systems improved security and health monitoring tools. Example- fall detection sensors and emergency alert systems. 3. Challenges such as system reliability and need for continuous advancements in smart technology to ensure accessibility for elderly and disabled persons.
5.	(Attar et al., 2024)	Saudi Arabia	To study the impact of Smart cities on improving the quality of life of PWDs	Qualitative methodology: 1. Literature review 2. Survey and interviews for data collection 3. Case study analysis 4. Stakeholder feedback – feedback from PWDs and experts in the field.	1. Positive impact of smart cities on enhancing accessibility to public services, healthcare, transportation etc. for people with disabilities. 2. Integration of smart traffic systems and intelligent public spaces and transportation made it easier for PWDs to interact with city environment. 3. Existing technology gaps such as awareness, non-inclusive designs etc. 4. Need for government policy and support.
6.	(Poli, 2021)	Greece	Access the impact of various smart technologies on the life of PWDs.	Qualitative and descriptive methodology focusing on literature review.	1. Smart technologies gold significant promise in improving accessibility and independence such as assistive technologies (screen reading), smart home technologies (voice activated devices) and wearable (smart watch). 2. Assistive devices like as mobility aid, smart glasses etc. 3. Barriers highlighted- Digital divide, usability and customization, coast and accessibility.

continued on following page

Table 3. Continued

S. No.	Author and Year	Country	Objective	Methodology	Outcome of the study
7.	(Kbar et al., 2015)	Multinational	Main objective is to design and evaluate smart systems that can help PWDs in the workplace –by SHW-PWD.	Applied approach which includes design, development and evaluation of the SHW-PWD system.	1. SHW-PWD system showed enhanced accessibility to workplaces by PWDs. 2. The system reduced the need for human assistance, allowing employees with disabilities to perform tasks independently. 3. Improved productivity by reducing physical barriers and enabling more efficient workflow management. 4. Feedback from users indicates a high level satisfaction with SHW-PWD system. It had positive impact on work environment and employee morale.
8.	(Ahmed et al., 2016)	Bangladesh	To explore how smart technologies can enhance the independent living of PWDS.	Designing and implementation.	1. Smart technologies in home environment allow individuals with disabilities to perform daily tasks independently. 2. Health monitoring features (e.g. tracking BP, sugar level etc.) helps people with disabilities manage their health. 3. Improved quality of life with ensuring independence and safety.

Intersectionality of Disability with Gender and Age

The intersectionality of disability with gender and age refers to how disability interacts with a person's gender and age to create unique experiences of advantage or disadvantage (Brown & Moloney, 2019). For instance, women with disabilities may face additional social, cultural, and economic barriers compared to men, while older adults with disabilities may encounter compounded physical, cognitive, and accessibility challenges. Considering these intersections is essential to design inclusive policies, technologies, and environments that address the diverse needs of all individuals (Matin et al., 2021).

Interventions and Technologies

Adaptive and Accessible Devices

Voice-activated or gesture-controlled devices for older adults with limited mobility. Hearing aids, screen readers, and wearable assistive devices for people with sensory impairments.

Inclusive Digital Platforms

Mobile apps and online services designed with easy navigation, local language options, and age-appropriate content. Telehealth and e-learning platforms that account for gender-specific and age-related accessibility needs.

Community and Social Support Tools

Social networks, peer-support apps, and caregiver coordination platforms to reduce isolation and provide practical assistance.

Smart Homes and Smart Cities Adaptations

Homes with automated lighting, fall detection, and emergency alerts. Public infrastructure designed for mobility, safety, and inclusive participation, ensuring accessibility for older adults and women with disabilities.

Training and Capacity-Building

Targeted digital literacy programs for older adults and women to improve confidence and independent technology use.

RESEARCH METHODOLOGY

Data Collection Methods

Surveys: To get quantitative data from a large sample of people with disabilities, structured surveys will be used. These surveys will evaluate perceived hurdles, experiences with smart technologies, and familiarity with digital tools

Sampling Technique

To guarantee that participants from a variety of urban, and rural backgrounds are included, a deliberate sampling technique will be used. To capture a range of experiences, the sample will comprise people with disabilities from various socio-economic backgrounds. The study plan to conduct 53 different type of disabilities people in various gender the study will conduct in Deharadun, Uttarakhand State. The study use for the interview schedule and used for tools and data collection. The study used for the descriptive statistics, simple frequency with support of SPSS.

Interoperability Between Assistive Technologies

Interoperability enables different assistive devices and systems—like screen readers, hearing aids, and speech-to-text software—to work seamlessly across smartphones, computers, and IoT devices. Standards (WCAG, ISO), integration with smart homes, digital learning, and telehealth, along with cloud and AI support, improve usability. Challenges include high costs, lack of standardization, and limited collaboration. Solutions involve universal design, cross-industry partnerships, and supportive regulations to create an inclusive ecosystem.

Ethical Safeguards

The study ensures informed consent, voluntary participation, data privacy, and human rights, while preventing algorithmic bias and promoting accessibility in research tools.

Data Security and Ethical Use of AI

Disability-related data is anonymized, encrypted, and restricted to authorized researchers. Ethical AI use emphasizes bias prevention, transparency, human oversight, and fairness.

Interoperability Challenges

Assistive devices often fail across platforms, limiting usability. Addressing this requires open standards, cross-platform compatibility, and collaboration among developers, policymakers, and disability advocates to build integrated, user-friendly ecosystems.

Data Analysis

The study will employ quantitative methods to identify trends, correlations related to the use of smart technologies among specially-abled individuals. Survey data will be systematically analyzed using statistical software like SPSS. Descriptive statistics will be used to summarize the demographic characteristics of the participants and to measure the extent of smart technology usage across different groups. Inferential statistics will be applied to examine relationships between variables such as geographic location, socioeconomic status, type of disability, and level of digital engagement. Comparative analysis of case study data will be used to identify optimal practices and transferable lessons across various contexts.

RESULT

Table 4. Demographic Details

Descriptions	Options	Frequency	%	Mean	SEM	SD	Variance	Rane
Age	18–25	*9*	*17*	2.830	0.169	1.236	1.52	4
	26–35	*13*	*24.5*					
	36–45	*14*	*26.4*					
	46–55	*12*	*22.6*					
	56 and above	*5*	*9.4*					
	Total	***53***	***100***					
Gender	Male	*44*	*83*	1.169	0.052	.0379	0.144	1
	Female	*9*	*17*					
	Total	*53*	*100*					
Level of Education	No formal education	*9*	*17*	2.735	0.168	1.227	1.50	4
	Primary education	*16*	*30.2*					
	Secondary education	*13*	*24.5*					
	Higher secondary education	*10*	*18.9*					
	Graduate or above	*5*	*9.4*					
	Total	***53***	***100***					

continued on following page

Table 4. Continued

Descriptions	Options	Frequency	%	Mean	SEM	SD	Variance	Rane
Employment Status	Employed	*17*	*32.1*	2.528	0.189	1.381	1.90	4
	Self-employed	*13*	*24.5*					
	Student	*5*	*9.4*					
	Unemployed	*14*	*26.4*					
	Retired	*4*	*7.5*					
	Total	***53***	***100***					
Living Status	Rural	*21*	*39.6*	1.603	.067	0.493	0.24	1
	Urban	*32*	*60.4*					
	Total	***53***	***100***					

Dominant age group is 36–45 (26.4%), followed by 26–35 (24.5%) and 46–55 (22.6%). The mean age group leans toward middle age (2.830), indicating most participants are mid-life adults, which may influence assistive tech needs. Majority of participants are male (83%) and female (17%). The sample is male-dominated (mean = 1.169), which may limit gender representation. Education levels are mainly primary (30.2%) and secondary (24.5%), with 17% having no formal education. The mean education level (2.735) suggests a need for simplified digital tools and training. Employment status includes employed (32.1%), unemployed (26.4%), and self-employed (24.5%), with some students (9.4%) and retirees (7.5%). This diversity points to different assistive technology needs based on occupational engagement. Most participants live in urban areas (60.4%) compared to rural (39.6%). The urban skew (mean = 1.603) may reflect better access to technology and services.

Most respondents are middle-aged, male, and live in urban areas. Hearing and physical disabilities are the most common. Education levels are moderate, with many having only primary or no formal schooling. Employment status varies, indicating a range of tech needs. Urban majority suggests easier access to services and digital solutions.

Figure 1. Type of Disability

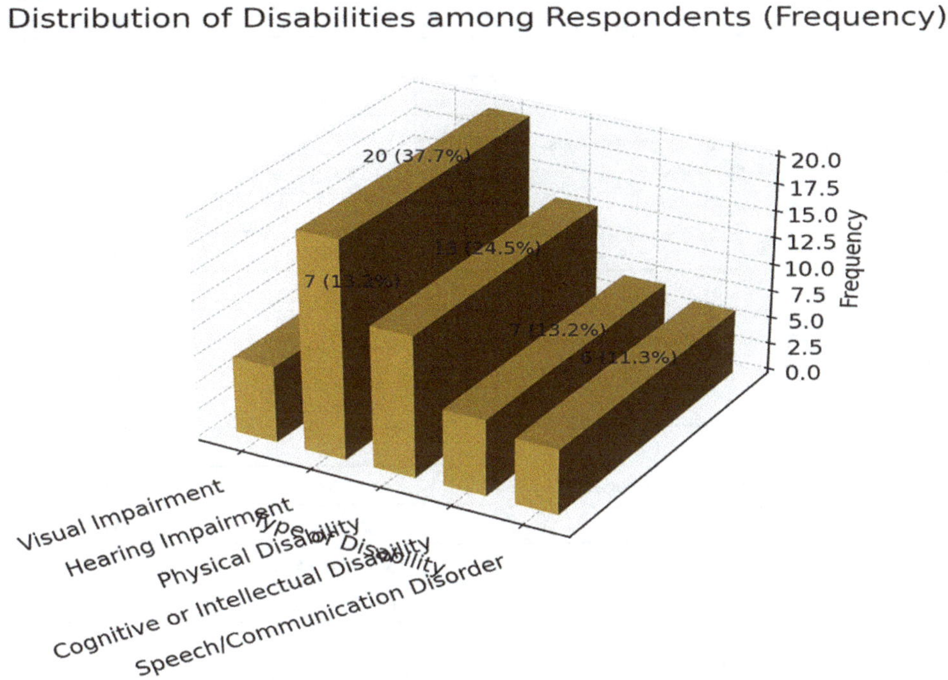

Most common disabilities are hearing impairment (37.7%) and physical disability (24.5%), followed by visual (13.2%), cognitive (13.2%), and speech/communication impairments (11.3%). Hearing and physical limitations are key areas for assistive tech focus.

Table 5. Digital Accessibility and Usage Profile of Respondents (N = 53)

Descriptions	Options	Frequency	%
Have Access to Digital Devices	Smartphone	*13*	*24.5*
	Tablet	*7*	*13.2*
	Laptop/Desktop	*9*	*17*
	Smart Home Devices	*10*	*18.9*
	Not using Any Digital Devices	*14*	*26.4*
	Total	***53***	***100***

continued on following page

Table 5. Continued

Descriptions	Options	Frequency	%
Frequently use Digital Services (e.g., mobile apps, websites, online banking, e-learning)?	Daily	*7*	*13.2*
	Weekly	*14*	*26.4*
	Monthly	*12*	*22.6*
	Rarely	*12*	*22.6*
	Never	*8*	*15.1*
	Total	***53***	***100***
Facing problem using online services (e.g., banking, e-learning, healthcare)	Yes	*20*	*37.7*
	No	*17*	*32.1*
	Sometimes	*16*	*30.2*
	Total	***53***	***100***
Received any training for Smart Technologies	Yes	*15*	*28.3*
	No	*38*	*71.7*
	Total	***53***	***100***
Confidently are you use digital services	Very confident	*10*	*18.9*
	Somewhat confident	*11*	*20.8*
	Neutral	*13*	*24.5*
	Not very confident	*12*	*22.6*
	Not confident at all	*7*	*13.2*
	Total	*53*	*100*
Current smart technologies meet your needs	Yes	*31*	*58.5*
	No	*11*	*20.8*
	Partially	*11*	*20.8*
	Total	***53***	***100***
Feature improvements would enhance for smart technologies	Better accessibility features	*13*	*24.5*
	Affordable pricing models	*11*	*20.8*
	User-friendly interfaces	*13*	*24.5*
	Improved compatibility with assistive devices	*8*	*15.1*
	More inclusive digital content	*8*	*15.1*
	Total	*53*	*100*
Like to participate in future research to improving digital accessibility	Yes	*42*	*79.2*
	No	*11*	*20.8*
	Total	*53*	*100*

continued on following page

Table 5. Continued

Descriptions	Options	Frequency	%
Are you regular using Internet	Yes, at home	*6*	*11.3*
	Yes, through mobile data	*33*	*62.3*
	Occasionally, at public places (e.g., cybercafé, library)	*7*	*13.2*
	No access	*7*	*13.2*
	Total	***53***	***100***

A considerable share of respondents reported no digital device use (26.4%), while smartphones (24.5%) were the most common, followed by smart home devices (18.9%), laptops/desktops (17%), and tablets (13.2%), showing reliance on mobile technology but a digital divide. Digital service use remained limited, with weekly (26.4%) being most frequent, while daily use was only 13.2%, and 15.1% never used such services. About 37.7% faced problems in online services, 30.2% sometimes, and 32.1% no issues, reflecting uneven experiences. Training gaps were clear, as 71.7% had no training, leading to low confidence, with only 18.9% very confident and 20.8% somewhat confident in digital use. While 58.5% said technologies met needs, 41.6% felt otherwise, pointing to scope for improvement. Key improvements sought were better accessibility (24.5%), user-friendly design (24.5%), and affordable pricing (20.8%). Most (79.2%) were willing to join future research, showing openness for better digital access. Internet use was dominated by mobile data (62.3%), with limited home access (11.3%), public access (13.2%), and 13.2% with no access. The findings show unequal access, lack of training, and low confidence as key barriers. Although smartphones dominate, regular digital engagement is limited. Accessibility, affordability, and inclusivity remain critical for improvement.

Figure 2. Difficulties to Use Smart Technologies

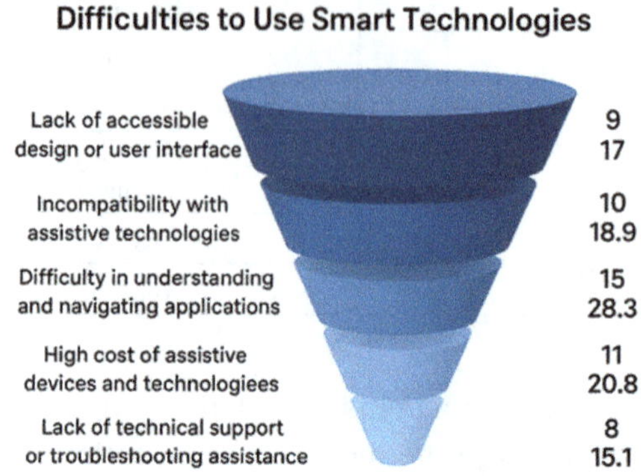

The findings show that the biggest challenge faced by users is *difficulty in understanding and navigating applications* (28.3%). This suggests that many assistive technologies are not user-friendly and require simpler, more intuitive design. The *high cost of devices* (20.8%) is another major barrier, limiting accessibility for low-income groups. *Incompatibility with existing assistive technologies* (18.9%) and *lack of accessible design or user interface* (17%) further reduce usability. Finally, *insufficient technical support or troubleshooting assistance* (15.1%) highlights the need for better aftercare services.

Figure 3. Facing problem using online services

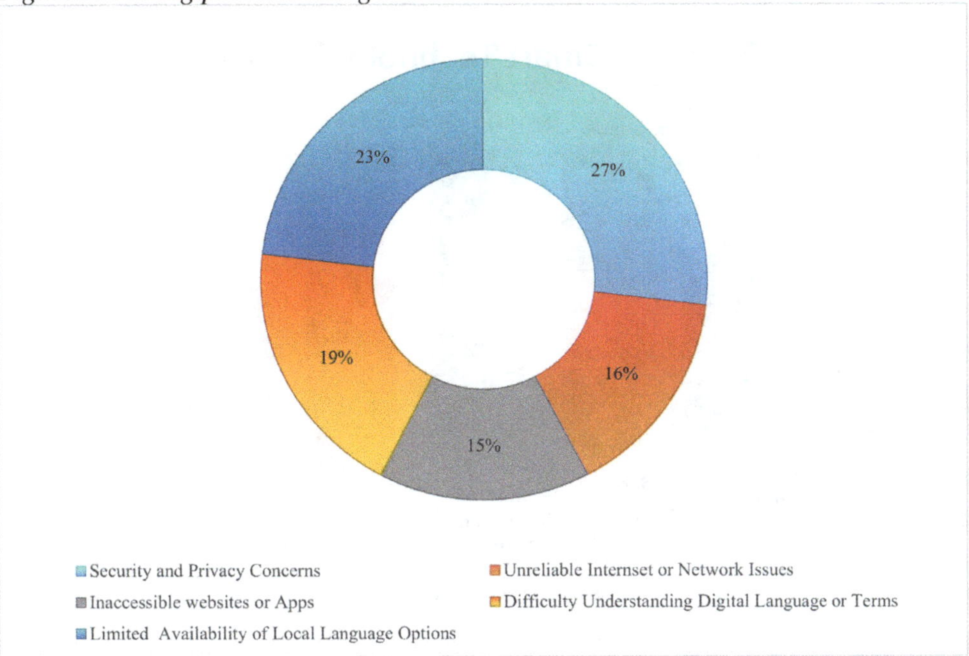

Among the respondents, the most common problem faced while using digital platforms is security and privacy concerns (26.9%), followed by limited availability of local language options (23.1%). A significant proportion also reported difficulty in understanding digital language or terms (19.2%). Issues such as unreliable internet or network (15.4%) and inaccessible websites or apps (15.4%) were also highlighted. This indicates that while technical barriers exist, concerns related to privacy, language accessibility, and digital literacy are the most pressing challenges.

Figure 4. Types of Smart Technologies Use

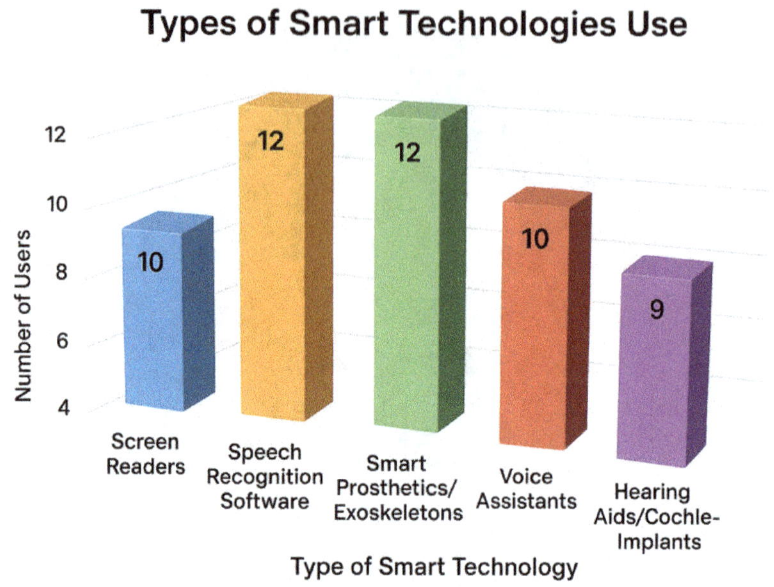

The data shows the distribution of smart technologies used by respondents. Speech Recognition Software and Smart Prosthetics/Exoskeletons are the most commonly used, each with **22.6%** (12 users). Screen Readers and Voice Assistants follow with **18.9%** (10 users each). Hearing Aids/Cochlear Implants account for **17%** (9 users). In total, 53 users participated, representing **100%** of the sample.

Table 6. Table Digital Literacy, Access, and Perception of Assistive Technologies among Respondents (N = 53)

Descriptions	*Very familiar*	*%*	*Somewhat familiar*	*%*	*Not familiar at all*	*%*	*Total*	*%*
Using digital devices	*25*	*47.2*	*18*	*34*	*10*	*18.9*	*53*	*100*
Computer/Laptop	*24*	*45.3*	*20*	*37.7*	*9*	*17*	*53*	*100*
Descriptions	***Yes***	*(%)*	***No***	*(%)*	***Total***		*%*	
Tablet	*31*	*22*	*58.5*	*41.5*	*53*		*100*	
Descriptions	***Yes***	*(%)*	***No***	*(%)*	***With Assistance***	*(%)*	***Total***	*(%)*
Send and receive emails	*22*	*41.5*	*23*	*43.4*	*8*	*15.1*	*53*	*100*

continued on following page

Table 6. Continued

Descriptions	*Very familiar*	*%*	*Somewhat familiar*	*%*	*Not familiar at all*	*%*	*Total*	*%*
Search information on the internet	*22*	*41.5*	*19*	*35.8*	*12*	*22.6*	*53*	*100*
Download and install apps	*23*	*43.4*	*18*	*34*	*12*	*22.6*	*53*	*100*
Use accessibility features	*21*	*39.6*	*25*	*47.2*	*7*	*13.2*	*53*	*100*
Descriptions	***Yes***	*(%)*	***No***	*(%)*	***Somewhat***	*(%)*	***Total***	*(%)*
Aware of basic online safety practices	*24*	*45.3*	*19*	*35.8*	*10*	*18.9*	*53*	*100*
Know how to protect personal information	*14*	*26.4*	*30*	*56.6*	*9*	*17*	*53*	*100*
Descriptions	***Very comfortable***	*(%)*	***Somewhat comfortable***	*(%)*	***Not comfortable***	*(%)*	***Total***	*(%)*
Social media platforms	*22*	*41.5*	*18*	*34*	*13*	*24.5*	*53*	*100*
E-learning Platforms	*11*	*20.8*	*18*	*34*	*24*	*45.3*	*53*	*100*
Online banking/financial services	*15*	*28.3*	*12*	*22.6*	*26*	*49.1*	*53*	*100*
Assistive technologies	*31*	*58.5*	*17*	*32.1*	*5*	*9.4*	*53*	*100*
Descriptions	***Very effective***	*%*	***Somewhat effective***	*%*	***Not effective***	*%*	***Total***	*%*
Screen readers/text-to-speech tools	*17*	*32.1*	*26*	*49.1*	*10*	*18.9*	*53*	*100*
Speech recognition/voice assistants	*13*	*24.5*	*21*	*39.6*	*19*	*35.8*	*53*	*100*
Smart prosthetics/mobility aids	*24*	*45.3*	*18*	*34*	*11*	*20.8*	*53*	*100*
Assistive mobile applications	*20*	*37.7*	*16*	*30.2*	*17*	*32.1*	*53*	*100*
Digital learning and education platforms	*24*	*45.3*	*17*	*32.1*	*12*	*22.6*	*53*	*100*
Digital learning/education platforms	*24*	*45.3*	*17*	*32.1*	*12*	*22.6*	*53*	*100*
Digital communication tools	*21*	*39.6*	*20*	*37.7*	*12*	*22.6*	*53*	*100*

Most respondents are familiar with using digital devices (47.2% very familiar) and computers/laptops (45.3% very familiar), though a notable portion remains only somewhat or not familiar, indicating uneven digital literacy. Only 58.5% have access to tablets, showing that device ownership is limited, especially for more specialized or secondary devices. Basic digital tasks such as sending/receiving emails (41.5%), searching information (41.5%), and downloading apps (43.4%) are done independently by fewer than half. A considerable number require assistance, especially for tasks like using accessibility features (47.2% do not use them), suggesting usability and awareness gaps. While 45.3% are aware of online safety practices, only 26.4% know how to protect personal information. This highlights a major vulnerability in digital security awareness. Comfort with digital platforms varies widely—respondents feel most comfortable with social media (41.5%), but discomfort is high for e-learning (45.3% not comfortable) and online banking (49.1% not comfortable), reflecting barriers in essential online services. Familiarity and confidence in assistive technologies are relatively strong—58.5% feel very comfortable using them, indicating their central role in users' digital experience. In terms of effectiveness, smart prosthetics/ mobility aids (45.3%) and digital learning platforms (45.3%) are rated very effective by nearly half the users. However, tools like speech recognition (35.8% not effective) and assistive mobile apps (32.1% not effective) show mixed responses, suggesting that functionality and customization still need improvement.

Table 7. Support, Usage, and Satisfaction with Digital and Assistive Technologies (N = 53)

Descriptions	Options	Frequency	%
Preferred Support to Improve Digital Literacy	Personalized training programs	*12*	*22.6*
	Accessible and easy-to-understand resources	*19*	*35.8*
	Free or low-cost internet services	*12*	*22.6*
	Mentoring and technical support	*10*	*18.9*
	Total	*53*	*100*
Satisfaction with Assistive Technologies	Completely meet my needs	*15*	*28.3*
	Meet some of my needs, but not all	*18*	*34*
	Do not adequately meet my needs	*14*	*26.4*
	Not applicable	*6*	*11.3*
	Total	*53*	*100*

The most preferred support for improving digital literacy is accessible and easy-to-understand resources (35.8%), followed by personalized training and free or low-cost internet (both at 22.6%), indicating a strong demand for practical, inclusive, and affordable learning tools. Use of assistive technologies is varied, with voice assistants (17%), hearing aids (15.1%), and speech-to-text software (13.2%) being the most commonly used. However, more advanced or niche tools like Braille devices, assistive apps, and accessible digital learning platforms are used by fewer individuals (7.5%), suggesting limited reach or availability. Satisfaction levels show that while 28.3% say assistive technologies completely meet their needs, a larger group (34%) find them only partially helpful. Additionally, 26.4% feel their needs are not adequately met, highlighting room for improvement in design, usability, or support features.

Figure 5. or Digital Solutions Assistive Technologies Used

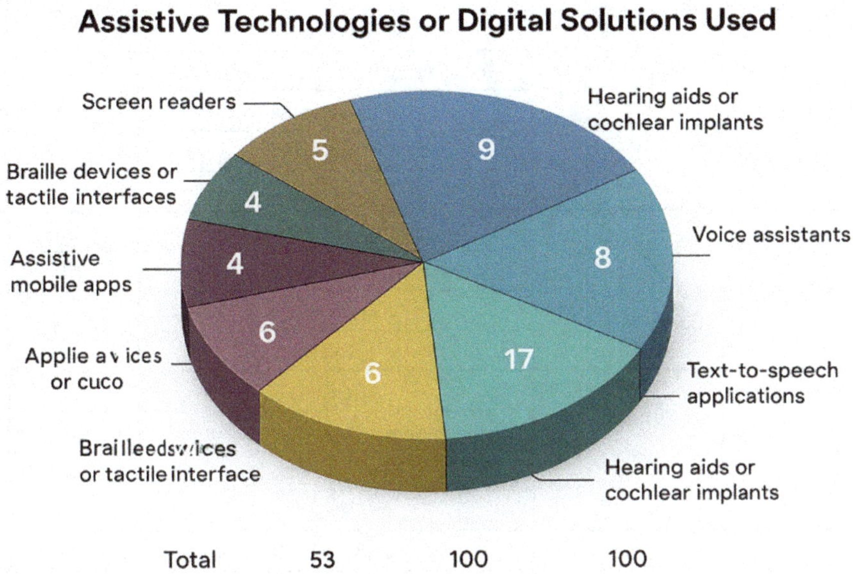

The voice assistants (17%) and hearing aids/cochlear implants (15.1%) are the most widely used assistive technologies. Speech-to-text software (13.2%) and text-to-speech applications (11.3%) also have significant use. Other solutions like smart prosthetics, Braille devices, assistive mobile apps, and digital learning platforms are used by smaller but important portions of users (7.5% each), reflecting diverse technological support for accessibility needs.

Table 8. Impact, Accessibility, and User Satisfaction on Assistive Technologies (N = 53)

Descriptions	*Options*	*Frequency*	*%*
Impact of Technologies	Mobility and accessibility	*10*	*18.9*
	Communication abilities	*9*	*17*
	Educational/professional growth	*9*	*17*
	Social inclusion	*8*	*15.1*
	Independence and autonomy	*6*	*11.3*
	Quality of life	*11*	*20.8*
	Total	*53*	*100*

continued on following page

Table 8. Continued

Descriptions	*Options*	*Frequency*	*%*
User-Friendliness	Very easy to use	22	41.5
	Moderately easy but requires assistance	16	30.2
	Difficult to use	9	17
	Not applicable	6	11.3
	Total	53	100
Cost Level	Affordable	25	47.2
	Somewhat expensive	19	35.8
	Very expensive	9	17
	Total	53	100
Affordability	Affordable	23	43.4
	Somewhat expensive	18	34
	Very expensive	12	22.6
	Total	53	100
Availability	Easily available	27	50.9
	Moderately available	15	28.3
	Difficult to access	11	20.8
	Total	53	100
Issues with Maintenance	Yes	16	30.2
	No	21	39.6
	Occasionally	16	30.2
	Total	53	100
Satisfaction Level	Very satisfied	18	34
	Somewhat satisfied	13	24.5
	Neutral	9	17
	Somewhat dissatisfied	8	15.1
	Very dissatisfied	5	9.4
	Total	53	100
Type of Support	Financial assistance or subsidies	20	37.7
	Better regulatory frameworks	20	37.7
	Awareness campaigns	13	24.5
	Total	53	100
Willingness to Participate in Research	Yes	40	75.5
	No	13	24.5
	Total	53	100

Technology has the greatest impact on quality of life most users (41.5%) find smart technologies very easy to use, though 30.2% need some assistance, and 17% find them difficult, suggesting a gap in usability for certain groups. Nearly half of respondents (47.2%) find current technologies affordable, but a significant portion (35.8%–43.4%) still feel cost is a barrier, emphasizing the need for more affordable solutions. Availability is generally good, with 50.9% stating technologies are easily available. However, 20.8% report difficulties in accessing them, pointing to regional or economic disparities. Maintenance is an issue for about 60% (30.2% regularly, 30.2% occasionally), which can affect long-term usability and satisfaction. Satisfaction is mixed: 34% are very satisfied, but around 24.5% express dissatisfaction or neutrality, showing room for improving effectiveness and user experience. Respondents prefer financial support and stronger regulatory frameworks (each at 37.7%), highlighting a demand for structural and policy-level improvements.Finally, 75.5% are willing to participate in future research, reflecting a strong interest in improving digital accessibility and inclusion.

Figure 6. Impact of Technologies

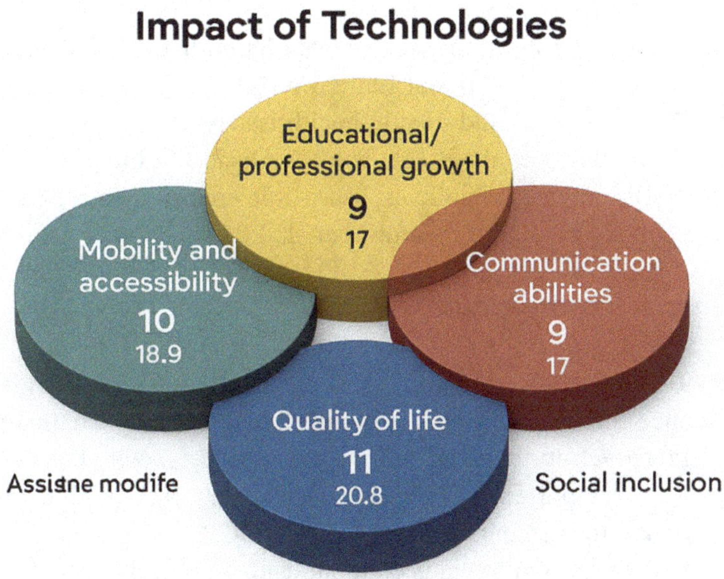

Technology has the greatest impact on quality of life (20.8%) and mobility and accessibility (18.9%), followed closely by communication abilities (17%) and educational/professional growth (17%). Social inclusion (15.1%) and independence and autonomy (11.3%) also play important roles. The overlaps illustrate how these domains are interconnected—improvements in mobility, communication, and education collectively enhance independence, social participation, and overall quality of life.

DISCUSSION

Digital Divide and Disability

Although over two billion people are online, nearly half the world remains disconnected (Citaristi, 2022). Persons with disabilities (PWDs) face greater challenges, as many digital innovations overlook their needs (Mavrou et al., 2017). The COVID-19 pandemic deepened this divide, limiting daily functioning and social participation (Blanck, 2023). Barriers such as poor access, limited skills, design flaws, and lack of trust restrict inclusion. Overcoming these requires public–private partnerships to expand opportunities in education, employment, finance, and independent living (Yadav et al., 2021).

Global Disability Context

WHO estimates that 16% of the world's population lives with disabilities, with 200 million facing severe functional limits (WHO, 2022). Prevalence increases with ageing, chronic illness, and mental health issues, raising both public health and rights concerns (Lang et al., 2011). The UN Disability Inclusion Strategy and SDG Report (2018) emphasize policies, accessible environments, and ICT-driven empowerment (Eberle et al., 2022; Jamwal et al., 2022).

Role of Smart Technologies

Industry 4.0 tools like AI, AR, and ML serve as assistive technologies, enhancing independence and participation. Cognitive and learning challenges benefit from reminders, speech-to-text, and specialized apps (Szabó et al., 2023; Ekepete, 2024). Mobility is supported by powered wheelchairs and exoskeletons (Mann, 2005), while visual impairments use smart canes, OCR, and screen readers (Rizzo et al., 2023). Speech recognition aids communication (Bhardwaj et al., 2024), and hearing devices improve access for the hearing-impaired (Rominger & Eiten, 2019). Elderly users rely on smart health monitors and GPS (Oladele et al., 2021). Socio-economic barriers are reduced through inclusive banking, subsidies, and digital services (Santoso, 2023).

AI, Smart Homes, and Smart Cities

AI strengthens healthcare, safety, and financial inclusion while reducing isolation. Smart homes use voice assistants, automation, and adaptive devices to support autonomy (Jamwal et al., 2022). Smart cities employ IoT-based infrastructure and inclusive transport to improve accessibility (Pearson & Shafik, 2024).

Robotics and Emerging Innovations

Robotics such as exoskeletons, manipulators, and social robots enhance mobility and companionship (Hillman, 2006; Chen et al., 2013). Self-driving cars promise inclusive transport, while AI wearables support health monitoring and independence. Telehealth services like India's *eSanjeevani* expand medical access (Srinivasan et al., 2025). Smart and assistive technologies are vital to bridging the disability divide, enhancing healthcare, mobility, education, and employment. They foster inclusion and dignity, but success depends on affordability, inclusive design, digital literacy, and global cooperation aligned with SDGs and human rights goals.

Most respondents are middle-aged (36–45 years, 26.4%), predominantly male (83%), and urban residents (60.4%). Education is generally primary (30.2%) or secondary (24.5%), with many having no formal schooling (17%), highlighting the need for simplified tools and training. Employment is diverse: employed (32.1%), unemployed (26.4%), and self-employed (24.5%), pointing to varied technology needs. The most common disabilities are hearing (37.7%) and physical impairments (24.5%), followed by visual, cognitive, and speech difficulties. Digital access is uneven—26.4% do not use devices, while smartphones (24.5%) dominate. Service use is low, with most engaging monthly or rarely. Key barriers include navigation (28.3%), cost (20.8%), and compatibility issues (18.9%). Over one-third face problems online, citing privacy concerns, language gaps, and technical terms.

A majority lack training (71.7%) and confidence, limiting effective use. Still, 58.5% say technologies meet their needs, though many remain only partially satisfied. Users prefer accessibility improvements, user-friendly interfaces (24.5% each), affordability (20.8%), and better compatibility Assistive technologies most used: voice assistants (17%), hearing aids (15.1%), and speech-to-text (13.2%). Tools like Braille devices and assistive apps (7.5%) remain underused. Effectiveness varies—prosthetics and digital learning are rated highly, while speech recognition and mobile apps face usability issues. Affordability, availability, and maintenance remain concerns, with 34% very satisfied but many neutral or dissatisfied. Respondents call for financial support and policy improvements (37.7% each). Technology most impacts quality of life (20.8%), mobility (18.9%), and communication (17%), showing that accessibility, affordability, and training are critical for inclusive adoption.

CONCLUSION

Persons with disability face challenges as a result of the growing reliance on digital platforms for basic services. In order to guarantee fair access to necessary services, this study emphasizes how urgent it is to close the disability divide. This study provides an extensive framework for intervention by identifying important obstacles, including limitations in technology, e- literacy, accessibility problems, and a lack of support networks. The path to inclusivity is further strengthened by the establishment of community support networks and the promotion of laws that prioritize accessibility. The study's mixed-methods methodology guarantees that suggestions are supported by empirical data and enables a detailed knowledge of the opportunities and difficulties. Working together with stakeholders like governmental organizations, non-profits, and IT companies guarantees that the solutions are workable, expandable, and long-lasting. This study does, however, recognize several limits, such as budget limitations, regional differences in digital infrastructure, and the speed at which technology is developing. The ultimate goal of this research is to promote a digitally inclusive society in which specially-abled citizens can easily and confidently access social and economic life. Policymakers, technologists, and communities working to achieve digital inclusion for all will find great value in the study's conclusions and suggestions.

Features and Implications of the Study

For starters, the emphasis on user-centered design ensures that smart technologies are accessible, straightforward, and adapted to the needs of people with disabilities. Second, the inclusion of digital literacy programs emphasizes the need of preparing the specially-abled to comfortably traverse digital platforms. Training modules built exclusively for the specially-abled will overcome technological impediments while also instilling a sense of independence and involvement in them. The report also emphasizes the use of assistive technology like voice recognition and screen readers to meet a variety of needs, making it more accessible to people with physical or cognitive disabilities. Another notable element is the emphasis on community support systems. Setting up digital kiosks and training staff to assist customers with disabilities at community centers can give instant, on-the-ground solutions.

Implementing the offered solutions can help governments improve service delivery, eliminate operational inefficiencies, and increase citizen happiness. Policymakers can use the study's findings to develop comprehensive frameworks that emphasize digital inclusion and accessibility. Finally bridging the disability divide improves social fairness by allowing the specially-abled citizens to actively engage in civic life. This openness strengthens community relationships and guarantees that specially-abled persons do not fall behind in an increasingly digital environment.

REFERENCES

Ahmed, E., Islam, A., Sarker, F., Huda, M. N., & Abdullah-Al-Mamun, K. (2016). A road to independent living with smart homes for people with disabilities. In *2016 5th International conference on informatics, electronics and vision (ICIEV)* (pp. 472-477). IEEE. DOI: 10.1109/ICIEV.2016.7760048

Al-Homoud, M. (2025). Aging in Place in Jordan: Assessing Home Modifications, Accessibility Barriers, and Cultural Constraints. *Buildings (Basel, Switzerland)*, *15*(17), 3125. DOI: 10.3390/buildings15173125

Attar, R. W., Habes, M., Almusharraf, A., Alhazmi, A. H., & Attar, R. W. (2024). Exploring the impact of smart cities on improving the quality of life for people with disabilities in Saudi Arabia. *Frontiers in Built Environment*, *10*, 1398425. DOI: 10.3389/fbuil.2024.1398425

Bhardwaj, A., Sharma, M., Kumar, S., Sharma, S., & Sharma, P. C. (2024). Transforming pediatric speech and language disorder diagnosis and therapy: The evolving role of artificial intelligence. *Health Sciences Review (Oxford, England)*, *100188*, 100188. Advance online publication. DOI: 10.1016/j.hsr.2024.100188

Blanck, P. (2023). On the importance of the Americans with Disabilities Act at 30. *Journal of Disability Policy Studies*, *34*(3), 176–198. DOI: 10.1177/10442073211036900 PMID: 39286446

Bricout, J., Baker, P. M., Moon, N. W., & Sharma, B. (2021). Exploring the smart future of participation: Community, inclusivity, and people with disabilities. [IJEPR]. *International Journal of E-Planning Research*, *10*(2), 94–108. DOI: 10.4018/IJEPR.20210401.oa8

Brown, R. L., & Moloney, M. E. (2019). Intersectionality, work, and well-being: The effects of gender and disability. *Gender & Society*, *33*(1), 94–122. DOI: 10.1177/0891243218800636

Chen, T. L., Ciocarlie, M., Cousins, S., Grice, P. M., Hawkins, K., Hsiao, K., & Takayama, L. (2013). Robots for humanity: Using assistive robotics to empower people with disabilities. *IEEE Robotics & Automation Magazine*, *20*(1), 30–39. DOI: 10.1109/MRA.2012.2229950

Citaristi, I. (2022). International telecommunication union—itu. In *The Europa Directory of International Organizations 2022* (pp. 365–369). Routledge., https://www.taylorfrancis.com/chapters/edit/10.4324/9781003292548-75/international-telecommunication-union%E2%80%94itu-ileana-citaristi DOI: 10.4324/9781003292548-75

Dev, P. S., Eljo, J. J. G., & Srinivasan, S. (2025). Navigating Mental Health Challenges in the Care of Elderly With Disabilities in Kerala: A Gerontological Social Work Perspective. In *Modern Digital Approaches to Care Technologies for Individuals With Disabilities* (pp. 33-56). IGI Global Scientific Publishing. DOI: DOI: 10.4018/979-8-3693-7560-0.ch003

Eberle, U., Wenzig, J., & Mumm, N. (2022). Assessing the contribution of products to the United Nations' Sustainable Development Goals: A methodological proposal. *The International Journal of Life Cycle Assessment*, *27*(7), 959–977. DOI: 10.1007/s11367-022-02063-8

Ekpete, O. H. (2024). Assistive listening devices for individuals with hearing impairment. *Faculty of Natural and Applied Sciences Journal of Mathematics, and Science Education, 5*(2), 78-81. https://fnasjournals.com/index.php/FNAS-JMSE/article/view/390

Gafoor, A., & Amilan, S. (2024). Fintech adoption and financial well-being of persons with disabilities: The mediating role of financial access, financial knowledge and financial behaviour. *International Journal of Social Economics*, *51*(11), 1388–1401. DOI: 10.1108/IJSE-08-2023-0596

Gell, N. M., Rosenberg, D. E., Demiris, G., LaCroix, A. Z., & Patel, K. V. (2015). Patterns of technology use among older adults with and without disabilities. *The Gerontologist*, *55*(3), 412–421. DOI: 10.1093/geront/gnt166 PMID: 24379019

Hillman, M. R. (2006). *Assistive robotics*. Wiley Encyclopedia of Biomedical Engineering., DOI: 10.1002/9780471740360.ebs1029

Humphry, J., & Chesher, C. (2021). Preparing for smart voice assistants: Cultural histories and media innovations. *New Media & Society*, *23*(7), 1971–1988. DOI: 10.1177/1461444820923679

Jamwal, R., Jarman, H. K., Roseingrave, E., Douglas, J., & Winkler, D. (2022). Smart home and communication technology for people with disability: A scoping review. *Disability and Rehabilitation. Assistive Technology*, *17*(6), 624–644. DOI: 10.1080/17483107.2020.1818138 PMID: 32924660

Joy, J., Balakrishnan, K., & M, S. (2019). SiLearn: An intelligent sign vocabulary learning tool. *Journal of Enabling Technologies*, *13*(3), 173–187. DOI: 10.1108/JET-03-2019-0014

Katsivelis, N., Anastasiou, A., Petropoulou, O., Lambrou, G., Giokas, K., & Koutsouris, D. (2017). Applied technologies and Smart Home applications in the health sector. In *2017 IEEE 30th International Symposium on Computer-Based Medical Systems (CBMS)* (pp. 544-549). IEEE. DOI: 10.1109/CBMS.2017.48

Kbar, G., Aly, S., Elsharawy, I., Bhatia, A., Alhasan, N., & Enriquez, R. (2015). Smart help at the workplace for persons with disabilities (SHW-PWD). *International Journal of Computer, Control. Quantum and Information Engineering*, *9*(1), 84–90. DOI: 10.1109/ICIEV.2016.7760048

Klingbeil, H., Baer, H. R., & Wilson, P. E. (2004). Aging with a disability. *Archives of Physical Medicine and Rehabilitation*, *85*, 68–73. DOI: 10.1016/j.apmr.2004.03.014 PMID: 15221734

Lang, R., Kett, M., Groce, N., & Trani, J. F. (2011). Implementing the United Nations Convention on the rights of persons with disabilities: Principles, implications, practice and limitations. *Alter (Paris)*, *5*(3), 206–220. DOI: 10.1016/j.alter.2011.02.004

Leal Filho, W., Tripathi, S. K., Andrade Guerra, J. B. S. O. D., Giné-Garriga, R., Orlovic Lovren, V., & Willats, J. (2019). Using the sustainable development goals towards a better understanding of sustainability challenges. *International Journal of Sustainable Development and World Ecology*, *26*(2), 179–190. DOI: 10.1080/13504509.2018.1505674

Liu, L., Stroulia, E., Nikolaidis, I., Miguel-Cruz, A., & Rincon, A. R. (2016). Smart homes and home health monitoring technologies for older adults: A systematic review. *International Journal of Medical Informatics*, *91*, 44–59. DOI: 10.1016/j.ijmedinf.2016.04.007 PMID: 27185508

Lynch, P., Singal, N., & Francis, G. A. (2024). Educational technology for learners with disabilities in primary school settings in low-and middle-income countries: A systematic literature review. *Educational Review*, *76*(2), 405–431. DOI: 10.1080/00131911.2022.2035685

Mahmoudi-Dehaki, M., Nasr-Esfahani, N., & Vasan, S. (2025). The Transformative Role of Assistive Technology in Enhancing Quality of Life for Individuals With Disabilities. In *Assistive Technology Solutions for Aging Adults and Individuals With Disabilities* (pp. 45–72). IGI Global Scientific Publishing., DOI: 10.4018/979-8-3693-6308-9.ch003

Mann, W. C. (2005). Aging, disability and independence: trends and perspectives. *Smart Technology for Aging, Disability, and Independence: The State of the Science*, 1-29. DOI: 10.1002/0471743941.ch1

Matin, B. K., Williamson, H. J., Karyani, A. K., Rezaei, S., Soofi, M., & Soltani, S. (2021). Barriers in access to healthcare for women with disabilities: A systematic review in qualitative studies. *BMC Women's Health*, *21*(1), 44. DOI: 10.1186/s12905-021-01189-5 PMID: 33516225

Mavrou, K., Meletiou-Mavrotheris, M., Kärki, A., Sallinen, M., & Hoogerwerf, E. J. (2017). Opportunities and challenges related to ICT and ICT-AT use by people with disabilities: An explorative study into factors that impact on the digital divide. *Technology and Disability*, *29*(1-2), 63–75. DOI: 10.3233/TAD-170174

Nam, S. J., & Park, E. Y. (2017). The effects of the smart environment on the information divide experienced by people with disabilities. *Disability and Health Journal*, *10*(2), 257–263. DOI: 10.1016/j.dhjo.2016.11.001 PMID: 27899268

Ojasalo, J., Suomalainen, N., Seppälä, H., & Moonen, R. (2010). Better technologies and services for smart homes of disabled people: empirical findings from an explorative study among intellectually disabled. In *2010 2nd International Conference on Software Technology and Engineering* (Vol. 1, pp. V1-251). IEEE. DOI: 10.1109/ICSTE.2010.5608845

Oladele, D. A., Markus, E. D., & Abu-Mahfouz, A. M. (2021). Adaptability of assistive mobility devices and the role of the internet of medical things: Comprehensive review. *JMIR Rehabilitation and Assistive Technologies*, *8*(4), e29610. DOI: 10.2196/29610 PMID: 34779786

Pearson, S. R., & Shafik, M. (2024). Smart Cities enhancing the lives of people with disabilities. MATEC Web of Conferences, 401, 07004. DOI: 10.1051/matecconf/202440107004

Poli, M. (2021). COVID-19 effects in people's daily life, social media's role and the power of emotions and mind. In *Strategic Innovative Marketing and Tourism in the COVID-19 Era: 9th ICSIMAT Conference 2020* (pp. 141-151). Springer International Publishing. DOI: 10.1007/978-3-030-66154-0_16

Poli, M. (2021). Smart Technologies and the Case of People with Disabilities: A Preliminary Overview. *NiDS*, 217-222. DOI: 10.3233/FAIA210096

Puli, L., Layton, N., Bell, D., & Shahriar, A. Z. (2024). Financial inclusion for people with disability: A scoping review. *Global Health Action*, *17*(1), 2342634. DOI: 10.1080/16549716.2024.2342634 PMID: 38726584

Rizzo, J. R., Beheshti, M., Hudson, T. E., Mongkolwat, P., Riewpaiboon, W., Seiple, W., Ogedegbe, O. G., & Vedanthan, R. (2023). The global crisis of visual impairment: An emerging global health priority requiring urgent action. *Disability and Rehabilitation. Assistive Technology*, *18*(3), 240–245. DOI: 10.1080/17483107.2020.1854876 PMID: 33332166

Rominger, A., & Eiten, L. R. (2019). Hearing loss and hearing-related factors: Technology and environmental interventions. *Assistive Technologies and Environmental Interventions in Healthcare: An Integrated Approach*, 306-3Santoso, B. (2023). Inclusive digital financial services for persons with disabilities: Impact on economic empowerment and financial inclusion. *Indonesian Journal of Disability Studies*, *10*(1), 105–124. DOI: 10.1002/9781394321759.ch18

Soar, J., & Croll, P. (2007). Assistive technologies for the frail elderly, chronic illness sufferers and people with disabilities-A case study of the development of a smart home. In *ACIS2007 Proceedings of the 18th Australasian Conference on Information Systems* (pp. 937–944). The University of Southern Queensland., https://eprints.qut.edu.au/14331/

Srinivasan, S., & Rajavel, N. (2025). Technology Improves the Quality of Life for Elderly People. In *Perspectives on the Economics of Aging* (pp. 109-150). IGI Global Scientific Publishing.dooi: DOI: 10.2139/ssrn.5277229

Srinivasan, S., Rajavel, N., & Mahmoudi-Dehaki, M. (2025). Elderly Inmates Living With Dementia in Central Prisons. In *Assistive Technology Solutions for Aging Adults and Individuals With Disabilities* (pp. 343–404). IGI Global Scientific Publishing., DOI: 10.4018/979-8-3693-6308-9.ch015

Srinivasan, S., Rajavel, N., & Sanchez, N. K. (2025). The Impact of AI on Elderly Inmates in Central Prison. In *Exploration of AI in Contemporary Legal Systems* (pp. 281–314). IGI Global Scientific Publishing., DOI: 10.4018/979-8-3693-7205-0.ch013

Stefanov, D. H., Bien, Z., & Bang, W. C. (2004). The smart house for older persons and persons with physical disabilities: Structure, technology arrangements, and perspectives. *IEEE Transactions on Neural Systems and Rehabilitation Engineering*, *12*(2), 228–250. DOI: 10.1109/TNSRE.2004.828423 PMID: 15218937

Szabó, P., Ara, J., Halmosi, B., Sik-Lanyi, C., & Guzsvinecz, T. (2023). Technologies designed to assist individuals with cognitive impairments. *Sustainability (Basel)*, *15*(18), 13490. DOI: 10.3390/su151813490

Tajadod, F. (2021). *Voice command android-based smart home system for controlling door lock, lights, and home appliance for physically disabled people based on iot* (Doctoral dissertation, California State University San Marcos). https://scholarworks.calstate.edu/downloads/4m90f171q

Techaraungrong, P., Suksakulchai, S., Kaewprapan, W., & Murphy, E. (2017). The design and testing of multimedia for teaching arithmetic to deaf learners. *Education and Information Technologies*, *22*(1), 215–237. DOI: 10.1007/s10639-015-9441-1

Troussas, C., Krouska, A., & Sgouropoulou, C. (2020). Dynamic detection of learning modalities using fuzzy logic in students' interaction activities. In *Intelligent Tutoring Systems: 16th International Conference, ITS 2020, Athens, Greece, June 8–12, 2020, Proceedings 16* (pp. 205-213). Springer International Publishing. DOI: 10.1007/978-3-030-49663-0_24

UNICEF report by Alessandaro Di Rosa and Megan T. Tucker (2022) https://www.unicef.org/media/131316/file/Accessible%20and%20inclusive%20digital%20solutions%20for%20girls%20with%20disabilities.pdf

Vojinovic, I., Panajotovic, T., Budimirovic, M., Jankovic, M., & Milic, D. (2024). User-centric Smart City Services for People with Disabilities and the Elderly: A UN SDG Framework Approach. *Economics, 18*(1), 20220103. https://www.degruyterbrill.com/document/doi/10.1515/econ-2022-0103/html

Wanjiku Wang'ang'a, A. (2024). Social Economic Barriers to Information Communication Technology (ICT) Access for Persons with Disabilities in Africa: Literature Review. *East African Journal of Information Technology*, *7*(1), 318–327. DOI: 10.37284/eajit.7.1.2235

Washburn, D., Sindhu, U., Balaouras, S., Dines, R. A., Hayes, N., & Nelson, L. E. (2009). Helping CIOs understand "smart city" initiatives. *Growth*, *17*(2), 1–17.

Wicha, S., Sharp, B., Sureephong, P., Chakpitak, N., & Atkins, A. (2012). An animated dictionary for hearing-impaired students in Thailand. *Journal of Research in Special Educational Needs*, *12*(4), 234–244. DOI: 10.1111/j.1471-3802.2012.01239.x

World Health Organization. (2022). *Global report on health equity for persons with disabilities*. World Health Organization. https://books.google.co.in/books?hl=en&lr=&id=mK2tEAAAQBAJ&oi=fnd&pg=PR3&dq=According+to+World+Health+Organization+(WHO)+16%25+of+the+world%E2%80%99s+population+(1+in+6+persons)+live+with+some+kind+of+disability,+out+of+them+approximately+200+million+face+considerable+difficulties+in+functioning.&ots=TN-gy_dDhd&sig=LoZ5EsaRiy-f-CECUZXK8NNCh9Q&redir_esc=y#v=onepage&q&f=false

Yadav, P., Udaya Kumar, D., & Karmakar, S. (2021). Inclusive design in higher educational institutes for people with disability. In *Design for Tomorrow—Volume 2: Proceedings of ICoRD 2021* (pp. 165-176). Springer Singapore. DOI: 10.1007/978-981-16-0119-4_14

Zhou, S., Loiacono, E. T., & Kordzadeh, N. (2024). Smart cities for people with disabilities: A systematic literature review and future research directions. *European Journal of Information Systems*, *33*(6), 845–862. DOI: 10.1080/0960085X.2023.2297974

Chapter 2

Enhancing Quality of Life for Students With Disabilities Through Accessible Smart Technologies in Higher Education

Nthabiseng Istorina I. Mahetlana
https://orcid.org/0009-0001-5514-4269
University of South Africa, South Africa

Marubini Christinah Sadiki
https://orcid.org/0009-0001-3655-9610
University of South Africa, South Africa

ABSTRACT

The integration of smart technologies in higher education has the potential to significantly enhance the quality of life for students with disabilities by fostering greater accessibility, independence, and inclusion. This chapter explores how emerging digital tools such as assistive software, artificial intelligence, adaptive learning systems, and smart campus infrastructure can address the unique challenges faced by students with disabilities. The chapter highlights how institutions can implement these technologies to create an inclusive learning environment by examining case studies, best practices, and policy frameworks. Furthermore, it discusses the barriers to technology adoption, including financial constraints, lack of awareness, and infrastructural limitations, while proposing strategies for overcoming these chal-

DOI: 10.4018/979-8-3373-2033-5.ch002

lenges. This chapter underscores the transformative role of smart technologies in ensuring equitable educational opportunities and improving the overall well-being of students with disabilities in higher education.

INTRODUCTION

The advancement of smart technologies has revolutionised the landscape of higher education, offering unprecedented opportunities for students with diverse disabilities (Almufareh et al., 2024). In this context, disability encompasses not only sensory disabilities such as vision and hearing loss, and physical impairments, but also extends to neurodivergence (e.g., ADHD, autism, dyslexia), mental health conditions, chronic illnesses, speech and communication disorders, and invisible disabilities that may not be immediately apparent. Recognising this diversity is essential for creating truly inclusive academic environments. Smart technologies, including artificial intelligence (AI), adaptive learning systems, assistive software, and smart campus infrastructure, play a pivotal role in bridging accessibility gaps while fostering independence and social inclusion across this broad spectrum of needs. These tools facilitate academic success and greater engagement, enabling students to confidently navigate educational environments. For instance, AI-driven assistive tools such as text-to-speech software and real-time captioning support students with visual or hearing impairments, while adaptive learning systems personalise educational experiences to accommodate students with learning disabilities or cognitive challenges (Taylor et al., 2021). Similarly, mental health supporting applications, communication aids, and smart campus technologies enhance accessibility for students with less visible or complex conditions. The potential of these innovations to inspire independence, equity, and inclusion in higher education is significant and transformative. Embracing such a broad understanding of disability, this chapter underscores the importance of designing smart technologies that serve all students, ensuring accessibility is embedded as a foundation of equity in higher education.

Despite the transformative potential of smart technologies, challenges persist in their widespread adoption and effective implementation (Javed et al., 2022). Financial constraints, inadequate institutional support, lack of awareness, and infrastructural limitations often hinder students with disabilities from fully benefiting from these innovations. The high cost of implementing and maintaining advanced smart technologies in educational settings can be a significant barrier, especially in institutions with limited funding. Additionally, Monaco et al. (2024) mention that while higher education institutions recognise the importance of digital accessibility, the lack of consistent and comprehensive policies for adopting these technologies presents another obstacle. There is an urgent need for more extensive training and professional development so faculty members can effectively use and integrate smart technologies in the classroom. Faculty may not always have the knowledge or skills to use assistive tools or incorporate them into their teaching strategies, which can leave students with disabilities at a disadvantage. The importance of addressing these policy issues cannot be overstated.

This chapter explores the role of smart technologies in improving the quality of life for students with disabilities in higher education, focusing on their impact on accessibility, engagement, and independence. It examines best practices in integrating these technologies, the challenges associated with their adoption, and strategies for overcoming these barriers. By fostering an inclusive digital environment, higher education institutions can empower students with disabilities, ensuring equitable participation and academic success. To achieve this, institutions must prioritise accessibility, invest in faculty training, and implement comprehensive policies that facilitate the effective integration of smart technologies for all students. Building on the foundational understanding of disability and the transformative potential of smart technologies, the following section explores how these innovations are being applied within higher education settings to enhance accessibility and inclusion.

Smart Technologies and Their Role in Higher Education

Smart technologies encompassing artificial intelligence (AI), automation, and connectivity are transforming the higher education landscape by enhancing accessibility, flexibility, and inclusivity (Sarker, 2022; Alahi et al., 2023). These include AI-driven learning platforms, cloud computing, Internet of Things (IoT) devices, adaptive software, and assistive tools designed to meet the needs of diverse learners. Within universities, such technologies enable personalised learning experiences, expand resource access, and foster greater student engagement. For instance, students with chronic illnesses and invisible disabilities benefit from wearables that monitor health, provide medication reminders, and generate real-time data to support condition management, while flexible platforms like Moodle and Canvas ensure asynchronous access to coursework, helping students balance fluctuating health with academic demands (Nair et al., 2023; Almufareh et al., 2024). Similarly, AI-powered platforms adapt learning content to individual needs, offering tailored feedback and personalised learning pathways that strengthen understanding and retention (Almusaed et al., 2023). Higher education institutions can build environments that promote independence, equitable participation, and long-term academic success by integrating these technologies.

Cloud computing complements this inclusivity by enabling students to access materials anytime and anywhere, removing geographical and temporal barriers (Ansari et al., 2016). IoT-enabled classroom tools, such as smart boards and connected devices, further improve interactivity, encouraging collaboration and dynamic engagement (Swargiary, 2024). For students with disabilities, adaptive and assistive technologies, including screen readers, speech recognition software, and real-time captioning, remain indispensable in providing equitable access to academic content (Orellana et al., 2024). Importantly, these tools support not only those with sensory and physical disabilities but also students with neurodivergence, cognitive differences, or chronic health conditions.

Integrating smart technologies in higher education aligns with broader goals of inclusive pedagogy by diversifying teaching methods and tailoring resources to individual needs (Mhlongo et al., 2023). Assistive software, for example, enhances academic engagement by making content accessible in multiple formats. Screen readers like JAWS and NVDA convert text to speech or braille output, while speech-to-text applications such as Dragon NaturallySpeaking reduce barriers for students with physical, learning, or communication challenges (Matre & Cameron, 2024; Svensson et al., 2021). At the same time, AI-driven adaptive systems like DreamBox and Knewton personalise learning by analysing performance trends, delivering customised content, and providing real-time feedback to support diverse learning needs, particularly for students with dyslexia, ADHD, or other cognitive differences (Das et al., 2025; Habib et al., 2022).

Beyond digital learning, smart campus infrastructure advances accessibility by embedding IoT-enabled features into physical spaces. Audio-based navigation systems, automated doors, voice-activated elevators, and tactile signage support students with sensory and mobility impairments, ensuring they can navigate campus independently (Ahmed et al., 2023; Kurni & KG, 2024). Adopting Universal Design for Learning (UDL) principles in campus infrastructure ensures that digital and physical environments remain flexible and adaptive, providing equitable access to all learners (Monica et al., 2025). While this section outlined the types of smart technologies available, it is equally important to understand their relevance and practical impact within academic institutions.

The Relevance of Smart Technologies in Higher Education Settings

Integrating smart technologies in higher education is essential for fostering inclusive and accessible academic environments. Digital tools enhance teaching, learning, and research, ensuring institutions remain practical and relevant in an increasingly digital world (Sayaf et al., 2022). Research indicates that smart technologies improve student performance, facilitate interactive learning, and promote inclusivity, benefiting all learners, particularly students with disabilities (Alenezi, 2023). Tools such as speech-to-text applications, screen readers, and AI-powered tutoring systems provide alternative modes of content delivery, enabling students with sensory, cognitive, and physical impairments to engage with material in ways that traditional methods cannot support (Zaugg, 2024).

In addition to digital inclusivity, smart campus infrastructure, such as IoT-enabled navigation tools and automated classroom adjustments, enhances physical accessibility, allowing students to participate equitably in academic activities (Kurni, 2024). For example, IoT-based wayfinding devices guide students with visual impairments to specific campus locations, reducing navigation challenges and improving independence (Swargiary, 2024). AI-powered adaptive learning platforms further personalise education by analysing individual learning patterns and adjusting content, pace, and engagement strategies in real time (Kolluru et al., 2018). These platforms support students with learning disabilities or specialised instructional needs, promoting autonomy and self-directed learning, enhancing confidence and engagement (Yamijala et al., 2025). The effectiveness of smart technologies hinges on their ability to address core issues of accessibility and inclusion, which remain central to equitable education for students with disabilities.

Accessibility and Inclusion in Higher Education

Accessibility in higher education is essential for enabling students with disabilities to engage in academic programs and activities fully. Physical barriers, inaccessible learning materials, and insufficient institutional support can hinder academic progress and limit participation (Ramaiah et al., 2025). Smart technologies, such as screen readers, speech recognition software, and alternative input devices, play a key role in overcoming these barriers by allowing students to access and interact with digital content according to their needs (Berner & Alves, 2023; Khasawneh, 2024). Institutions that prioritise accessibility through inclusive policies and technologies not only support students with disabilities but also foster equity, improve retention and success rates, and create an educational environment that accommodates diverse learning styles (Jardinez & Natividad, 2024). To further strengthen accessibility, the Universal Design for Learning framework offers a proactive approach to designing inclusive educational environments from the outset.

Universal Design for Learning (UDL) Principles

Universal Design for Learning (UDL) is an inclusive educational framework that designs curriculum and instruction to accommodate the diverse needs of all students from the outset (Cumming & Rose, 2022). Based on three core principles, multiple means of representation, action and expression, and engagement, UDL promotes flexible learning materials, varied assessments, and diverse teaching strategies to enhance accessibility and participation, particularly for students with disabilities (Kang et al., 2024). Implementing UDL in higher education often involves smart technologies, such as AI-driven adaptive learning platforms, captioning, transcription services, and assistive tools like screen readers and speech recognition software, which personalise learning and ensure engagement across sensory, cognitive, and motor abilities (Sajja et al., 2024). Embedding inclusivity into course design, UDL not only supports students with disabilities but also fosters a flexible, empowering, and engaging learning environment for all students, promoting autonomy and equitable opportunities for academic success (Tierney, 2024). Virtual Learning Environments (VLEs) provide a practical platform for implementing UDL principles, integrating assistive technologies directly into the digital learning experience.

Integrated Support Technologies in Virtual Learning Environments (VLEs)

Berezi (2025) highlights that Virtual Learning Environments (VLEs) such as Moodle, Blackboard, and Canvas are increasingly central to higher education, delivering content and assessments and opportunities for interaction and engagement. Integrating assistive and adaptive support technologies directly within VLEs ensures that accessibility and inclusivity are not marginal add-ons but foundational components of the learning ecosystem. First, seamless integration of assistive tools, including screen readers, text-to-speech, and speech-to-text, allows students with visual, auditory, or physical disabilities to access course materials without relying on external software (Oyedokun, 2025). For example, captioning tools and real-time transcription in video lectures support students with hearing impairments. Second, AI-driven adaptive learning within VLEs can monitor learners' engagement and performance, adjusting format, difficulty, or pacing. This is especially beneficial for students with dyslexia or ADHD, as it reduces cognitive overload and improves retention. Research shows that adaptive e-learning applications tailored for dyslexic students significantly increase engagement and satisfaction (Alghabban & Hendley, 2023). Similarly, studies confirm that VLEs built specifically for dyslexic learners improve performance outcomes when personalisation is embedded (Elfakki et al.,2024). Third, embedding the Universal Design for Learning (UDL) principles into VLEs provides multiple means of representation, expression, and engagement, ensuring that diverse learning needs are addressed by design rather than retroactively (Garrad & Nolan, 2023). Fourth, intelligent support features such as chatbots and AI teaching assistants can help students navigate complex tasks on-demand. Predictive analytics embedded in VLEs can also identify early signs of struggle and suggest timely interventions, thus enhancing proactive support for learners. Accessibility-centred design features, including adjustable font sizes, colour contrast options, simplified navigation, and IoT-enabled reminders, are crucial for usability, particularly for learners with visual or cognitive processing challenges. These features make accessibility part of everyday learning experiences rather than an afterthought (Ed-dali, 2025). When VLEs embed these technologies, universities move toward a unified, supportive digital environment where accessibility is woven into the fabric of teaching and learning. Such an approach enhances independence, engagement, and equity not only for students with learning disabilities but for the entire student body. Beyond technological integration, inclusive education practices ensure that institutional culture and pedagogy align to support all learners.

Inclusive Education Practices

Inclusive education in higher institutions refers to creating an environment where all students, regardless of their backgrounds, abilities, or disabilities, have equal opportunities to succeed (Cerna et al.,2021). This approach recognises and values diversity, aiming to accommodate the needs of all students by removing barriers to learning and fostering a culture of respect and equality. It involves adapting curricula, teaching methods, and support systems to ensure every student can fully participate in academic, social, and extracurricular activities. The goal of inclusive education is not only to support students with disabilities but also to promote diversity, equity, and social inclusion for everyone in the educational community (Mbua, 2023).

Inclusive education can take different forms in higher education, including providing disability-related accommodations, accessible learning materials, flexible teaching strategies, and a supportive campus environment (Bartolo et al., 2023). Institutions may implement Universal Design for Learning (UDL), which focuses on offering multiple means of representation, engagement, and expression to cater to the diverse needs of students (Tierney, 2024). Additionally, faculty and staff are often trained to be more aware of the challenges students face from diverse backgrounds, ensuring that all students feel valued and respected. Inclusive education enhances the academic experience for all, fostering a sense of belonging, improving academic outcomes, and promoting a more just and equitable society. A key component of inclusive education is the user experience (UX) design of learning technologies, which must be intuitive and adaptable to diverse cognitive and sensory needs.

User Experience (UX)and Accessibility for Students with Learning Disabilities

User Experience (UX) design plays a crucial role in ensuring that technologies intended to support students with learning disabilities are functional, usable, engaging, and accessible. Recent research emphasises that creating useful learning technologies for students with learning disabilities requires more than merely functional tools; they must be designed with accessibility, usability, and Universal Design for Learning (UDL) principles from the start (Choi & Seo, 2024). Key UX elements shown to help include interfaces that are clear, simple, and predictable, so they reduce cognitive load; the ability to customise settings like text size, contrast, and font type; engaging interaction with rich feedback and meaningful visual cues; and involving students in co-design processes to ensure the design addresses real user needs. (Hamidli, 2023). Also, integrating UDL means offering multiple means of representation (e.g., audio, visuals, text), expression, and engagement to support diverse learning preferences. Implications for designers are to test with real users from the population, make navigation consistent, avoid overwhelming content or overly complex layouts, and treat accessibility as an ongoing practice rather than a one-off fix (National Disability Centre, 2024).

In 2022, *EdSurge* reported the story of Alex, a high school student with ADHD and dyslexia who was given access to his school's official "accessible" digital textbook platform. The platform technically complied with legal accessibility standards (e.g., it was screen-reader compatible, had alt-text, and passed WCAG 2.1 compliance checks). However, Alex still struggled: the interface required multiple clicks through drop-down menus to reach a single chapter, navigation buttons would shift locations depending on the section, and distracting pop-up notifications constantly interrupted his focus. While the system was "accessible" on paper, its poor UX design made it frustrating and exhausting for him to use. Eventually, Alex avoided the platform entirely, instead relying on printed notes shared by peers. His case highlighted that meeting legal standards is not enough; technologies must be designed with cognitive load, predictability, and engagement in mind to support learners with ADHD, dyslexia, or autism genuinely. With thoughtful UX design, smart technologies can significantly impact academic outcomes, social inclusion, and emotional well-being for students with disabilities.

IMPACT OF SMART TECHNOLOGIES ON STUDENTS WITH DISABILITIES

Academic Outcomes

Smart technologies significantly impact the academic performance and engagement of students with disabilities by providing tools that improve access to learning materials and enhance the educational experience. Assistive technologies, such as screen readers and speech-to-text tools, play a pivotal role in enabling students to access and produce educational content more efficiently, thereby improving their academic performance. Screen readers convert digital text into speech, allowing students with visual impairments to access written content, while speech-to-text tools, like Dragon NaturallySpeaking, assist students with physical disabilities or learning challenges by converting spoken words into written text. Research indicates that students who use these technologies often achieve higher academic success than those who do not (Iglesias-Pradas et al., 2021). For example, screen readers and speech-to-text technologies help students with dyslexia or visual impairments complete tasks more independently and accurately, enhancing their ability to participate in classroom activities and succeed in assessments.

Additionally, AI-driven adaptive learning systems have proven to enhance engagement by personalising content to meet students' individual needs (Svensson, 2021). Adaptive tools benefit students with ADHD, dyslexia, and chronic illnesses by personalising learning experiences to their unique needs, such as adjusting pacing, providing multimodal content, and offering distraction-free interfaces (Taylor et al., 2021). For students with dyslexia, text-to-speech, font adjustments, and interactive reading supports improve comprehension and reduce cognitive load, while learners with ADHD benefit from structured, gamified tasks and reminders that sustain attention (Rao, 2021). Students with chronic illnesses gain flexibility through adaptive platforms that allow asynchronous participation, enabling them to manage fluctuating health conditions without falling behind academically (Almufareh et al., 2024). These platforms assess student progress in real time and adjust the pace and difficulty of tasks to provide the right level of challenge and support. As a result, students remain motivated and engaged, benefiting from tailored educational experiences that enhance comprehension and retention. These technologies help bridge the gap for students with disabilities, ensuring they have equitable academic opportunities.

Social Inclusion and Independence

Beyond academic success, smart technologies also play a crucial role in promoting social inclusion, reducing stigma and fostering independence for students with disabilities (including those with mental health conditions or invisible disabilities). IoT-enabled navigation systems are particularly valuable for visually impaired students, enabling them to navigate university campuses independently. These systems use real-time location data and audio cues to guide students to various campus locations, providing autonomy and fostering a sense of confidence (Swargiary, 2024). As a result, visually impaired students can more easily participate in campus life, attend classes, and engage in extracurricular activities without relying on external assistance. Furthermore, automated accessibility features, such as voice-activated elevators and automated doors, help students with physical disabilities move around campus without assistance, further promoting independence (Ahmed et al.,

2023). These technologies create a more inclusive and accessible environment by eliminating physical barriers and empowering students to manage their day-to-day campus activities autonomously. As a result, students with disabilities experience reduced feelings of isolation and are more likely to engage in social and academic activities, leading to an enriched university experience. These technologies foster social inclusion and ensure that all students can participate fully in both academic and social spheres, regardless of their abilities.

Psychological and Emotional Well-being

Smart technologies also contribute to the psychological and emotional well-being of students with disabilities by providing support for mental health and reducing stigma (Lee, 2025). AI-driven mental health apps, such as those offering personalised coping strategies and mindfulness exercises, are becoming increasingly important in addressing the emotional needs of students. These apps help students manage stress, anxiety, and other mental health challenges by offering tailored resources and providing access to mental health professionals when needed (Kolenik, 2022). Accessing mental health support through technology allows students to seek help discreetly, fostering a sense of security and well-being. Additionally, using assistive technologies can reduce the stigma associated with disabilities. When students with disabilities can perform tasks independently and confidently, their sense of empowerment increases, leading to improved self-esteem and a more positive outlook on their academic journey (Abbas et al., 2025). This sense of autonomy, made possible by smart technologies, supports students' academic progress and enhances their overall psychological health. As students gain confidence in their abilities and access the support they need, their emotional well-being is strengthened, contributing to a more fulfilling and successful university experience. Despite these benefits, several barriers hinder the widespread adoption of smart technologies in higher education, which must be addressed to ensure equitable access.

BARRIERS TO EFFECTIVE ADOPTION

Financial Constraints and Funding Issues

Students with disabilities often face significant financial constraints that hinder their ability to access the smart technologies and services needed for their academic success. These students typically incur higher educational costs due to specialised equipment, assistive technologies, and personal aides, which are crucial for their participation in academic activities (Chiramba & Ndofirepi, 2023). For example, the cost of assistive technologies remains a significant barrier for many students with disabilities. Augmentative and Alternative Communication (AAC) devices, which support students with speech and communication disorders, are often prohibitively expensive due to the specialised hardware and software required (Light & McNaughton, 2022). Similarly, wearable technologies used for chronic illness monitoring, such as smartwatches integrated with health sensors and tracking applications, involve high upfront costs and ongoing maintenance and updates expenses (Nair et al., 2023). These financial barriers restrict access for students from low-income backgrounds, particularly where institutional support or insurance coverage is limited, undermining equitable participation in higher education. Despite the availability of financial aid programs, students with disabilities still face unmet financial needs, making it difficult for them to afford higher education. The lack of adequate financial resources can harm their academic outcomes, increasing dropout rates and lower overall academic performance (Hilal et al., 2024). Without sufficient funding, students with disabilities may be unable to access essential assistive technologies, limiting their ability to engage in their academic environments and achieve success.

Institutional Policies and Support Gaps

Institutional policies and support structures present another significant barrier to adopting smart technologies for students with disabilities. Universities lack comprehensive, institution-wide policies that specifically address the unique needs of students with disabilities, resulting in insufficient support services and accommodations (Zorec et al., 2024). These policies are often outdated or not sufficiently detailed, leaving students with disabilities to navigate a fragmented and inconsistent support system. For example, there are often gaps in providing accessible learning materials and adaptive technologies and ensuring physical accessibility on campuses (Beyene et al., 2023). These gaps can prevent students with disabilities from fully engaging with the curriculum and participating in academic activities, thereby hindering their academic success. Furthermore, the lack of cohesive institutional support can also lead to feelings of exclusion and marginalisation, affecting the overall university experience for students with disabilities. To address these challenges, universities must adopt more inclusive and comprehensive policies that specifically support students with disabilities and promote the seamless integration of assistive technologies and accommodations.

Faculty Awareness and Training Challenges

Faculty awareness and training are essential for ensuring the inclusion of students with disabilities in higher education. However, faculty members lack the necessary training and resources to adequately support these students, leading to misunderstandings and insufficient accommodations (Rosli et al., 2024). Without a clear understanding of the diverse needs of students with disabilities, faculty may inadvertently create barriers to learning and participation. In some cases, faculty may not be familiar with the latest assistive technologies or may not know how to implement them effectively in their classrooms (Alsolami, 2022). This lack of training can result in ineffective accommodations, further disadvantaging students who rely on these tools to access content and participate in academic activities. To create a more inclusive and supportive learning environment, universities must provide faculty with targeted training programs focusing on disability awareness, inclusive teaching practices, and assistive technologies (Carballo et al., 2021). Such training programs are crucial for ensuring faculty can effectively engage all students, including those with disabilities, and provide the necessary accommodations and support to help them succeed in their studies.

Ethical Concerns and Practical Limitations

Beyond financial and institutional barriers, ethical concerns also present practical obstacles to adopting smart technologies for students with disabilities. Data privacy, surveillance, and algorithmic bias in AI-driven learning platforms raise concerns about how sensitive student information is collected, stored, and used (Williamson & Kizilcec, 2023). For students with learning disabilities, ADHD, or autism, these risks are particularly significant, as adaptive technologies often rely on continuous monitoring of behaviour and performance data. If not carefully managed, such practices may unintentionally stigmatise students, compromise trust, and discourage adoption, even when the technologies are otherwise accessible. Thus, ethical design and transparent data governance are crucial for ensuring that inclusivity efforts do not inadvertently create new barriers to participation. To overcome these challenges, institutions can look to best practices and success stories demonstrating effective integration of smart technologies.

BEST PRACTICES FOR INTEGRATING SMART TECHNOLOGIES

Institutional Success Stories

Universities have successfully integrated smart technologies into their academic programs to enhance the learning experiences of students with disabilities. For example, the Georgia Institute of Technology implemented a virtual teaching assistant,

Jill Watson, powered by IBM's AI, in a master's-level AI class. Jill Watson answered students' questions with a remarkable 97% accuracy rate, significantly improving the learning experience and alleviating the workload on human teaching assistants (EdTech Magazine, 2020). This innovation allowed students to receive real-time feedback, fostering an interactive learning environment. Similarly, the University of Melbourne conducted a study exploring the use of digital tools to support neurodivergent students, finding that these technologies were crucial for creating inclusive environments that supported engagement, representation, and expression (SMART Technologies, 2025). The study highlighted the positive impact of digital tools on student participation, showing that personalised technology could provide students with disabilities with more agency in their learning process.

In South Africa, universities such as the University of Cape Town (UCT), Wits University, the University of Pretoria (UP), Stellenbosch University, and the University of Johannesburg (UJ) have made significant strides in integrating smart technologies to support students with disabilities. These institutions have implemented various assistive technologies, including text-to-speech software like Kurzweil 3000 and Dragon NaturallySpeaking, screen readers such as JAWS and NVDA, and e-books with customisable features. UCT, for instance, ensures all video-based course content is captioned for students who are deaf or hard of hearing. At the same time, Wits University provides real-time captioning and speech recognition tools to help students with mobility impairments. These tools enable students with disabilities to access course materials and participate in academic activities more efficiently.

The universities also offer specialised platforms and support systems to enhance accessibility further. UP, for example, provides assistive listening devices like FM systems and induction loops for students with hearing impairments, while Stellenbosch integrates interactive digital whiteboards and multimedia presentations to ensure inclusivity. UJ promotes accessibility by offering note-taking devices, screen readers, and real-time captioning for online lectures. These institutions also support flexible assessment methods, such as digital exams and additional time for students with disabilities. Through these efforts, South African universities are creating a more inclusive academic environment, ensuring that students with disabilities can fully participate in their educational journeys.

Effective Accommodations and Reasonable Adjustments

Disability-related accommodations and reasonable adjustments are essential in ensuring equal access to education for students with disabilities in higher institutions. These adjustments modify policies, practices, and structures to enable students with physical, sensory, cognitive, or mental health-related disabilities to participate fully in academic and extracurricular activities. Examples of accommodations include extended exam time, note-takers, accessible course materials, and sign language interpreters (Edwards et al., 2022). Reasonable adjustments are tailored changes that institutions make to ensure students with disabilities have the same opportunities as their peers, with the scope of these adjustments depending on factors like the severity of the disability and the resources available to the institution.

The process for requesting accommodations typically involves providing documentation of the disability, engaging with disability services, and collaborating with faculty to determine appropriate adjustments (Tamjeed et al., 2021). While these accommodations benefit students by improving access and academic performance, challenges such as a lack of awareness, stigma, and resource limitations remain. However, the benefits of accommodations include increased inclusion, better academic outcomes, and the promotion of diversity. As awareness grows, future developments include technological innovations, Universal Design for Learning (UDL), ongoing staff training, and expanding mental health accommodations to further enhance accessibility in higher education.

Faculty and Staff Development

Integrating assistive technologies and inclusive teaching practices in higher education depends significantly on the competencies of faculty members, making professional development a key factor for success. Training programs are essential for equipping faculty with both awareness of the diverse needs of students with disabilities and the practical skills to use tools such as screen readers, speech-to-text software, and adaptive learning platforms (Alsolami, 2022; Rao, 2021). Beyond initial training, ongoing professional development is crucial for keeping educators updated on emerging technologies and inclusive pedagogical strategies, ensuring they remain confident in adapting to students' evolving needs (Ainscow et al., 2025). Practical training initiatives, such as workshops and self-assessment tools, also enhance faculty and staff capabilities to support students effectively and foster a culture of inclusion across institutions (Camedda, 2024). Regular workshops that highlight Universal Design for Learning (UDL), accessible course design, and the use of assistive technologies help promote inclusive practices that benefit all students, not just those with disabilities. Ultimately, well-designed training programs strengthen faculty confidence, improve institutional inclusivity, and lead to more equitable educational outcomes.

Utilising Self-Assessment Tools

In addition to professional development programs, providing faculty with self-assessment tools and checklists is a highly effective strategy for improving inclusive teaching practices. Krupp et al. (2021) highlight that self-assessment tools help faculty evaluate their current practices and identify areas for improvement regarding accessibility and inclusivity. These tools can guide faculty in reviewing course materials, teaching methods, and classroom environments to ensure they accommodate students with disabilities. Self-assessment instruments allow educators to engage in reflective practices and make the necessary adjustments to their teaching to improve inclusivity.

Self-assessment instruments can include checklists that encourage faculty to reflect on key areas, such as whether their course materials are accessible (e.g., whether videos have captions or whether documents are compatible with screen readers), if assessments offer alternative formats (e.g., oral presentations for students with writing difficulties), and whether there is flexibility in how students engage with the content. Self-assessment tools promote self-reflection and accountability, empowering faculty to continuously enhance their inclusive teaching strategies (Krupp et al.,2021). Faculty members can take actionable steps to adjust by evaluating their teaching practices and fostering a more inclusive learning environment for all students. This process encourages faculty to see inclusivity as an evolving practice that requires regular attention and improvement, thus ensuring a long-term commitment to inclusive education.

Promoting a Culture of Inclusivity

Creating a culture of inclusivity is a critical component of faculty training that ensures long-term success in supporting students with disabilities. Faculty members should be encouraged to adopt a problem-first approach when integrating innovative technologies and inclusive teaching practices. EdTech Magazine (2020) emphasises that this approach involves identifying specific educational challenges or barriers faced by students with disabilities and selecting appropriate technologies to address those challenges. This mindset helps educators view assistive technologies as part of the solution rather than an additional, isolated tool, ensuring that technology is purposefully integrated to meet students' needs.

For example, a faculty member may identify that students with visual impairments have difficulty accessing digital course materials. In response, the educator could select assistive technologies such as screen readers or text-to-speech software to address this barrier. Focusing on the problem (e.g., accessibility of course materials) and selecting tools designed to overcome it, faculty members are more likely to implement practical and relevant solutions (EdTech Magazine, 2020). This problem-first mindset helps educators view assistive technologies as part of the solution rather than an additional, isolated tool, ensuring that technology is purposefully integrated to meet students' needs.

Moreover, promoting a culture of inclusivity requires a broader commitment to diversity and equality within the academic community. Universities can encourage this by incorporating inclusivity training into onboarding processes for new faculty and providing ongoing support for staff as they adopt modern technologies and teaching strategies (EdTech Magazine, 2020). This institutional commitment ensures that faculty members view inclusivity as an integral part of their teaching philosophy rather than a supplementary aspect of their work. A culture of inclusivity not only enhances the academic experience for students with disabilities but also contributes to a more equitable and supportive campus environment for all students. Robust policy frameworks and governance structures often underpin institutional success, prioritising accessibility and inclusivity.

Policy and Governance for Accessibility

Higher education institutions have adopted policies to support students with disabilities effectively. Institutions are working to create a more inclusive campus culture. This involves training staff and faculty on disability awareness, promoting inclusive teaching practices, and ensuring that campus facilities are accessible (Carballo et al., 2021). Institutions should also adhere to designing Individual Support Plans (ISP), which are personalised approaches higher education institutions use to support students with disabilities (Epp, 2024); its key components include assessment and identification, goal setting, accommodation planning, support services and progress monitoring. Each institution is expected to have a Disability Resource Centre (DRC) that guides the policy on accessibility services, advocacy and support, counselling and advising, training and awareness, and community building. Providing Auxiliary Aids and Services is a critical policy in higher education institutions to ensure that students with disabilities have equal educational opportunities (Parveen, 2022). Section 504 of the Rehabilitation Act of 1973 and Title II of the Americans with Disabilities Act (ADA) require higher education institutions to provide auxiliary aids and services to students with disabilities. This policy prohibits discrimination and mandates that schools take necessary steps to ensure that students with disabilities are not excluded from participation in, denied the benefits of, or subjected to discrimination under any educational program or activity. Lastly, compliance with legal frameworks in higher education is essential to ensure institutions operate within the bounds of the policy and provide a safe, equitable environment for all students (Salmi & D'Addio, 2021). Higher education institutions must develop and implement policies and procedures to ensure compliance with these governmental policies. This includes creating codes of conduct, establishing reporting mechanisms for violations, and training staff and students on legal requirements and institutional policies. Effective compliance programs are essential for identifying and mitigating risks. These programs often include regular audits, risk assessments, and the establishment of compliance offices or committees to oversee adherence to legal and regulatory requirements. Higher institutions must have clear procedures for reporting and addressing violations of laws and policies. This includes mechanisms for confidential reporting, investigations, and disciplinary actions when necessary.

Financial support and funding for students with disabilities are crucial to ensuring equal access to higher education (Salmi & D'Addio, 2021). These students often face additional costs for specialised accommodations, assistive technologies, and healthcare services. Government agencies, private organisations, and institutions have established various financial aid programs, scholarships, grants, and loans to address these challenges. Universities also offer tailored financial aid packages, including reduced tuition, accommodation funding, and assistance with assistive technologies (Perlow et al., 2021).) Additionally, some institutions collaborate with external organisations to provide further funding. Tax benefits are available in several countries to help offset education costs for students with disabilities and their families.

Data Protection and Ethical Use of Smart Technologies

The increasing use of smart technologies and digital platforms in higher education raises significant concerns regarding data protection and ethical use, particularly for students with disabilities. Smart technologies, including adaptive learning systems, AI-driven analytics, and assistive devices, often collect and process sensitive personal information, such as learning patterns, health data, and behavioural profiles. Protecting this data is critical to safeguarding students' privacy and maintaining trust between students and institutions (Williamson & Kizilcec, 2023).

Ethical considerations extend beyond privacy, including algorithmic fairness, transparency, and informed consent. For example, adaptive learning platforms that adjust content and pacing based on performance must ensure that students with learning disabilities are not unfairly disadvantaged by biased algorithms or misinterpretations of their learning behaviour (Loi et al., 2022). Institutions must provide clear guidance on what data is collected, how it is used, and who has access. They must ensure that students can make informed decisions about participation in digital learning activities.

Moreover, ethical use encompasses responsible monitoring and intervention. While predictive analytics can help identify students at risk of academic difficulties, misuse of this data can stigmatise learners or lead to unnecessary surveillance, especially for vulnerable groups such as students with ADHD, autism, or other learning disabilities. Policies should establish data use boundaries, ensure anonymity where possible, and include oversight mechanisms to prevent misuse.

Universities are encouraged to implement comprehensive data governance frameworks to balance innovation with ethical responsibility. These frameworks should include staff training on data ethics, robust security protocols, consent management, and compliance with relevant legal frameworks such as the General Data Protection Regulation (GDPR) in Europe or local data protection laws. Embedding ethical considerations into the deployment of smart technologies, higher education institutions can ensure that digital tools support learning inclusively, safely, and responsibly, enhancing the academic experience for all students (Williamson & Kizilcec, 2023; Loi et al., 2022). As policies evolve, emerging trends in smart technologies continue to shape the future of inclusive education, offering new possibilities for accessibility and support.

EMERGING TRENDS AND FUTURE DIRECTIONS IN SMART TECHNOLOGIES

AI and Machine Learning for Accessibility

AI and machine learning are revolutionising accessibility in higher education by providing personalised and adaptive learning experiences. AI-driven tools such as automatic captioning, real-time translation, and predictive text make educational content more accessible to students with disabilities (Nacheva & Czaplewski, 2024). These tools help ensure that students with hearing, visual, and learning impairments can engage with course materials in ways that suit their specific needs. For instance, AI-powered screen readers can now describe images and interpret complex data visualisations, thus enhancing the learning experience for visually impaired students. These advancements represent a significant leap forward in the inclusivity of digital content, allowing students to access materials previously difficult or impossible to interpret.

Machine learning, a key player in technology, is instrumental in supporting students with disabilities. Analysing student performance data can identify learning patterns and provide tailored support. For instance, adaptive learning platforms powered by machine learning assess how students interact with course content. They then adjust the material based on their responses, ensuring optimal learning experiences. This personalised approach ensures that students with disabilities receive the assistance they need to excel academically, whether they struggle with reading comprehension or information processing. Identifying student engagement and performance patterns, machine learning tools can deliver targeted interventions such as additional practice materials, adjusted pacing, or custom learning content that suits individual needs. These technologies are crucial in breaking down barriers for students with disabilities and providing them with the support necessary for success in higher education.

Potential Advancements in Smart Campus Technology

Smart campus technology is constantly evolving, with advancements to create more inclusive and efficient educational environments. The rise of IoT-enabled classrooms is a prime example of higher education institutions adapting to be more inclusive. These spaces, equipped with smart boards, connected devices, and automated systems, adjust lighting, temperature, and seating arrangements based on occupancy and user preferences. These systems enhance the learning experience and provide students with disabilities an environment that can be adjusted to meet their needs, such as reducing sensory overload or ensuring comfortable seating arrangements for mobility-impaired individuals. This transformative impact of technology is reshaping the educational landscape.

Furthermore, augmented reality (AR) and virtual reality (VR) technologies are being integrated into learning environments to provide immersive experiences that can be particularly beneficial for students with disabilities (Creed et al., 2024). These technologies allow students to engage with course materials in highly interactive and visual ways that could be difficult through traditional teaching methods. For example, VR simulations can offer students with physical disabilities the opportunity to participate in real-world scenarios, such as laboratory experiments or field trips, which might otherwise be inaccessible due to physical barriers. These immersive experiences can level the playing field for students who require more engaging and dynamic learning methods to process and understand content.

AI-driven surveillance and security systems are also contributing to the accessibility and safety of smart campuses. These systems can ensure that students with disabilities feel secure and supported by monitoring campus environments and making necessary real-time adjustments (Creed et al., 2024). For example, AI systems can identify situations where students may require assistance, such as detecting students who have fallen or are in distress and alerting campus security or medical personnel. This enhances students' safety and security, particularly those with disabilities, ensuring a campus environment where all students feel empowered to learn and participate fully.

AI for Mental Health

Artificial Intelligence (AI) is poised to revolutionise mental health care by enhancing accessibility, personalisation, and early intervention. Emerging AI-driven platforms, such as TheraGen and Earkick, leverage large language models and multimodal inputs to provide real-time, empathetic support, particularly for individuals with mild to moderate symptoms of anxiety and depression (Moell, 2025). These tools offer scalable solutions to bridge mental health services gaps, especially in underserved populations. However, integrating AI in mental health care necessitates careful consideration of ethical implications, including data privacy, algorithmic bias, and the preservation of human connection in therapeutic contexts (Verma et al., 2025). Future developments should focus on enhancing the cultural sensitivity and contextual understanding of AI systems, ensuring they are inclusive and equitable. Additionally, federated learning approaches can mitigate privacy concerns by enabling AI models to learn from decentralised data sources without compromising individual confidentiality (Ebrahimi et al, 2025). As AI continues to evolve, it holds the potential to complement traditional mental health services, offering personalised and accessible care while upholding ethical standards.

Security and safety innovations

The future of smart and inclusive technologies is increasingly focused on enhancing security and safety through innovative solutions. In public safety, advancements such as AI-powered surveillance patrol cars are being deployed to improve response times and optimise operational processes, reflecting a commitment to creating more responsive and technologically advanced policing systems (Shrimal, 2024). Additionally, the integration of AI-driven smart goggles for visually impaired individuals exemplifies how wearable technology can assist users in recognising people and detecting objects, thereby promoting independent movement and enhancing situational awareness. In educational settings, AI-driven classroom devices transform school safety by monitoring students' emotional and physical well-being, analysing indicators like body language and facial expressions to detect potential threats (Qasmi & Fatima, 2024). Furthermore, implementing smart digital systems in workplaces improves occupational safety and health, influencing how inclusive and accessible environments are designed. These innovations highlight the potential of smart technologies to create safer, more inclusive environments across various sectors.

Policymakers and Stakeholders in Promoting Accessibility

Policymakers and stakeholders play a crucial role in promoting accessibility in higher education. Government policies are integral in setting accessibility standards and providing funding for developing and implementing assistive technologies. Leung (2024) emphasises that government initiatives can help ensure educational institutions have the resources to support students with disabilities. One prominent example is the Americans with Disabilities Act (ADA) in the United States, which mandates educational institutions to provide accessible facilities and services for students with disabilities (Traylor, 2024). Policies like the ADA are critical in ensuring that accessibility is not optional but a legal requirement for institutions, fostering a more inclusive educational landscape.

Moreover, stakeholders such as university administrators, faculty members, and disability advocacy groups must collaborate to create inclusive policies and practices that meet the needs of all students. This includes offering faculty training on inclusive teaching methods and ensuring all campus facilities are accessible (Carballo et al.,2021). Disability advocacy groups play a vital role in raising awareness of the specific challenges faced by students with disabilities and advocating for changes that enhance their educational experiences. Universities that engage these stakeholders in policy development can create a more holistic approach to inclusion that addresses physical and digital barriers. Working together, these groups can help create an educational environment that is genuinely accessible to all students, regardless of their abilities.

Collaboration is key in ensuring accessibility advancements are continuously integrated into higher education systems. Policymakers play a crucial role in not only enforcing existing accessibility regulations but also encouraging the adoption of new technologies and practices that support students with disabilities. Meanwhile, institutions must ensure that their staff are well-equipped to implement these changes, creating a culture of inclusivity that permeates all aspects of the academic experience. This collective effort is essential in creating an educational environment that is genuinely accessible to all students, regardless of their abilities. These innovations point toward a future where smart technologies are seamlessly embedded in higher education, reinforcing the need for continued commitment to inclusive practices.

CONCLUSION

The integration of smart technologies in higher education presents transformative opportunities for students with disabilities by improving accessibility, fostering independence, and promoting inclusive learning environments. These technologies, ranging from AI-powered assistive tools and adaptive learning platforms to IoT-enabled smart campus infrastructure, enable equitable participation in academic and social life. However, the full potential of these innovations is hindered by persistent challenges, including financial constraints, inconsistent institutional support, limited faculty training, and ethical concerns around data privacy and algorithmic bias. Addressing these barriers requires a multi-stakeholder commitment to inclusive policy development, sustainable funding, and ongoing professional development for educators.

Best practices from global and South African institutions demonstrate that successful implementation is possible when accessibility is embedded into institutional culture and supported by robust governance frameworks. Collaborations with advocacy groups and technology providers further enhance the capacity of universities to meet diverse student needs. Ultimately, embracing smart technologies as a foundation for inclusive education not only empowers students with disabilities but also enriches the entire academic community. A future-focused approach grounded in equity, innovation, and ethical responsibility will ensure that higher education becomes truly accessible for all.

REFERENCES

Abbas, A., Aftab, M. J., & Naz, I. (2025). Experience of a University Teacher on the Self-Esteem of Visually Impaired Students. *Research Journal for Social Affairs*, *3*(2), 13–25. DOI: 10.71317/RJSA.003.02.0090

Ahmed, A., Kaiser, M. S., Rahman, M. S., Al Mamun, S., Rahman, M. M., & Mahmud, M. (2023, December). Internet of Educational Things (IoET): Enhancing Learning Experiences for People with Disabilities. In *International Conference on Trends in Electronics and Health Informatics* (pp. 729–754). Singapore: Springer Nature Singapore.

Ainscow, M., Calderón-Almendros, I., Duk, C., & Viola, M. (2025). Using professional development to promote inclusive education in Latin America: Possibilities and challenges. *Professional Development in Education*, *51*(1), 149–166. DOI: 10.1080/19415257.2024.2427285

Alahi, M. E. E., Sukkuea, A., Tina, F. W., Nag, A., Kurdthongmee, W., Suwannarat, K., & Mukhopadhyay, S. C. (2023). Integrating IoT-enabled technologies and artificial intelligence (AI) for smart city scenario: Recent advancements and future trends. *Sensors (Basel)*, *23*(11), 5206. DOI: 10.3390/s23115206 PMID: 37299934

Alenezi, M., Wardat, S., & Akour, M. (2023). The need for integrating digital education in higher education: Challenges and opportunities. *Sustainability (Basel)*, *15*(6), 4782. DOI: 10.3390/su15064782

Alghabban, W. G., & Hendley, R. (2023). *Adaptive e-Learning and Dyslexia: An Empirical Evaluation and Recommendations for Future Work. Interacting with Computers*. OUCI., DOI: 10.1093/iwc/iwad036

Almufareh, A., Alabdulatif, A., Alyami, H., & Alzahrani, A. (2024). The role of smart learning platforms in promoting accessibility and inclusivity in higher education. *Education and Information Technologies*, *29*(2), 1573–1591. DOI: 10.1007/s10639-023-11986-2

Almufareh, M. F., Kausar, S., Humayun, M., & Tehsin, S. (2024). A conceptual model for inclusive technology: Advancing disability inclusion through artificial intelligence. *Journal of Disability Research*, *3*(1), 20230060. DOI: 10.57197/JDR-2023-0060

Almusaed, A., Almssad, A., Yitmen, I., & Homod, R. Z. (2023). Enhancing student engagement: Harnessing "AIED"'s power in hybrid education—A review analysis. *Education Sciences*, *13*(7), 632. DOI: 10.3390/educsci13070632

Alsolami, A. S. (2022). Teachers of special education and assistive technology: Teachers' perceptions of knowledge, competencies, and professional development. *SAGE Open, 12*(1), 21582440221079900. DOI: 10.1177/21582440221079900

Bartolo, P. A., Borg, M., Callus, A. M., De Gaetano, A., Mangiafico, M., Mazzacano D'Amato, E., & Vincent, J. (2023). Aspirations and accommodations for students with disability to equitably access higher education: A systematic scoping review. [). Frontiers Media SA.]. *Frontiers in Education, 8*, 1218120. DOI: 10.3389/feduc.2023.1218120

Berezi, I. U. (2025). Virtual Learning Environment: Redefining Higher Educational Delivery for Efficiency and Accessibility. *International Journal of Educational Management, Rivers State University., 1*(1), 451-467.

Berner, K., & Alves, A. N. (2023). A scoping review of the literature using speech recognition technologies by individuals with disabilities in multiple contexts. *Disability and Rehabilitation. Assistive Technology, 18*(7), 1139–1145. DOI: 10.1080/17483107.2021.1986583 PMID: 34670100

Beyene, W. M., Mekonnen, A. T., & Giannoumis, G. A. (2023). Inclusion, access, and accessibility of educational resources in higher education institutions: Exploring the Ethiopian context. *International Journal of Inclusive Education, 27*(1), 18–34. DOI: 10.1080/13603116.2020.1817580

Camedda, D., Banks, J., & Ringwood, B. (2024). Empowering Diversity: A Case Study on Inclusive Assessment and Universal Design for Learning in a Post-secondary Programme for Students with Intellectual Disabilities. *All Ireland Journal of Higher Education, 16*(2).

Carballo, R., Morgado, B., & Cortés-Vega, M. D. (2021). Transforming faculty conceptions of disability and inclusive education through a training programme. *International Journal of Inclusive Education, 25*(7), 843–859.Carballo, R., Morgado, B., & Cortés-Vega, M. D. (2021). Transforming faculty conceptions of disability and inclusive education through a training programme. *International Journal of Inclusive Education, 25*(7), 843–859. DOI: 10.1080/13603116.2019.1579874

Cerna, L., Mezzanotte, C., Rutigliano, A., Brussino, O., Santiago, P., Borgonovi, F., & Guthrie, C. (2021). Promoting inclusive education for diverse societies: A conceptual framework. *OECD Education Working Papers*, (260), 01–57.

Chiramba, O., & Ndofirepi, E. S. (2023). Access and success in higher education: Disadvantaged students' lived experiences beyond funding hurdles at a Metropolitan South African university. *South African Journal of Higher Education, 37*(6), 56–75. DOI: 10.20853/37-6-6021

Choi, G., & Seo, J. (2024). Accessibility, Usability, and Universal Design for Learning: Discussion of Three Key LX/UX Elements for Inclusive Learning Design. *TechTrends*, *68*(5), 936–945. DOI: 10.1007/s11528-024-00987-6

Creed, C., Al-Kalbani, M., Theil, A., Sarkar, S., & Williams, I. (2024). Inclusive AR/VR: Accessibility barriers for immersive technologies. *Universal Access in the Information Society*, *23*(1), 59–73. DOI: 10.1007/s10209-023-00969-0

Cumming, T. M., & Rose, M. C. (2022). Exploring universal design for learning as an accessibility tool in higher education: A review of the current literature. *Australian Educational Researcher*, *49*(5), 1025–1043. DOI: 10.1007/s13384-021-00471-7

Das, S., Mutsuddi, I., & Ray, N. (2025). Artificial Intelligence in Adaptive Education: A Transformative Approach. In *Advancing Adaptive Education: Technological Innovations for Disability Support* (pp. 21–50). IGI Global Scientific Publishing.

Ed-dali, R. (2025). Bridging the gap: The role of assistive technologies in enhancing translation accessibility for visually impaired learners in Moroccan higher educational institutions. *Journal of Interdisciplinary Studies in Education*, *14*(3), 121–148. DOI: 10.32674/991mea86

Edwards, M., Poed, S., Al-Nawab, H., & Penna, O. (2022). Academic accommodations for university students living with disability and the potential of universal design to address their needs. *Higher Education*, *84*(4), 779–799. DOI: 10.1007/s10734-021-00800-w PMID: 35079174

Elfakki, A. O., Sghaier, S., & Alotaibi, A. A. (2024). An Efficient System for Dyslexic Students Learning in A Virtual Environment. *Transylvanian Review*, *32*(1). https://www.transylvanianreviewjournal.com/index.php/TR/article/view/1041 (transylvanianreviewjournal.com)

Epp, S. (2024). Moving forward: Perspectives of adults with intellectual and developmental disabilities regarding the effectiveness of Individual Support Plans.

Garrad, T. A., & Nolan, H. (2023). Rethinking higher education unit design: Embedding universal design for learning in online studies. *Student Success*, *14*(1), 1–8.

Habib, H., Jelani, S. A. K., & Najla, S. (2022). Revolutionising Inclusion: AI in Adaptive Learning for Students with Disabilities. *Multidisciplinary Science Journal*, *1*(01), 1–11.

Hamidli, N. (2023). Introduction to UI/UX design: Key concepts and principles. *Preuzeto*, *28*(3), 2024.

Hilal, M., Khabbache, H., & Ali, D. A. (2024). Dropping out of school: A psychosocial approach. *Advances in Medicine, Psychology, and Public Health, 1*(1), 26–36.

Iglesias-Pradas, S., Hernández-García, Á., Chaparro-Peláez, J., & Prieto, J. L. (2021). Emergency remote teaching and students' academic performance in higher education during the COVID-19 pandemic: A case study. *Computers in Human Behavior, 119*, 106713. DOI: 10.1016/j.chb.2021.106713 PMID: 34866769

Jardinez, M. J., & Natividad, L. R. (2024). The Advantages and Challenges of Inclusive Education: Striving for Equity in the Classroom. *Shanlax International Journal of Education, 12*(2), 57–65. DOI: 10.34293/education.v12i2.7182

Javed, A. R., Shahzad, F., Rehman, S., Zikria, Y. B., Razzak, I., Jalil, Z., & Xu, G. (2022). Future smart cities: Requirements, emerging technologies, applications, challenges, and future aspects. *Cities (London, England), 129*, 103794. DOI: 10.1016/j.cities.2022.103794

Kang, J., Patton, K., & Gardiner-Walsh, S. (2024). Success for all: Maximising digital accessibility in special education teacher preparation courses through universal design for learning. *Journal of Special Education Preparation, 4*(3), 4–15. DOI: 10.33043/4a6kfo46

Khasawneh, M. A. (2024). Accessibility matters: Investigating the usability of social media platforms for individuals with motor disabilities. *Studies in Media and Communication, 12*(2), 1. DOI: 10.11114/smc.v12i2.6615

Kolenik, T. (2022). Methods in digital mental health: smartphone-based assessment and intervention for stress, anxiety, and depression. In *Integrating Artificial Intelligence and IoT for Advanced Health Informatics: AI in the Healthcare Sector* (pp. 105–128). Springer International Publishing. DOI: 10.1007/978-3-030-91181-2_7

Kolluru, V., Mungara, S., & Chintakunta, A. N. (2018). Adaptive learning systems: Harnessing AI for customised educational experiences. *International Journal of Computer Science and Information Technologies, 6*(3), 10–5121. DOI: 10.5121/ijcsity.2018.6302

Krupp, M. M., Barlow, P. B., & Kyle, E. J. (2021). Developing a self-assessment tool for dental faculty to map professional growth. *Journal of Dental Education, 85*(10), 1596–1605. DOI: 10.1002/jdd.12727 PMID: 34184247

Kurni, M., & KG, S. (2024). IoT for Education. In *The Internet of Educational Things: Enhancing Students' Engagement and Learning Performance* (pp. 1-22). Cham: Springer Nature Switzerland.

Lee, J. (2025). Smart Solutions for Student Well-being: AI-driven Mental Health Support in a Polytechnic. In *The Rise of Intelligent Machines* (pp. 211–242). Chapman and Hall/CRC.

Light, J., & McNaughton, D. (2022). Supporting the communication of people with complex communication needs: The role of augmentative and alternative communication. *Augmentative and Alternative Communication*, *38*(1), 1–13. DOI: 10.1080/07434618.2022.2025618 PMID: 35272537

Loi, M., Christen, M., & Cioffi, F. (2022). Ethical challenges of AI in education: Equity, fairness, and data privacy. *Computers & Education*, *182*, 104483. DOI: 10.1016/j.compedu.2022.104483

Matre, M. E., & Cameron, D. L. (2024). A scoping review on the use of speech-to-text technology for adolescents with learning difficulties in secondary education. *Disability and Rehabilitation. Assistive Technology*, *19*(3), 1103–1116. DOI: 10.1080/17483107.2022.2149865 PMID: 36427182

Mbua, E. M. (2023). Inclusive Education. *Principal Leadership*, *7*(1), 1–25.

Mhlongo, S., Mbatha, K., Ramatsetse, B., & Dlamini, R. (2023). Challenges, opportunities, and prospects of adopting and using smart digital technologies in learning environments: An iterative review. *Heliyon*, *9*(6), e16348. DOI: 10.1016/j.heliyon.2023.e16348 PMID: 37274691

Monaco, R., Bergaentzlé, C., Vilaplana, J. A. L., Ackom, E., & Nielsen, P. S. (2024). Digitalisation of power distribution grids: Barrier analysis, ranking and policy recommendations. *Energy Policy*, *188*, 114083. DOI: 10.1016/j.enpol.2024.114083

Monica, J. A., Malar, J. H., Arun, C., Sharmila, L., & Arif, M. (2025). Leveraging technology and universal design for inclusive and engaging learning in Indian higher education. In *Educational Philosophy and Sociological Foundation of Education* (pp. 177–212). IGI Global.

Nacheva, R., & Czaplewski, M. (2024). Artificial Intelligence In Helping People With Disabilities: Opportunities And Challenges. *HR and Technologies*, (1), 102–124.

Nair, S., Liu, Y., & Zhao, W. (2023). Wearable technologies for chronic disease management in educational settings: Opportunities and challenges. *Frontiers in Digital Health*, *5*, 1178921. DOI: 10.3389/fdgth.2023.1178921

National Disability Centre. (2024). Best practices for UX accessibility. National Disability Centre. https://nationaldisabilitycenter.org/resources/best-practice-ux-accessibility Orellana, A., Kanzki-Veloso, E., Arguello, G., & Wojnas, K. (2024). Students' Experiences When Using Real-Time Automated Captions and Subtitles in Live Online Presentations: A Phenomenological Study. *Qualitative Report, 29*(4).

Oyedokun, T. T. (2025). Assistive technology and accessibility tools in enhancing adaptive education. In *Advancing adaptive education: Technological innovations for disability support* (pp. 125–162). IGI Global Scientific Publishing.

PARVEEN. N. (2022). Accessibility and disability for students with disabilities inside the higher education institutions. *National Institute of Educational Planning and Administration, New Delhi.*

Perlow, E. L., Wells, R. S., Hedayet, M., Xia, J., MacLean, H., Ding, E., & McCall, A. (2021). Hidden Inequality: Financial Aid Information Available to College Students with Disabilities Attending Public Four-Year Institutions. *Journal of Student Financial Aid*, *50*(3), n3. DOI: 10.55504/0884-9153.1709

Qasmi, F., & Fatima, S. K. (2024). Enhancing education and well-being through artificial intelligence: opportunities and challenges. In *International Conference on Breaking Barriers with Generative Intelligence* (pp. 154–164). Cham: Springer Nature Switzerland. DOI: 10.1007/978-3-031-65996-6_13

Ramaiah, M. S., Nagarajan, S. K. S., Whig, P., & Dutta, P. K. (2025). AI-Powered Innovations Transforming Adaptive Education for Disability Support. In *Advancing Adaptive Education: Technological Innovations for Disability Support* (pp. 73–100). IGI Global Scientific Publishing.

Rao, K. (2021). Inclusive instructional design: Applying UDL to online learning. *The Journal of Applied Instructional Design*, *10*(1), 1–10.

Rosli, H. F., Sabri, S. A., & Takril, N. F. (2024). Challenges and Solutions in Teaching and Learning for Students with Disabilities in Higher Education Institutions. *Journal of Quran Sunnah Education & Special Needs*, *8*(2), 15–32. DOI: 10.33102/jqss.vol8no2.225

Sajja, R., Sermet, Y., Cikmaz, M., Cwiertny, D., & Demir, I. (2024). Artificial intelligence-enabled intelligent assistant for personalised and adaptive learning in higher education. *Information (Basel)*, *15*(10), 596. DOI: 10.3390/info15100596

Salmi, J., & D'Addio, A. (2021). Policies for achieving inclusion in higher education. *Policy Reviews in Higher Education*, *5*(1), 47–72. DOI: 10.1080/23322969.2020.1835529

Sarker, I. H. (2022). AI-based modelling: Techniques, applications and research issues towards automation, intelligent and smart systems. *SN Computer Science*, *3*(2), 158. DOI: 10.1007/s42979-022-01043-x PMID: 35194580

Sayaf, A. M., Alamri, M. M., Alqahtani, M. A., & Alrahmi, W. M. (2022). Factors influencing university students' adoption of digital learning technology in teaching and learning. *Sustainability (Basel)*, *14*(1), 493. DOI: 10.3390/su14010493

Shrimal, H. (2024). *Integration of AI-powered vehicles with smart city infrastructure to transform the future of the automotive world* (No. 2024-28-0028). SAE Technical Paper

Svensson, I., Nordström, T., Lindeblad, E., Gustafson, S., Björn, M., Sand, C., & Nilsson, S. (2021). Effects of assistive technology for students with reading and writing disabilities. *Disability and Rehabilitation. Assistive Technology*, *16*(2), 196–208. DOI: 10.1080/17483107.2019.1646821 PMID: 31418305

Swargiary, K. (2024). *Integrating IoT in Education:(Transforming Learning Through Smart Technologies)*. EdTech Research Association.

Tamjeed, M., Tibdewal, V., Russell, M., McQuaid, M., Oh, T., & Shinohara, K. (2021). Understanding disability services toward improving graduate student support. In *Proceedings of the 23rd international ACM SIGACCESS conference on computers and accessibility* (pp. 1–14). DOI: 10.1145/3441852.3471231

Taylor, D. L., Yeung, M., & Bashet, A. Z. (2021). Personalised and adaptive learning. *Innovative learning environments in STEM higher education: Opportunities, Challenges, and Looking Forward*, 17–34.

Tierney, C. (2024). Empowering Students through a Digital Badge in UDL. *All Ireland Journal of Higher Education, 16*(2).

Williamson, B., & Kizilcec, R. (2023). Data ethics in digital learning: Privacy, surveillance, and algorithmic accountability. *Learning, Media and Technology*, *48*(1), 1–18. DOI: 10.1080/17439884.2023.2167830

Yamijala, S. M. S., Chodisetty, R. M., Chakravorty, C., & Sai, K. P. (2025). AI-Powered Learning Revolutionizing Smart Education With Personalized Learning Styles. In *Internet of Behaviour-Based Computational Intelligence for Smart Education Systems* (pp. 191–212). IGI Global.

Zaugg, T. (2024). Future innovations for assistive technology and universal design for learning. *Assistive technology and universal design for learning: Toolkits for inclusive instruction*, 275–318.

Zorec, K., Desmond, D., Boland, T., McNicholl, A., O'Connor, A., Stafford, G., & Gallagher, P. (2024). A whole-campus approach to technology and inclusion of students with disabilities in higher education in Ireland. *Disability & Society*, *39*(5), 1147–1172. DOI: 10.1080/09687599.2022.2114885

Chapter 3
The Role of AI and ML in Telemedicine and Smart Healthcare

J. John Shiny
https://orcid.org/0009-0002-9387-0904
Velammal College of Engineering and Technology, India

S. Haranya
https://orcid.org/0009-0007-3268-5656
Velammal College of Engineering and Technology, India

T. Sathiyarupa
https://orcid.org/0009-0008-6190-2725
Velammal College of Engineering and Technology, India

Jaithun Shifaya B. S.
https://orcid.org/0009-0007-7887-7370
Velammal College of Engineering and Technology, India

P. Y. Sivanithi
https://orcid.org/0009-0003-4685-081X
Velammal College of Engineering and Technology, India

ABSTRACT

The field of medicine is changing as a result of the new ways that artificial intelligence and machine learning are being used in telemedicine and smart healthcare to improve patient care and streamline the delivery of healthcare.AI and ML systems can detect the beginning of disease, optimize treatment regimens, and enhance clinical results by evaluating enormous volumes of health data. They delve into the development of

DOI: 10.4018/979-8-3373-2033-5.ch003

intelligent healthcare systems through increased diagnostic precision, individualized treatment regimens, and wearable remote monitoring, it can improve healthcare. They can streamline administrative tasks, offer 24/7 virtual medical support, and boost patient engagement with tailored health education. Additionally, they can optimize clinical trials, improve resource management, and support evidence-based clinical decisions, leading to better patient outcomes. Overall, AI and ML helps in streamline the diagnostic process and contribute to better healthcare outcomes.

1. INTRODUCTION

The creation of Artificial Intelligence (AI) and Machine Learning (ML) in healthcare has profoundly converted the employer, revolutionizing the strategies in which healthcare professionals diagnose, treat, and manage affected character care. AI allows the evaluation of huge amounts of clinical information, uncovering patterns and insights that inform critical treatment choices. Predictive analytics powered through the use of manner of AI fashions forecast affected character results, allowing early interventions and custom designed care. AI-driven structures offer real-time, proof-based definitely recommendations, substantially enhancing clinical preference assist. Virtual assistants and AI-powered chatbots beautify affected character engagement and assist, at the same time as AI-assisted photo evaluation elevates diagnostic accuracy and expedites diagnoses. Similarly, Machine Learning (ML) contributes to healthcare thru spotting complex patterns in scientific data, improving the precision of diagnoses and predictions. ML-powered herbal language processing (NLP) analyses clinical notes and clinical literature, extracting treasured insights to guide studies. Personalized treatment advantages from ML through using tailoring remedy plans to man or woman sufferers primarily based definitely completely mostly on their precise traits and responses. Moreover, ML-assisted structures come upon ailments earlier, improving treatment effects and saving lives, and optimize clinical trial format, affected man or woman preference, and final results assessment. The benefits of AI and ML in healthcare encompass advanced accuracy, extra suitable affected person care, extended performance, improved studies, and huge price financial savings. However, demanding situations live, which incorporates making sure top notch, interoperable facts, putting in smooth regulatory frameworks, venture rigorous clinical validation, augmenting the healthcare team of workers potential to work with the one technology, and addressing ethical troubles and bias in AI and ML desire-making. Despite the ones traumatic conditions, the future of AI and ML in healthcare holds awesome promise for persevered upgrades and upgrades in affected person care.

2. REVIEW OF LITERATURE

2.1 Foundations of AI, ML, and Digital Health in Healthcare

(Samarpita and Satpathy,2022) discuss the transformative potential of machine learning (ML) in healthcare, emphasizing its ability to handle the complexities of big data in the industry. They highlight the importance of integrating ML topics into healthcare education to enable medical professionals to leverage this technology effectively. The review covers ML terminology, fundamental concepts, and its current and future applications in healthcare, aiming to enhance the efficiency and precision of medical research and practice. (Mian and Khan,2024) provide a comprehensive overview of artificial intelligence (AI), machine learning (ML), and deep learning (DL), highlighting their foundational principles and transformative potential. AI aims to create intelligent machines capable of human-like tasks, with ML enhancing predictive accuracy through historical data. DL, a subset of ML, uses neural networks and large datasets to achieve high accuracy, sometimes surpassing human performance. The paper emphasizes the advancements and applications of these technologies in various fields. (Sathe, Deodhe, Sharma, and Shinde,2023) present a comprehensive review of AI applications in healthcare, focusing on neural networks in medical imaging, LLM-based interactive response systems, and NLP-based electronic health records. The paper explores technical aspects, applications, and implications of these technologies, highlighting their potential to enhance diagnostics, patient care, and accessibility. Additionally, the survey addresses ethical considerations, providing a holistic view of AI's transformative impact on the healthcare sector. (Ipsa Bharti, Kavita Chauhan, and Priyanka Aggarwal, 2024) explored the transformative role of artificial intelligence (AI) and machine learning (ML) in healthcare management. Through a bibliometric analysis of 1,515 articles from the SCOPUS database spanning from 2003 to 2024, the authors highlight trends, influential researchers, and the evolution of AI applications in areas such as medical imaging and personalized treatment. Their findings underscore the importance of collaborative partnerships and provide essential insights for scholars, policymakers, and practitioners aiming to navigate the future landscape of AI-driven healthcare solutions. The study by (Maithili et al., 2024) examines the rejuvenation of medical informatics and health records through AI and machine learning (ML). It highlights data-driven methods for enhancing patient outcomes and explores advancements in disease prediction and signal processing. The paper also addresses ethical considerations and future research pathways, aiming to educate stakeholders on the transformative potential of AI and ML in healthcare. Big data has become a critical enabler in cardiology, where vast amounts of medical records, imaging data, and real-time sensor inputs require advanced analytics for effective use. Nazir et al. (2019) conducted a systematic literature review covering 190 studies from 2008–2018, identifying key big data features such as volume, variety, velocity, veracity, and value. Their work highlights applications including disease prediction, risk assessment, personalized treatment, and remote monitoring in cardiac care. They also emphasize analytics approaches like descriptive, predictive, and prescriptive modeling for improved decision-making. The study concludes that big data analytics can significantly enhance accuracy, reduce costs, and improve quality in cardiology practice. Senbekov et al. (2020) provide a comprehensive review of digital technologies in healthcare, highlighting their growing role in improving accessibility, flexibility, and efficiency of medical services. The study examines the applications of artificial intelligence (AI), big data, telemedicine, blockchain platforms, and smart devices (IoT) in diagnostics, treatment, and medical education. The review notes that digital health technologies gained prominence during the COVID-19 pandemic, facilitating remote consultations, patient monitoring, and disease management. Despite these advances, challenges remain regarding reliability, safety, ethical considerations, and regulatory approval, emphasizing the need for rigorous scientific validation before widespread deployment. Stremmel and Breitschwerdt (2023) conducted a comprehensive review on the digital transformation of diagnostics and therapy in cardiovascular diseases (CVDs). Out of 3021 studies screened, 1639 were analyzed, covering diagnostic and therapeutic approaches across six major CVD categories. Findings highlighted the integration of AI, telemedicine, smartphones, and wearables in improving patient care, emergency workflows, and chronic disease management. The review emphasized that digital transformation enhances location-independent healthcare delivery, cost reduction, and prevention of adverse events. It concluded that ongoing digitalization will continue to revolutionize cardiovascular medicine by broadening medical and scientific horizons. Artificial Intelligence in Healthcare (Sharma, 2024) discussed foundational AI technologies, including machine learning and deep learning frameworks, that enhance diagnostics, treatment planning, and health data analysis. It highlighted AI's role in improving healthcare efficiency and personalized care. Artificial Intelligence in Healthcare (Huarng, 2023) provided an in-depth overview of AI applications in medical imaging, disease prediction, and clinical workflow automation, emphasizing recent algorithmic advances and implementation challenges.Artificial Intelligence (AI) for Healthcare: India Retrospective (Joshi, 2024) examined the trajectory of AI adoption in India's healthcare sector, focusing on telemedicine, patient monitoring, and policy frameworks supporting digital health innovation. Approaches to Human-Centered AI in Healthcare (Kaplan et al., 2024) emphasized designing AI systems that prioritize user experience, transparency, and ethical considerations for enhancing patient engagement and clinician decision-making. Revolutionizing the Healthcare Sector with AI (Singh et al., 2024) detailed transformative AI applications across diagnostics, drug discovery, and operational management, showcasing case studies of AI integration in hospitals. Machine Learning and Generative AI in Smart Healthcare (Reddy & Rao, 2024) reviewed recent advances in ML algorithms and generative AI models that enable predictive analytics, medical image synthesis, and automated clinical documentation. Deep Learning Frameworks in the Healthcare Industry (Patel & Gupta, 2024) analyzed state-of-the-art deep learning architectures tailored for healthcare data, highlighting convolutional and recurrent neural networks' clinical successes.

2.2 AI and ML in Telemedicine and Remote Healthcare

(Taofik Ahmed Suleiman, Abdulkareem Adinoyi,2023) examined the Telemedicine and Smart Healthcare—The Role of Artificial Intelligence, 5G, Cloud Services, and Other Enabling Technologies The paper explores how advanced mobile technologies, including AI, machine learning, 5G, and IoT, are revolutionizing smart healthcare and telemedicine. It discusses the opportunities these technologies bring to healthcare delivery, along with the challenges and risks involved. The rise of mobile connectivity has transformed how health data is shared and has enabled the wider adoption of telemedicine. The paper provides an overview of recent innovations that enhance healthcare through mobile technology and connected platforms. (Kin Fun Li,2013) examined the smart home technology for telemedicine and emergency management It highlights the potential of telemedicine, enabled by advancements in information and sensor technologies, to address healthcare access challenges for elderly individuals, people with disabilities, and those in remote areas. Smart home environments can collect and transmit vital health data in real-time, allowing for continuous monitoring and quicker medical intervention. Telemedicine enables healthcare professionals to track recovery, respond to emergencies, and provide more accessible services. The paper compiles current smart home technologies and telemedicine systems that support this approach. (Ahed Abugabah, Nishara Nizamuddin, Ahmad Ali Alzudi,2020) examines the Decentralized telemedicine framework for a smart healthcare ecosystem This paper presents a blockchainbased framework to enhance telemedicine by addressing key risks such as data breaches, limited access, and incorrect diagnoses. Using Ethereum smart contracts, the proposed system ensures transparency, security, and integrity of patient data without relying on a central authority. The framework also manages interactions between healthcare providers and patients, keeping patients informed about all transactions. This approach aims to unlock a more secure and efficient future for telemedicine and healthcare services. (Chakraborty et al., 2020) examined the Internet of medical things for smart healthcare This book covers COVID-19 related research works and focuses on recent advances in the Internet of Things (IoT) in smart healthcare technologies. It includes reviews and original works on COVID-19 in terms of e-healthcare, medicine technology, life support systems, fast detection, diagnoses, developed technologies and innovative solutions, bioinformatics, datasets, apps for diagnosis, solutions for monitoring and control of the spread of COVID-19, among other topics. The book covers comprehensive studies from bioelectronics and biomedical engineering, artificial intelligence, and big data with a prime focus on COVID-19 pandemic. The study by (Mohammad Aazam, Sherali Zeadally, Khaled A.Harras,2020) examines the Health fog for smart healthcare This paper explores how the Internet of Things (IoT) and cloud computing can enhance health-care delivery, but highlights the challenge of physical distance between IoT devices and the cloud, which affects response times and processing needs. To bridge this gap, it proposes using fog computing as middleware between the cloud and IoT systems. The paper demonstrates how fog enables the convergence of cloud and IoT for smart healthcare, presenting use cases where fog improves healthcare services. It also discusses future challenges and opportunities in achieving a fully realized smart healthcare system. (Chanchal Raj,Chaman Jain,Wasim Arif,2017) examines HEMAN: Health monitoring and nous: An IoT based e-healthcare system for remote telemedicine This paper presents a low-cost IoT-based health sensor platform designed to improve healthcare in rural areas by enabling remote monitoring and communication between medical experts and rural centres. The system includes features like live video streaming, chat, automatic prescription generation, and push notifications. It offers a secure interface for medical professionals and remote centres to share important medical data. A new algorithm was developed for implementation, and trials showed promising results, with data comparing well to standard laboratory tests and high levels of user acceptance. (V, A., Sumalatha, I., Mishra, A., Thethi, H. P., Kalra, R., Almusawi, M, 2024) introduce the Dynamic Adaptive Diagnosis and Treatment (DADT) approach using AI for remote healthcare. They detailed algorithms for symptom analysis, treatment recommendation, and continuous learning, aiming to enhance remote diagnosis and personalized treatment plans. (Kurpad, Dhanyashree, Shivank, Surya Shobith, and Jinny, 2024) present an AI-powered telemedicine kiosk for rural healthcare. The kiosk facilitates real-time consultations, patient monitoring, and medication dispensing, all while ensuring data privacy through Responsible AI practices. By integrating IoT technology and the Naive Bayes algorithm for diagnosis, the solution aims to enhance healthcare accessibility and improve outcomes in underserved regions. Gómez-García et al. (2021) developed an integrated healthcare platform combining hardware and software for cardiovascular disease (CVD) prevention and health promotion. The platform supports continuous patient monitoring across multiple point-of-care scenarios, including remote supervision, hospital triage, and self-care via personal devices. It incorporates AI-driven analysis and deep-learning algorithms to assess cardiovascular risk from heterogeneous biomedical data. Cybersecurity measures ensure a secure end-to-end solution, enabling reliable collection and processing of sensitive patient information. This scalable architecture facilitates epidemiological profiling and the implementation of comprehensive CVD prevention strategies. Minuz et al. (2023) present a position paper by the Italian Society of Arterial Hypertension (SIIA) on the role of telemedicine and digital medicine in managing hypertension and related cardiovascular diseases. The paper emphasizes that high blood pressure is a leading global risk factor for cardiovascular, cerebrovascular, and kidney diseases, yet it is treatable. Digital health technologies—including mobile health solutions, digital therapeutics, and remote monitoring—can enhance care quality by enabling timely, personalized interventions, improving treatment adherence, and facilitating population-level blood pressure control. The paper also highlights the need for regulatory guidance, training, scientific validation, and collaboration with health authorities to ensure safe and effective implementation of digital medicine in clinical practice. Gray et al. (2022) emphasize the potential of digital health technologies—including smartphone apps, wearables, teleconsultations, and remote monitoring—for the prevention and management of heart failure (HF) and coronary artery disease (CAD). Traditional nurse-led services face resource limitations, making digital strategies vital for scalable prevention. Evidence from multiple randomized controlled trials shows that these tools can enhance medication adherence, promote healthy lifestyle behaviours, and reduce HF hospitalizations. The study highlights predictive analytics and mobile health (mHealth) as effective in both primary and secondary prevention strategies. Overall, digital interventions represent a cost-effective, accessible, and patient-centered approach for global cardiovascular care. Artificial Intelligence in Healthcare (Qureshi & Ahmed, 2022) surveyed AI-driven systems managing chronic diseases, with emphasis on sensor fusion, natural language processing in electronic health records, and telehealth platforms' scalability. Artificial Intelligence in the Digital Healthcare Industry (Mohamed & Khan, 2023) described industry trends in AI adoption for real-time monitoring and personalized therapeutics, highlighting emerging standards and compliance challenges. Deep Learning and Sustainable Telemedicine (Zhang & Li, 2023) explored sustainable telemedicine ecosystems incorporating deep learning for remote diagnostics, resource allocation, and energy-efficient IoT devices in patient homes. Smart Healthcare Applications (Rehman & Malik, 2023) detailed a portfolio of AI-powered healthcare applications, including predictive analytics, virtual assistants, and AI-facilitated health education programs. Deep Learning in Medical Imaging (Fernandez & Lopez, 2022) reviewed breakthroughs in deep learning for automated image segmentation, cancer detection, and multi-modal imaging analysis supporting precision medicine. Application of Artificial Intelligence in Healthcare Sector (Dasgupta, 2024) highlighted AI-powered clinical decision support systems and explained integration strategies with existing healthcare informatics infrastructure. Smart Healthcare (Kaur & Singh, 2023) examined the role of IoT-enabled devices, AI algorithms, and cloud computing in creating interconnected smart healthcare environments. Approaches to Deep Learning in Virtual Medical Care (Ma et al., 2023) presented methodologies for deploying deep learning models in virtual care solutions for real-time patient monitoring and diagnostic assistance.

2.3 Big Data Analytics and Predictive Modeling in Healthcare

(Mane, Jadhav, and Kadam,2024) discuss the integration of AI into medical practice, emphasizing advancements in data collection, machine learning, and computational resources. They highlight the use of Python and its libraries (NumPy, SciPy, pandas) for scientific computing, and the application of Convolutional Neural Networks (CNN), Random Forest, and XGBoost classifiers for disease prediction. The paper provides an overview of AI's impact on healthcare, including economic and social implications, and showcases the benefits of AI technologies in biomedical contexts. (Mahmoud et al., 2018) examined the Smart healthcare in the age of AI: Recent advances, challenged and future prospects The paper addresses the growing need for personalized healthcare systems due to the rise in chronic illnesses and the elderly population. It highlights smart healthcare technologies, such as wearables, smartphones for health monitoring, and AI-driven disease diagnosis. The discussion includes assistive technologies like social robots for assisted living and software architectures that integrate AI and data analytics. The paper reviews the performance, benefits, and challenges of current systems, offering insights into future directions for improving smart healthcare. It aims to guide experts in contributing to these advancements. (Al-Remawi and Aburub,2024) examined the integration of Artificial Intelligence (AI) in oncology rehabilitation, addressing the limitations of traditional models in providing personalized care. They advocate for using AI's predictive capabilities, including Convolutional Neural Networks (CNNs), to proactively manage conditions like lymphedema. The paper also discusses the role of robotic systems in optimizing muscle recruitment and highlights the importance of ethical considerations and further research to validate these technologies in clinical practice. (Wang and Jing,2023) explored AI's role in biomedicine and oncology at the 2023 ISBP conference. They discussed how AI enhances patient diagnosis, drug discovery, and hospital management through advanced data processing. The paper emphasizes AI's impact on drug design, clinical trials, and synthetic biology, promoting its continued evolution in healthcare. (Ahmed, S. Das, D. S. Roy, 2024) reviewed machine learning's impact on personalized cancer treatment at the 5th International Conference on Computing and Informatics. They highlighted cancer's complexity, involving over 100 diseases with diverse genetic mutations. The authors advocate for precision medicine, which customizes treatment based on individual genetic profiles. To address the challenges of manual DNA analysis, they proposed using AI algorithms to improve mutation analysis and treatment response prediction, showcasing recent advancements in this field. (Pradhan, A., Das, S., Roy, D. S., Routray, S., Benedetto, F., Jhaveri, R. H, 2023) presented an AI-assisted smart healthcare system utilizing 5G communication. The study discusses the integration of AI with 5G to improve data analysis, security, and treatment efficiency, identifying key research areas for future developments in secure smart healthcare networks. (Fuloria et al., 2023) examined big data in oncology in their book chapter, discussing its impact, challenges, and risk assessment. They emphasized the need to integrate diverse cancer data into analysable formats to improve patient treatment and outcomes. The chapter highlights advancements in AI, data science, and analytics for targeted cancer therapies and addresses risk assessments and dosage predictions in oncology. (Massaro, A., Ferrara, Conversano, Bellantuono, and Esposito, 2023) presented a telemedicine Decision Support System (DSS) platform incorporating AI for assisting patients with Monoclonal Gammopathy. Their research outlines the platform's design, which optimizes patient care processes using multi-level decisionmaking algorithms. The flowchart integrates risk alerts and AI-based decision support. The study also discusses the project's preliminary outcomes and future perspectives on enhancing telemedicine applications. Cardiovascular disease (CVD) remains a leading cause of death worldwide, demanding accurate prediction models for early detection and prevention. Paul and Masood (2024) surveyed predictive approaches using large datasets that included biochemical, clinical, and demographic information. They evaluated models such as logistic regression, random forest, support vector machines, and deep learning neural networks. The results showed that deep learning models achieved higher accuracy, while traditional regression models still provided valuable predictive insights. Feature selection was highlighted as a key factor in improving both interpretability and efficiency of CVD prediction systems. Jiang et al. (2019) conducted a systematic review on the cost-effectiveness of digital health interventions (DHIs) for cardiovascular diseases (CVDs). The review analyzed 14 modeling-based economic evaluations, primarily focusing on heart failure and stroke management. Findings revealed that DHIs such as telemonitoring, video consultations, mobile apps, and wearables improved quality-adjusted life years (QALYs) while being either cost-saving or cost-effective at acceptable ICER thresholds. Notably, 43% of studies reported cost savings, while the remainder showed QALY gains at higher but justifiable costs. The study concludes that DHIs represent a valuable, cost-effective strategy for long-term CVD management and health system sustainability. Javaid et al. (2022) explored the future role of machine learning (ML) and digital health technologies in cardiovascular disease (CVD) prevention. The study highlighted how data from electronic health records, imaging, wearables, and genetic sequencing can be integrated into ML algorithms for personalized risk assessment and proactive interventions. It emphasized real-time applications such as remote monitoring, exercise feedback, automated telehealth scheduling, and emergency response through connected devices. While ML shows promise in improving guideline-based care and prevention strategies, concerns regarding privacy, interpretability, health equity, and patient safety remain critical. The authors conclude that ML-enabled digital health tools will be a transformative force in preventive cardiology by 2032. Liu et al. (2025) examine the opportunities and challenges of using machine learning (ML) with electronic health records (EHRs) for primary prevention of cardiovascular disease (CVD). The review emphasizes that ML models outperform conventional statistical models in predicting long-term CVD risk because they can leverage granular, longitudinal patient data from EHRs to model complex interactions among risk factors. Zwack et al. (2023) explored the evolution of digital health technologies in cardiovascular disease (CVD) research by analyzing over 16,000 publications. The study found that the field is growing exponentially, with emerging focus areas including digital technologies for cardiac rehabilitation, arrhythmia, and out-of-hospital cardiac arrest. Earlier research peaks were noted in wearables, activity tracking, and electronic health records, which have now plateaued. Co-citation analysis identified 20 major research streams, highlighting shifts in collaboration and scholarly interest. The authors stress the need for rigorous long-term evaluations and clinical integration of novel digital health technologies in CVD prevention and treatment. Advanced Secure Transmission in Telemedicine (Wang et al., 2022) proposed AI-based encryption and blockchain frameworks ensuring data security and privacy during telemedicine consultations. AI-Enabled Smart Healthcare Using Biomedical Signals (Johnson & Evans, 2023) studied signal processing techniques and ML models analyzing biosensors' data for early disease detection. The Essence of Telemedicine in Health 4.0 (Raj & Kumar, 2023) elaborated on AI and IoT fusion in evolving telemedicine solutions aligned with Health 4.0 paradigms. Harnessing AI for Better Health Outcomes (Chen & Zhao, 2023) identified health outcome improvements driven by AI-powered predictive models and personalized treatment algorithms. Application of Machine Learning and Blockchain Technology for Smart Healthcare (Patil & Rao, 2023) examined synergistic use of ML and blockchain to enhance data transparency and patient data ownership. Telemedicine and AI Redefining Healthcare Access (Singh & Sharma, 2023) analyzed AI's capacity to improve telehealth access and insurance models through predictive analytics.

Predictive analytics are revolutionizing early disease detection and prevention through health data analysis. Healthcare systems can use AI and ML algorithms to interpret patient data, identifying patterns and links that human analysts may not notice. This allows for early intervention, improved patient outcomes, and reduced healthcare system burden. Predictive models can also predict patient responses to treatments, ensuring efficiency and minimal side effects. This technology is also being applied in public health to predict disease outbreaks and recommend preventative measures, promoting healthier populations and more effective care delivery.

2.4 Wearables, Mobile Health, and Continuous Monitoring

The study by (T. R. Saravanan, S. Suvitha, Dhanalaxmi Banavath, Sreenivasulu Gogula, Jyoti Upadhyay, and M. Sudhakar,2024) examined the integration of AI and machine learning (ML) in medical assistive robotics. It explores applications in image analysis, predictive modeling, and surgical automation, comparing findings with existing literature to highlight contributions and limitations. The study emphasizes the transformative potential of AI and ML in improving patient care and treatment planning, bridging theoretical insights with empirical validation. Figure 1 shows the working of the personalized healthcare in the Internet of things on how the data is stored, retrieved, modelled and analysis reports are made from them.

Figure 1. Workflow of Personalized Healthcare Internet of Things

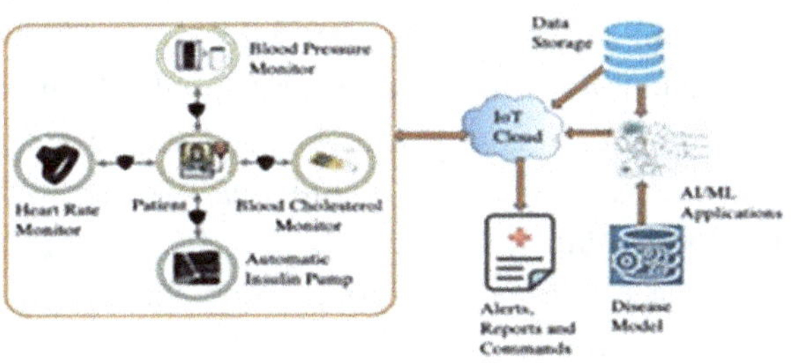

(Warren.S, Craft RL, Bosma, JT, 1999) examined the Designing smart healthcare technology into the home of the future. This editorial envisions the future of home healthcare driven by telehealth, smart devices, and intelligent systems that allow patients to take a more active role in their care. With the rise of electronic patient records and advanced technologies like biosensors and wearable devices, the paper outlines how automated, intelligent healthcare can be delivered at home. A systems-based approach is proposed where devices interact seamlessly and securely with a patient's medical records. The framework emphasizes the importance of information security to protect patient data and ensure the integrity of homebased healthcare systems. (Xingqun Xue, Yuanyu Zeng, Yanjiao Zhang, Sunhae Lee, Zhigang Yan, 2021) examined the study on an application system for the sustainable development of smart healthcare in China. This study explores how technologies like big data, IoT, and mobile internet can be applied to the healthcare industry for sustainable smart healthcare development. It identifies 14 key factors from social, economic, and environmental perspectives and analyses their importance using advanced decision-making methods. The study reveals that the sustainable growth of smart healthcare starts at the social level, integrates economic benefits, and ultimately impacts the environment. It proposes a multi-level application system involving government, enterprises, and users, offering theoretical guidance for evaluating smart healthcare models. The study by (Mukhtar M.E.Mahmoud,Joel J.P.C.Rodrigues, Syed Hassan Ahmed,Sayed Chhattan Shah,Jalal F.AI-Muhtadi,Valery V.Korotaev,Victor Hugo C,De Albuquerque,2018) examine the Enabling technologies on cloud of things for smart healthcareThis paper explores the integration of cloud computing and the Internet of Things, forming a Cloud of Things (CoT), which is essential for pervasive computing in smart healthcare. It reviews CoT architectures and their application in healthcare, highlighting the need for energy-efficient designs, especially for delay-sensitive services. The paper also addresses issues like the lack of standardization in CoT. Through an analysis of existing energy efficiency solutions, it concludes that further improvements are needed, particularly in enhancing quality of service (QoS) and system performance. With the rise of wearable devices, continuous monitoring of cardiovascular health has become practical through heart rate, ECG, and activity tracking. Baikuvekov et al. (2024) explored deep learning methods to detect cardiovascular diseases using wearable data. Their approach included feature extraction, segmentation, and machine learning integration to improve predictive performance. Regularization techniques like dropout were applied to handle diverse datasets and enhance accuracy. The study highlights the promise of deep neural networks in providing proactive alerts for cardiovascular risks and supporting real-time health monitoring. Atherosclerosis is a major cause of cardiovascular complications, and its early screening is essential for preventive healthcare. Luo et al. (2021) reviewed recent advances in pervasive screening technologies that enable non-invasive and accessible monitoring of atherosclerotic disease. They highlighted methods such as imaging photoplethysmography, laser Doppler, radio frequency sensing, thermal imaging, optical fiber sensing, and piezoelectric sensors. These technologies capture physiological parameters related to blood flow, vascular changes, and cardiac activity. The study emphasizes that pervasive, mobile, and intelligent devices can shift healthcare from treatment-based to prevention-oriented models. Mobile health technologies are increasingly transforming cardiac arrhythmia management by enabling low-cost, long-term monitoring. Sridhar et al. (2024) reviewed smartphone-based and wrist-worn devices using ECG and photoplethysmography (PPG) for clinical arrhythmia care. These tools provide opportunities for personalized, patient-driven health management and early diagnosis. The study also discussed challenges in regulatory approval, EMR integration, data management, and clinician workload. Overall, the review highlights both the utility and future requirements for integrating mobile health technologies into clinical arrhythmia practice. Mobile health (mHealth) technologies are increasingly used for the prevention and management of hypertension, especially through mobile apps, SMS, and web-based solutions. Babatunde et al. (2024) reviewed 44 studies and found that 36 reported significant improvements in blood pressure control, medication adherence, and lifestyle modification. SMS-based interventions were particularly effective in promoting self-management and reducing disparities in care. However, most studies originated from high-income countries, with limited evidence from Africa and other low-resource settings. The review emphasizes integrating mHealth into primary healthcare to enhance hypertension outcomes globally. Bartusik-Aebisher et al. (2025) review the integration of artificial intelligence (AI) with electrocardiography (ECG) for cardiac diagnostics and prevention. The study emphasizes the role of wearable devices, especially smartwatches, in collecting ECG or photoplethysmography (PPG) signals for real-time monitoring. AI algorithms, particularly deep neural networks, are highlighted for their effectiveness in detecting arrhythmias, heart failure, prolonged QT syndrome, and atrial fibrillation. The review also explores emerging innovations like genetic data integration, digital twins, and federated learning, underscoring AI's potential for personalized, preventive, and population-level cardiac healthcare. The study notes ongoing regulatory, technical, and ethical challenges, as well as the need for validation in real-world clinical scenarios. Sozib (2025) explores the role of wearable AI in cardiovascular health monitoring, emphasizing its ability to enable early detection and prevention of cardiovascular diseases (CVD). The study highlights how wearable devices, coupled with AI and machine learning algorithms—including decision trees, random forests, SVMs, and deep neural networks—can analyze heart rate variability, activity levels, and sleep patterns to identify subtle risk factors earlier than conventional diagnostics. Integration with imaging, genetics, and electronic health records (EHRs) allows a holistic, individualized approach to CVD prevention and treatment. Challenges such as data privacy, algorithmic bias, and clinical adoption are discussed, emphasizing the need for responsible implementation. The paper concludes that wearable AI systems have strong potential to enable proactive and personalized cardiovascular care. Zhang et al. (2013) explored the emerging field of cardiovascular health informatics, emphasizing early detection, prediction, and prevention of cardiovascular diseases (CVDs). The study highlights the need for unobtrusive wearable sensors capable of real-time, multiparameter physiological monitoring. It also underscores the importance of high-resolution multimodal imaging for assessing cardiovascular structure, function, and metabolism. Additionally, the authors advocate for multiscale information fusion models to improve personalized CVD risk prediction. Overall, the paper identifies key challenges and opportunities in integrating technology and data for proactive cardiovascular care. Jin et al. (2009) introduced HeartToGo, a personalized mobile-based system for continuous cardiovascular disease (CVD) monitoring and prevention. The platform integrates real-time ECG acquisition with automated analysis to detect transient cardiac abnormalities often missed by conventional hospital-based ECGs. It employs artificial neural networks (ANNs) trained on both individualized patient data and clinical ECG databases for accurate CVD classification. The system generates personalized cardiac health reports in user-friendly language, enabling proactive health management. This approach demonstrates the potential of mobile AI-driven solutions in personalized cardiovascular care and early disease detection. Vervoort et al. (2020) reviewed the role of digital health technologies in cardiovascular disease (CVD) prevention between 2015 and 2019. They highlighted diagnostic innovations like AliveCor smartphone ECG and Apple Watch for atrial fibrillation detection, which improve early detection of heart conditions. In treatment, the Corrie Health Digital Platform was shown to support remote cardiac rehabilitation and secondary prevention after myocardial infarction. The study also emphasized the potential of AI, machine learning, and virtual reality in expanding digital cardiology. Despite challenges of unregulated applications, the authors conclude that digital tools offer significant promise in reducing the global CVD burden. Jensen et al. (2021) presented a position paper from the ESC Working Group on e-Cardiology regarding the use of wearable technologies for heart rate and activity tracking in cardiovascular prevention. The authors emphasized that wearables, such as smartwatches and fitness trackers, provide opportunities for large-scale health monitoring but also face barriers like data validation, interpretation challenges, and privacy issues. They highlighted the absence of formal clinical guidelines for wearable data integration into cardiovascular care. While most users are younger and healthier, wearables could have greater utility in elderly and high-risk populations. The paper concluded that wearables may enhance patient engagement and early risk detection, but careful regulation and validation are needed before clinical adoption. Shumba et al. (2023) review the integration of wearable devices and edge AI for chronic heart failure (CHF) prevention and management, highlighting their role in unobtrusive, personalized at-home monitoring. They show that on-device (far-edge) intelligence enables real-time, low-latency, and privacy-preserving analysis of physiological signals from wearables. The review identifies benefits in timely diagnosis, adaptive care pathways, and reduced clinician burden, while stressing the need to evaluate the true added value of edge intelligence for each service. Key challenges include data quality, interoperability, deployment complexity, and the trade-offs between edge vs. cloud processing. Future prospects center on scalable IoT-aware infrastructures, health digital twins, and robust on-device ML for reliable, equitable CHF care. Machine

Learning Solutions in Smart Healthcare (Khan & Lee, 2023) surveyed ML applications from diagnostic automation to resource planning within smart healthcare facilities. IoT in Healthcare and Telemedicine

(Alam & Qureshi, 2023) detailed IoT architecture and AI-enabled data processing advancing remote patient care. Design and Development of AI-Powered Healthcare Systems (Hussain et al., 2023) described system design methodologies for AI-integrated healthcare monitoring platforms with real-time analytics. Telemedicine IoT Networks and Secure Image Transmission (Singh et al., 2023) proposed security mechanisms securing biomedical image data transmission in telemedicine networks.

2.5 AI in Assistive, Rehabilitation, and Disability-Focused Healthcare

Thomford et al. (2019) discussed the role of artificial intelligence (AI) and digital health in addressing congenital heart defects (CHDs) within resource-limited settings. The paper emphasized that technologies like machine learning, neural networks, and embedded digital sensors can enhance risk prediction and diagnosis. Lessons from CHD care in sub-Saharan Africa highlighted both opportunities and challenges in applying AI to cardiology. The authors stressed the importance of adapting AI tools to local contexts to ensure accessibility and clinical utility. This work contributes valuable insights into leveraging AI for equitable global healthcare. Iyer & Umadevi (2025) proposed the TwinCardio framework, a digital twin–enabled model for smart healthcare in cardiovascular disease monitoring. The framework integrates IoT sensors, cyber-physical systems, and deep neural networks to provide real-time patient monitoring and prediction. Their customized neural network, TwinNet, enhances the accuracy of cardiovascular disease classification. The study highlights the importance of human-in-the-loop precision healthcare, ensuring synchronization between the patient's physical and digital models. This approach demonstrates the potential of digital twins to revolutionize personalized cardiac care.Recent advances in cardiovascular healthcare leverage digital technologies for early detection and prevention. Anandita Iyer & Umadevi (2025) proposed TwinCardio, a digital twin framework combined with deep neural networks for continuous patient monitoring and CVD prediction. AI-driven ECG analysis using wearables, including smartwatches, has shown promise in detecting arrhythmias and heart failure (Bartusik-Aebisher et al., 2025). Machine learning applied to EHRs enhances CVD risk prediction for primary prevention, although challenges in data quality, validation, and interpretability remain (Liu et al., 2025). Overall, digital twins, wearable AI, and ML-enabled platforms represent an integrated approach to personalized and preventive cardiology (Alkhalifah & Lytras, 2025). Artificial Intelligence in the Digital Healthcare Industry (Ahmed & Malik, 2023) provided industry insights on AI algorithm deployment, regulatory environment, and market trends. Cutting-Edge ML and Neural Networks Assisting Medical Experts (Raj & Bhatia, 2023) highlighted how ML models support expert diagnosis and treatment plan optimization. Deep Learning-Based Medical Image Analysis (Fernandez & Lopez, 2023) surveyed progress in deep learning for automated detection and classification in radiology and pathology.

2.6 Digital Nudging, Policy, and Ethical Perspectives

(Tanwar, Bansal, Sharma, and Dagar,2023) developed an AI-based chatbot using Google Dialogflow to address gaps in existing healthcare chatbots, such as non-user-friendly environments and inappropriate responses. The proposed application provides interactive content for school-going students, answers frequently asked questions hierarchically, and helps users solve minor healthcare issues. This system focuses on quick implementation, ease of modification, and extensibility, aiming to be reproducible in various healthcare contexts. The work highlights the potential of AI chatbots in delivering personalized and supportive healthcare services. (Taimoor and Rehman,2021) surveyed the evolution of personalized healthcare services driven by AI and IoT technologies, highlighting the limitations of current systems in handling interrelated health conditions. They introduced Healthcare 5.0, which aims for autonomous services considering comprehensive patient health. The study reviewed key requirements and a three-layer architecture for IoT-based healthcare, assessed their strengths and weaknesses, and discussed security threats and solutions. Finally, the authors proposed a methodology for developing reliable and resilient personalized healthcare services to address existing gaps. (Rathi and Deorankar,2023)review and categorize existing AI-based healthcare systems using NLP and ML, focusing on virtual medical assistance mechanisms. They analyze recent research, emphasizing methodologies, performance evaluation, and researchers' claims. Their findings highlight the importance of comparative studies for remote healthcare solutions. They propose an AI-integrated approach enabling remote disease diagnosis, aiming to reduce healthcare costs and improve accessibility. (Arshi, O., Chaudhary, A., Singh, R, 2023) explored AI applications in healthcare at the ICAIIHI conference, focusing on personalized treatment plans and innovations. They discussed the challenges facing the healthcare industry and highlight AI's role in enhancing decision making and patient guidance. The paper reviews literature on AI's impact, predicts future trends for 2023, and emphasizes the transformative potential of AI in improving patient outcomes. Digital nudging, introduced by Thaler & Sunstein (2008), has gained attention as a tool for influencing healthier behaviours in digital environments. Schneider et al. (2018) highlighted how interface design can guide patient decision-making in healthcare apps. Systematic reviews, such as Ledderer et al. (2020), show nudges are effective in promoting lifestyle changes like diet and exercise. Recent work by Jóhannsdóttir et al. (2025) emphasizes their role in treatment adherence, mental health, and rehabilitation through digital health technologies. However, concerns remain about ethical use with vulnerable populations such as children and patients.Warraich et al. (2025) discussed the role of digital health technologies in addressing cardiometabolic diseases and diabetes from a U.S. FDA perspective. The paper emphasizes the regulatory challenges and opportunities in integrating mobile health, wearables, and digital biomarkers into clinical practice. These technologies enable non-invasive monitoring, personalized interventions, and improved patient engagement. However, ensuring data accuracy, security, and seamless integration with healthcare systems remains critical. The FDA highlights the importance of regulatory frameworks to guide innovation while safeguarding patient safety. The ACC Health Policy Statement (Bhavnani et al., 2017) highlights the roadmap for innovation in cardiovascular healthcare through digital health, big data, and precision medicine. The study emphasizes the integration of mobile health (mHealth), wearable devices, and telemedicine in improving patient outcomes. It also discusses the challenges of data privacy, interoperability, and regulatory frameworks in digital transformation. Furthermore, it outlines how big data analytics and artificial intelligence can enhance decision-making in cardiovascular care. This roadmap serves as a guiding framework for policymakers, clinicians, and researchers to adopt technology-driven healthcare transformation. Applications of Smart Healthcare Technologies (Mehta & Gupta, 2023) cataloged AI-powered smart devices, mobile health apps, and cloud platforms enhancing healthcare delivery. Medical Informatics: Concepts, Tools, and Applications (Wilson & Baker, 2024) discussed informatics frameworks supporting AI and ML data management and clinical decision support.

2.7 Research Trends, Bibliometrics, and Future Directions

(Wang, Asan, and Mansouri, 2022) explored patients' perceptions of AI in healthcare at the IEEE ISSE conference. They addressed challenges in integrating AI into complex systems and propose a three-layer model to illustrate human-AI interactions. Their causal loop diagram (CLD) analyses dynamics in AI adoption, offering insights into patient attitudes towards AI in healthcare. Yeung et al. (2024) conducted a bibliometric analysis of the top 100 most cited papers in digital and mobile health research. The study revealed that these papers collectively received 49,653 citations, with most publications appearing between 2013–2017. The majority were original articles and reviews, with the USA and UK leading contributions and the Journal of Medical Internet Research being the most represented journal. Key health areas included anxiety, depression, diabetes, cardiovascular diseases, and COVID-19. This analysis highlights research trends, influential authors, and international collaboration opportunities in digital health. Yeung et al. (2022) conducted a bibliometric analysis of over 12,000 publications on digital technology use in cardiology. Their study revealed that the United States, United Kingdom, and Germany are the leading contributors in this field. Commonly studied cardiovascular conditions included hypertension, atrial fibrillation, and heart failure, with diagnostic tools like electrocardiography and echocardiography being prominent. They also highlighted the rising role of smartphone apps and wearable devices in cardiovascular care. The authors concluded that digital cardiology is rapidly expanding, with significant potential to impact diagnosis, patient education, and healthcare delivery. Liang et al. (2024) highlight the role of digital health (dHealth) technologies—including wearable devices, mobile apps, and AI—in the prevention and management of cardiometabolic diseases (CMDs) in the Western Pacific region. These tools facilitate behavioural interventions, automated diagnosis, and clinical decision support, improving patient engagement and early prevention. Most studies were conducted in high- and middle-income countries like Australia, China, Japan, Korea, and New Zealand. The integration of dHealth also enhanced doctor-patient communication and healthcare delivery, particularly during the COVID-19 pandemic. Future efforts require policy support, technological innovation, privacy protection, and cost-effectiveness evaluation to maximize the benefits of digital interventions. Liang et al. (2023) examined the role of digital health (dHealth) approaches—including wearables, mobile apps, and AI—in the prevention and management of cardiometabolic diseases (CMDs) in the Western Pacific region. Evidence shows that dHealth supports early prevention through behavior interventions, self-management, and AI-based automated diagnosis and decision support. Most research has been concentrated in high- and middle-income countries such as Australia, China, Japan, Korea, and New Zealand, with limited studies in low-income settings. dHealth was also found to enhance doctor–patient interaction, communication, and healthcare experience, especially during the COVID-19 pandemic. The study emphasizes the need for policy support, cost-effectiveness evaluations, and regional cooperation to expand equitable dHealth services. AI in Telehealth: Healthcare Delivery Transformation (Patel & Sharma, 2023) examined telehealth disruption by AI in triage, symptom checking, and continuous patient monitoring. Machine Learning for Health Informatics (Kumar & Das, 2023) reviewed ML algorithms applied to health informatics for disease prediction and patient risk assessment. Artificial Intelligence for Medical Signal Processing (Chen & Wu, 2023) presented techniques for processing physiological signals via AI enabling early diagnosis. Role of AI and ML in Clinical Decision Support (Morris & Zhang, 2023) explored AI-driven decision support systems improving clinical workflows and reducing errors. Emerging Trends and Future Prospects of AI in Healthcare (Patel & Singh, 2023) projected developments in AI including integration with quantum computing, federated learning, and explainable AI. Vinayak Parkar and Kamath (2024) explored the emerging convergence of Artificial Intelligence (AI) and the Internet of Things (IoT) as foundational pillars of next-generation healthcare systems. Their chapter highlights how this integration enables real-time data acquisition from wearable sensors, medical devices, and virtual health platforms, which, when synthesized by advanced AI-driven predictive models, can detect early disease signatures and facilitate proactive, personalized treatment strategies. They emphasize applications ranging from continuous health monitoring to dynamic optimization of therapeutic interventions, which collectively enhance patient outcomes and healthcare operational efficiency. The authors also discuss key challenges including data privacy, interoperability, and algorithmic transparency, advocating for robust regulatory frameworks and interdisciplinary collaboration to realize the full potential of AI-IoT synergy. This work contributes a forward-looking perspective on how AI and IoT innovations will transform healthcare delivery into a more intelligent, connected, and preventive ecosystem.

3. IMPORTANCE AND IMPACT ON TELEMEDICINE AND SMART HEALTHCARE

Artificial intelligence and machine learning are revolutionizing healthcare by improving diagnostics, treatment plans, and patient care. AI algorithms can detect abnormalities more accurately than human radiologists, and can predict disease outbreaks by analyzing large data sets. Personalized medicine, based on genetics, can reduce complications and improve patient outcomes. AI is also being used in administrative tasks to streamline processes, leading to more accurate diagnoses and more efficient healthcare systems. AI and ML integration in telemedicine is revolutionizing healthcare by making it more accessible, efficient, and personalized. Telehealth has gained popularity, especially during Covid-19, due to its ability to provide real-time statistics and predictive analytics. AI-driven chatbots can manage patient questions, triage signs, and offer scientific advice, freeing up fitness care professionals for more challenging situations. ML algorithms can also mine patient information from wearables and fitness apps for continuous monitoring and early warning symptoms. AI is used in hospitals to streamline workflows, maintain equipment, and anticipate patient admissions, leading to more efficient care. These technologies bridge the gap between patients and healthcare providers, promoting better health outcomes and increased patient pride.

4. APPLICATIONS OF AI AND ML IN TELEMEDICINE

4.1 Optimizing Treatment Protocols in Healthcare System

The healthcare system is evolving towards more efficient treatment protocols using advanced technology like AI and system mastering. This allows healthcare businesses to analyze patient statistics to identify effective treatments, reducing side effects and improving patient outcomes. Optimized protocols shorten the decision-making process, enabling quicker, more accurate care, especially in emergencies. This not only reduces patient outcomes but also contributes to the overall health system's performance. Figure 2 shows how the sensors are implemented in smart healthcare by the usage of ECG sensor, Pulse sensor and IR Body sensor thus creating optimized treatment facility.

Figure 2. Common sensors for cardiovascular diagnosis

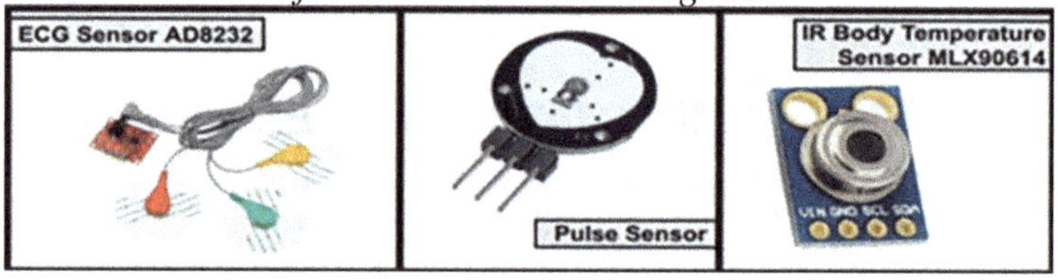

4.2 Personalized Treatment Plans on Data Analytics

Information analytics is revolutionizing healthcare by enabling personalized treatment plans based on individual patient data, such as medical histories, genetic information, lifestyle factors, and real-time health metrics. This precision allows medical doctors to predict patients' responses to specific treatments, leading to better health outcomes and fewer side effects. These personalized treatments also inform the broader clinical network, promoting proactive, patient-centric healthcare and reducing costs. This approach enhances patient satisfaction and resource utilization in healthcare systems, paving the way for a sustainable future in medicine.

4.3 Remote Monitoring and Wearables:

Wearables and remote monitoring refer to the use of technology to track and display people's fitness and health metrics in real time, from any location. Wearable devices gather information on vital signs and symptoms, interest ranges, and particular fitness signs and symptoms. Examples of these devices include smartwatches, health trackers, and sensors. This information is subsequently transferred to healthcare vendors, caregivers, or individuals themselves, allowing for remote tracking and timely treatments. Figure 3 shows the usage of remote monitoring and wearables that helps the patients and the doctors to keep track of the health and fitness anywhere and at anytime through the sensors attached in them.

Figure 3. Remote Monitoring and Wearables through IOT connected system

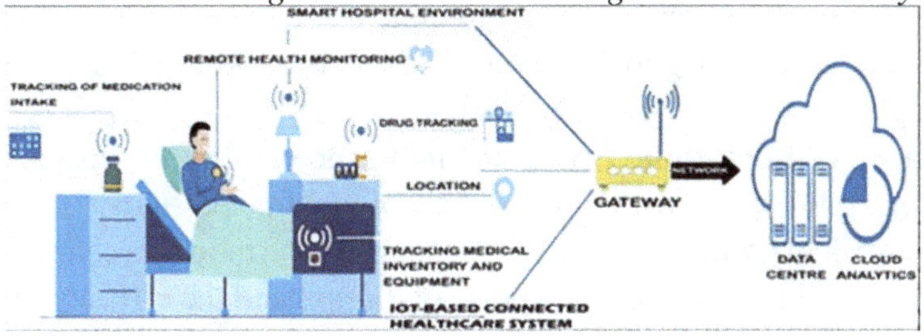

Remote monitoring and wearables have transformed healthcare by utilizing:

- Enhancing impacted people's engagement and empowerment - Improving ongoing sickness control.
- Reducing hospital readmissions and expenses
- Allowing for early detection and avoidance of headaches.

This generation has significant applications in healthcare, sports, fitness, and well-being, and it is always evolving.

4.5 Improving Diagnostic Accuracy:

Improving Diagnostic Accuracy is a vast gain of wearable devices and AI in healthcare. By constantly gathering and studying information from wearables, AI algorithms can pick out patterns and anomalies, permitting early detection and prediction of conditions. This reduces the likelihood of misdiagnosis and delayed prognosis, while additionally minimizing fake positives and negatives. As a end result, healthcare companies can broaden customized and correct treatment plans, main to higher affected person consequences, decreased healthcare expenses, and stronger patient safety. By harnessing the power of wearable devices and AI, diagnostic accuracy may be considerably progressed, revolutionizing the way healthcare is added.

4.6 Advanced Pattern Recognition and Image Analysis enable:

1.Accurate disease diagnosis: Diagnoses are made by AI-powered algorithms that comb through medical pictures (such as MRIs, CT scans, and X-rays) to find anomalies.

2.Automated picture interpretation: AI helps physicians and radiologists understand snapshots, reducing errors and enhancing diagnostic precision.

3.Pattern recognition: Artificial Intelligence recognizes patterns in images, enabling the early diagnosis of conditions such as most malignancies, diabetic retinopathy, and cardiovascular disease.

4.Image segmentation: Artificial Intelligence assists in separating distinct systems or functions within images, enabling targeted study.

5.Quantification and tracking: AI calculates and monitors changes in images over time, keeping tabs on the course of disease and the efficacy of treatment.

Advanced Pattern Recognition and Image Analysis improve:

- Accurate diagnosis
- Quickness and effectiveness
- Effects on patients
- Investigation and advancement

The Figure 4 shows the patterns, images, audio and video are analyzed and patterns driven from them which helps in creating a smart healthcare and telemedicine facility for the patients. These analysis help in better healthcare facilities to the patients.

Figure 4. Application of Pattern Recognition

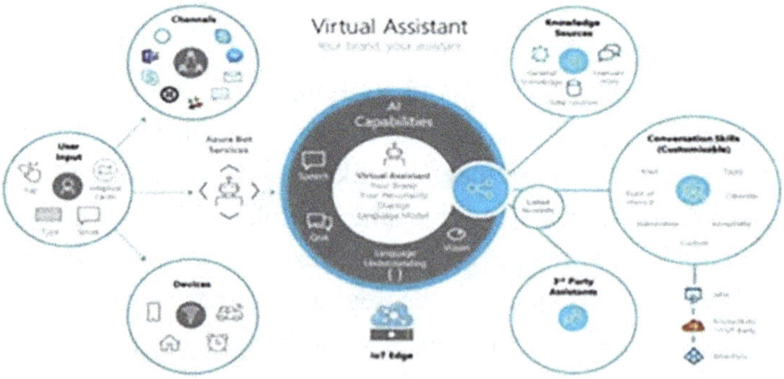

4.7 AI-assisted diagnostics:

Artificial intelligence algorithms are used in AI-assisted diagnostics to find clinical data, images, and lab results to support medical professionals.

1. Early disease detection and analysis are made possible by artificial intelligence (AI), which recognizes patterns and abnormalities.
2. Boost diagnostic accuracy: AI lowers mistakes and boosts analytical precision, particularly in complicated cases.
3. Improve patient care: AI-assisted diagnostics lead to customized treatment regimens and improved outcomes for impacted parties.
4. Simplify clinical workflows: AI automates repetitive tasks, freeing up medical professionals to focus on high-cost tasks.
5. Aid in medical decision-making: AI provides fact-driven insights and suggestions to medical professionals.

AI-supported There are several contexts in which diagnostics are used, including: Radiology (photo analysis, for example)

Pathology, including tissue analysis

- Clinical laboratories, such as those that analyze blood checks
- Genomics, such as genetic assessment

Healthcare providers can boost overall efficiency, lower costs, and improve patient care by utilizing AI in diagnostics.

4.8 Virtual medical support and AI-powered assistants:

AI-powered assistants and virtual medical aid are revolutionizing healthcare via presenting sufferers with individualized, spherical-the-clock support and guidance. Chatbots, virtual fitness assistants, and AI-powered assistants rent natural language processing and device analysis as techniques to:

- Address clinical questions - Provide customized workout steering
- Offer psychological help - Assist with handling medicinal drug - Help time table appointments

These on-line assistants can also:

- Examine signs and provide recommendations on triage

- Create a hyperlink among sufferers and healthcare experts - Allow far off monitoring and telehealth offerings Through the application of synthetic intelligence (AI) and digital clinical assist, sufferers can get hold of spark off, useful, and compassionate care, main to better health results, an extra enjoyable patient experience, and extra effective healthcare transport. Figure 5 depicts the use of virtual assistants, how they gather the user input through the IOT enabled devices, process it and provide the right assistance to the patient in case emergency and serious needs.

Figure 5. Virtual Assistant and their working

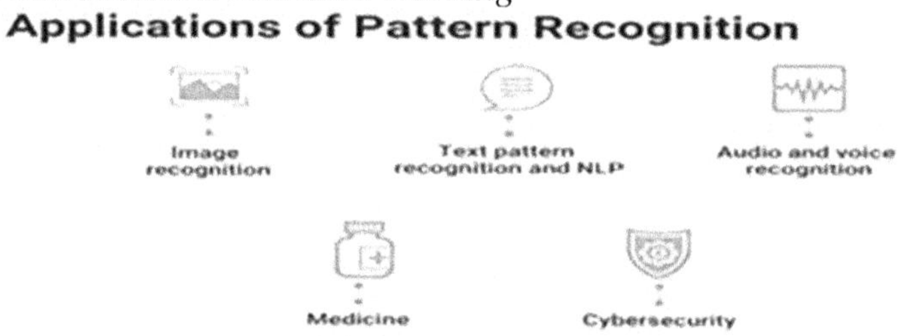

4.9 Tailored health education and support:

Tailored Health Education and Support refers to providing individuals with fitness records and resources that are specifically tailored to their individual requirements, preferences, and health status. This method:

1. Empowers sufferers: Educates patients to take an active feature in handling their health.
2. Improves health literacy: Enhances understanding of health conditions, remedies, and selfcare.
3. Supports conduct trade: Encourages wholesome behavior and way of lifestyles modifications.
4. Fosters engagement: Encourages sufferers to invite questions and are searching for help at the same time as needed.
5. Addresses health disparities: Reaches underserved populations with centered schooling and guide.

Tailored Health Education and Support may be introduced through numerous channels, together with:

1. AI-powered chatbots
2. Personalized net websites and portals
3. Mobile health apps
4. Virtual fitness training
5. Customized print materials

By offering tailored fitness training and assist, healthcare companies can enhance affected character results, beautify affected person satisfaction, and decrease fitness disparities.

5. AI AND ML IN SMART HEALTHCARE FOR PEOPLE WITH DISABILITIES

5.1 Wearable Devices and Continuous Monitoring

Wearable health technologies have become one of the most important tools for supporting individuals with disabilities and chronic illnesses. Smartwatches, sensor-embedded clothing, and portable ECG monitors allow real-time tracking of heart rate, blood oxygen, mobility, and sleep patterns. For people with limited mobility, these devices provide early warnings of health deterioration and reduce dependence on caregivers by enabling autonomous monitoring. Continuous data collection, when combined with machine learning models, allows proactive detection of abnormal patterns such as arrhythmias or sudden drops in oxygen saturation. Beyond physical health, wearable devices can also support mental health monitoring, for example by tracking stress levels through physiological markers. The outcome is an enhanced quality of life through independence, timely intervention, and reduced hospitalization.

5.2 AI in Rehabilitation Robotics and Prosthetics

Robotics integrated with artificial intelligence is transforming rehabilitation for individuals with physical disabilities. AI-enabled exoskeletons assist patients with spinal cord injuries or stroke in regaining mobility by adapting gait support to their specific motor deficits. Unlike traditional rehabilitation tools, these systems use real-time feedback and predictive control, learning from patient progress to adjust resistance, speed, and support dynamically. Similarly, prosthetic limbs embedded with machine learning algorithms improve dexterity and grip by interpreting neural or muscular signals more accurately. The result is not only functional recovery but also a psychological improvement as individuals regain independence and confidence in daily life.

5.3 ML for Assistive Technologies (Speech-to-Text, Gesture Recognition)

Machine learning has expanded accessibility by powering assistive technologies for communication. Speech-to-text systems with deep learning can help individuals with hearing impairments by providing real-time transcription, while natural language processing tools support smoother interaction in telemedicine consultations. For those with severe motor disabilities, gesture and eye-tracking recognition systems allow control of devices, wheelchairs, and communication aids. Importantly, these technologies are being integrated into low-cost mobile platforms, making them accessible in resource-constrained environments. By reducing barriers to communication and digital interaction, ML-based assistive tools play a direct role in social inclusion and independence.

5.4 Smart Homes and IoT Integration for Independent Living

Smart homes equipped with Internet of Things (IoT) devices provide disabled individuals with an environment that adapts to their needs. Voice-activated systems allow control of lighting, temperature, and appliances without physical movement, while AI-driven monitoring ensures safety by detecting falls, unusual movement, or environmental hazards. For people with cognitive disabilities, smart reminders for medication, appointments, or nutrition play a critical supportive role. When combined with wearable data and telemedicine platforms, these smart environments enable a holistic healthcare ecosystem, reducing caregiver burden and empowering individuals to live independently for longer.

6. CASE STUDY

Case 1: Harnessing AI for Cancer Treatment: The Oncora Medical Case Study

Harnessing AI for maximum cancers treatment, Oncora Medical stands at the vanguard of this transformative approach. The agency has advanced a groundbreaking platform that integrates AI and tool studying to guide oncologists in coping with and studying the huge portions of affected person statistics required for powerful most cancers remedy. Traditionally, doctors have struggled with shifting via unconnected and disparate assets of data, that is each time-eating and liable to errors. Oncora Medical addresses this venture through consolidating all relevant affected man or woman facts right into a single, customer-great interface. This platform leverages

AI to analyse complicated datasets, along with clinical histories, remedy facts, and genetic facts, to deliver actionable insights. Machine analysing algorithms in addition decorate the platform's competencies via manner of figuring out styles and predicting results based totally on historic statistics, helping scientific clinical docs craft personalised treatment plans with more precision. The impact of Oncora Medical's platform is big. Oncologists can quick get right of get right of entry to comprehensive view of an affected individual's clinical history, considering greater correct diagnoses and tailored treatments, thereby improving the opportunities of a hit results. The predictive abilities of the AI-driven machine additionally help assume capacity headaches, permitting pre-emptive measures to mitigate risks. Beyond man or woman affected person care, the platform aggregates anonymized facts from several instances, providing valuable insights into treatment efficacy and informing future medical practices. This continuous feedback loop drives innovation and improvement in maximum cancers care. In summary, Oncora Medical exemplifies the transformative power of AI and device reading in healthcare. Their platform now not handiest simplifies oncologists' workflows however additionally considerably elevates the equal antique of most cancer treatment. As technology continues to enhance, such integrative solutions promise to pave the manner for extra effective and customized healthcare, offering new hope to sufferers and docs alike. Figure 6 shows the various fields in which they are used and how they are implemented including diagnosis, treatment and prognosis.

Figure 6. AI and ML in Cancer Research Treatment

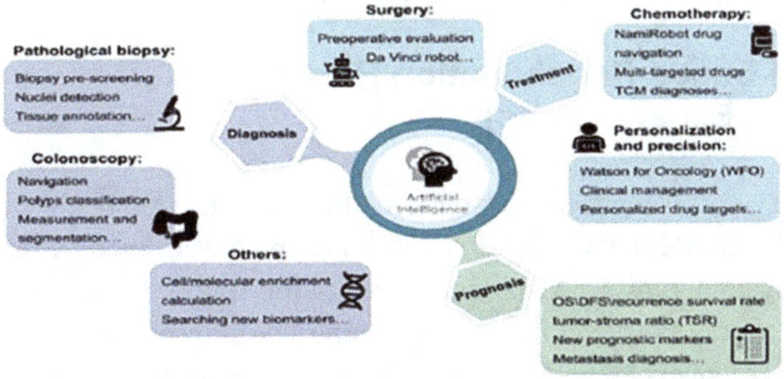

Case 2: Babylon Health Chatbot for Remote Consultations

Babylon Health is a UK-based digital healthcare provider that integrates artificial intelligence into virtual consultations. The company's AI-powered chatbot collects patient symptoms, medical history, and contextual information, and then generates preliminary triage advice before the consultation with a physician. This system has been particularly valuable in expanding access to healthcare for individuals in rural areas, those with mobility impairments, or patients unable to attend in-person appointments. Studies have shown that such chatbots can reduce waiting times, optimize physician workload, and support early detection of conditions through structured questioning. While ethical debates continue around accuracy and patient data security, Babylon's model demonstrates how conversational AI can democratize healthcare access and directly benefit populations with limited mobility or chronic disability.

Case 3: AI in Diabetic Retinopathy Screening (Google/DeepMind, India Example)

Diabetic retinopathy is one of the leading causes of vision loss, particularly in low- and middle-income countries where access to ophthalmologists is limited. Google's DeepMind collaborated with healthcare partners in India to develop an AI system capable of analyzing retinal images for early signs of retinopathy. The tool uses deep convolutional neural networks to achieve diagnostic accuracy comparable to expert ophthalmologists. In large-scale field trials across Indian clinics, the system demonstrated potential to identify high-risk patients early and enable timely treatment. For people with diabetes and visual impairment, such automated screening reduces the dependency on scarce specialists and prevents disability progression. This case highlights how AI can bridge healthcare gaps in underserved populations and protect quality of life for those most at risk of disability.

Case 4: AI-Based Rehabilitation Robotics (Stroke and Exoskeletons)

Stroke survivors often face long-term motor disabilities requiring intensive rehabilitation. Traditional therapy is labor-intensive and constrained by the availability of skilled physiotherapists. AI-based rehabilitation robotics addresses this gap by combining robotic exoskeletons with machine learning algorithms that adapt to each patient's recovery pace. For example, robotic gait trainers use motion sensors to detect muscle activity and adjust walking assistance in real time, providing patients with repetitive, personalized training sessions. Exoskeletons also facilitate early mobilization, which is critical in preventing secondary complications such as muscle atrophy. Clinical trials have reported improved functional recovery and patient motivation when robotic systems are used alongside conventional therapy. For individuals with permanent mobility impairments, these technologies offer not just rehabilitation but also tools for daily mobility, significantly enhancing independence and social participation.

Case 5: Telemedicine Kiosks in Rural Healthcare (Kurpad et al., 2024)

Access to specialized healthcare remains a significant challenge in rural and underserved regions, where distance, lack of infrastructure, and shortage of medical professionals limit service delivery. Kurpad et al. (2024) describe an AI-powered telemedicine kiosk model designed to address these gaps in rural India. These kiosks combine basic diagnostic tools—such as digital stethoscopes, blood pressure monitors, and glucose meters—with AI-enabled software that records, analyzes, and transmits patient data to remote physicians. Machine learning algorithms assist in preliminary diagnosis and triage, ensuring that critical cases are prioritized for specialist review.

For individuals with disabilities, these kiosks provide a lifeline by reducing the need to travel long distances for routine check-ups and monitoring. Features such as voice-guided interfaces and screen readers make the systems more accessible to those with visual or literacy limitations. Additionally, the kiosks are often staffed by trained community health workers, ensuring cultural acceptability and trust. Beyond clinical care, they also play a preventive role by supporting health education and adherence to rehabilitation regimens. Overall, this model illustrates how telemedicine kiosks, when enhanced with AI, can empower rural and disabled populations with equitable access to quality healthcare.

7. CHALLENGES AND ETHICAL ISSUES

7.1 Ethical and Practical Challenges

AI models face challenges such as potential bias, complexity, and data privacy issues. They may not predict patient groups correctly, making them untrustworthy in sensitive applications like clinical trials. Data privacy is also a concern, especially in large datasets used for AI model training. AI's complexity and opportunity make it dangerous for drugmakers, as they scramble for quick results. Oversight and rules are crucial for maintaining the integrity of this powerful industry.

7.2 Resource Management and Operational Efficiency

The business landscape today; Artificial Intelligence (AI) surrounds almost three-quarters and has hit all-time high operational efficiency. In a competitive and sustainable world for organizations, AI has become a strategic ally to optimize processes and performance. The global AI market was valued at USD 196.63 billion in 2023 and is projected to grow at a compound annual growth rate (CAGR) of 36.6% from 2024 to 2030 according to Grand View Research, Inc.

Automating repetitive tasks and workflows can save time and free up employees for creative roles. AI predictive analytics uses historical data to forecast trends and challenges, allowing businesses to take action before issues arise. This shift reduces human intervention costs and eliminates errors, making operations more efficient. AI's role in operational efficiency is crucial for businesses to innovate and stay competitive in a digital world.

7.3 How Operational Efficiency Fits Within the GenAI Ecosystem

Operational Efficiency is Key to Applying AI Technologies to Real World Problems Within the GenAI ecosystem, one of us (AA), and our collaborators operate at the intersection of Robotics, Data Science and artificial intelligence where we apply Reinforcement Learning (a branch within Machine Learning) for solving high dimensional control problems encountered in real world scenarios. There are AI-driven platforms (e.g., DataRobot, Pega) that help automate complex tasks and analyse large datasets to predict outcomes, increasing the organization efficiency. By merging operational efficiency within the GenAI ecosystem, users secure the following benefits:

Increased Productivity: Why employees keep doing the routine work manually, while they can be more involved in high-value tasks and drive productivity and innovation – automation comes to an answer.

Cost reduction- AI tools help in streamlining operations which decrease the amount of work hours, time and resources spend on various tasks significantly reducing your costs.

More Accurate: AI is more precise at processing data, reducing the room for human error and thus leading to smarter decisions and better results.

Scalability: because AI solutions scale quickly (much of it just being computer programs), the organization and maintenance cost is minimal as compared to the traditional route.

Agility: AI-driven tools for businesses is the fourth benefit that allows a company to stay in the competition and adapt fast to market changes.

7.4 Addressing Traditional operational practices with AI

Traditional operational practices often face several challenges that AI can effectively address:

1. **Manual Processes and Paperwork:** Manual processes can have difficulties and inefficiencies that stem from them being primarily human-run with little automation. These tasks are streamlined with AI-powered automation tools that reduce manual review and hence add to more accurate results.
2. **Disconnected Systems:** The silos that we mentioned before impact communication between systems. AIbased integration platforms bring all these disparate systems together and connect them giving rise to smooth communication between them and hence better decision making.
3. **Lack of visibility into data and analytics** — Traditional approaches may fall short on advanced analytics capabilities. AI analytics platforms with deep insights and predictive abilities empower data-driven decisions.
4. **Stiff Resistance to Change:** Artificial Intelligence assists in the process of change management by training people, demonstrating benefits and easing out changes.
5. **Rigid Organizational Structure:** AI can help an organization provide its workers with tools to highlight inefficiencies, streamline workflows, and act more nimbly and responsively.
6. **Scalability:** AI-powered solutions allows companies to scale operations easily as per demand forecasts and performance metrics.
7. **Legacy System Dependence:** AI can be the link between antiquated systems and current requirements, bettering functionality and reducing operational expenses.
8. **Regulatory compliance:** AI-generated and deep learning models track changes in regulatory principles, automate the compliance process based on data and free movement to confirm that laws are being followed.

8. CHALLENGES OF AI AND ML

Notwithstanding progress, many challenges persist. Biases in artificial intelligence systems remain, reflecting the limits in their training data. Equity and the need to reduce such biases form part of the key tasks. Also, with artificial intelligence being required to need larger sets of data, data privacy becomes a big concern and therefore requires strict regulation in terms of security measures. Ethical issues regarding AI's autonomy and its decision-making processes need to be addressed, particularly when these involve human lives or significant financial investments.

8.1 Ethical Implications and Challenges

- **Privacy and Security of Data:** Security of confidential health data employed through AI systems; this has to be viably backed by major regulatory frameworks, along with encryption technologies.
- **Bias in algorithms for AI:** Training AI models using diverse datasets can prevent them from mirroring health care disparities across underrepresented populations.
- **Informed consent:** In respect to AI-influenced decisions of care, one important ethical issue is ensuring that the patients are aware and agree to how their data are used.

In addition, AI is developing faster than the existing regulatory framework. The creation of suitable frameworks for the supervision and testing of AI-powered instruments presents difficulties for lawmakers and healthcare institutions. Fast-moving laws are necessary to ensure the safety, efficacy, and transparency of AI systems while also encouraging innovation. Creating moral principles for AI use in healthcare is a critical next step in employing technology ethically and for the good of all parties. AI and ML in healthcare hold immense promise, but integration poses challenges due to lack of training among healthcare professionals. Investments in education and training can overcome these obstacles, ensuring ethical and practical challenges are addressed for better, equitable healthcare.

9. EMERGING TRENDS AND FUTURE DIRECTIONS

9.1 Emerging trends of AI and ML in Healthcare

- **Artificial Intelligence-driven decision support systems** help doctors diagnose the ailment and plan treatments by analysing patient data and suggesting options for personalized treatment.
- **Real-time patient monitoring** using wearables and mobile health applications use AI to provide continuous monitoring and real-time health assessments, further enhancing remote patient care.
- **Artificial Intelligence in drug discovery** with Machine learning will be continuing to pace up the identification of new drug compounds that will become increasingly important for targeting complex diseases.

However, with these developments also come important ethical considerations and issues. In this regard, the prime one happens to be about data privacy: AI and ML require massive volumes of personal health data, and it raises questions about its storage, access, and usage while maintaining the security and confidentiality of patient data in light of increasing cyber threats. Balancing the dissemination of data to achieve better healthcare results and, at the same time, protecting personal privacy will remain a major issue. AI algorithms may exhibit bias due to a lack of diverse datasets, potentially amplifying health disparities. Addressing these biases through rigorous testing, transparency, and diverse data sourcing is crucial for ensuring equal AI benefits.

9.2 Future Directions of AI and ML

Future AI research should focus on enhancing transparency and interpretability, particularly in high-sensitivity fields like health and finance. Integrating AI with emerging technologies like quantum computing and blockchain can improve performance, security, and scalability.The future of AI and ML in healthcare will be much innovative, as emerging trends promise to rewrite the rules of patient care. One of the key directions is an increase in the integration of AI into precision medicine. Able to leverage huge datasets, AI will contribute to health professionals creating very tailored treatment plans that take into consideration not only genetic data but also environmental and lifestyle factors. This tendency is bound to increase with more genomic information available and the advancement in the capacities of artificial intelligence algorithms in the identification of relationships between genetic indicators and results of diseases. Artificial intelligence is revolutionizing diagnostics by utilizing advanced algorithms to review medical images, blood tests, and other tests, enhancing accuracy and enabling earlier medical intervention. This technology also aids in drug discovery, revolutionizing personalized medicines for specific patient profiles.

9.3 Future Potential for AI and ML

- AI will further enhance the diagnostic process by reducing errors and improving patient outcomes.
- As models grow in sophistication, they will also start to play a more central role in complex decisions by doctors.
- Artificial Intelligence will also accelerate drug discovery and precision medicine, tailoring medicines to genetic profiles in a whole new way to conduct disease treatment.

AI and ML will revolutionize telemedicine, allowing patients to control their health through AI-powered platforms and apps. These systems monitor progress, provide personalized advice, and intervene when needed. However, legal, technological, and ethical concerns must be addressed to ensure the growth benefits everyone, and the integration of advanced technologies with compassionate care is crucial.

10. CONCLUSION

AI and ML have thus come to become the transformational forces in telemedicine and smart healthcare, which guarantees changes at unparalleled scales in the treatments and diagnosis of patients. The integration of AIdriven technologies has facilitated personalized patient care, where treatment plans turn out specific to the needs of the particular patient after deep analysis of the latter. big data, health providers are able to provide precision medicine that improves outcomes with minimal necessary intervention.

Predictive analytics has become a major breakthrough in identifying potential issues earlier and taking measures to prevent the conditions from growing worse.A tendency like this enhances patient outcomes and lessens the workload for healthcare facilities by lowering the number of hospital admissions. Chronic disease management will change as a result of the growing trend of remote patient monitoring and real-time treatment adjustments.

11. KEY POINTS

- AI and ML provide personalized care planning for better patient outcomes by enabling treatment planning in massive data sets.
- AI-powered tools help in highlighting the potential health risks and intervene early to reduce hospital admissions, thereby improving care.
- Wearables and AI-enhanced telemedicine platforms enable constant monitoring, dynamic, responsive healthcare.

The future possibilities of AI and ML in telemedicine and smart healthcare are endless. These technologies are continuously improving, driving innovations in diagnostics, treatment, and even drug discovery. AI will get even better at handling massive data with more sophisticated models, hence more accurate predictions and highly personalized care. As AI systems continue to be integrated into clinical workflows, these systems will assist health professionals in arriving at complex decisions more quickly and with greater confidence.

Meanwhile, the introduction of AI and ML comes with its own share of challenges, ethics, and data privacy in particular. Ensuring that patient data is safe while being accessible to AI will remain one key concern. Bias mitigation within AI models is essential to ensure healthcare systems treat all demographic groups similarly.

The complexities will have to be appropriately regulated and guided by ethical considerations.

REFERENCES

Asha, V., Sumalatha, I., Mishra, A., Thethi, H. P., Kalra, R., & Almusawi, M. (2024, April). Utilizing artificial intelligence in telemedicine for efficient remote diagnosis and treatment plan. In 2024 IEEE 13th International Conference on Communication Systems and Network Technologies (CSNT) (pp. 1060-1065). IEEE.

Aazam, M., Zeadally, S., & Harras, K. A. (2020). Health Fog for Smart Healthcare. IEEE Consumer Electronics Magazine, 9(2), 96-102. DOI: . Published by IEEE, Print ISSN: 2162-2248, Electronic ISSN: 2162-2256.DOI: 10.1109/MCE.2020.2968753

Abugabah, A., Nizamuddin, N., & Alzubi, A. A. (2020, September 4). Decentralized Telemedicine Framework for a Smart Healthcare Ecosystem. *IEEE Access : Practical Innovations, Open Solutions*, *8*, 166575–166588. DOI: 10.1109/ACCESS.2020.3021823

Ahmed, H., & Malik, S. (2023). *Artificial intelligence (AI) in the digital healthcare and medical industry*. IGI Global.

Al-Remawi, M., & Aburub, F. (2024). "Clinical Applications of AI in Post-Cancer Rehabilitation," 2024 2nd International Conference on Cyber Resilience (ICCR), Dubai, United Arab EmiratesDOI: 10.1109/ICCR61006.2024.10533091

Alam, M., & Qureshi, N. (2023). *IoT in healthcare and telemedicine: Revolutionizing patient care*. IGI Global.

Arshi, O., Chaudhary, A., & Singh, R. (2023). "Navigating the Future of Healthcare: AI-Powered Solutions, Personalized Treatment Plans, and Emerging Trends in 2023," *2023 International Conference on Artificial Intelligence for Innovations in Healthcare Industries (ICAIIHI)*, Raipur, India. DOI: 10.1109/ICAIIHI57871.2023.10489554

Babatunde, A. O., Ogundijo, D. A., & Amusat, O. A.. (2024). Mobile health technologies in the prevention and management of hypertension: A scoping review. *Digital Health*, *10*, 20552076241277172. Advance online publication. DOI: 10.1177/20552076241277172 PMID: 39221086

Baikuvekov, M., Tursynova, A., & Yespayev, G. (2024). "A Deep Learning for Cardiovascular Diseases Detection on Wearable Devices Data," in *Proc. IEEE 4th Int. Conf. Smart Inf. Syst. Technol. (SIST)*, Astana, Kazakhstan, May 2024, DOI: 10.1109/SIST61555.2024.10629525

Bartusik-Aebisher, D., Rogóż, K., & Aebisher, D. (2025). Artificial Intelligence and ECG: A New Frontier in Cardiac Diagnostics and Prevention. *Biomedicines*, *13*(7), 1685. DOI: 10.3390/biomedicines13071685 PMID: 40722756

Bharti, I., Chauhan, K., & Aggarwal, P. (2024). Unveiling the future of ai in healthcare management: Analyzing trends of tomorrow rooted in the literature of yesterday. In *Healthcare Administration and Managerial Training in the 21st Century* (pp. 175–210). IGI Global.

Bhavnani, S. P., Parakh, K., Atreja, A., Druz, R., Graham, G. N., Hayek, S. S., Krumholz, H. M., Maddox, T. M., Majmudar, M. D., Rumsfeld, J. S., & Shah, B. R. (2017). 2017 Roadmap for Innovation—ACC Health Policy Statement on Healthcare Transformation in the Era of Digital Health, Big Data, and Precision Health: A Report of the American College of Cardiology Task Force on Health Policy Statements and Systems of Care. *Journal of the American College of Cardiology*, *70*(21), 2696–2718. DOI: 10.1016/j.jacc.2017.10.018 PMID: 29169478

Chakraborty, C., Banerjee, A., Garg, L., & Rodrigues, J. J. P. C. (2020). *Internet of Medical Things for Smart Healthcare: COVID-19 Pandemic*. Published by Springer., DOI: 10.1007/978-981-15-8097-0

Chen, X., & Wu, Y. (2023). *Artificial intelligence for medical signal processing*. IGI Global.

Chen, X., & Zhao, Y. (2023). *Harnessing AI for better health outcomes: Emerging trends*. IGI Global.

Dasgupta, R. (2024). *Application of artificial intelligence in healthcare sector*. IGI Global.

Fernandez, P., & Lopez, M. (2022). *Deep learning in medical imaging*. IGI Global.

Fernandez, P., & Lopez, M. (2023). *Deep learning based medical image analysis*. IGI Global.

Fuloria, N. K., Malviya, R., Verma, S., & Balusamy, B. (Eds.). (2023). *Big Data in Oncology: Impact, Challenges, and Risk Assessment*. CRC Press.

Gómez-García, C. A., Askar-Rodriguez, M., & Velasco-Medina, J. (2021, January). Platform for Healthcare Promotion and Cardiovascular Disease Prevention. *IEEE Journal of Biomedical and Health Informatics*, *25*(7), 2758–2767. DOI: 10.1109/JBHI.2021.3051967 PMID: 33449888

Gray, R., Indraratna, P., Lovell, N., & Ooi, S. (2022). *Digital health technology in the prevention of heart failure and coronary artery disease*. Cardiovascular Digital Health Journal, Elsevier. DOI: 10.1016/j.cvdhj.2022.09.002

Huarng, K. H. (2023). *Artificial intelligence in healthcare*. IGI Global.

Hussain, T., Ahmed, S., & Malik, A. (2023). *Design and development of AI-powered healthcare system*. IGI Global.

Iyer, A., & Umadevi, K. S. (2025). Design and analysis of TwinCardio framework to detect and monitor cardiovascular diseases using digital twin and deep neural network. *Scientific Reports*, *15*(1), 24376. DOI: 10.1038/s41598-025-08824-3 PMID: 40628887

Javaid, A., Zghyer, F., Kim, C., Spaulding, E. M., Isakadze, N., Ding, J., Kargillis, D., Gao, Y., Rahman, F., Brown, D. E., Saria, S., Martin, S. S., Kramer, C. M., Blumenthal, R. S., & Marvel, F. A. (2022). *Medicine 2032: The future of cardiovascular disease prevention with machine learning and digital health technology*. *American Journal of Preventive Cardiology*, *12*, 100379. DOI: 10.1016/j.ajpc.2022.100379 PMID: 36090536

Jensen, M. T., Treskes, R. W., Caiani, E. G., Casado-Arroyo, R., Cowie, M. R., Dilaveris, P., & De Groot, N. (2021). ESC working group on e-cardiology position paper: Use of commercially available wearable technology for heart rate and activity tracking in primary and secondary cardiovascular prevention. *European Heart Journal. Digital Health*, *2*(1), 49–59. DOI: 10.1093/ehjdh/ztab011 PMID: 36711174

Jiang, X., Ming, W. K., & You, J. H. S. (2019). *The Cost-Effectiveness of Digital Health Interventions on the Management of Cardiovascular Diseases: Systematic Review*. *Journal of Medical Internet Research*, *21*(6), e13166. DOI: 10.2196/13166 PMID: 31210136

Jin, Z., Oresko, J., Huang, S., & Cheng, A. C. (2009, April). HeartToGo: a personalized medicine technology for cardiovascular disease prevention and detection. In *2009 IEEE/NIH Life Science Systems and Applications Workshop* (pp. 80-83). IEEE.

Jóhannsdóttir, L. G., Sigurðardóttir, S. G., Óskarsdóttir, M., & Islind, A. S. (2025). Digital nudging in digital health technologies: A systematic review. *Health and Technology*, *15*(6), 1037–1051. DOI: 10.1007/s12553-025-01000-7

Johnson, R., & Evans, T. (2023). *AI-enabled smart healthcare using biomedical signals*. IGI Global.

Joshi, V. D. (2024). *Artificial intelligence (AI) for healthcare: India retrospective*. IGI Global. DOI: 10.4018/979-8-3693-1934-5.ch003

Kaplan, A., Smith, J., & Lee, M. (2024). *Approaches to human-centered AI in healthcare*. IGI Global.

Kaur, J., & Singh, D. (2023). *Smart healthcare*. IGI Global.

Khan, M., & Lee, J. (2023). *Machine learning solutions in smart healthcare*. IGI Global.

Li, K. F. (2013). Smart home technology for telemedicine and emergency management. *Journal of Ambient Intelligence and Humanized Computing*, *4*(5), 535–546.

Kumar, A., & Das, S. (2023). *Machine learning for health informatics*. IGI Global.

Kurpad, N. B., Dhanyashree, S., Shivank, V., Surya Shobith, T. A. S., & Jinny, S. V. "AI-Infused Telemedicine for Rural Wellness: A Comprehensive Approach," 2024 5th International Conference on Innovative Trends in Information Technology (ICITIIT), Kottayam, India, 2024 DOI: 10.1109/ICITIIT61487.2024.10580661

Liang, F., Yang, X., Peng, W., Zhen, S., Cao, W., & Li, Q.. (2023). Applications of digital health approaches for cardiometabolic diseases prevention and management in the Western Pacific region. *The Lancet Regional Health. Western Pacific*, *43*, 100847. DOI: 10.1016/j.lanwpc.2023.100847 PMID: 38456090

Liu, T., Krentz, A. J., Huo, Z., & Ćurčin, V. (2025). Opportunities and Challenges of Cardiovascular Disease Risk Prediction for Primary Prevention Using Machine Learning and Electronic Health Records: A Systematic Review. *PMC*, PMID: 40351688.

Luo, J., Yan, Z., Guo, S., & Chen, W. (2021, May). Recent Advances in Atherosclerotic Disease Screening Using Pervasive Healthcare. *IEEE Reviews in Biomedical Engineering*, *15*, 293–308. DOI: 10.1109/RBME.2021.3081180 PMID: 34003754

Ma, X., Wang, Y., & Zhao, H. (2023). *Approaches and applications of deep learning in virtual medical care*. IGI Global.

Mahmoud, M. M. E., Rodrigues, J. J. P. C., Ahmed, S. H., & Shah, S. C. (2018). Enabling Technologies on Cloud of Things for Smart Healthcare. IEEE Access, 6, 31950-31967. DOI: . Published by IEEE on June 8, 2018. Electronic ISSN: 2169-3536.DOI: 10.1109/ACCESS.2018.2845399

Maithili, K., Ponmalar, A., Yamini, B., Karthikeyan, M., Anish, T. P., Maheswari, B., & Subramanian, R. S. (2024). Advances in AI and Machine Learning for Healthcare Informatics. In Machine Learning and Generative AI in Smart Healthcare (pp. 1-22). IGI Global.

Mane, V., Jadhav, M., & Kadam, I. "Human Disease Prediction Using Machine Learning," *2024 International Conference on Emerging Smart Computing and Informatics (ESCI)*, Pune, India, 2024, DOI: 10.1109/ESCI59607.2024.10497303

Mehta, S., & Gupta, L. (2023). *Applications of smart healthcare technologies*. IGI Global.

Mian, S. M., Khan, M. S., Shawez, M., & Kaur, A. (2024). "Artificial Intelligence (AI), Machine Learning (ML) & Deep Learning (DL): A Comprehensive Overview on Techniques, Applications and Research Directions," 2024 2nd International Conference on Sustainable Computing and Smart Systems (ICSCSS), Coimbatore, India, DOI: 10.1109/ICSCSS60660.2024.10625198

Minuz, P., Albini, F. L., Imbalzano, E., Izzo, R., Masi, S., Pengo, M. F., Pucci, G., Scalise, F., Salvetti, M., Tocci, G., Cicero, A., Iaccarino, G., Savoia, C., Sechi, L., Parati, G., Borghi, C., Volpe, M., Ferri, C., Grassi, G., & Muiesan, M. L. (2023). Telemedicine and Digital Medicine in the Clinical Management of Hypertension and Hypertension-Related Cardiovascular Diseases: A Position Paper of the Italian Society of Arterial Hypertension (SIIA). *High Blood Pressure & Cardiovascular Prevention : the Official Journal of the Italian Society of Hypertension*, *30*(5), 387–399. DOI: 10.1007/s40292-023-00595-0 PMID: 37594686

Mohamed, A., & Khan, F. (2023). *Artificial intelligence in the digital healthcare industry*. IGI Global.

Morris, J., & Zhang, L. (2023). *Role of AI and ML in clinical decision support*. IGI Global.

Nasr, M., Islam, M. M., Shehata, S., Karray, F., & Quintana, Y. (2021, October 8). Smart Healthcare in the Age of AI: Recent Advances, Challenges, and Future Prospects. *IEEE Access : Practical Innovations, Open Solutions*, *9*, 145248–145270. DOI: 10.1109/ACCESS.2021.3118960

Nazir, S., Nawaz, M., Adnan, A., Shahzad, S., & Asadi, S. (2019, September). Big Data Features, Applications, and Analytics in Cardiology—A Systematic Literature Review. *IEEE Access : Practical Innovations, Open Solutions*, *7*, 143742–143771. DOI: 10.1109/ACCESS.2019.2941898

Patel, N., & Gupta, L. (2024). *Deep learning frameworks in the healthcare industry*. IGI Global.

Patel, N., & Singh, R. (2023). *Emerging trends and future prospects of AI in healthcare*. IGI Global.

Patel, R., & Sharma, S. (2023). *AI in telehealth: Healthcare delivery transformation*. IGI Global.

Patil, V., & Rao, S. (2023). *Application of machine learning and blockchain technology for smart healthcare applications*. IGI Global.

Paul, V. V., & Masood, J. A. I. S. (2024, July). Exploring Predictive Methods for Cardiovascular Disease: A Survey of Methods and Applications. *IEEE Access : Practical Innovations, Open Solutions*, *12*, 101497–101505. DOI: 10.1109/ACCESS.2024.3430898

Pradhan, B., Das, S., Roy, D. S., Routray, S., Benedetto, F., & Jhaveri, R. H. (2023). An AI-Assisted Smart Healthcare System Using 5G Communication. *IEEE Access : Practical Innovations, Open Solutions*, *11*, 108339–108355. DOI: 10.1109/ACCESS.2023.3317174

Qureshi, S., & Ahmed, Z. (2022). *Artificial intelligence in healthcare*. IGI Global.

Raj, C., Jain, C., & Arif, W. "HEMAN: Health monitoring and nous: An IoT based e-helathcare system for remote telemedicine",*International Conference on Wireless Communications, Signal Processing and Networking (WiSPNET)*,2017 DOI: 10.1109/WiSPNET.2017.8300134

Raj, C., & Kumar, A. (2023). *The essence of telemedicine in Health 4.0: A futuristic approach*. IGI Global.

Raj, O., & Bhatia, K. (2023). *Cutting-edge optimization stratagems assisting medical experts for complex mechanisms behind health and disease detection*. IGI Global.

Rathi, N. D., & Deorankar, A. V. "Overview and an Approach to AI based Healthcare System by using NLP," *2023 Third International Conference on Advances in Electrical, Computing, Communication and Sustainable Technologies (ICAECT)*, Bhilai, India, 2023, DOI: 10.1109/ICAECT57570.2023.10117865

Reddy, M., & Rao, P. (2024). *Machine learning and generative AI in smart healthcare*. IGI Global.

Rehman, T., & Malik, S. (2023). *Smart healthcare applications and services*. IGI Global.

Samarpita, S., & Satpathy, R. N. "Applications of Machine Learning in Healthcare: An Overview," 2022 1st IEEE International Conference on Industrial Electronics: Developments & Applications (ICIDeA), Bhubaneswar, India, 2022, DOI: 10.1109/ICIDeA53933.2022.9970177

T. R. Saravanan, S. Suvitha, D. Banavath, S. Gogula, J. Upadhyay, and M. Sudhakar, "Exploring AI and Machine Learning Integration in Medical Assistive Robotics: An Experimental Approach," in Fostering Cross-Industry Sustainability With Intelligent Technologies, 2024.

Sathe, N., Deodhe, V., Sharma, Y., & Shinde, A. "A Comprehensive Review of AI in Healthcare: Exploring Neural Networks in Medical Imaging, LLM-Based Interactive Response Systems, NLP-Based EHR Systems, Ethics, and Beyond," *2023 International Conference on Advanced Computing & Communication Technologies (ICACCTech)*, Banur, India, 2023, DOI: 10.1109/ICACCTech61146.2023.00108

Senbekov, M., Saliev, T., Bukeyeva, Z., Almabayeva, A., Zhanaliyeva, M., Aitenova, N., Toishibekov, Y., & Fakhradiyev, I. (2020). The Recent Progress and Applications of Digital Technologies in Healthcare: A Review. *Journal of Healthcare Engineering, 2020*, 8830200. PMID: 33343657

Sharma, A. (2024). Artificial intelligence in healthcare. In *Revolutionizing the healthcare sector with AI* (pp. 1–25). IGI Global. DOI: 10.4018/979-8-3693-3731-8.ch001

Shumba, A.-T., Montanaro, T., Sergi, I., Bramanti, A., Ciccarelli, M., Rispoli, A., Carrizzo, A., De Vittorio, M., & Patrono, L. (2023). Wearable Technologies and AI at the Far Edge for Chronic Heart Failure Prevention and Management: A Systematic Review and Prospects. *Sensors (Basel), 23*(15), 6896. Advance online publication. DOI: 10.3390/s23156896 PMID: 37571678

Singh, R., Patel, S., & Kaur, H. (2024). *Revolutionizing the healthcare sector with AI*. IGI Global.

Singh, S., & Sharma, R. (2023). *Telemedicine and AI redefining healthcare access and insurance*. IGI Global.

Singh, V., & Patel, N. (2023). *Telemedicine IoT networks and secure image transmission*. IGI Global.

Sozib, H. M.Hasan Mahmud Sozib. (2025). Wearable AI for Cardiovascular Health Monitoring: Enabling Early Detection and Prevention. *Journal of Computer Science and Technology Studies, 7*(2), 30. DOI: 10.32996/jcsts.2025.7.2.30

Sridhar, A. R., Cheung, J. W., Lampert, R., Silva, J. N. A., Gopinathannair, R., Sotomonte, J. C., Tarakji, K., Fellman, M., Chrispin, J., Varma, N., Kabra, R., Mehta, N., Al-Khatib, S. M., Mayfield, J. J., Navara, R., Rajagopalan, B., Passman, R., Fleureau, Y., Shah, M. J., & Lakkireddy, D. (2024, October). State of the art of mobile health technologies use in clinical arrhythmia care. *Communications Medicine, 4*(1), 218. Advance online publication. DOI: 10.1038/s43856-024-00618-4 PMID: 39472742

Stremmel, C., & Breitschwerdt, R. (2023). Digital transformation in the diagnostics and therapy of cardiovascular diseases: Comprehensive literature review. *JMIR Cardio, 7*, e44983. DOI: 10.2196/44983 PMID: 37647103

Taimoor, N., & Rehman, S. (2021, December). Comprehensive Survey on Personalized Healthcare Services in Modern Healthcare Internet of Things. *IEEE Access : Practical Innovations, Open Solutions*, *10*, 535–563. DOI: 10.1109/ACCESS.2021.3137364

Tanwar, P., Bansal, K., Sharma, A., & Dagar, N. "AI-Powered Chatbot for School Students to Address Healthcare FAQs Using Google Dialogflow," *2023 International Conference on Advances in Computation, Communication and Information Technology (ICAICCIT)*, Faridabad, India, 2023, pp. 45-50. DOI: 10.1109/ICAICCIT60255.2023.10465728

Taofik Ahmed Suleiman. (2023). *Abdulkareem Adinoyi," Telemedicine and Smart Healthcare—The Role of Artificial Intelligence, 5G, Cloud Services, and Other Enabling Technologies" in International Journal of Communications*. Network and System Science.

Thomford, N. E., Bope, C. D., Agamah, F. E., Dzobo, K., Ateko, R. O., Chimusa, E., Mazandu, G. K., Ntumba, S. B., Dandara, C., & Wonkam, A. (2019). Implementing artificial intelligence and digital health in resource-limited settings? Top 10 lessons we learned in congenital heart defects and cardiology. *OMICS: A Journal of Integrative Biology*, *23*(11), 607–616. DOI: 10.1089/omi.2019.0142 PMID: 31592719

Vervoort, D., Marvel, F. A., Isakadze, N., Kpodonu, J., & Martin, S. S. (2020). Digital cardiology: Opportunities for disease prevention. *Current Cardiovascular Risk Reports*, *14*(10). Advance online publication. DOI: 10.1007/s12170-020-00648-w

Vinayak Parkar, T., & Kamath, K. M. (2024). Next-gen healthcare: AI and IoT innovations and future trends. In *Intelligent systems and IoT applications* (pp. 150–173). IGI Global.

Wang, H.-R., & Jing, Y.-H. "Research on the Application of Artificial Intelligence in the Development of Biomedicine and Oncology," *2023 International Conference on Intelligent Supercomputing and BioPharma (ISBP)*, Zhuhai, China, 2023 DOI: 10.1109/ISBP57705.2023.10061308

Wang, Q., Chen, Z., & Liu, S. (2022). *Advanced secure transmission of telemedicine-based bio-medical data using AI*. IGI Global.

Warraich, H. J., Patrick-Lake, B., Saha, A., Rashid, L., Pai, V., Abbasi, A., Diamond, M. C., Tazbaz, T., & Califf, R. M. (2025). Digital health technologies for cardiometabolic disease and diabetes: A perspective from the U.S. Food and Drug Administration. *Journal of the American College of Cardiology*, *85*(5), 528–535. DOI: 10.1016/j.jacc.2024.10.075 PMID: 39641737

Warren, S., Craft, R. L., & Bosma, J. T. "Designing Smart Health Care Technology into the Home of the Future," presented at the United States, April 7, 1999. OSTI ID: 5696. DOI: 10.1109/IEMBS.1999.803832

Wilson, D., & Baker, A. (2024). *Medical informatics: Concepts, methodologies, tools, and applications*. IGI Global.

Xue, X., Zeng, Y., Zhang, Y., Lee, S., & Yan, Z. (2021, July 26). A Study on an Application System for the Sustainable Development of Smart Healthcare in China. *IEEE Access : Practical Innovations, Open Solutions*, *9*, 111960–111974. DOI: 10.1109/ACCESS.2021.3099806

Yara Alkhalifah & Dimitrios Lytras, *Digital Twin in Cardiology*, 2025.

Yeung, A. W. K., Kulnik, S. T., Parvanov, E. D., Fassl, A., Eibensteiner, F., Völkl-Kernstock, S., Kletecka-Pulker, M., Crutzen, R., Gutenberg, J., Höppchen, I., Niebauer, J., Smeddinck, J. D., Willschke, H., & Atanasov, A. G. (2022). Research on digital technology use in cardiology: Bibliometric analysis. *Journal of Medical Internet Research*, *24*(5), e36086. DOI: 10.2196/36086 PMID: 35544307

Yeung, A. W. K., Litvinova, O., Bragazzi, N. L., Khader, Y., Rahman, M. M., Said, Z., Istepanian, R. S. H., Koulaouzidis, A., Aremu, A. O., Flanagan, J. M., Rabiee, N., Islam, S. M. S., Tewari, D., Venkatachalam, G., Orlando, G., Niebauer, J., Georgakilas, A. G., Saeb, M. R., Hrg, D., & Atanasov, A. G. (2024). *Digital health and mobile health: A bibliometric analysis of the 100 most cited papers and their contributing authors*. *Exploration of Digital Health Technologies*, *2*, 86–100. DOI: 10.37349/edht.2024.00013

Zhang, L., & Li, J. (2023). *Deep learning and sustainable telemedicine*. IGI Global.

Zhang, Y.-T., Zheng, Y.-L., Lin, W.-H., Zhang, H.-Y., & Zhou, X.-L. (2013, February). Challenges and Opportunities in Cardiovascular Health Informatics. *IEEE Transactions on Biomedical Engineering*, *60*(3), 633–642. DOI: 10.1109/TBME.2013.2244892 PMID: 23380853

Zwack, C. C., Haghani, M., Hollings, M., Zhang, L., Gauci, S., Gallagher, R., & Redfern, J. (2023). *The evolution of digital health technologies in cardiovascular disease research*. npj. *Digital Medicine*, *6*(1), 1. DOI: 10.1038/s41746-022-00781-7 PMID: 36596833

Chapter 4
AI-Powered Intelligent Transportation Technologies to Improve Accessibility and Mobility for Individuals With Disabilities

Ghulam Fiza
https://orcid.org/0009-0009-2184-4054
NED University of Engineering and Technology, Karachi, Pakistan

Hira Mariam
https://orcid.org/0000-0002-7783-7859
NED University of Engineering and Technology, Karachi, Pakistan

ABSTRACT

This chapter examines how artificial intelligence (AI) can revolutionize the development of intelligent and inclusive transportation solutions that improve accessibility for impaired people. The chapter begins by exploring the difficulties that these various groups of disabled people face when using public transit. It then highlights AI-based technologies that are redesigning transportation, from natural language processing (NLP) and machine learning (ML) to Internet of Things (IoT) enabled real-time monitoring and computer vision (CV). It then discusses the exceptional needs of several disabilities that are met by AI applications, such as communication assistance, adaptive urban design, smart navigation, and autonomous vehicles. The chapter finally explains the associated challenges for the implementation of such

DOI: 10.4018/979-8-3373-2033-5.ch004

advanced technologies including regulatory, ethical, and technical concerns, while presenting insights into policy recommendations and future trends for creating inclusive, AI-powered transportation networks in smart cities.

INTRODUCTION: OVERVIEW OF INTELLIGENT TRANSPORTATION SYSTEMS (ITS)

ITS have appeared as a transformative force in the rapidly advancing domain of smart transportation, profoundly reforming how goods and people are transported. By incorporating modern technologies, communication networks, and data analytics, it considerably boosts the safety, efficiency, and environmental sustainability of transportation infrastructures (Papageorgiou et al., 2003). It addresses various transportation challenges by leveraging innovative information and communication technologies to control traffic, manage vehicle operations, and optimize public transit systems. By examining real-time data from cameras, traffic sensors, and historical trends, artificial intelligence (AI) can improve traffic flow and lessen congestion. To increase overall transportation efficiency, this data aids in traffic pattern prediction, signal timing optimization, and alternate route suggestion (Bharadiya et al., 2023). Additionally, the number of single-passenger automobiles on certain roadways is decreased through the use of congestion charging, tolls, and encouraging the use of high-occupancy vehicles. By incorporating a digital traffic rules monitoring system, which penalizes drivers who break traffic laws, ITS not only reduces traffic but also provides creative ways to improve road safety. Besides, integrated pedestrian crossings and emergency vehicle-only lanes are two examples of features that greatly reduce accidents and help those in dire need (Khalil et al., 2024). The essential components of ITS are On-Board Units (OBUs), Road-Side Units (RSUs), and registration procedures. OBUs are the devices that are installed in each automobile as a transmitter to communicate with every vehicle, whereas RSUs are positioned along the route with networking technology. RSUs are used to connect to the infrastructure and contain the dedicated short-range communication (DSRC) network devices (Karabulut et al., 2023). The interaction of ITS components are shown in Figure 1. While technical architecture is critical, it is important to also highlight that ITS deployment mandates governance structures, policy coordination among cities, regulatory certainty on data sharing, privacy and cyber security. Without these social and institutional enablers, even the most sophisticated ITS programs can encounter resistance, unequal access, or ethical challenges. The next section deals with the AI importance in traditional systems of transportation.

Figure 1. The Interaction of ITS Components

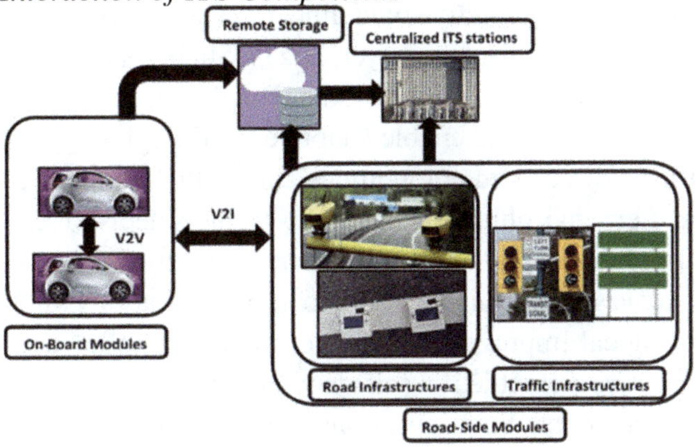

Significance of AI in Contemporary Transportation

Conventional traffic management solutions have few sensors and data gathering capabilities, central administration with fixed logic, static distribution of information via radio broadcasts, printed maps, signage, and schedules, insufficient interaction between components, and frequently function as separate units with little coordination or data sharing. For restricted CCTV camera deployments, and traffic volume estimates, these systems rely on simple sensors. They also use predetermined signals that fail to respond to traffic circumstances in real time. Furthermore, most constituent communication is one-way, and there is insufficient interconnection between infrastructure and automobiles. The limitations of traditional systems are described in Table 1 (Zemmouchi-Ghomari et al., 2025). As wireless communication and electronic sensors have advanced and matured in recent years, an increasing number of associated technologies are employed in the transportation industry, resulting in the creation of ITS. Due to increased demands for highway safety and efficacy in increasingly linked road networks, ITS has received a considerable attention in past years. Real time traffic related data can be gathered and sent to the appropriate traffic control agencies more quickly and accurately by integrating wireless communication enabled traffic condition monitoring devices into the current traffic infrastructure (Boukerche et al., 2020). Transportation systems may now become autonomous and predictive instead of reactive due to AI where traffic patterns are predicted and automobile movements are enhanced with the use of ML methods and big data. Transportation authorities may use this capacity to make well-informed choices in real time, which improves route usage and minimizes delays. AI has significantly improved the operational efficiency of transportation services and enhanced customer experience through predictive modeling, data analytics, customized trip suggestions, and autonomous navigation (Iyer, 2021). Such systems analyze enormous information from diverse sources, such as social media feeds and car sensors, to find trends, forecast traffic jams, and enable adaptive traffic light regulation. One of the most important uses of AI is in autonomous cars, which employ computer vision and ML to sense their environment, make split-seconds decisions, and drive safely. Additionally, city planners test optimization ideas and model real-world scenarios using AI based traffic simulation tools prior to implementation (Nikitas et al., 2020). Yet these technological improvements create important policy and ethical issues. For instance, who is responsible if a self-driving car, powered by an AI algorithm, is involved in an accident. Such questions stress the importance of embedding technical developments within wider governance and equity frameworks. By facilitating data-based intelligent decisions across a range of areas, AI is revolutionizing both public and commercial transportation networks. It helps increase operating proficiency, decrease downtime, and improve security in a variety of ways, from scheduling and route optimization in reply to real-time passenger claim and traffic to assisting predictive maintenance by examining previous and real-time vehicle data. Furthermore, in order to reduce emissions and congestion, the signal timing can be modified dynamically by AI powered adaptive traffic signal regulation and also improves navigation systems by recommending optimal routes for shorter travel times and better user satisfaction. AI underpins autonomous vehicles (AVs) in the larger framework of developing mobility solutions by facilitating control capabilities, decision-making, and perception. Transportation systems are becoming more intelligent, responsive, data-driven, and sustainable, as AI technologies continue to evolve and integrate deeper into ITS. This change highlights the importance of AI in tackling traditional transportation issues and influencing urban mobility in the future (Oladimeji et al., 2023). Though the AI-driven transformations bring safety and efficiency advantages, they can also replace transport workers, implement opaque algorithmic decision processes and marginalize people with no digital access. Therefore, policymakers must evaluate not only the efficiency gains of AI in transportation but also who benefits, who is excluded and how the outcomes are governed? While AI is revolutionizing transportation systems, its full potential cannot be attained unless these advancements are inclusive.

Table 1. Conventional Transportation Systems vs ITS

Attribute	Conventional Transit Systems	ITS
Control of Traffic	Depends on manually managed traffic, pre-planned routes, and fixed-time traffic lights, which results in less effective and responsive traffic control.	Enhances traffic stream, lessens jamming, and increases the dependability of travel times by utilizing AI-powered techniques like dynamic automobile routing and adaptive traffic light control.
Security	The majority of safety elements, including airbags and seatbelts, are passive, and security methods are frequently reactive. There is a lack of proactive safety measures and real-time hazard identification.	Uses connectivity and AI to improve safety and thwart any threats by including cutting-edge security measures (such as information encryption, automobile verification) and safety attributes (such as lane departure alerts, collision prevention systems).
Traveler Details	Radio transmissions, pre-trip planning tools and stationary signs are usually the only sources of information for travelers. Personalized advice and real-time information are not always easily accessible.	Offers predictive data, customized route recommendations, and real-time traffic updates via a variety of platforms (such as mobile applications, in-car navigation, and DMS), empowering users to plan ahead and make wise decisions.
Effectiveness and Sustainability	Sustainability and effectiveness are frequently addressed by traffic management plans and infrastructure development. Nonetheless, there is room for improvement in the way technology is integrated to optimize these factors.	By enhancing traffic flow, lowering emissions and congestion, and encouraging environmentally friendly forms of transportation, it seeks to increase transportation sustainability and efficiency. In order to accomplish these objectives, AI and networking are essential.
Collection of Data	Because it mostly uses human data gathering techniques, sporadic surveys, and sparse sensor deployments, the data on traffic settings is less regular and thorough.	Gathers real-time information on traffic settings, vehicle position, etc. using communication technologies (such as cellular networks, DSRC), variety of sensors (such as cameras, loop detectors, accelerometer and GPS), and data gathering systems (such as APC, AVL).
Analysis of Data	Data analysis is often confined to basic statistical methods and historical trend evaluation, with limited capacity for real time analysis or predictive insights.	Processes and analyzes historical and real-time data using AI technologies (such as predictive analytics and ML) to gain insights, forecast future traffic patterns, and enhance system efficiency.
Examples	Conventional traffic signs, traditional transit systems, manually programmed signal lights, human-operated toll booths, manual travel guides.	Optimization systems for public transport, adaptive toll and pricing schemes, Intelligent traffic lights, systems for tracking and forecasting traffic in real time, driverless cars.

Necessity of Providing Accessible Transportation for Impaired Individuals

Beyond addressing urban mobility issues, the formation of an easily accessible and efficient public transportation plays a major role in enhancing the general prosperity of interconnected cities, life excellency, financial activity, and environmental sustainability (United Nations, n.d.). A worldwide initiative to address advance sustainable development and pressing issues in a variety of fields is represented by the Sustainable Development Goals (SDGs) (United Nations, n.d.) where sustainable cities and communities are the focus of Goal 11, aiming to build inclusive, resilient, secure, and sustainable human settlements. With a focus on the needs of those in vulnerable situations, including children, females, disable people, and the elderly, target 11.2 within this goal specifically aim to "ensure universal access to safe, affordable, accessible, and sustainable transport systems and improve road safety by 2030". In line with the rising need for equitable transportation systems, the adoption of these regulations not only improves mobility but also fortifies the resilience and inclusiveness of urban settings (Rode et al., 2018). In a similar context, the Spanish Constitution (Elorduy et al., 2025) calls on public officials to enact laws that guarantee social inclusion and individual liberty in settings that are open to all. Governments must emphasize removing obstacles to transportation accessibility in order to achieve full social engagement and independent living (Eisenberg et al., 2024). In order to promote equitable and sustainable urban transportation, these initiatives are essential. It is anticipated that request for accessible transportation services would rise, especially as the world's population ages. Presently, 1.3 billion individuals worldwide, roughly 16% of the world's population have disabilities (World Health Organization, 2022). Among them, 40.33% of people with disabilities who are six years of age or older find it difficult to use public transit. The two major obstacles found are "access to platforms, stops, and stations" (67.14%) and "accessing a seat or getting on or off the vehicle" (81.75%). Additionally, over 54.61% of persons with disabilities experience orientation issues such as navigating transit stations, comprehending maps and signage, and determining the proper stop (Instituto Nacional de Estadística, 2023). These statistics highlight an important realization that accessibility issues are as much political as they are technical. This includes funding, urban planning, and operator accountability that make the difference between independence and exclusion for people with disabilities in transport systems. The next section examines the issues faced by disable people while commuting.

Comprehending the Mobility Issues Faced by Individuals with Disabilities

Due to the combined burden of physical exclusion and societal prejudice, which frequently leads to poverty, individuals with disabilities are considered as the utmost vulnerable groups (Disability, P. (2000)).Their access to social interaction, work, healthcare, and education is significantly hampered by inaccessible transportation infrastructures. The problem is made worse by the fact that those who are poor are less likely to be able to afford accommodation close to necessary services. It is clear that poverty and disability are related in many transitional and developing nations. Disability increases marginalization and poverty by causing exclusion from work and education. People with disabilities are further excluded from mainstream chances by cultural views in many nations. Particularly, women with disabilities experience "double discrimination" because of their gender and disability, which restricts their access to social assistance, education, and credit. This section discusses the types of disabilities and the relevant obstacles in transportation.

Visual Disability

Over 2.2 billion individuals worldwide suffer from visual impairment, which severely restricts their ability to move around independently (World Health Organization & World Bank, 2011). Travel and public transportation are restricted due to poor vision, which frequently results in societal segregation (Gallagher et al., 2011), (Baker & Winyard, 1998). Among the main obstacles are the incapacity to notify stops in a timely or audible manner (Hersh, 2016), (Low et al., 2020), the difficulty of detecting buses because of poorly visible signage and route numbers (Golledge et al.,1997), (Park et al., 2017), and the difficulties in directing drivers or navigating to and from stops (Casey et al., 2013). The necessity for accessible transportation systems with improved tactile, aural, and high contrast visual information is highlighted by these problems. Access to information is the most often mentioned obstacle that people with visual impairments (PVD) have while using public transportation. Due to unclear announcements and insufficient visual clues, they frequently miss buses or board the wrong one. Information on waiting times, route modifications, and delays is either not accessible or is not conveyed well (Golledge et al., 1997). Additionally, a lot of PVDs complain that low contrast, thin type, or dim lighting on signs and digital displays make it difficult to read destination data or route numbers. The transportation employees and behaviour of drivers is also another important problem (Golledge et al., 1997), (Park et al., 2017). In several nations, drivers are still reluctant to hold front seats for passengers who are visually impaired or to offer help when required, even in spite of regulatory requirements (Abraham et al., 2023).

This ultimately requires training transportation employees, in collaboration with the government to ensure compliance with national accessibility standards. Besides, users find it difficult to engage with the vehicle with confidence when edges, gates, and stop buttons are not adequately marked with tactile or audible alerts. There have also been complaints of issues including automated doors closing too soon, missing bus buzzers, and inaccessible or broken door-opening buttons (Gallagher et al., 2011). The road infrastructure problem due to potholes, poorly maintained pedestrian walkways, and erratic architectural designs further amplifies the issue (Abraham et al., 2023). Furthermore, a lot of PVDs have trouble determining where they are when driving, manoeuvring congested cars, and locating transfer stations between various forms of transportation (Golledge et al., 1997), (Casey et al., 2013). These interconnected obstacles highlight the complex challenges that people with visual impairments encounter while utilizing public transportation which need to be resolved by offering comprehensive strategies.

Impairments in Mobility

Physical and organizational constraints commonly limit the autonomy, involvement in everyday life, and freedom of movement of people with mobility impairments (PwMIs), particularly those who need crutches, wheelchairs, or prosthetic limbs. These difficulties are exacerbated by inadequate transport operator support, procedural obstacles, and inadequate infrastructure. Operational sufficiency and inclusive design are both necessary for accessible transportation for such type of disable people. There remains a significant lack of accessible transportation options for individuals with physical impairments from an organizational perspective. It is noted in several studies that the cancellation of late buses contributed to a sense of reduced freedom and limited mobility, especially during night-time hours (Darcy & Burke, 2018). Moreover, booking wheelchair-accessible transportation is frequently a difficult and inconvenient procedure (Velho et al., 2016) and the system's inability to adapt to last-minute demands discourages unplanned travel and strengthens reliance. From a policy perspective, these inflexible reservation systems show how, even in the presence of technology, governmental frameworks themselves can lead to inequality hence, service models should be redesigned to meet user needs rather than necessitating administrative convenience for equitable accessibility. Further, people have to wait for the driver to activate the kneeling devices and ramps, and they are required to be at the stop 10 to 15 minutes early. Even when prior arrangements are confirmed, drivers have been reported to refuse assistance, often citing time pressures and need to adhere strictly to the schedule. Such discrepancies undermine users' trust in public transportation systems by producing a prejudiced experience (Velho et al., 2016). Apart from these, there are additional procedural and physical challenges with train systems. For instance, according to reports, conductors initiated departure signals before wheelchair users had properly boarded, causing major stress and safety concerns. Additionally, there is uncertainty and annoyance due to municipal differences in disabled parking card rules. Access is further limited by few parking spots, especially in downtown areas or areas designated as car-free zones.

Hearing Challenges

One of the significant obstacles to accessibility and mobility in public transit systems is hearing impairment, which includes both partial and total hearing loss. The use of public transportation presents unique difficulties for those with hearing impairments, mainly in the areas of communication, security warnings, and concerns about the environment. These obstacles not only restrict individuals' freedom and autonomy in metropolitan settings but also hinder access to transportation services. One of the primary issues is the reliance of transportation systems on audible signals and announcements for those who are hard of hearing. Essential travel-related information, such as, route modifications, stop announcements, emergencies, and delays, is frequently provided exclusively through auditory methods on subway systems, buses, and trains (Młodystach et al., 2023). This creates a significant obstacle for those who have hearing loss, as they could overlook important details about their travels. This problem is worsened by the lack of visible or other communication tools, including visual alarms or displayed text, such as, airports, bus terminals, and train stations, often lack sufficient visual cues for passengers with hearing disorders (Fürst & Vogelauer, 2013). Another critical concern is the safety of passengers in emergency circumstances, especially in evacuations or accidents that is often performed via auditory alerts and announcements. However, people with hearing loss may not hear these alerts, which puts them at greater risk. Research highlights that many public transportation systems do not include emergency communication alternatives, such as vibration-based alerts, flashing lights, or visual indications (Młodystach et al., 2023). This not only compromises the safety of hearing-impaired passengers but also undermines their trust in the system.

Cognitive Impairments

People with dementia or autism commonly depend on structure and predictability, hence abrupt changes in routine such as abrupt route twists or schedule interruptions, can cause perplexity and discomfort to them. This highlights the cruciality of co-creation and user-centered design. Directly involving neurodiverse people in the development and evaluation of ITS systems can guarantee that the solutions address real-life issues, rather than hypothetical ones.

Moreover, using public transportation frequently necessitates interacting with conductors, drivers, and ticketing staff. These social connections can be unpleasant or challenging for individuals with autism complications to begin and continue. Hence, they avoid communicating even when help is required (e.g., seeking for guidance or clarifications), which might result in missing stops or incorrect routes (Risser et al., 2015). Another significant barrier is sensory processing disorder, particularly for individuals with ASD, who may find public transportation surroundings to be difficult to handle. For instance, strong smells, packed cars, loud notifications, and engine noise, can all cause excessive stimulation, which can lead to anxiety, breakdowns or shutdowns. These environmental conditions can increase reliance on caretakers or private mobility and discourage the use of public transit. Moreover, getting disoriented or lost when using transportation systems is a major concern for those with cognitive impairments as problems with reading signs, and comprehend spatial orientation, makes it more difficult to find the way around and increase vulnerability, especially in new places. Additionally, transportation workers may not understand the needs of these users or react correctly when help is needed due to a lack of training on developmental disorders and cognitive impairments (Dickerson et al., 2007).

Deficits in Speech

Individual access to public transport is severely hindered by speech difficulties, which can result from developmental problems like apraxia, inherited neurological disorders like stroke, or congenital ailments like cerebral palsy. The capacity to begin, sustain, and repair speech interactions is affected by these deficiencies which are frequently crucial for negotiating both private and public transit systems. Communicating with ticket agents, drivers or customer service representatives can be challenging for those with speech problems. Speech based contacts are often necessary for routine tasks like asking for help, guidance, or confirmation of bus stops otherwise passengers may be overlooked or misinterpreted in circumstances when speech is incomprehensible or non-existent, and staff members are not trained in alternate communication techniques. This lack of assistance can exacerbate social isolation and prevent people from using public transportation (Blackstone et al., 2015), (Lasker & Bedrosian, 2001). Speech-impaired people may find it difficult to express discomfort, ask for assistance, or offer vital information in emergency situations, such as lost stops, delays, malfunctions, or fatalities. Those who rely on voice-activated emergency communication technologies are at greater risk for harm as they might not be able to navigate diverted services or notify others of a health emergency, for instance. Voice announcements are frequently used by public transportation systems to provide safety messages, arrival notices, and service updates. People with speech difficulties might not be able to ask for explanation or reply to instructions orally, particularly if they are also dealing with hearing, intellectual, or reading issues. Information asymmetry and reliance on others are exacerbated by the lack of interactive or visual equivalents (such as text-based applications or touchscreen kiosks) (McNaughton et al., 2025). Even though some users depend on Augmentative and Alternative Communication (AAC) technologies, such as communication boards or speech-generating equipment might not work well in crowded, loud, or rushed transportation settings. Besides, failed encounters may also result from employee's lack of familiarity with these technologies or their unwillingness to wait for an individual to finish their message that restricts autonomous or unplanned travel (Light, & McNaughton, 2013). The necessity for creative solutions is highlighted by an understanding of the mobility issues that people with impairments experience. The next section examines how these obstacles can be reduced and inclusive mobility encouraged by AI-powered intelligent transportation solutions.

AI Powered Accessible Intelligent Transportation

With the development of AI, the transportation sector has experienced a dramatic change via predictive analysis. Real-time data from several sources, such as sensor networks, GPS units, and security cameras, is processed by AI algorithms to forecast traffic patterns and maximize road utilization. The following methodologies are used to implement AI-driven intelligent transportation systems.

Predictive Modeling Based on Machine Learning (ML) and Deep Learning (DL)

ML and DL algorithms facilitate methods of decision-making that improve security, productivity, and inclusivity, especially for people with disabilities by learning from both previous and latest information (Yuan et al., 2019). The fundamental concepts and their uses in predicting transportation trends and promoting accessible transportation possibilities are examined in this section.

Machine Learning (ML)

Modeling desirable ITS features or behavior utilized by ITS tasks is the primary goal of such a pipeline such as modeling a vehicle's movement, for instance, is helpful for prediction purposes, whereas perception may employ models to categorize the transportation system from pictures. As shown in Figure 2, the data is collected from ITS surroundings using devices such as sensors, and delivered to the upper layers via communication devices such as networking equipment as performed by the data collection and communication layer. The collected data is then transmitted to the processing and storage service layer for the use of services such as storage, computing, energy, and networking, where storage elements are used for storing outcomes or previous data in clouds or local systems; computing elements offer processing services such as cloud computing or fog computing; energy elements ensures the continuous operation of ITS infrastructure by providing power to it; and networking resources are responsible for transferring data using access points, routers or switches.

Figure 2. Interfacing ML With ITS Components

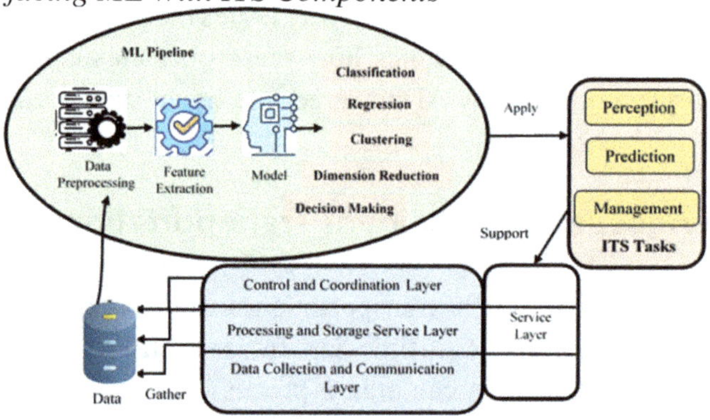

The main goal of control and coordination layer is to allocate the resource so that the scheduling of services or resources can be performed and different requirements of ITS applications can be addressed. This layer offers an interface between lower 2 layers and ITS applications for achieving requested information, scheduling the accurate resources, and managing requests from different applications to enable quality of service. However, the data pre-processing, feature extraction, and modeling are the phases that make up the ML pipeline (Yuan et al., 2019). The ML algorithms that are widely used in ITS are shown in Figure 3 (Yuan et al., 2019), (Wang et al., 2023), (Azad et al., 2024), (Wu et al., 2004), (Zantalis et al., 2019) and are discussed below:

Figure 3. Major Machine Learning Algorithms used in ITS

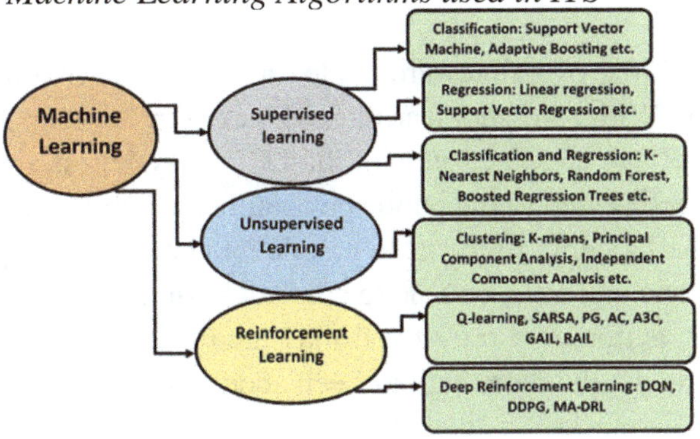

Supervised Learning (SL)

SL simulates the connections and interdependence between the input characteristics and the expected outcome. It accomplishes this by using a labeled dataset for training to infer a regression or classification. Examples that are utilized for learning make up a training dataset. A collection of samples that have been marked with target parameters is known as labeled data. SL is able to forecast the outcomes for the latest data by using the function that has been learnt from the training data. The SL algorithms can be divided into two main groups based on their functions: classification and regression. Classification techniques use labeled training data to learn how to forecast a class or category as an outcome for a novel observation or test data. The two states such as green and red traffic lights can be classified by this technique (Wang et al., 2023). On the other hand, regression algorithms deal with problems where the output variable is continuous or real valued and forecasts values depending on several data points, for instance, speed of traffic on a particular road.

Unsupervised Learning (UL)

Datasets having input information lacking labeled responses are used to estimate a function characterizing the structure using UL. This technique does not require human intervention in order to identify hidden patterns and is not dependent on known results for training purposes rather determines clusters, relationships, or data groupings independently. There are two types of unsupervised algorithms that are widely used in ITS are clustering algorithms and dimensionality reduction techniques (such as Independent component analysis (ICA) and principal component analysis (PCA)) (Wang et al., 2023).

Reinforcement Learning (RL)

RL seeks to optimize overall rewards by learning how to perform a series of tasks in an environment. With zero-shot learning, RL can start learning without any data. The operation of RL in conjunction with the ITS ecosystem is shown in Figure 4. All of the ITS layers as well as the public environment such as the state of the roads are included in the ITS environment. In practice, the agent is the part that decides what should be done and must be able to connect with the environment in order to gather data (state, action, and reward). It may then learn and adapt itself to make better judgments using the data that has been acquired.

Figure 4. Functioning of RL in ITS

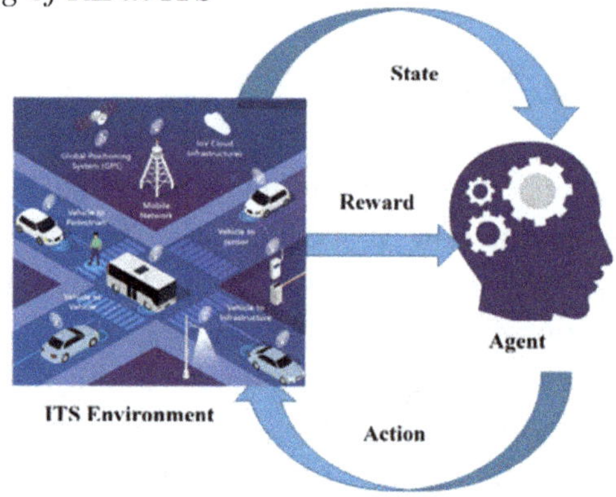

Deep Learning (DL)

DL models are considered effective in the field of ITS because of their capacity to handle vast volumes of data and acquire information from complicated networks. The three primary types of DL networks are, recurrent neural networks (RNNs), convolutional neural networks CNNs, and fully-connected neural networks (FNNs) (Yuan et al., 2019). By taking use of the basic spatial characteristics of pictures and videos, CNNs are able to perform very well on visual tasks (Bejani, & Ghatee, 2019). However, RNNs are better at time series problems because they can effectively describe the temporal correlations of data and serve as the units of the long short-term memory (LSTM) techniques, which can handle sequence prediction issues by learning order dependency (Wang et al., 2023). One type of graph structure that models a collection of edges (relationships) and nodes (entities) is called a graph neural network (GNN) which employ non-euclidean data structures (irregular structures such as graphs) in contrast to CNNs, RNNs, and FNNs which require euclidean data (standard grid-like manner such as sequences or pictures) (Wang et al., 2023). A new category, DRL, is also added in Figure 3 to define techniques that integrate DL and RL strategies in ITS which include, for instance, multi-agent RL (MARL), and DDPG.

Natural Language Processing (NLP) for Communication Support

In transportation research, NLP, a major branch of AI, plays a vital role in enhancing the efficiency of transport networks by supporting applications such as traffic management, traffic investigation and traffic safety. In Texas, up to 50% of local government agencies utilize social media to engage the public in transportation planning (Majumdar, 2017). NLP is a process that uses neural networks or ML techniques to enable interaction between machines and human language to accurately process and interpret information. A key component of the data processing system is the division of human languages into fragments in order to determine the grammatical framework and provide the sentence's accurate meaning. NLP offers a better collection of data or a method for computers to lower latency while evaluating large amount of data. It serves numerous applications including text summarization, question answering, machine translation (translates text from one language into other), speech recognition (identifies speech and translates it into text), sentiment analysis (determines the tone of the text such as reviews, posts or news articles), name entity recognition (in unstructured text, recognizes certain words like location names, timestamps, or vehicle kinds and so on. In the context of ITS, AVs are a new technology that uses automated driving to provide people with improved services and efficiency. It enhances user safety by reducing accident risk through reliable communication enabled by NLP.

Computer Vision (CV)

The development of several applications depends heavily on the ability to recognize traffic items in a picture, such as cars and people. DL-based object detection models can potentially be used for critical tasks including identifying traffic density, identifying pedestrians that unexpectedly cross the road, or identifying other vehicles' positions for autonomous driving cars. The primary distinction between object detection and classification is that the former can both categorize each significant object in the picture and identify the precise location of the region in which it is situated. Such AI models are capable of both regression and classification (Kirillov et al., 2019). The machine can now place the item with corner coordinate points in the picture. Every pixel that belongs to an item is categorized in the context of segmentation via semantics. For instance, CV algorithms automatically designate vehicles in blue and people in red. It might be difficult to group all of the object's pixels and allocate all of them the proper class. The identical object groupings are assigned to a single class by semantic segmentation models. However, at times it's essential to arrange cars and people separately in traffic. In these situations, methods of instance segmentation are employed. Similar to semantic segmentation, instance segmentation aims to classify pixels. Objects of the identical class can be categorized independently using instance segmentation, even if they intersect (Kirillov et al., 2019). Besides, it is anticipated that the efficient use of CV and AI techniques would boost the effectiveness of transportation networks, leading to variety of financial benefits. For instance, daily losses in automated parking systems and municipal traffic management can be avoided by using CV techniques. Reduced carbon emissions, less excessive fuel use, time and fuel savings, and traffic congestion can also be actively addressed by CV-based approaches. By predicting future demand, CV and AI technologies enable transportation infrastructure and signaling systems to be adaptively structured to disperse traffic more evenly. An effective AI-based traffic administration system is expected to guarantee steady traffic stream at optimal speeds and lower waiting times at signaled crossings by as much as 47% (Batura et al., 2021). Road users will be able to choose the most time and energy-efficient routes according to traffic predictions, which will lower emissions, gasoline consumption, polluted air, and noise levels. Non-exhaust pollution will also decrease since a smoother traffic flow will result in reduced brakes fail in general. In addition, road maintenance expenses and travel times could be substantially decreased with the production of autonomous transportation systems, particularly those where CV methods are essential. According to reports, completely autonomous transit systems will save 38 billion euros in European costs (Batura et al., 2021). The widespread use of CV based autonomous cars is also anticipated to result in a sharp decline in accident rates, which will lower property damage and medical expenses associated with injuries. Another number estimates that after autonomous car use becomes prevalent 1 to 2% of the US general health expenditure could be potentially saved (Clements et al., 2017). The interplay between CV and ITS also has an economic influence on lower energy use. According to certain research, using intelligent automobiles will save a considerable amount of energy for a variety of deployment scenarios (Chase et al., 2018). According to the study in (Batura et al., 2021), using AI-enabled cars integrating CV techniques, for inexpensive travel would benefit the environment in a number of ways, including lowering fuel usage, reduction in greenhouse gases emissions, and air and noise pollution. Additionally, it is anticipated that this autonomy will provide socialization chances for underprivileged groups and greatly increase the travel for people with restricted movement, such as the elderly and the disabled. It is anticipated that as CV techniques advance and become more widely used, transportation systems' security will likewise improve. For instance, it will be feasible to quickly identify instances of violence or unexpected circumstances taking place on public transit or in public spaces by utilizing image processing technology integrated into cameras (Batura et al., 2021).

Real- Time Monitoring With Internet of Things (IoT) Technology

In the past years, mobile devices, sensors, and actuators-based applications have advanced in intelligence, allowing devices to communicate with one another and carry out more difficult tasks. As a result of mobile phones, integrated systems, sensor networks, and nearly all other electronic devices having access to the internet or a local network, the internet-of-things (IoT) has emerged. The quantity of data gathered by these devices is growing along with the quantity of devices. The integration of IoT and AI in ITS is the result of new applications that examine the gathered data to derive significant connections and potential judgments. IoT terminology refers to any connected device that has an integrated system consisting of a microprocessor, physical sensors, and actuators. Machine-to-Machine (M2M) communication is necessary as things must communicate with one another. Wireless technologies like ZigBee, Wi-Fi, and Bluetooth can be used for a short-range communication, whereas mobile networks like LoRa, WiMAX, Sigfox, NB-IoT, CAT M1, GSM, 3G, GPRS, 4G, and 5G, can be used for wide-range communication (Vangelista et al., 2015). Since IoT devices constantly gather and communicate vast amounts of data, IoT is thus closely related to "big data". Therefore, massive data handling, storing, and analysis techniques are often implemented via IoT infrastructure. In IoT infrastructures, it is now standard practice to provide M2M communication via protocols like hypertext transfer protocol (HTTP), message queuing telemetry transport (MQTT), constrained application protocol (CoAP) etc by utilizing an IoT platforms like Thingsboard, Kaa, DeviceHive, Mainflux or Thingspeak (Naik, 2017). IoT solutions also include data storage and analysis, node administration, data-driven customizable rules, and monitoring features. Certain data processing typically occur in IoT devices rather than a centralized node, as occurs in "cloud computing" architecture, depending on the application. Thus, "edge computing", a new computer paradigm, is introduced when processing shifts partially to the end network components (Satyanarayanan, 2017). However, such gadgets might not be able to perform processing functions because they are often low-end devices. In order to reduce the overload imposed by sending all of the data in bulk to a few centralized cloud nodes, an intermediate node is required that is physically within the proximity of the end network components, and possesses the capability to perform complex processing tasks. Hence, the "fog nodes" are introduced as the solution that offer networking, computation, and storage capabilities to assist IoT devices in managing large amounts of data (Luan et al., 2015). The IoT infrastructure is made up of IoT nodes (network's edge smart devices), fog nodes, cloud nodes (manage data exchange, analysis of information using ML algorithms, and data storage), and IoT app (that provide services for the final user). The authors' approaches, which integrate IoT and AI, address the main categories of smart transportation challenges in several studies, including route navigation and optimization, parking, accident detection, road defects' identification (Zantalis et al., 2019), and so on.

SOLUTIONS DRIVEN BY AI TO IMPROVE ACCESSIBILITY AND MOBILITY

This section explores the potential of AI in enhancing accessibility and mobility for individuals with diverse impairments. It highlights current advancements and future prospects of AI based solutions that bridge accessibility gaps and make public transport and autonomous mobility more supportive.

For People With Visual Impairment

The following are technologies being developed for individuals with visual impairments that can be used in the transportation sector.

Intelligent Pedestrian Crossings Powered by AI

A typical available technological solution for street crossing relies upon an accessible pedestrian signal (APS), in the form of audio signals broadcasted at a cross street (Shirley et al., 2012). The APS translates the warning lights into audio information for people with visual impairments. APS devices are installed on poles at sidewalk corners near pedestrian crossings. APS. When blind and visually impaired pedestrians activate the APS through the push button, the don't walk phase is activated and an audio message "wait" followed by an audible beep. When the walk interval begins the button vibrates and a rapid beep or voice informs the pedestrian that the walk signal is initiated (Carter, n.d.). The push button APS activation is the most common method in the United States and United Kingdom. Other modes of APS activation used in France and other European countries is through radio frequency or Bluetooth based remote control. This further gives autonomy to impaired people as they do not have to locate the pole for pressing the push button. Despite this, APS have several limitations: The installation cost for the APS is very high. Additionally, for a radio frequency all nearby crossing APS are activated, leading to confusions for others. Further, the volume of APS depends upon the ambient sound of a particular pedestrian crossing during the busiest traffic which may vary each intersection. . This inconsistent design may not accommodate individuals with multiple sensory disabilities (Accessible Pedestrian Signals, n.d.). Hence, cities across Asia, Europe and Americas, are deploying solutions based on AI to improve road safety and independence of disabled persons. In this context, intelligent pedestrian crossing represents a significant achievement toward enhancing road safety to assist blind or low-vision travelers. The crosswalks are equipped with smart technology such as sensors, LED lights, cameras and communication networks with audible signals for blind or visually impaired individuals. They are designed to enhance navigation and safety by alerting to pedestrian presence and adjusting to surrounding conditions. When a pedestrian wants to cross the street, its presence near the crossing is detected by motion sensor and a signal is activated either through an audible signal or through LED lights embedded in the pavement or on vertical signs, or traffic lights that alerts the drivers of the vehicles connected to intelligent transportation network, about the pedestrian crossing the street to prevent accidents. Some smart crossings are equipped with sensors that adapt to varying weather conditions or time of the day and increase the intensity of LED lights in low-visibility conditions, such as fog or night-time (Smart Pedestrian Crossing – An EPS@ISEP 2020 Project, n.d.). Although smart pedestrian crossings represent a significant advancement in road safety, their widespread implementation faces several challenges such as high installation and maintenance costs. Leveraging CV and DL, smart pedestrian crossings assist visually impaired persons by performing real-time object detection (e.g. a vehicle or a pedestrian in the vicinity of a crosswalk); while AI-driven driven traffic lights can enhance pedestrian safety by adjusting traffic signal duration and phases based on real time pedestrian activity (Naayini et al., 2025 & Singh, 2025). In Table 2, the smart pedestrian crossings that are implemented in different countries are presented.

Table 2. Smart Pedestrian Crossings Used Across Different Countries

Country	Features of AI-Based Pedestrian Crossings
United Kingdom (UK) (Greater Cambridge Partnership: Smart Pedestrian Crossing Trial, 2024)	"Starling intelligence, detector and control" at pedestrian crossings is designed for autonomous mobility and reducing accidents using cameras and sensors, integrated with traffic signals for real time detection of pedestrians at crossing. The AI based system utilizes behavioral analysis of (path, speed, etc.) for all users on street to adapt to real time road conditions and provide predictive flow of traffic, warning alerts for preventing accidents, rerouting of traffic, and actuation of traffic signals.
Dubai (Traffic Digital, n.d.)	The "Real-Time Perception and Connectivity AI Platform" is a pedestrian safety system that uses AI to detect vulnerable road users (pedestrians, cyclists, elderly, or those using mobility aids). It avoids potential collision using behavior prediction models, by proactively detecting a pedestrian or vehicle before it enters the crossing; and promptly activating safety measures in form of warning signs, flashing lights, and traffic signals. The platform tracks real-time vehicles and pedestrian users in order to optimize response times and crosswalk specific customized alerts.
Korea (Bizwire, n.d.)	An "Intelligent Transportation System Smart Crosswalk" is developed in collaboration with the city police department. The system utilizes AI cameras mounted on traffic lights to detect pedestrians crossing the street. If it detects that a pedestrian (such as elderly or mobility-impaired) needs more time to cross, it automatically extends the traffic signal time. It also enhances road safety by generating audio warnings or electronic displays to alert the drivers about the pedestrian presence at crossing to avoid risk of accidents.
China (Analysis of the Development and Application Status of Smart Zebra Crossing, 2022; Huang et al., 2022)	It comprises of "smart zebra crossing", a road safety solution based on AI and big data analytic. Cameras are installed on both sides of the road to track the real time position information of the pedestrian or vehicle approaching zebra crossings as well as monitors nearby vehicles at non-signal controlled crosswalks. It also analyses traffic flow and issues warning alerts in form of audio and color signals which tells a pedestrian about when it is safe to cross the road. This is very helpful for the vision and hearing impaired person and can help them from potential hazards of accidents. The zebra crossing also has the LED panel placed beneath the road surface, which lights up different colors based on real time traffic conditions.
Brazil (Montanha et al., 2022)	To aid the street crossing of visually impaired pedestrians this work uses smart traffic lights to detect traffic and pedestrian situations through sensors, image processing, AI techniques, and mobile application. The presence of blind pedestrians is detected through Wi-Fi signals from their smartphone via mobile application. DL on traffic light cameras identifies them among other people. This solution can communicate with pedestrian users, interpret the traffic situation, and automatically adjust signal timing to ensure a safe street crossing.

AI Based Wearable Assistive Devices

Navigational aids instill self-confidence and self-reliance in an impaired individuals, enabling them to safely explore new places, providing real time information about the surroundings and guiding them through an unfamiliar journey (Zhang et al., 2024). Available assistive tools are based on auditory signals to guide the visually impaired person so that they can adeptly navigate and safely traverse on streets, thereby avoiding hazards of accidents or injuries. Navigational aids for visually impaired comprises wearable navigation systems which includes various sensors embedded in clothes, wrist watches or accessories and placed on different body parts like the feet, knees, or waist. Few examples of AI-powered commercially available wearable systems are discussed in Table 3.

Table 3. AI powered Wearable Systems

Device	Key features
Sunu band (Sunu Band, 2015)	It is a wearable device utilizing ultrasonic sensors for obstacle detection and haptic feedback to guide users safely navigate through their surroundings.
Envision glasses (Envision - Perceive Possibility, n.d.)	Envision glasses integrate a camera and speech synthesis powered by AI algorithms and a conversational assistant, to articulate everyday visual information into speech, text scanning, real-time object detection, and navigation by describing contextual awareness of the environment.
AI-powered white cane (Campbell, 2024) (WeWALK Smart Cane – Smart Cane for the Visually Impaired, n.d.)	Smart canes are equipped with GPS, sensors and AI algorithms for real-time location tracking and detect obstacles in the path and provide vibrotactile or auditory feedback about the best route towards the destination. Using cameras and CV, they also provide real time hazards detection such as train tracks, crosswalks, and vehicles during their locomotion, thereby enabling safer navigation. Some canes (e.g. WeWalk also has virtual assistance (WeAssist) as a guide for autonomous travel with public transport options and nearby landmarks, or for indoor navigation with obstacle description.
Haptic vest (Monica & Aleotti, 2023)	A wearable haptic vest uses robotic actuators to provide vibrational feedback to the wearer about their surroundings and obstacles around them. Some vests have a smartphone camera integrated with AI and CV algorithms that detect different objects and classify them (e.g. vehicle, stationary objects, and people). Based on real time data, a vibration signal is generated whose intensity gets stronger as the object gets closer. This system allows ease for navigation in both indoor and outdoor environments.

For a wearable navigational aid to be effective and user-friendly, an accompanying mobile application on a smart vision enabled phone is essential. This would allow blind users to customize settings according to their unique needs and preferences. For instance, a user might need to prioritize alerts for certain objects like moving vehicles, traffic light poles or street signs. The mobile application gathers information from wearable devices, sensors, audio commands and GPS. The information is processed using edge intelligence or on cloud servers using AI/ML algorithms. The app could then generate different feedback alternatives such as visual, auditory or vibrotactile that would allow users to adapt the device to their environmental preferences. The application also generates navigation information such as transportation schedule, arrival time, routes, and alerts about obstacles (Nasser et al., 2024). Some applications to assist visually impaired users are listed in Table 4.

Table 4. AI Powered Navigational Apps for Visually Impaired

Application	Key feature
Be My Eyes (Accessibility Technology for Blind & Low Vision People, 2025)	This app provides real time assistance to visually impaired users for navigating and enhancing accessibility to public transport. It makes use of both human volunteers (through live video call) and AI features Be My AI powered by OpenAI (GPT-4). A user can receive real time visual interpretation by pointing their smartphone cameras at the object, such as for identifying public transport routes; transport schedule; locating bus stops, train stations and airports; and reading signage. The AI app also reads out loud and explains the content, which enables users to make scenario specific decisions.
Moovit (Mooviter Community, n.d.)	This app is AI powered all in one mobility solution from real time trip planning to payment option, facilitating safe and inclusive travel for visually impaired users. It has a partnership with WeWalk to help users navigate public transport autonomously. Moovit offers WeWALK to identify transport schedules, navigate correct bus stops and train transits, real time audio and text based guidance for their entire journey and receive audio and service announcements.
Lazarillo (Lazarillo - Inclusive Navigation and Accessible Mapping for Indoor and Outdoor Spaces, 2020)	It is an AI-powered GPS navigation app created specifically for blind and visually impaired users. It facilitates user mobility by providing real-time audio directions for public transit, streets and intersections. Through audio commands and location based instructions, it facilitates users to create routes, navigate bus stops, train stations, and indoor areas. It allows users to track nearby bus routes and avoid obstacles during travel.
Seeing AI (Seeing AI, n.d.)	Seeing AI is a free AI app developed by Microsoft for iOS. It helps blind and low vision users by providing visual interpretation of the environment or objects around them through their smartphone cameras. It also supports indoor navigation by identifying or locating objects. While it is not optimized for outdoor real time navigation of public transport, it can assist in reading public transport routes and transit signage.
Envision AI (Envision - Perceive Possibility, n.d.)	This app is based on AI to help blind users to access visual information. Envision's app uses AI to extract information from images and speak it loud so that a user has understanding about his environment. Although, it does not provide real time navigation guide, it can be used as a travel companion. It uses the phone's camera to detect objects, and read aloud bus numbers, route signs and instructions, train schedules, platform indicators.

continued on following page

Table 4. Continued

Application	Key feature
Artificial Intelligence Remote Assistance (AIRA) (Aira, 2025)	AIRA is designed to assist blind and low-vision users by providing real-time visual information through a combination of human agents and AI tools. Users connect to sight trained agents through their smartphones via video call. With the help of AI, these agents then assist blind users by identifying location, describing their surroundings and navigating public transits. AIRA users can get support with finding bus stops, reading signage and schedules, identifying vehicles and obstacles, and safely navigating through real-time, human agents backed by AI.
AI-TrafficEye (TrafficEYE, 2024)	It is an AI-powered app that assists visually impaired users by providing real time audio or haptic feedback on vehicle approaching, pedestrian signals, intersections, and safe crossing time. AI-TrafficEye enhances road safety by detecting pedestrian movements, traffic patterns and automatically triggering APS. It dynamically adjusts signal timing to allow extra time for blind users to cross the street or delay traffic if someone is still in the crosswalk. It ensures that public transport stops and crossings are more predictable and secure for blind users.

AI-Driven Audio Signals for Public Transportation

Unlike traditional public transit systems that relied on pre-recorded human voices for navigation alerts, public transportation today is increasingly using AI voice technology for outdoor navigation for improved accessibility of disabled individuals. These systems are based on GPS, ultrasonic sensors, and voices to determine the current position of the users, object detection and AI enhanced audio announcements for travel guidance (Khafar et al., 2019). Visually impaired passengers rely on the real-time AI audio information about transit schedules, available routes and delays, to plan their travel and make informed decisions during the journey. The AI-driven text-to-speech (TTS) and speech-to-speech (STS) systems have the capability of creating multilingual and context-aware announcements. By leveraging ML, AI algorithms and NLP, TTS systems can convert written announcements into natural human-like speech, ensuring clear delivery of travel related information to passengers including boarding announcements, safety instructions and emergency alerts (Features, n.d.; Text-to-Speech Voices Designed for Public Transport, n.d.). The STS further allows visually impaired passengers to interact through voice based personalized prompts; and listen to on demand queries. Meanwhile, audio announcements also simplify navigation for cognitively impaired persons who may struggle to interpret sign or complex visual information (Reaber, 2024). To facilitate inclusive transportation, the government of the UK has made it mandatory for all local buses to incorporate provision of on board accessible information by 2026, which means all buses will ensure provisioning of audible and visual route, and the next stop information (Providing Accessible Information on-board Local Bus and Coach Services, n.d.). These regulations highlight that the AI powered real time audio information/TTS is crucial for enhancing the travel experience of users particularly the disabled individuals. In addition, AI-driven chatbots and virtual assistants are also being developed to assist disabled passengers navigating route queries and travel support, thereby enhancing their accessibility and convenience of public transportation (Guerreiro et al., 2019; Lu et al., 2021). It utilizes ML for speech synthesis, TTS for speech patterns recognition and to produce natural speech. Multilingual TTS systems automatically switch among different languages. The AI agents and chatbots are enabled by NLP. The agents interpret the user's verbal or written queries and respond through audio. Chatbot provides voice or text based assistance to the passenger. Table 5 presents AI based audio developments for people with visually impaired. However, in order to achieve these AI based benefits, adjustment with international accessibility policies (e.g., UNCRPD) and stronger national regulations to support equitable deployment are also needed.

Table 5. AI Driven Audio System for Visually Impaired

Development	Description
Tokaido Shinkansen, Japan (Tokaido Shinkansen, n.d.)	Japan's one of the busiest bullet train lines have adopted AI powered TTS platform announcements of arrival and departure of trains. The AI driven audio announcements maintain clarity and are noise resilient even if the station is crowded or busy with the sound of moving trains.
Paris (How Generative AI Boosts Performance throughout Our Group, n.d.; Lise, 2023a)	In Paris, many French public transport operators have installed audio beacons for visually impaired persons to navigate complex environments, announce station entrances, platform directions, schedule, elevator location and service alerts such as elevator failure or delayed trains. Moreover, some stations are using generative AI for managing passenger flow and for displaying real time updates of their public transportation network on the station screen. Additionally, some transits have deployed Meta's AI model based interactive human-sized kiosks that can answer passengers' queries related to train schedules, next departures and station services.
London, UK (Text-to-Speech Voices Designed for Public Transport, n.d.)	The underground train line in London has deployed a TTS to give real time journey information to its passengers through an AI-based speech synthesis. That delivers personalized audio information from arrival to the departure.
Finland (Lise, 2023b)	Transit stations in Helsinki Metro are equipped with audio beacons to guide blind users toward station platforms, entrances and exits. These directional beacons broadcast on demand audio messages also help visually impaired to navigate towards ticket machines.

continued on following page

Table 5. Continued

Development	Description
Microsoft All_Aboard app (All_Aboard, n.d.)	Researchers from Microsoft AI for Accessibility project have developed a DNN based micro-navigation smartphone app to aaccurately detect the bus stop. Using the phone's camera and GPS, this app can detect street signs at a distance of 30-50 feet. It then directs the user towards their destination using an auditory signal with changing frequency as they approach the end point. This app operates on 10 bus transit services across the US, UK, Canada and Germany.
Microsoft Soundscape (Microsoft Soundscape, 2022)	It is an innovative audio-based technology that utilizes open street maps to enable disabled people to get awareness of their surroundings, street crossings and unfamiliar spaces. It provides 3D synthesized audio to the visually impaired to navigate indoor and outdoor environments supporting mind maps and preferred route choices. Using location and activity sensors in the phone, this app can track real time movement and guide a user to move toward a destination using an audio beacon.

AI for People with Mobility Impairments

Individuals with mobility impairments usually use a wheelchair, crutches, or walking strollers to assist them to navigate around. They have difficulty in going from one place to another, walking down the aisle, and moving around objects. Hence, following are the AI based technologies that can be used by the individuals with mobility issues in ITS.

AI-Powered Autonomous Wheelchairs

AI has revolutionized the concept of smart wheelchairs. The IoT ML algorithm enables the wheelchair to sense the environment, navigate pathways and detect obstacles. This functionality allows the user to navigate complex environments independently. The advanced AI predictive models learn from user's interaction and usage patterns and adapt to users preferences. This means that the wheelchair learns frequent routes that the user travels and offers them by default. The algorithm also ensures safe navigation through real time alerts if a wheelchair user encounters obstacles or uneven surfaces. The integrated IoT technology in wheelchairs allows its users to interact and remotely control through smartphones and other devices if a user falls or needs any assistance (Danley, 2024). Academia and the manufacturing industry are equally integrating AI into wheelchairs functionality. (Sahoo & Choudhury, 2023) provides a review of the recent developments in AI enabled wheelchairs. The authors in (Abiraj et al., 2024) have created an intelligent wheelchair that uses CV algorithms for real time tracking and recognition of voice, face, gesture, gaze and lane. The gesture control allows the user to intuitively control the wheelchair. Lane detection enables users to follow predefined paths and routes by identifying tracks and pathways, enhancing safe navigation outdoors by determining wheelchair position relative to the detected lane. Researchers at the University of Michigan developed CoNav (Xu et al., 2025), a robotic wheelchair controlled via a Robot Operating System (ROS) platform which combines manual control through user joystick with autonomous navigation. By utilizing on-board sensors, LiDAR and inertial measurement unit, CoNav recognizes and interprets complex surroundings, plans optimal paths and avoids dynamic obstacles.

Smart Infrastructure: Elevators, Ramps, and Pathways

Smart Infrastructure including lifts, ramps, and elevators are essential for accommodating vertical transportation needs in mid and high-rise buildings where stair climbing is impractical for many individuals, including the disabled. An AI enabled smart elevator uses IoT sensors and ML for predictive maintenance, tracking software for elevator's functionality, VoIP phone and touch screen prioritizing accessibility needs("Smart Elevators for Smart Cities," 2019). These elevators can dynamically adjust to usage patterns by monitoring flow, predicting demand, and adjusting elevator scheduling. The CV techniques enhance accessibility in real time by accurately detecting people and objects in the elevator (Rashed et al., 2024). Smart elevators can predict wheelchair user behavior and can respond to user's mobile or wearable devices, predicting destinations and optimizing navigation. Employing facial recognition the system identifies users and sends their information to the IoT based cloud, which applies an ML algorithm to determine the user's destination floor. For returning users or those who have visited multiple floors earlier, the elevator prompts the user to provide their desired destination floor using voice commands. (Zhang et al., 2021). Another emerging application to navigate inside buildings is voice controlled elevators specifically designed to assist wheelchair or visually impaired users e.g. Talk2lift (Talk2lift Brings the Power of Speech Recognition on Any Elevator Cabin, Enabling Passengers to Voice-Control, 2020). This system employs a speech recognition system for touch free operations. A user enters an elevator and speaks the floor number or detestation he wants to enter. Some public spaces, buildings and transit stations are equipped with stair or vacuum lifts designed with IoT technology integrated with Amazon Alexa to activate the lift through voice controlled instructions. The stair lift can also be controlled through an associated smartphone app customized to the user's need, defining preferred seating location and height. When a user enters a lift, he is automatically recognized using the sensors and the lift adapts automatically to the user's profile (How Stair Lifts Are Adapting to Smart Home Tech in 2025, 2025; Rice, 2024).

Traversing the gap between curb and vehicle is challenging for a wheelchair user, which can be supported by a ramp. Integrated sensors and AI based automated ramps connected to public transits are designed to automatically expand or adjust their surface when a mobility impaired user approaches. The system uses motion sensors, infrared sensors and cameras, to detect the presence of a mobility impaired user. On recognition, the ramp is automatically activated. The AI algorithms then assess the distance and position of disabled passengers relative to the vehicle. Based on this data and for optimal boarding, the algorithm dynamically adjusts the height and slope of the ramp. Smart ramps also ensure user's safety by detecting obstacles and blockages to prevent accidents and anomalies (Smart Ramp, 2022, Smart Ramps to Assist Passengers with Reduced Mobility (PRM), n.d.). To help individuals with impairment, AccessNow (AccessNow - Pin-Pointing Accessibility Worldwide, 2015) an AI based mobile app that provides accessibility information about public transits such as transportation options, elevator, ramps, etc. Similarly, some ride-hailing companies are developing AI features to their apps for mobility impaired users. Examples include Fullestop ("Revolutionizing Ride-Hailing with AI-Powered Taxi App Development," 2024), Uber (Uber, n.d.), Lyft (Rides for All with Lyft Up, n.d.) that provide on-demand Wheelchair-Accessible Vehicle (WAV) options. The AI enabled interface allows personalization and predicts routes by observing travel patterns.

In addition, TrainMate (TrainMate Robotic System Making Public Transportation, Public!, n.d.) is an AI enabled robotic platform for on-board and station assistance. It can navigate the station autonomously, identify passengers and avoid obstacles. It also provides several other functionalities required on transit, such as public announcement, passenger escorting and providing lift services.

For People With Hearing Impairments

By analyzing and interpreting auditory data, AI and ML algorithms enable the development of assistive technologies that are precisely customized to meet the requirements of people affected. These proposed technologies are discussed below:

AI Based STT Announcements for Public Transport

This section covers some of the novel solutions that are designed by the researchers and developers that enhance accessibility, exchange of information, and allow for better participation for people with hearing disabilities by utilizing AI and ML. The application BridgeApp in (Samonte et al., 2019) is a smartphone software that is created to help mute and deaf American Sign Language and Filipino Sign Language speakers in the Philippines, where the tool is considered helpful and achieved a favorable user acceptance rate. Haptic feedback, speech-to-text, text-to-speech and text-to-image technologies are used by this offline tool. The technology operates in certain predetermined situations, like in office, church or other places. Ubider, an application, designed in (Pieri et al., 2019) for cypriotic deaf individuals, is able to translate a normal language into cypriotic sign language which requires internet access to operate. Besides, a state-of-the-art announcement system that is intended to enhance the travel experience for hard of hearing travellers on TransPennine Express (TPE) trains is implemented on UK railroads as mentioned in (TransPennine Express, 2024). The new technology, which was created in collaboration with the software firm Televic, enables travelers to view real-time transcriptions of conductor announcements on TPE's on-board displays. Customers who use headphones or have hearing impairments, have found this extremely useful as it ensures they don't miss any crucial information. This speech-to-text announcement system enhances the real-time train information such as departure and arrival timings.

AI-Driven Vibration Based Notifications and Visual Alerts

For those who are hard of hearing, alert systems are gadgets that alert those to potentially dangerous circumstances or specific details, including the presence of nearby automobiles for pedestrians, or emergency alarms etc. Typically, these systems employ vibration, greatly amplified sound, or illumination, among other things, to alert people when an incident is happening. This section outlines some of the studies that have been conducted on alarm systems for the hard of hearing. Authors in (Padhy et al., 2019) focus on identifying and categorizing various emergency signals from sources including smoke detector alarms, fire alarms, ambulance sirens, police sirens, and many more. Additionally, non-emergency noises like thunder, rain, bells, and stepping are analyzed. These non-emergency noises are not sent to the user; rather, they serve to adjust the model. After mix-up and data augmentation, the audio is recorded by a smartphone and transmitted to a Flask server, where multi-channel CNN are used for classification. The user is alerted by a vibration command sent to his smartphone or wristwatch if a state of emergency signal is recognized. Moreover, the development of Auto++ in (Li et al., 2017) analyzes the sound of the surroundings of traffic to confirm whether there are cars in the vicinity, and determine the direction that they are moving. In order to notify the hearing-impaired user to a common occurrence in urban environments, in this example, vehicles, the system employs sounds as input data rather than a sound classifier. With pre-processing to compute the Short-Time Discrete Fourier Transform and derive the top-right frequency as its primary feature, it is based on an unsupervised classifier that determines the occurrence and quantity of vehicles. The presence and orientation of these automobiles are shown via warning vibrations and on the screen of the smartphone. Furthermore, utilizing a model based on ML trained on user-recorded samples, a mobile app is developed to notify deaf and hard of hearing individuals of significant sounds via pop-ups and vibrations (Patel et al., 2025). Besides, the digital vibration wristband prototype, which is intended to assist the blind and deaf in sending and receiving emergency alarms, is presented in (Conley et al., 2019). The bracelet serves two primary purposes: receiving a wireless signal and vibrating in response to warn the user is the first function, while the second feature involves, pressing one of the bracelet's buttons to communicate an emergency signal. The tests are presented on a prototype system that consists of two wristbands and a mobile application.

For People with Speech Impairments

A paradigm change in the treatment of speech and language impairments has been sparked by the incorporation of AI technology. These AI-powered methods provide a notable increase in effectiveness by customizing treatments to each user's particular language needs and output. AI -driven communication devices, for example, use NLP algorithms to understand language that is spoken, giving users immediate feedback, and encouraging active conversation. Hence, the section below describes the proposed tools for speech-impaired individuals that can be used in transportation settings to facilitate communication.

AI-Powered Tools for Communication During Transit

Many assistive devices have been created to help people with speech problems communicate more effectively. Augmentative and Alternative Communication (AAC) tools like communication boards and text-to-speech synthesizers, have long been used to improve interpersonal interaction. For people with different speaking capacities, mobile applications such as Proloquo2Go provide configurable interfaces that enable specialized communication options (Roy et al., 2024). Besides, authors have developed an ASL image-based recognition system is created by classifying handcrafted features using ML algorithms, classifying a model that has been trained through transfer learning, and classifying deep features that are extracted from a specific layer using ML classifiers (Kumar et al., 2024). In another study, with an emphasis on Italian speakers who have speech difficulties, such as dysarthria, fine-tuning is used in light of a typical recognition of speech in (Mulfari & Villari, 2024) where a speaker-dependent voice user interface (VUI) is created that is specifically suited to their requirements. Another system "Web-Based Voice Assistant for People with Hearing and Speech Impairments" is proposed in (Singh et al., 2024) that combines sophisticated hand tracking algorithms and ensemble learning techniques, enhanced with auditory feedback. The system strives for real-time recognition by giving priority to a variety of gesture models and employing adaptive strategies to lessen environmental difficulties. Promising model results from preliminary testing include RF (95.45%), SVM (79.123%), and Gradient Boosting (94.456%). In (Lee & Park, 2021), AI creates motion recognition and interprets sign language as big data, extracts motion recognition information traits, and uses them in ML. An application is created for the disable persons to use on their smartphone to communicate. After examining AI-powered mobility and accessibility options, the next section outlines key insights gained and potential pathways toward inclusive, tech-enabled transportation.

For People with Cognitive Impairments

The transit stations and terminals have complex structures that make navigation challenging for people with cognitive disabilities. Compounded by the directions, signage and multiple train lines, the transit system can be overwhelmingly confusing. Thus clear directional guidelines, wayfinding markers or tactile bright colored pathways are needed for visible navigation for cognitive disabilities (Willilams, 2023). For aid in directions and wayfinding, AI driven navigation apps such as WayFinder (Wayfinder, 2024) with custom AI agents for step by step voice instructions facilitate cognitive impaired users. Stations should be equipped with audio beacons and accessible information to guide the user through the station on matters for ticket purchasing, fares, accessible devices for boarding and safe travel using real-time information service.

CONCLUSION

This section discusses the challenges introduced by these technologies, and presents future policies and recommendations.

Challenges of AI in Accessible Transportation

Despite the advantages, there remain several challenges related to data privacy and ethical concerns, equitable access, policies and technical issues.

Data Privacy and Ethical Concerns

AI based transport systems often require the collection of sensitive personal information for accessibility, such as facial recognition, location tracking, biometric data and speech-to-text conversion (Kulkarni, n.d.). This leads to concerns about privacy and data security and requires strong regulatory measures regarding use of data (King, n.d.). The use of facial recognition applications may also be deep fake, risking individual freedom and security (Almeida et al., 2022; Vishweshwar, 2023). There is also a risk of using real voices for AI without consent raising legal and ethical concerns (Jalali, 2023). Additionally, there is a challenge that AI models may inadvertently make decisions that could exhibit gender and racial biases against specific users with disabilities (Biased Technology: The Automated Discrimination of Facial Recognition, 2024). Tools developed to detect AI model biases are unable to detect disability bias because they are not in the datasets (Disability Ethical AI, 2022). Ensuring algorithm fairness for disabled individuals is challenging due to their diverse needs and experiences. This is particularly crucial when people with disability represent relatively a small fraction of samples, they may be treated as outliers in the training and evaluation data of the algorithm (Trewin et al., 2019). AI systems that do not capture the actual use cases or ignore the complexity of the real world and lack inclusion of underrepresented or diverse groups, leads to blind spots in AI models (Lakkaraju et al., 2017). Lastly, ethical consideration arise in decision making of AI algorithm in a complex scenario for inclusive access. For example, in case of a crash whether a self-driving car should consider safety of a disabled passenger or a pedestrian; or in case of an accident, whom to blame, the manufacturer, the disabled vehicle owner, or the AI developer (Bezrukov, 2025).

Equitable and Affordable Access

The significant cost of these devices hinders wide adoption of AI based assisted devices, especially in low income and resource limited countries. As reported by the UN, one billion disabled individuals do not have access to affordable assistive solutions in low and middle income countries (WHO-UNICEF, 2022). Moreover, the internet coverage or the lack of stable connectivity in remote areas, particularly in developing nations further exacerbate the disparity. Without reliable internet, a user cannot access cloud based AI services that rely on high-speed internet for frequent real time updates and data-intensive content. On the other hand, establishing and expanding an AI based infrastructure for transportation requires a high initial investment for logistics, software programs and tools. (Smita, 2025) estimates an investment of $74,000 – $210,000+ for deploying AI based transportation from project planning to quality assurance testing and compliance. The cost depends upon a number of factors, including project features and complexity, AI systems and data requirements.

Infrastructure and technical challenges

Due to rapidly changing environments such as construction sites, the AI algorithm faces significant complexity in decision making and convergence. In a dynamic urban transportation network, the AI algorithm has to interpret vehicle speed and direction from constantly changing real time spatial data. The complexity is further exacerbated by the presence of occlusion, traffic density, high pedestrian flow and frequent infrastructure changes (Zhou et al., 2012). Another significant barrier to outdoor mobility is the built environment or the environmental factors/features. Focusing to improve the built environment is necessary for enhanced transportation accessibility through infrastructure design, urban planning and assistive technology (Bastola et al., 2025). The built environment includes poor pathways, potholes, uneven surfaces and street layouts. For instance, poor curb ramps not only cause difficulty for mobility impaired individuals to use wheelchairs or crutches, but also pose risk for visually impaired in street crossings. Similarly, poor APS and ambient lightening conditions (day and night), inadequate lightening and weather conditions like rain and hail, hinders the use of built features such as landmarks and signage, causing trip hazards for low vision users (Seetharaman et al., 2024). The perceptron in AI networks may fail to update their internal representations as quickly as the dynamic environment leading to inaccurate localization due to changing visual patterns, and false object detection. The performance of AI algorithms in some situations, such as construction related problems, improper signage or obstructions may even cause the person to turn around (Jevinger et al., 2024). Moreover, the AI based audio signal for navigation and accessibility is also limited by background noise and echoes particularly due to crowded crossings and busy roadway (Jenkins et al., 2015). Under such uncertainty, the decision making of the algorithm becomes computationally complex, leading to no recognition or timed out announcements confusing passengers with memory or attention disability. Another critical bottlenecks in transportation is identifying frequency and duration of traffic congestion (Saki & Soori, 2025). Spatial and temporal uncertainty—such as moving crowds or penetration of connected vehicles, limits the reliability of predictive models like Kalman filters or LSTMs, to incorporate real time traffic patterns (Aljebreen et al., 2024). In addition, the AI based object detection struggles to exploit semantic regularities and contextual information (Sünderhauf et al., 2018), i.e. if they detect an object, wall or a ramp, they often fail to recognize their context in a specific situation such as recognizing that a blocked path means a wheelchair user needs rerouting.

Policy and Regulatory Barriers

Although the improvements in urban transportation has been discussed in several research, there is a significant need of proposing policies that promote safe, inclusive and accessible public transportation infrastructure (Anthony Jnr et al., 2021; Azevedo et al., 2021). The security vulnerabilities, privacy and ethical concerns issues that arise from the use of AI, necessitate transparency in data collection and usage, regulations and governance policies for robust security measures (Lamssaggad et al., 2021; Zemmouchi-Ghomari, 2025). Currently the accessible infrastructure is fragmented with technologically advanced nations adopting diverse infrastructures, data security, and privacy regulations (Breaking Barriers: Global Accessibility in Public Transportation Systems, 2025). For instance, bike services, public buses and metro operators, ride hailing companies, use proprietary systems and softwares, that can hinder real-time communication, coordination and integrated planning (Olayinka, 2021, 12(03), 711-726). Thus, standardization of ethical AI use, data format and interoperability are needed to scale up accessibility worldwide.

Future Trends and Recommendations

This section discusses future advancements in AI-based systems, outlines policy recommendations, and presents a vision for an AI-driven transportation system aimed at supporting individuals with disabilities.

Advancements in AI-Driven Transportation Accessibility

There is a need for prioritizing ethical considerations and inclusivity in future AI systems to ensure algorithm fairness and responsible deployment respecting the rights and interests of the disabled person. Researchers and AI developers must ensure that systems and algorithms are designed on fairness that avoid biases and protect privacy. There is a need for creating diverse and contextual training datasets so that the system responds to real world variability. Furthermore, robust data anonymity techniques must be implemented to safeguard privacy and identity of a user. AI solutions must emphasize trustworthiness and assurance. In addition, there is a need for inclusive transport design for equitable and accessible solutions. AI-driven accessible transportation should be designed to address the needs of vulnerable groups and individuals with disabilities. Without accurate and reliable data, even the most sophisticated AI algorithms will struggle to make informed decisions about pedestrian safety.

Policy Recommendations for AI-Enabled Transportation Systems

Implementing a disability inclusive public transportation system requires active involvement of different stakeholders. Including consultations and feedback regarding unique challenges the disabled communities encounter, would highlight the accessibility barriers and can help to overcome these challenges with user centric system design. In addition, engagement of urban planners and policy makers is essential for unified design incorporating participatory planning and regulatory policies for improved accessibility and inclusivity for disabled individuals.

REFERENCES

Abidi, M. H., Noor Siddiquee, A., Alkhalefah, H., & Srivastava, V. (2024). A comprehensive review of navigation systems for visually impaired individuals. *Heliyon*, *10*(11), e31825. DOI: 10.1016/j.heliyon.2024.e31825 PMID: 38841448

Abiraj, S., Janney, B., Prince, P. G. K., Sudhakar, T., & Jebaraj, E. (2024). AI-powered automated wheelchair with Lane detection. 2024 International Conference on Emerging Smart Computing and Informatics (ESCI), 1–5. DOI: 10.1109/ESCI59607.2024.10497306

Abraham, C. H., Ocansey, S., Boadi-Kusi, S. B., Faheem, F., Gyan, B. O., Nti, Y. A., Berchie, M., & Abu, E. K. (2023). Knowledge and practice of drivers on the provision of service to persons with visual disability: A survey of public transport drivers in a tertiary inclusion school in West Africa. *British Journal of Visual Impairment*, *41*(2), 414–424. DOI: 10.1177/02646196211044969

Accessibility Technology for blind & low vision people. (2025, January 30). Be My Eyes. https://www.bemyeyes.com/

Accessible pedestrian signals. (n.d.). Retrieved June 27, 2025, from https://www.okeenea.com/en/accessible-pedestrian-signal

AccessNow - pin-pointing accessibility worldwide. (2015, July 29). AccessNow. https://accessnow.com/

Aira. (2025, February 14). Aira | Access Is a Human Right; Aira. https://aira.io/aira-app/

Aljebreen, M., Alamro, H., Al-Mutiri, F., Othman, K. M., Alsumayt, A., Alazwari, S., Hamza, M. A., & Mohammed, G. P. (2024). Enhancing traffic flow prediction in intelligent cyber-physical systems: A novel bi-LSTM-based approach with Kalman filter integration. *IEEE Transactions on Consumer Electronics*, *70*(1), 1889–1902. DOI: 10.1109/TCE.2023.3335155

All_Aboard. (n.d.). "all_aboard" app effectively aids blind and visually impaired commuters in finding bus stops. Mass Eye and Ear. Retrieved June 27, 2025, from https://masseyeandear.org/news/press-releases/2024/01/all-aboard-app-effectively-aids-blind-and-visually-impaired-commuters

Almeida, D., Shmarko, K., & Lomas, E. (2022). The ethics of facial recognition technologies, surveillance, and accountability in an age of artificial intelligence: A comparative analysis of US, EU, and UK regulatory frameworks. *AI and Ethics*, *2*(3), 377–387. DOI: 10.1007/s43681-021-00077-w PMID: 34790955

Analysis of the development and application status of smart zebra crossing. (2022, August 26). https://www.trafficsolution.cn/analysis-of-the-development-and-application-status-of-smart-zebra-crossing/

Anthony Jnr, B., Abbas Petersen, S., Helfert, M., Ahlers, D., & Krogstie, J. (2021). Modeling pervasive platforms and digital services for smart urban transformation using an enterprise architecture framework. *Information Technology & People*, *34*(4), 1285–1312. DOI: 10.1108/ITP-07-2020-0511

Azad, A. K., Atkison, T., & Shah, A. F. M. (2024). A Review on Machine Learning in Intelligent Transportation Systems Applications. The Open Transportation Journal, 18(1).

Azevedo, G. A., Sampaio, R. R., Filho, A. S. N., Moret, M. A., & Murari, T. B. (2021). Sustainable urban mobility analysis for elderly and disabled people in São Paulo. *Scientific Reports*, *11*(1), 1–10. DOI: 10.1038/s41598-020-80906-w PMID: 33436990

Baker, M., & Winyard, S. (1998). *Lost vision: older visually impaired people in the UK*. Royal National Institute for the Blind.

Bastola, A., Wang, H., Boroujeni, S. P. H., Brinkley, J., Moshayedi, A. J., & Razi, A. (2025). Driving toward inclusion: A systematic review of AI-powered accessibility enhancements for people with disability in autonomous vehicles. *IEEE Access : Practical Innovations, Open Solutions*, *13*, 61384–61415. DOI: 10.1109/ACCESS.2025.3555923

Batura, O., Regeczi, D., Vassilev, A., Yagafarova, A., Bani, E., Bonneau, V., ... & DE STREEL, A. (2021). Artificial intelligence in road transport: annex to cost of non-Europe report.

Bejani, M. M., & Ghatee, M. (2019). Convolutional neural network with adaptive regularization to classify driving styles on smartphones. *IEEE Transactions on Intelligent Transportation Systems*, *21*(2), 543–552. DOI: 10.1109/TITS.2019.2896672

Bezrukov, O. (2025, May 28). AI in transportation: Ethical balance between safety and privacy. Blog. https://tech-stack.com/blog/ai-in-transportation/

Bharadiya, J. P. (2023). Artificial intelligence in transportation systems a critical review. *American Journal of Computing and Engineering*, *6*(1), 35–45. DOI: 10.47672/ajce.1487

Biased technology: The automated discrimination of facial recognition. (2024, February 29). ACLU of Minnesota. https://www.aclu-mn.org/en/news/biased-technology-automated-discrimination-facial-recognition

Bizwire, K. (n.d.). Gwangju launches smart crosswalk system to assist elderly and mobility-impaired pedestrians. Be Korea-Savvy. Retrieved June 27, 2025, from http://koreabizwire.com/gwangju-launches-smart-crosswalk-system-to-assist-elderly-and-mobility-impaired-pedestrians/285633

Blackstone, S. W., Beukelman, D. R., & Yorkston, K. M. (2015). *Patient-provider communication: Roles for speech-language pathologists and other health care professionals*. Plural Publishing.

Bocarejo, J. P., & Urrego, L. F. (2022). The impacts of formalization and integration of public transport in social equity: The case of Bogota. *Research in Transportation Business & Management*, *42*, 100560. DOI: 10.1016/j.rtbm.2020.100560

Boukerche, A., Tao, Y., & Sun, P. (2020). Artificial intelligence-based vehicular traffic flow prediction methods for supporting intelligent transportation systems. *Computer Networks*, *182*, 107484. DOI: 10.1016/j.comnet.2020.107484

Breaking barriers: Global accessibility in public transportation systems. (2025, June 9). KNOW-THE-ADA. https://know-the-ada.com/examining-accessibility-in-global-public-transportation-systems/

Building an accessible future for all: AI and the inclusion of Persons with Disabilities. (2024, December 2). United Nations Western Europe; United Nations. https://unric.org/en/building-an-accessible-future-for-all-ai-and-the-inclusion-of-persons-with-disabilities/

Campbell, P. (2024, July 1). Johns Hopkins researchers develop AI-enhanced navigation system for visually impaired. Johns Hopkins University Applied Physics Laboratory. https://www.jhuapl.edu/news/news-releases/240701-johns-hopkins-creates-navigation-system-for-the-visually-impaired

Carter, D. L. H. D. (n.d.). Accessible Pedestrian Signals: A Guide to Best Practices. https://onlinepubs.trb.org/onlinepubs/nchrp/nchrp_w117a.pdf

Casey, H., Brady, N., & Guerin, S. (2013). 'Is seeing perceiving?'Exploring issues concerning access to public transport for people with sight loss. *British Journal of Visual Impairment*, *31*(3), 217–227. DOI: 10.1177/0264619613495023

Chase, N., Maples, J., & Schipper, M. (2018, June). Autonomous vehicles: Uncertainties and energy implications. In *2018 EIA Energy Conference* (Vol. 5, p. 2018).

Clements, L. M., & Kockelman, K. M. (2017). Economic effects of automated vehicles. *Transportation Research Record: Journal of the Transportation Research Board*, *2606*(1), 106–114. DOI: 10.3141/2606-14

Conley, K., Foyer, A., Hara, P., Janik, T., Reichard, J., D'Souza, J., ... & Ababei, C. (2019). Vibration alert bracelet for notification of the visually and hearing impaired. Journal of Open Hardware.

Danley, K. (2024, October 25). Developments that will shape the future of smart wheelchairs. https://straitsresearch.com/article/key-advancements-in-smart-wheelchairs

Darcy, S., & Burke, P. F. (2018). On the road again: The barriers and benefits of automobility for people with disability. *Transportation Research Part A, Policy and Practice*, *107*, 229–245. DOI: 10.1016/j.tra.2017.11.002

Dickerson, A. E., Molnar, L. J., Eby, D. W., Adler, G., Bedard, M., Berg-Weger, M., Classen, S., Foley, D., Horowitz, A., Kerschner, H., Page, O., Silverstein, N. M., Staplin, L., & Trujillo, L. (2007). Transportation and aging: A research agenda for advancing safe mobility. *The Gerontologist*, *47*(5), 578–590. DOI: 10.1093/geront/47.5.578 PMID: 17989400

Digital, A. C. L. (2024, January 4). IoT enabled elevator system – A big lift ahead in smart elevator technology. ACL Digital. https://www.acldigital.com/blogs/smart-elevator-technology

Digital, T. (n.d.). DIEZ and derq launch AI-powered smart pedestrian crossing system in DSO. Government of Dubai Media Office. Retrieved June 27, 2025, from https://mediaoffice.ae/en/news/2023/august/02-08/diez-and-derq-launch

Disability, P. (2000). *Development: Issues Paper*. Dept. For International Development.

Disability ethical AI. (2022, March 17). Disability Ethical AI. https://disabilityethicalai.org/

Eisenberg, Y., Heider, A., Labbe, D., Gould, R., & Jones, R. (2024). Planning accessible cities: Lessons from high quality barrier removal plans. *Cities (London, England)*, *148*, 104837. DOI: 10.1016/j.cities.2024.104837

Elorduy, J. L., Pino, Y., & Gento, Á. M. (2025). Assessing public transport accessibility for people with physical disabilities in burgos, spain: A user-centered approach to inclusive urban mobility. *PLoS One*, *20*(4), e0322068. DOI: 10.1371/journal.pone.0322068 PMID: 40299992

Features, C. (n.d.). Voice Systems Solutions. https://www.redbooks.ibm.com/redbooks/pdfs/sg246884.pdf

Fürst, E., & Vogelauer, C. (2013). Best and bad practices in public transport: approaches to a barrier-free design for the visually and hearing impaired. In *Proc. European Transport Conference 2013*.

Gallagher, B. A., Hart, P. M., O'Brien, C., Stevenson, M. R., & Jackson, A. J. (2011). Mobility and access to transport issues as experienced by people with vision impairment living in urban and rural Ireland. *Disability and Rehabilitation*, *33*(12), 979–988. DOI: 10.3109/09638288.2010.516786 PMID: 20846055

Golledge, R. G., Marston, J. R., & Costanzo, C. M. (1997). Attitudes of visually impaired persons toward the use of public transportation. *Journal of Visual Impairment & Blindness*, *91*(5), 446–459. DOI: 10.1177/0145482X9709100505

Greater Cambridge partnership. Smart pedestrian crossing trial. (2024, April 15). GOV.UK. https://www.gov.uk/algorithmic-transparency-records/greater-cambridge-partnership-smart-pedestrian-crossing-trial

Guerreiro, J., Sato, D., Asakawa, S., Dong, H., Kitani, K. M., & Asakawa, C. (2019). CaBot: Designing and evaluating an autonomous navigation robot for blind people. *Proceedings of the 21st International ACM SIGACCESS Conference on Computers and Accessibility*, 68–82. DOI: 10.1145/3308561.3353771

Hersh, M. A. (2016). Improving deafblind travelers' experiences: An international survey. *Journal of Travel Research*, *55*(3), 380–394. DOI: 10.1177/0047287514546225

How generative AI boosts performance throughout our Group. (n.d.). SNCF Group. Retrieved June 27, 2025, from https://www.groupe-sncf.com/en/innovation/emerging-technologies/generative-ia

How stair lifts are adapting to smart home tech in 2025. (2025, May 8). Smart G Home. https://smartghome.com/smart-stair-lifts-in-2025/

Huang, C.-Y., Wu, C.-K., & Liu, P.-Y. (2022). Assistive technology in smart cities: A case of street crossing for the visually-impaired. *Technology in Society*, *68*(101805), 101805. DOI: 10.1016/j.techsoc.2021.101805

Instituto Nacional de Estadística. (2023). Survey on Disability, Personal Autonomy and Dependency Situations [Online]. Retrieved June 10, 2025, from: https://www.ine.es/dyngs/INEbase/es/operacion.htm?c=Estadistica_C&cid=1254736176782&menu=resultados&idp=1254735573175#!tabs-1254736195764

Iyer, L. S. (2021). AI enabled applications towards intelligent transportation. *Transportation Engineering*, *5*, 100083. DOI: 10.1016/j.treng.2021.100083

Jalali, D. (2023, September 5). The ethics of artificial intelligence: Are AI voices legal? Voices. https://www.voices.com/blog/are-ai-voices-legal/

Karabulut, M. A., Shah, A. S., Ilhan, H., Pathan, A. S. K., & Atiquzzaman, M. (2023). Inspecting VANET with various critical aspects–a systematic review. *Ad Hoc Networks*, *150*, 103281. DOI: 10.1016/j.adhoc.2023.103281

Khafar, N. H. B. A., Soomro, D. M., Rahman, R. A., Abdullah, M. N., Soho, I. A., & Rahimoon, A. A. (2019). Intelligent navigation system using ultrasonic sensor for visually impaired person (VIP). 2019 IEEE 6th International Conference on Engineering Technologies and Applied Sciences (ICETAS), 1–4. DOI: 10.1109/ICETAS48360.2019.9117297

Khalil, R. A., Safelnasr, Z., Yemane, N., Kedir, M., Shafiqurrahman, A., & Saeed, N. (2024). Advanced learning technologies for intelligent transportation systems: Prospects and challenges. *IEEE Open Journal of Vehicular Technology*, *5*, 397–427. DOI: 10.1109/OJVT.2024.3369691

King, J. (n.d.). Privacy in an AI era: How do we protect our personal information? Retrieved June 26, 2025, from https://hai.stanford.edu/news/privacy-ai-era-how-do-we-protect-our-personal-information

Kirillov, A., He, K., Girshick, R., Rother, C., & Dollár, P. (2019). Panoptic segmentation. In *Proceedings of the IEEE/CVF conference on computer vision and pattern recognition* (pp. 9404-9413).

Kulkarni, M. P. (n.d.). Innovations Challenges Managing Cab Aggregators.

Kumar, S. A., Sasikala, S., & Arun, N. (2024). Enhancing the Communication of Speech-Impaired People Using Embedded Vision-based Gesture Recognition through Deep Learning. In *Exploration of Artificial Intelligence and Blockchain Technology in Smart and Secure Healthcare* (pp. 179–198). Bentham Science Publishers. DOI: 10.2174/97898151654321240700011

Lakkaraju, H., Kamar, E., Caruana, R., & Horvitz, E. (2017). Identifying unknown unknowns in the open world: Representations and policies for guided exploration. Proceedings of the ... AAAI Conference on Artificial Intelligence. AAAI Conference on Artificial Intelligence, 31(1). DOI: 10.1609/aaai.v31i1.10821

Lamssaggad, A., Benamar, N., Hafid, A. S., & Msahli, M. (2021). A survey on the current security landscape of intelligent transportation systems. *IEEE Access : Practical Innovations, Open Solutions*, *9*, 9180–9208. DOI: 10.1109/ACCESS.2021.3050038

Lasker, J., & Bedrosian, J. (2001). Promoting acceptance of augmentative and alternative communication by adults with acquired communication disorders. *Augmentative and Alternative Communication, 17*(3), 141–153. DOI: 10.1080/aac.17.3.141.153

Lee, H., & Park, D. (2021). AI TTS smartphone app for communication of speech impaired people. Data Science and Digital Transformation in the Fourth Industrial Revolution, 219-229.

Lee, R. J. T. (n.d.). Usability challenges assistive technologies: Bridging gap between innovation accessibility.

Li, S., Fan, X., Zhang, Y., Trappe, W., Lindqvist, J., & Howard, R. E. (2017). Auto++ detecting cars using embedded microphones in real-time. *Proceedings of the ACM on Interactive, Mobile, Wearable and Ubiquitous Technologies, 1*(3), 1–20. PMID: 30417164

Li, X., & Dang, A. (2025). The disruptive effect of AI on urban planning. Nature Cities, 1-3.

Lise. (2023a, February 17). 7 good reasons to install audio beacons at public transport. Inclusive City Maker. https://www.inclusivecitymaker.com/install-audio-beacons-public-transport-network/

Lise. (2023b, March 10). Our audio beacons guide blind users at the Helsinki subway. Inclusive City Maker. https://www.inclusivecitymaker.com/audio-beacons-blind-visually-impaired-helsinki-subway/

Low, W. Y., Cao, M., De Vos, J., & Hickman, R. (2020). The journey experience of visually impaired people on public transport in London. *Transport Policy, 97*, 137–148. DOI: 10.1016/j.tranpol.2020.07.018

Lu, C.-L., Liu, Z.-Y., Huang, J.-T., Huang, C.-I., Wang, B.-H., Chen, Y., Wu, N.-H., Wang, H.-C., Giarré, L., & Kuo, P.-Y. (2021). Assistive navigation using deep reinforcement learning guiding robot with UWB/voice beacons and semantic feedbacks for blind and visually impaired people. *Frontiers in Robotics and AI, 8*, 654132. DOI: 10.3389/frobt.2021.654132 PMID: 34239900

Luan, T. H., Gao, L., Li, Z., Xiang, Y., Wei, G., & Sun, L. (2015). Fog computing: Focusing on mobile users at the edge. arXiv preprint arXiv:1502.01815.

Majumdar, S. R. (2017). The case of public involvement in transportation planning using social media. *Case Studies on Transport Policy, 5*(1), 121–133. DOI: 10.1016/j.cstp.2016.11.002

McNaughton, D., Rackensperger, T., & McLemore, L. (2025). Supporting meaningful participation in society by adults with developmental disabilities who need and use AAC: Lived experiences, key research findings, and future directions. *Augmentative and Alternative Communication, 41*(3), 1–14. DOI: 10.1080/07434618.2025.2504497 PMID: 40464637

Messaoudi, M. D., Menelas, B.-A. J., & Mcheick, H. (2022). Review of navigation assistive tools and technologies for the visually impaired. *Sensors (Basel), 22*(20), 7888. DOI: 10.3390/s22207888 PMID: 36298237

Młodystach, Ł., Orczyk, M., & Tomaszewski, F. (2023). Evaluation of public transport in Poland form the perspective of the deaf and hard of hearing people towards the improvement of mobility. Archives of transport, 66(2), 61-76.

Monica, R., & Aleotti, J. (2023). Improving virtual reality navigation tasks using a haptic vest and upper body tracking. *Displays, 78*(102417), 102417. DOI: 10.1016/j.displa.2023.102417

Montanha, A., Oprescu, A. M., & Romero-Ternero, M. (2022). A context-aware artificial intelligence-based system to support street crossings for pedestrians with visual impairments. *Applied Artificial Intelligence, 36*(1), 2062818. Advance online publication. DOI: 10.1080/08839514.2022.2062818

Mulfari, D., & Villari, M. (2024). A voice user interface on the edge for people with speech impairments. *Electronics (Basel), 13*(7), 1389. DOI: 10.3390/electronics13071389

Naayini, P., Myakala, P. K., Bura, C., Jonnalagadda, A. K., & Kamatala, S. (2025). AI-powered assistive technologies for visual impairment. In arXiv [cs.HC]. arXiv. https://arxiv.org/abs/2503.15494

Naik, N. (2017, October). Choice of effective messaging protocols for IoT systems: MQTT, CoAP, AMQP and HTTP. In 2017 IEEE international systems engineering symposium (ISSE) (pp. 1-7). IEEE.

Nasser, N., Ali, A., Karim, L., & Al-Helali, A. (2024). Enhancing mobility for the visually impaired with AI and IoT-enabled mobile applications. In ScienceOpen. DOI: 10.14293/PR2199.000775.v1

Nikitas, A., Michalakopoulou, K., Njoya, E. T., & Karampatzakis, D. (2020). Artificial intelligence, transport and the smart city: Definitions and dimensions of a new mobility era. *Sustainability (Basel), 12*(7), 2789. DOI: 10.3390/su12072789

Oladimeji, D., Gupta, K., Kose, N. A., Gundogan, K., Ge, L., & Liang, F. (2023). Smart transportation: An overview of technologies and applications. *Sensors (Basel), 23*(8), 3880. DOI: 10.3390/s23083880 PMID: 37112221

Olayinka, O. H. (2021, 12(03), 711-726). Data driven customer segmentation and personalization strategies in modern business intelligence frameworks. World Journal of Advanced Research and Reviews, 12(03), 711–726. https://wjarr.com/content/data-driven-customer-segmentation-and-personalization-strategies-modern-business

Padhy, S., Tiwari, J., Rathore, S., & Kumar, N. (2019, December). Emergency signal classification for the hearing impaired using multi-channel convolutional neural network architecture. In *2019 IEEE Conference on Information and Communication Technology* (pp. 1-6). IEEE. DOI: 10.1109/CICT48419.2019.9066252

Papageorgiou, M., Diakaki, C., Dinopoulou, V., Kotsialos, A., & Wang, Y. (2003). Review of road traffic control strategies. *Proceedings of the IEEE, 91*(12), 2043–2067. DOI: 10.1109/JPROC.2003.819610

Park, J., Bamford, J., Byun, H., & Chowdhury, S. (2017, November). Journey by visually impaired public transport users: Barriers and consequences. In Australasian Transport Research Forum (pp. 27-29).

Patel, P., Pampaniya, S., Ghosh, A., Raj, R., Karuppaih, D., & Kandasamy, S. (2025). Enhancing Accessibility Through Machine Learning: A Review on Visual and Hearing Impairment Technologies. *IEEE Access : Practical Innovations, Open Solutions, 13*, 33286–33307. DOI: 10.1109/ACCESS.2025.3539081

Pieri, K., & Cobb, S. V. G. (2019). Mobile app communication aid for Cypriot deaf people. *Journal of Enabling Technologies, 13*(2), 70–81. DOI: 10.1108/JET-12-2018-0058

Providing accessible information onboard local bus and coach services. (n.d.). GOV.UK. Retrieved June 28, 2025, from https://www.gov.uk/government/publications/providing-accessible-information-onboard-local-bus-and-coach-services/providing-accessible-information-onboard-local-bus-and-coach-services

Rashed, A. N. Z., Yarrarapu, M., Prabu, R. T., Raj Antony, G. S., Edeswaran, L., Kumar, E. S., Aswitha, K., Snehith, N., & Ahammad, S. H. (2024). Connected smart elevator systems for smart power and time saving. *Scientific Reports, 14*(1), 19330. DOI: 10.1038/s41598-024-69173-1 PMID: 39164299

Reaber, G. (2024, May 2). From stations to exhibits: Enhancing public spaces with AI voice technology. https://www.respeecher.com/blog/enhancing-public-spaces-with-ai-voice-technology

Revolutionizing ride-hailing with AI-Powered Taxi App Development. (2024, December 18). Fullestop Blogs. https://www.fullestop.com/blog/ai-powered-taxi-app-development-revolutionizing-ride-hailing

Rice, P. (2024, September 11). Alexa integration, elevate your home with voice-controlled convenience: The PVE vacuum elevator. Anglian Lifts. https://anglian-lifts.co.uk/alexa-integration-pve-vacuum-lifts/

Rides for all with Lyft Up. (n.d.). Retrieved June 29, 2025, from https://www.lyft.com/lyftup/programs

Risser, R., Lexell, E. M., Bell, D., Iwarsson, S., & Ståhl, A. (2015). Use of local public transport among people with cognitive impairments–A literature review. *Transportation Research Part F: Traffic Psychology and Behaviour*, *29*, 83–97. DOI: 10.1016/j.trf.2015.01.002

Rode, P., & da Cruz, N. F. (2018). Governing urban accessibility: Moving beyond transport and mobility. *Applied Mobilities*, *3*(1), 8–33. DOI: 10.1080/23800127.2018.1438149

Roy, A., Karim, E., Bin Farukee, M., & Makedon, F. (2024, June). ChatGPT as an Assistive Technology: Enhancing Human-Computer Interaction for People with Speech Impairments. In *Proceedings of the 17th International Conference on PErvasive Technologies Related to Assistive Environments* (pp. 63-66). DOI: 10.1145/3652037.3663956

Sahoo, S., & Choudhury, B. (2023). AI advances in wheelchair navigation and control: A comprehensive review. *Journal of Process Management New Technologies*, *11*(3-4), 115–132. DOI: 10.5937/jpmnt11-45181

Saki, S., & Soori, M. (2025). Artificial intelligence, machine learning and deep learning in advanced transportation systems, A review. *Multimodal Transportation*, *100242*(1), 100242. DOI: 10.1016/j.multra.2025.100242

Samonte, M. J. C., Gazmin, R. A., Soriano, J. D. S., & Valencia, M. N. O. (2019, October). BridgeApp: An assistive mobile communication application for the deaf and mute. In *2019 International Conference on Information and Communication Technology Convergence (ICTC)* (pp. 1310-1315). IEEE. DOI: 10.1109/ICTC46691.2019.8939866

Satyanarayanan, M. (2017). The emergence of edge computing. *Computer*, *50*(1), 30–39. DOI: 10.1109/MC.2017.9

Shinkansen, T. (n.d.). Retrieved June 27, 2025, from https://www.readspeaker.com/resources/tokaido-shinkansen/

Shirley, B., Thomas, J., & Roche, P. (2012, September). VoIPText: Voice chat for deaf and hard of hearing people. In 2012 IEEE Second International Conference on Consumer Electronics-Berlin (ICCE-Berlin) (pp. 19-23). IEEE.

Singh, H. K., Yadav, A. K., & Claret, S. A. (2024, April). Voice Assistant for Hearing and Speech-Impaired Individuals Using Web framework. In 2024 2nd International Conference on Networking and Communications (ICNWC) (pp. 1-7). IEEE. DOI: 10.1109/ICNWC60771.2024.10537426

Singh, V. (2025). AI-Powered Assistive Technologies for People with Disabilities: Developing AI Solutions that Aid Individuals with Various Disabilities in Daily Tasks. *Journal of Engineering Research and Reports*, *27*(2), 292–309. DOI: 10.9734/jerr/2025/v27i21410

Smart elevators for smart cities. (2019, October 27). Imdaad. https://www.imdaad.ae/case-studies/smart-elevators-for-smart-cities/

Smart Pedestrian Crossing – An EPS@ISEP 2020 Project. (n.d.). https://www.eps2020-wiki6.dee.isep.ipp.pt/lib/exe/fetch.php?media=smart_pedestrian_crossing_t6_eps_isep_2020.pdf

Smart ramp. (2022, March 15). DIGIFED. https://digifed.org/portfolio-item/smart-ramp/

Smart ramps to assist passengers with reduced mobility (PRM). (n.d.). Retrieved June 28, 2025, from https://danova-next-toolkit.com/smart-ramps-to-assist-passengers-with-reduced-mobility-prm/

Smita. (2025, June 16). AI in Transportation industry: Everything you need to know. ScalaCode. https://www.scalacode.com/guides/ai-in-transportation/

Soundscape, M. (2022, June 7). Microsoft Research. https://www.microsoft.com/en-us/research/product/soundscape/

Sünderhauf, N., Brock, O., Scheirer, W., Hadsell, R., Fox, D., Leitner, J., Upcroft, B., Abbeel, P., Burgard, W., Milford, M., & Corke, P. (2018). The limits and potentials of deep learning for robotics. *The International Journal of Robotics Research*, *37*(4-5), 405–420. DOI: 10.1177/0278364918770733

Sunu band. (2015). National Federation of the Blind. National Federation of the Blind Jernigan Institute Research Collaboration: Sunu Band. https://nfb.org/blog/national-federation-blind-jernigan-institute-research-collaboration-sunu-band

Talk2lift brings the power of speech recognition on any elevator cabin, enabling passengers to voice-control. (2020, September 14). Talk2Lift; bmjwu. https://talk2lift.com/

Text-to-speech voices designed for public transport. (n.d.). Acapela Group. https://www.acapela-group.com/tts-voices-for-transport/

TrainMate Robotic System Making Public Transportation. Public! (n.d.). Retrieved June 29, 2025, from https://onlinepubs.trb.org/onlinepubs/IDEA/FinalReports/Transit/Transit100.pdf

TransPennine Express. (2024, Sep, 20). TransPennine Express tests UK-first AI speech-to-text announcements designed to improve journeys for hearing-impaired passengers [Press release]. Mediacentrefile. Retrieved June 28, 2025, from: https://mediacentre.tpexpress.co.uk/news/video-transpennine-express-tests-uk-first-ai-speech-to-text-announcements-designed-to-improve-journeys-for-hearing-impaired-passengers

Trewin, S., Basson, S., Muller, M., Branham, S., Treviranus, J., Gruen, D., Hebert, D., Lyckowski, N., & Manser, E. (2019). Considerations for AI fairness for people with disabilities. *AI Matters*, *5*(3), 40–63. DOI: 10.1145/3362077.3362086

Uber. (n.d.). Retrieved June 29, 2025, from https://www.uber.com/us/en/about/accessibility/

United Nations. (n.d.). Transforming our world: The 2030 Agenda for Sustainable Development [Online]. Retrieved June 10, 2025, from: https://sdgs.un.org/2030agenda

Vangelista, L., Zanella, A., & Zorzi, M. (2015). Long-range IoT technologies: The dawn of LoRa™. In Future Access Enablers for Ubiquitous and Intelligent Infrastructures: First International Conference, FABULOUS 2015, Ohrid, Republic of Macedonia, September 23-25, 2015. Revised Selected Papers 1 (pp. 51-58). Springer International Publishing.

Velho, R., Holloway, C., Symonds, A., & Balmer, B. (2016). The effect of transport accessibility on the social inclusion of wheelchair users: A mixed method analysis. *Social Inclusion (Lisboa)*, *4*(3), 24–35. DOI: 10.17645/si.v4i3.484

Vishweshwar, S. M. (2023). Implications of Deepfake Technology on Individual Privacy and Security [St. Cloud State University]. https://repository.stcloudstate.edu/cgi/viewcontent.cgi?article=1199&context=msia_etds

Wang, Y., Cui, Z., & Ke, R. (2023). *Machine learning for transportation research and applications*. Elsevier.

Wayfinder. (2024). https://paper.wayfinder.ai/wayfinder_paper_v1.pdf

WeWALK smart cane – smart cane for the visually impaired. (n.d.). Retrieved June 27, 2025, from https://wewalk.io/en/

WHO-UNICEF. (2022, May). Global report on assistive technology. https://www.unicef.org/reports/global-report-assistive-technology#:~:text=Highlights,replacements

Willilams, J. D. (2023). Creating an Equitable Transit System for New York City. Metropolitan Transit Authority (MTA), New York City. https://advocate.nyc.gov/resources/reports/MTA-Accessibility-Report-PRINT-YR9jvk9Z6b9x.pdf

World Health Organization. (2022). Global report on health equity for persons with disabilities [Online]. Retrieved June 10, 2025, from: https://www.who.int/publications/i/item/9789240063600

World Health Organization. (2023, August 10). Blindness and vision impairment. https://www.who.int/news-room/fact-sheets/detail/blindness-and-visual-impairment

World Health Organization, & World Bank. (2011). World report on disability [Online]. Geneva: World Health Organization; 2011 Retrieved June 10, 2025. Available from: https://iris.who.int/handle/10665/44575

Wu, C. H., Ho, J. M., & Lee, D. T. (2004). Travel-time prediction with support vector regression. *IEEE Transactions on Intelligent Transportation Systems*, *5*(4), 276–281. DOI: 10.1109/TITS.2004.837813

Xu, Y., Wang, Q., Lillie, J., Kamat, V., & Menassa, C. (2025). CoNav Chair: Design of a ROS-based smart wheelchair for shared control navigation in the built environment. In arXiv [cs.RO]. arXiv. https://arxiv.org/abs/2501.09680 DOI: 10.22260/ISARC2025/0046

Yuan, T., da Rocha Neto, W. B., Rothenberg, C., Obraczka, K., Barakat, C., & Turletti, T. (2019). Harnessing machine learning for next-generation intelligent transportation systems: a survey. *Proceedings of the computational intelligence, communication systems and networks (CICSyN).*

Zantalis, F., Koulouras, G., Karabetsos, S., & Kandris, D. (2019). A review of machine learning and IoT in smart transportation. *Future Internet*, *11*(4), 94. DOI: 10.3390/fi11040094

Zemmouchi-Ghomari, L. (2025). Artificial intelligence in intelligent transportation systems. Journal of Intelligent Manufacturing and Special Equipment.

Zemmouchi-Ghomari, L. (2025). Artificial intelligence in intelligent transportation systems. *Journal of Intelligent Manufacturing and Special Equipment*, *6*(1), 26–42. DOI: 10.1108/JIMSE-11-2024-0035

Zhang, X., Huang, X., Ding, Y., Long, L., Li, W., & Xu, X. (2024). Advancements in smart wearable mobility aids for visual impairments: A bibliometric narrative review. *Sensors (Basel)*, *24*(24), 7986. Advance online publication. DOI: 10.3390/s24247986 PMID: 39771730

Zhou, H., Hou, K.-M., Zuo, D., & Li, J. (2012). Intelligent urban public transportation for accessibility dedicated to people with disabilities. *Sensors (Basel)*, *12*(8), 10678–10692. DOI: 10.3390/s120810678 PMID: 23112622

KEY TERMS AND DEFINITIONS

Intelligent Transportation System: A cutting-edge, data-driven approach for enhancing the sustainability, efficiency, and safety of transportation networks. It is composed of modern technologies including sensors, wireless networks, analysis of data, and monitoring in real time for improved administration of automobiles and transportation infrastructure.

Artificial Intelligence: The term artificial intelligence describes computer programs that are able to carry out sophisticated operations that were previously restricted to humans, such as problem-solving, thinking, and decision-making.

Natural Language Processing: The field of creating machines that can control the language of humans, or information that mimics human language, in its spoken, written, and structured forms.

Internet of Things: The Internet of Things (IoT) is the broad category of physical devices that have sensors and software installed that allow them to communicate with one another by gathering and sharing data across a network.

Computer Vision: The artificial intelligence discipline that teaches systems and machines how to extract useful information from video clips, digital images, and other optical inputs.

Machine Learning: A branch of artificial intelligence called machine learning employs algorithms that have been trained on sets of data to build models that can perform tasks like picture classification, data analysis, and price prediction that would normally only be feasible for humans.

Deep Learning: Deep learning is a technique that allows machines to automatically find patterns and make logical conclusions from huge volumes of unorganized data by simulating the neural networks seen in the human brain.

Chapter 5
Machine Learning to Enhance Road and Traffic Safety for Senior and Disabled Citizens

Soorya Sathish
https://orcid.org/0009-0000-7692-2165
Heriot-Watt University, Dubai, UAE

Cristina Turcanu
https://orcid.org/0009-0003-2018-4935
Heriot-Watt University, Dubai, UAE

ABSTRACT

Machine learning (ML) models have the potential to improve road safety by predicting and preventing accidents. Building on this idea, this study examines how ML can enhance safe transportation for the elderly and people with disabilities, who often face significant mobility challenges. Traditional transport safety strategies tend to react to accidents rather than proactively address risks, further disadvantaging these vulnerable road users. This chapter explores how predictions based on specific ML models can analyse accident patterns and inform specific safety measures. By integrating AI-based accident prediction with intelligent traffic systems, adaptive signals, and accessibility-focused solutions, this research explores solutions and recommendations to guide urban planning and create safer and more inclusive transport networks tailored to those who need them most.

DOI: 10.4018/979-8-3373-2033-5.ch005

INTRODUCTION

Road traffic accidents are a public safety concern on the increase, resulting in thousands of deaths and millions of injuries globally every year. Older people and individuals with disabilities are primarily vulnerable in such accidents due to poor mobility, slower reflex, and increased dependence on accessible infrastructure. This research is significant in promoting public security and assisting the authorities in controlling traffic for the citizens whose mobility is certainly not their strong suit. As traditional measures of security continue to fail these groups, there is a pressing need for technology-based, preventive measures. This chapter explores the use of Machine learning to predict traffic crashes and contribute to more responsive, inclusive transportation systems that secure better and protect their peace of mind whilst their journey.

Motivation

Traffic crashes are a major cause of death and severe injury, high economic and personal expenses across the world. The World Health Organization reports that millions of people get injured or paralyzed every year from road accidents, which are among the top causes of death globally. Some of the most vulnerable populations are older citizens and those with disabilities, who are already posed at a greater risk due to limited mobility, weaker senses, and slower reactions. Traditional road safety systems are not necessarily designed with these groups in consideration. Because there are a lot of various contributory causes of traffic accidents, anticipating them precisely remains still a challenging job in spite of improvement in automobile safety technologies and traffic control technologies. There are some factors leading to car accidents, that includes weather conditions (such as rain or fog), lighting conditions (such as day or night), road surface type (such as dry, wet, or slippery), and the driver's demographics. The relationship between each of these factors can often be too complex for traditional methods to handle. Nevertheless, machine learning can potentially identify patterns in large datasets and better predict traffic crashes.

Aim and Scope

The aim of this chapter is to explain theoretically how machine learning can be utilised to improve road safety, with a special emphasis on its implications for elderly citizens and individuals with disabilities. The content is structured to elaborate on relevant literature, methods, theoretical concepts, and emerging technologies pertinent to this field and explores a case study on the use of ML in transportation.

This analysis discusses how road traffic crashes affect vulnerable groups, highlighting more equitable transportation planning. It also investigates key environmental and demographic factors widely applied in crash prediction research, including weather, traffic counts, and population data. The review also looks at the ways machine learning models have been applied or suggested to improve the accuracy of crash prediction. Its possible application to real-time city infrastructure, e.g., Intelligent Transportation Systems (ITS), is also discussed. Finally, the larger implications of incorporating machine learning into transport systems are assessed, specifically its ability to promote more responsive, equitable, and inclusive mobility solutions.

Contributions

This chapter contributes to ongoing scholarly and real-world discussions on the use of AI for public safety, especially at the intersection of predictive analytics and inclusive transportation planning. The main contributions of the chapter are detailed below:

Conceptual Framework for Inclusive Crash Prediction: The chapter proposes a conceptual foundation for how ML algorithms like Random Forest, CAT Boost and XGBoost can be applied to predict road crashes in scenarios where vulnerable populations are disproportionately affected.

Mapping of Risk-Relevant Variables: A review-based synthesis that identifies and categorizes critical environmental and demographic variables (e.g., weather, light conditions, road surface, age) that influence crash likelihood, specifically among the elderly and disabled.

ITS Integration Pathways: It explores how predictive crash models can conceptually feed into adaptive Intelligent Transportation Systems, enabling real-time and location-sensitive interventions to better serve mobility-impaired road users.

Equity-Centered Design and Policy Insight: The chapter advocates for embedding ML-derived insights into urban planning and transportation policy, offering forward-thinking recommendations that align predictive safety measures with universal accessibility and inclusive mobility goals.

Organisation

The content is organised to build a logical and holistic understanding of how machine learning can support inclusive transportation systems. It begins with an introductory section that lays out the motivation behind the research and defines the chapter's aims, scope, and key contributions.

Following the introduction, the literature review provides a thorough analysis of existing research on crash prediction and the application of machine learning in transportation safety, particularly focusing on its potential to improve conditions for senior citizens and individuals with disabilities. It also highlights gaps in current systems and the pressing need for adaptive solutions.

The chapter then delves into the core focus of the article, structured into subsections that emphasize the centrality of vulnerable road users, the role of predictive ML models, and the importance of embedding these insights into real-time ITS infrastructure. A dedicated section explores actionable solutions and recommendations, ranging from smart city applications and inclusive design principles to community feedback mechanisms and public-private collaborations. Subsequently, a comprehensive future research section outlines key limitations, ethical considerations, and opportunities for scaling ML-based transport safety systems. The chapter concludes with a summary of knowledge achievements and reflections on societal implications thus laying a robust foundation for continued academic and policy-driven work in inclusive mobility.

BACKGROUND

The literature review analyses key concepts and prior research on predicting road traffic crashes with help of machine learning, providing a strong conclusive foundation to help understand the potential of improving the transport accessibility and security of vulnerable users. Road accidents are escalating globally, leading to millions of fatalities each year and imposing severe financial and economic burdens on society. According to the World Health Organization (World Health Organization, 2021), approximately 1.35 million people die annually due to road accidents, with an additional 20 to 50 million sustaining severe injuries. The socio-economic costs are staggering, affecting not only individuals but also healthcare systems, insurance companies, and governments. In countries like New Zealand (NZ), road accidents cost nearly 3% of the country's gross domestic product (GDP) (Ministry of Transport, 2020). According to the NZ Ministry of Transport, the average social cost per fatality is NZD 4.46 million, and the Value of Statistical Life (VSL) is NZD 4.42 million per fatality as of June 2020.

It is well understood that the geriatric age group is particularly vulnerable to road traffic injuries. Research indicates geriatric patients often suffer from collision-related injuries more frequently and severely compared to younger populations due to physiological changes associated with aging, such as decreased muscle strength and reduced bone density (Yıldırım et al., 2021). Despite global policies and strategic efforts aimed at mitigating road crashes, there is a need to explore advanced approaches, such as machine learning, to proactively predict, manage, and ultimately reduce traffic incidents especially for senior and disabled individuals where mobility is not their strong suit.

The subsequent sections provide a comprehensive review of global road safety challenges; further detail the specific vulnerabilities faced by senior citizens and disabled individuals and explore the application of machine learning and intelligent transportation systems (ITS) to enhance road safety and mobility.

Importance of Understanding Contributing Factors

Several studies have explored the importance of different contributing factors in road accidents and their severity. However, only a limited number of studies have investigated the performance of a subset of ensemble ML models in predicting road accidents, particularly using the New Zealand Road accident dataset (Williams Zhou, 2020). The challenge lies in the lack of straightforward or linear relationships between the contributing factors and accident severity. Understanding these factors is essential not only for building predictive models but also for designing safer roads and policies that can reduce accident occurrences and minimize their impact. Poorly designed intersections, lack of pedestrian crossings, and in- adequate road signage all which are part of influence of road design contribute significantly to the likelihood of accidents. Poorly designed roads, inadequate signage, and lack of pedestrian infrastructure are significant contributors to road accidents (Infrastructure Australia, 2018).

Prediction Factors

The effectiveness of predicting road accidents and their severity largely depends on under- standing a range of environmental, infrastructural, and situational factors. In this study, we focus on key factors that contribute to accident prediction and severity. Traffic accident data may miss key factors affecting injury severity, making variability and heterogeneity crucial in analyses (Li et al., 2024).

Climate Conditions

Weather plays a crucial role in road safety and accident occurrence. Dry weather characterized by clear skies and no precipitation, offers optimal driving conditions. Windy conditions, how- ever, can destabilize vehicles. Snow and icy surfaces significantly reduce traction, increasing accident risks. Mist and fog obstruct visibility, making driving more hazardous. Sunny weather can cause glare, impairing driver vision, while extreme heat can lead to vehicle malfunctions or driver fatigue. Rainy conditions extend braking distances and reduce visibility, resulting in a higher likelihood of accidents compared to sunlit days (Zou et al. 2023).

Light Conditions

Light conditions greatly influence visibility and reaction time, which are crucial for accident prevention. Daylight typically offers better visibility, while night driving is more dangerous due to limited visibility, even with high-beam headlights. Night driving is dangerous because, even with high-beam headlights on, visibility is limited to about 500 feet (250 feet for normal headlights) creating less time to react to something in the road, especially when driving at higher speeds (National Safety Council, n.d.). For Street lighting Residents, pedestrians, and drivers can obtain or lose visual acuity depending on the physical characteristics of street lighting such as the light level and uniformity. Street lighting provides illumination to maintain visual acuity, surveillance, and a sense of safety in nighttime environments, but unshielded or poorly designed street lighting can reduce human's nighttime vision, decrease levels of safety, and create roadway hazards (Suk and Walter, 2018).

Road Surface Condition

Road safety can be understood as the result of the safe interaction of participants of traffic between themselves and the environment. The condition of road surfaces plays a critical role in influencing the risk of accidents. Dry surfaces provide optimal traction, offering better control over vehicles. However, wet surfaces reduce friction, leading to longer stopping distances. Icy or snowy surfaces are especially hazardous, as they offer minimal traction, increasing the chances of skidding. Gravel or uneven surfaces can cause instability, making vehicles harder to control. When these conditions combine with high-speed driving, the likelihood of accidents rises significantly, highlighting the importance of maintaining safe speeds in challenging environments (Batrakova and Gredasova, 2016).

Speed Limit of the Road

Speed is one of the most critical factors in road accident severity. Roads with higher speed limits tend to result in more severe accidents. The study considers the speed limit as an important predictive factor, since lower speeds can reduce accident severity while higher speeds often lead to more serious injuries or fatalities. For example, an adult pedestrian hit by a car travelling at 50 kilometres per hour will be seriously injured but most likely survive; whereas, that same pedestrian hit by the same car travelling at 80 kilometres per hour will likely suffer severe injuries and quite possibly die. Reducing average travelling speeds by just 5 percent could reduce fatal road crashes by 30 percent, according to studies (World Health Organization, 2017).

Output Variable: Accident Severity

In this chapter's case study, accident severity, the model's outcome, is classified into three levels. Level 1 refers to minor accidents where injuries may not require hospitalization. Level 2 covers moderate accidents, where medical attention is needed for 1–2 days. Finally, Level 3 represents severe accidents that result in hospitalization or fatalities, with recovery times exceeding three days. By analyzing these predictive factors, we aim to develop an accurate model to assess the risk and severity of road accidents under various conditions. "Accident severity is typically classified based on the extent of injuries, which can range from minor cuts to life-threatening trauma requiring hospitalization" (Department of Transport, 2019).

Evolution and Role of Intelligent Transportation Systems (ITS)

As cities grow and traffic conditions become more challenging, traditional road safety methods just aren't enough anymore, especially for people who need extra support, like senior citizens or those with disabilities. That's why there's been a growing shift inclining towards using Intelligent Transportation Systems (ITS). At its core, ITS means bringing technology together like sensors, communication systems, live data, and automation to help manage traffic in smarter, more adaptive ways. However, traditional detection methods, especially those relying on 2D imagery, often struggle with accuracy, real-time responsiveness, and occlusion in complex urban environments. A recent study by (Wang et al., 2025) highlights that these limitations can be significantly addressed by using 3D point cloud-based detection methods, which offer better real time perception and recognition performance under challenging conditions. Additionally, the economic growth and investment in ITS reflect its global importance. In 2020, the estimated market for the global intelligent transportation system was USD 29.69 billion, and it is expected to grow at a CAGR of 6.3%, reaching nearly USD 47.89 billion by 2030 (Chakraborty et al., 2025).

What once used to be a reactive process is now turning into a proactive system that can adjust in real-time based on what's happening on the roads.

Figure 1. Intelligent Transport System

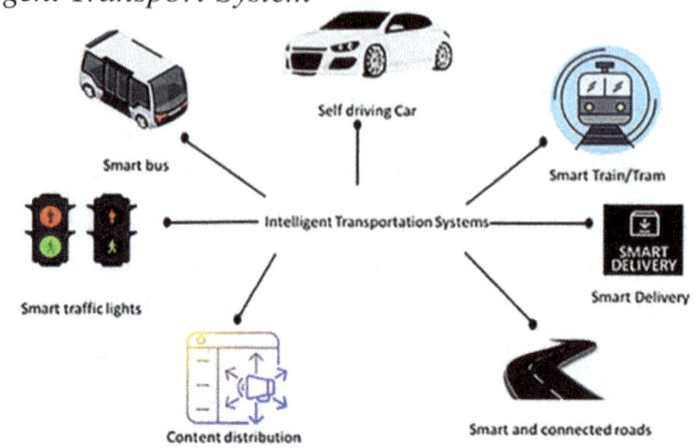

Figure 1 illustrates a few areas the ITS is integrated in, giving a simple understanding of it. The advanced technology and machine learning makes it possible for integrating its in such a way that it helps drivers as well as pedestrians and especially vulnerable users like senior and disabled citizens.

Defining ITS and Its Core Components

When we talk about ITS, we're talking about a collection of advanced technological tools that help monitor and manage transportation networks traffic in real time. This may include things like adaptive traffic lights that respond to congestion, GPS-based routing, vehicle-to-infrastructure communication, and dynamic signs that change based on traffic conditions. In rail networks, ITS technologies can include AI-driven scheduling, predictive maintenance, and crowd monitoring systems that help optimise travel experience and improve the safety across stations. By using real-time data, ITS can give cities the opportunity to act with immediate effect instead of waiting for problems to build up. This contributes to creating a pro-active system all around. The goal of ITS, whether for roads or rails, is to make traffic flow better, reduce congestions, cut emissions, and above all, make roads safer for everyone.

ITS and Inclusive Mobility

ITS has its fair share of advantageous features. But one that is significant enough to stand out is show it can help make cities more inclusive. Crosswalks can now have sensors that detect if someone's moving slower than the average person and automatically give them more time to cross. Intersections can use sounds and vibrations to guide visually impaired individuals. If you take it a step further and connect these systems with wearable tech or mobile apps, people can even get alerts and navigation guidance that fits their specific needs. Furthermore, AI's impact extends to enhancing the safety of non-motorized road users by improving detection systems for pedestrians and cyclists, which is important for integrating active mobility into comprehensive urban transportation planning (Papageorgiou et al., 2024).

ITS Alongside Machine Learning: A Synergistic Approach

With the expansion of transportation networks and the advancement of embedded and communication technologies, research on intelligent transportation systems has gained immense interest from the research community, especially utilizing the potential of machine learning techniques for increasing efficiency, safety, and travel experience. One of the most potential developments in transportation safety is the integration of machine learning with ITS. While ITS provides the real-time infrastructure and responsive systems, machine learning brings in the predictive power through its high-level analysis approach. In my own research project, for example, I trained models like Random Forest and CAT Boost on historical crash data to predict accident risks. These predictions can be fed directly into ITS frameworks like adaptive traffic lights, pedestrian alerts, or emergency routing systems to enhance their real-time decision-making (Azad et al., 2024).

The idea of combining machine learning and ITS goes far beyond automation; it's about using data not just to react to problems, but to prevent them altogether.

Machine Learning and Predictive Analytics in Traffic Safety

Introduction to Machine Learning in Crash Prediction

In recent years, machine learning (ML) has emerged as one of the most promising tools in the effort to enhance road safety. Traditional statistical methods, as useful as they are, struggle to face the complexity and non-linearity that underlie crash data. Machine learning, however, is specifically geared towards uncovering delicate patterns in large, high-dimensional datasets and hence well-suited for modeling the multifactorial causes of road accidents.

Figure 2. ML in ITS

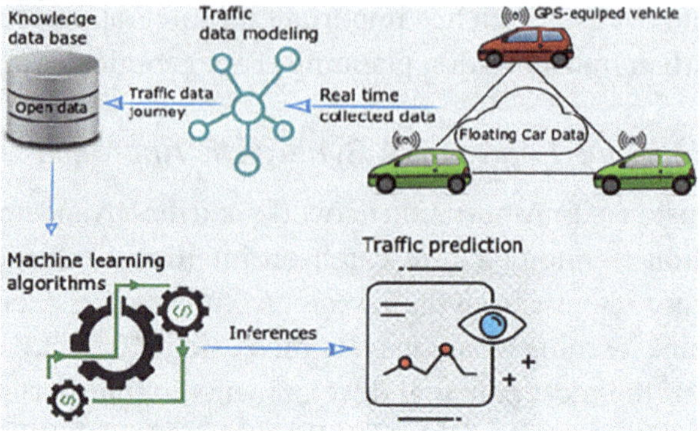

Figure 2 illustrates how machine learning collaborates with ITS to gather real-time data from GPS-equipped cars, deposit it in a central database, and subsequently utilise it to provide traffic forecasts. These predictions help the system take smarter actions like adjusting routes or triggering alerts which in turn helps in making the roads safer and more accessible, especially for senior citizens and people with disabilities who might struggle with mobility and are vulnerable to accidents.

Applications and Real-World Implementations

Various research demonstrated the value of such ML models. For example, researchers have used Random Forest to predict crash-prone locations by training models on geographic, infrastructural, and environmental features. Some have used XGBoost to analyse accident severity, integrating temporal and vehicle-related features. Others are also being constructed to run in real-time, offering predictive inputs into adaptive traffic signal control or pedestrian warning systems.

Challenges in ML-Based Crash Prediction

Depiste their popularity, there are some limitations to these models. Data quality is one of the larger limitations of crash prediction. Publicly accessible data might have missed, imbalanced, or poorly labeled records, which might have a negative impact on model performance. Moreover, most of these models are not interpretable, especially ensemble methods like XGBoost with consequences for interpretability and accountability in safety-critical applications.

Generalisability is another weakness. A model trained from urban crash data in one region of the world may not generalize to a different setting, e.g., rural settings or countries with varying traffic conventions. In addition, one of the biggest challenges faced by most machine learning algorithms lies in attempting to establish correlations between the many interdependent factors that influence traffic accident risk

(Banerjee et al., n.d.). While tools like Random Forest classifiers can help uncover these relationships, the mutual dependencies between variables further complicate model design and validation.

Considerations for Inclusivity

To solve these challenges, scholars have begun exploring hybrid alternatives that combine ML with domain expertise and simulation packages. Others are integrating real-time sensor data from Intelligent Transportation Systems (ITS) to increase the precision and responsiveness of forecasts. As technology advances, the focus is gradually being put on models that are not just accurate but also interpretable, flexible, and fair particularly when deployed to benefit vulnerable groups like elderly citizens and people with disabilities.

AI and ML Solutions Tailored for Senior and Disabled Mobility

Ensuring equitable access to safe mobility has become a core consideration in modern urban design. With growing recognition of the challenges faced by senior citizens and individuals with disabilities, artificial intelligence (AI) and machine learning (ML) are being increasingly applied to develop solutions tailored to their specific mobility needs. These technologies offer the potential to create smarter, more inclusive transportation environments by accounting for different levels of physical ability, sensory limitations, and mobility aids.

Adaptive Pedestrian Infrastructure

One of the most visible and impactful applications of AI for inclusive mobility is in pedestrian infrastructure. Adaptive traffic signals, powered by sensors and AI algorithms, can detect slower-moving individuals and automatically extend crossing times to ensure they can safely reach the other side. These systems often incorporate infrared sensors, pressure-sensitive mats, or LiDAR technology to assess movement patterns in real-time. For visually impaired users, audible pedestrian signals that adjust in intensity based on ambient noise levels are also being developed. Additionally, sensors play a critical role in Intelligent Transportation Systems (ITS). Vehicle detection, tracking, classification, and road safety analysis are commonly conducted using both intrusive and non-intrusive sensors, where intrusive sensors are embedded beneath the road surface and non-intrusive ones are mounted above it (Santhiya et al., 2021).

AI in Public Transportation Accessibility

Certain pilot schemes are exploring the use of computer vision to determine whether priority seats are available for use or if the boarding ramps are clear. Coupled with real-time location of vehicles, this data can be utilised by passengers to select the most convenient travel options on a demand basis. For example, BRIDJ, a smart bus service launched in Boston, uses real-time traffic big data and passenger inputs to optimise routes based on user demand, helping minimize fleet size while maximizing efficiency and accessibility (Ushakov et al., 2022). AI has also proven effective in tracking vehicles and improving service performance across transportation networks.

Ethical and Social Considerations in AI-driven Transportation

As AI becomes more integrated into transportation systems, it poses important ethical and social questions particularly when it comes to the safety and rights of vulnerable populations. While predictive modeling and real-time automation can enhance traffic safety, these benefits must be balanced with the need for privacy, fairness, transparency, and public trust. AI in traffic management can be instrumental in easing congestion and improving flow, but it must be implemented with responsible data handling and inclusive system design to ensure long-term societal acceptance and trust (Koch, n.d.).

Privacy and Surveillance

Most Artificial Intelligence systems rely on data collected through cameras, sensors, GPS, and mobile applications. While these inputs enable valuable safety functions, they also pose privacy concerns. Continuous data collection, especially in public spaces, can lead to unwanted surveillance and misuse of information. There are various regulatory reasons accessing demographics for debiasing is not always possible. "The General Data Protection Regulation (GDPR) in the European Union and the California Consumer Privacy Act (CCPA) in the U.S. protect consumer privacy rights regarding digital products and services, setting the groundwork for global best practices" (Erickson, 2025). The risk is especially high for individuals who may already face marginalization or limited access to legal resources, such as people with disabilities or elderly individuals.

To address these concerns, ethical design principles must prioritize anonymization, encryption, and clearly defined data retention policies. Consent mechanisms and opt-out options should be standard features, and regulations must be enforced to ensure data is not repurposed without user knowledge.

Fairness and Inclusivity

Another critical issue in AI-driven transportation is algorithmic fairness. Models trained on non-representative datasets can unintentionally reinforce bias, leading to unequal treatment of users. AI systems have the risk of exhibiting discriminatory behaviour. Without intervention, AI training algorithms may learn and perpetuate biases in data, leading to discriminatory predictions (Erickson, 2025). For example, a crash prediction model that fails to consider wheelchair users or older adults with different mobility patterns may result in infrastructure or safety measures that overlook their needs. To tackle this, developers can institute algorithmic fairness checks, perform bias audits on a scheduled basis, and apply interpretable AI approaches that enable tracking model decisions. Training datasets must also be grown and diversified so that underrepresented user segments are represented and prioritized equally in predictive precision.

Fairness starts with representative data collection that reflects wide physical, cognitive, and situational circumstances. Developers must also engage a variety of stakeholders, particularly from disability and aging advocacy organizations, in design and testing. Such participation may reduce the threat of exclusion and improve the reliability of AI solutions.

Trust and Public Acceptance

Adoption of AI in public systems depends largely on public trust. When users feel that AI is opaque, biased, or invasive, they are unlikely to embrace it even if the system promises real safety benefits. Transparency in algorithmic decision-making, clear communication of risks and benefits, and accessible explanations for system behaviour are all crucial for trust-building with citizens.

Governments and transit authorities must lead with transparency, publishing impact assessments and opening systems up to third-party audits where relevant. Educational and awareness campaigns can also help users better understand the purpose and limits of AI systems, reducing resistance and promoting informed participation.

FOCUS OF THE ARTICLE

Why Senior and Disabled Citizens are at the Center of this Research

The focus of this chapter is to understand how machine learning (ML) could best assist complementing the comprehensive band of artificial intelligence (AI) solutions aimed at providing a safer, more inclusive mode of transport particularly through road networks for senior citizens and individuals with disabilities. These groups often face significant mobility challenges due to age-related physical limitations, sensory impairments, or long-term disabilities. Yet, despite being among the most vulnerable road users, their specific needs are frequently overlooked in the design and deployment of modern transportation systems.

Machine Learning as the First Step to Safer Mobility

Machine Learning can be the base layer upon which danger detection is initiated. Thus, comprehending how ML algorithms actively identify threats and how they are interpreted into actionable predictions starts with the procurement of multi-dimensional data: traffic volume, environmental conditions, pedestrian activity, environmental indicators, and live feed from smart sensors. Algorithms such as CAT boost, random forest, etc., are explored to determine if they can handle such data and provide prompt judgments of the probability of crashes.

SOLUTIONS AND RECOMMENDATIONS

This chapter identifies key pathways through which machine learning (ML) can be harnessed to address safety inequities in urban transportation, particularly for senior citizens and individuals with disabilities. While previous sections have outlined the conceptual foundations and ethical imperatives of inclusive design, this section presents a set of actionable solutions and practical recommendations to help researchers, policymakers, and urban planners bridge the gap between theory and implementation.

Integrate ML Risk Predictions into ITS

Machine learning models have shown significant potential in forecasting crash-prone zones, high-risk time windows, and environmental triggers associated with road accidents. These models must be deeply embedded into Intelligent Transportation Systems (ITS) to create a truly adaptive urban mobility environment. When integrated correctly, predictive outputs can automate adjustments in traffic signal behaviour, pedestrian alerts, and vehicle routing in real time.

Potential Algorithms for Crash Prediction in ITS

Several AI algorithms provide foundational methods for incorporating machine learning into traffic risk prediction, specifically aiming to enhance safety for senior citizens and disabled individuals. Utilizing these algorithms involves systematically analyzing data to identify vulnerable locations and effectively addressing associated risks, ultimately benefiting ITS design and application.

CatBoost, which stands for Categorical Boosting, is a robust gradient boosting algorithm with outstanding support for categorical variables. Unlike most other standard models that need heavy preprocessing, e.g., one-hot encoding CatBoost naturally deals with categorical features while retaining information and lowering the chances of overfitting. This makes it particularly effective in road accident prediction tasks where variables such as road type, light conditions, or time of day are categorical in nature. It is particularly well-suited for large-scale datasets with many independent features. Unlike other gradient boosting algorithms, CatBoost is specially designed to handle both categorical and numerical features seamlessly without requiring manual feature encoding (GeeksforGeeks, 2025). Furthermore, CatBoost is also very accurate and resistant to imbalanced datasets, which is a regular problem in traffic safety analysis. Nevertheless, its added sophistication and longer training time compared to more basic models can be a factor when working in resource-scarce applications.

Random Forest, an ensemble learning decision tree algorithm, has shown superior performance in the majority of crash prediction studies. It achieves this through training many decision trees and giving the mode of classes for classification problems. Random Forest performs best in handling missing values, huge sets of features, and overfitting due to its intrinsic cross-validation. It also provides some insight into feature importance, so it is easier to know which such features as light conditions or road surface status are most crucial in producing crashes.

XGBoost (Extreme Gradient Boosting), another ensemble method, builds upon the principles of gradient boosting and offers improved accuracy, efficiency, and scalability. It has been especially effective in competitions and real-world applications that involve imbalanced datasets such as those where crashes are rare events compared to normal traffic flow. In the context of crash prediction, XGBoost models have been trained on national and regional traffic datasets to predict both the likelihood and severity of incidents.

Translating ML Predictions into Actionable ITS Strategies

Successfully integrating ML crash predictions into ITS requires clear and effective translation from predictive analytics to actionable strategies. ML models identify high-risk zones and scenarios through comprehensive data analysis, but the practical impact of these predictions relies on timely, targeted, and context-sensitive implementation within ITS.

Once ML algorithms pinpoint critical risk areas, ITS can automatically adjust traffic signals, pedestrian crosswalk timings, and variable message signs to mitigate these identified risks. For example, if ML predictions indicate increased crash risk during evening peak hours due to reduced visibility and higher pedestrian density, ITS could proactively extend pedestrian crossing durations, intensify street lighting, or provide automated visual and auditory alerts to both pedestrians and drivers approaching the intersection.

Moreover, real-time ML predictions can dynamically inform emergency services, triggering preemptive deployments or heightened readiness near identified high-risk locations. ITS integrated with ML can continuously update routing recommendations for public transportation, directing vehicles away from identified high-risk zones, particularly during adverse conditions or peak vulnerability periods.

For these integrations to be effective, municipalities and transportation agencies must ensure seamless data interoperability between ML prediction models and ITS infrastructure. Establishing standardized communication protocols, continuous data exchanges, and real-time feedback loops will be essential. This integration creates a proactive safety environment, significantly enhancing mobility security and comfort for senior citizens and individuals with disabilities.

Flowchart of different communications

1. ML Engine → ITS → Police

As machine learning algorithms process real-time traffic and accident data, their predictions like mapped high-risk zones or real-time probabilities of accidents are integrated to the Intelligent Transportation System (ITS). The ITS uses this information to control traffic signals and give public warnings. Meanwhile, it can forward important alerts to police patrols or emergency services, initiating instant deployment or traffic control in the targeted areas.

Figure 3. ML to Police

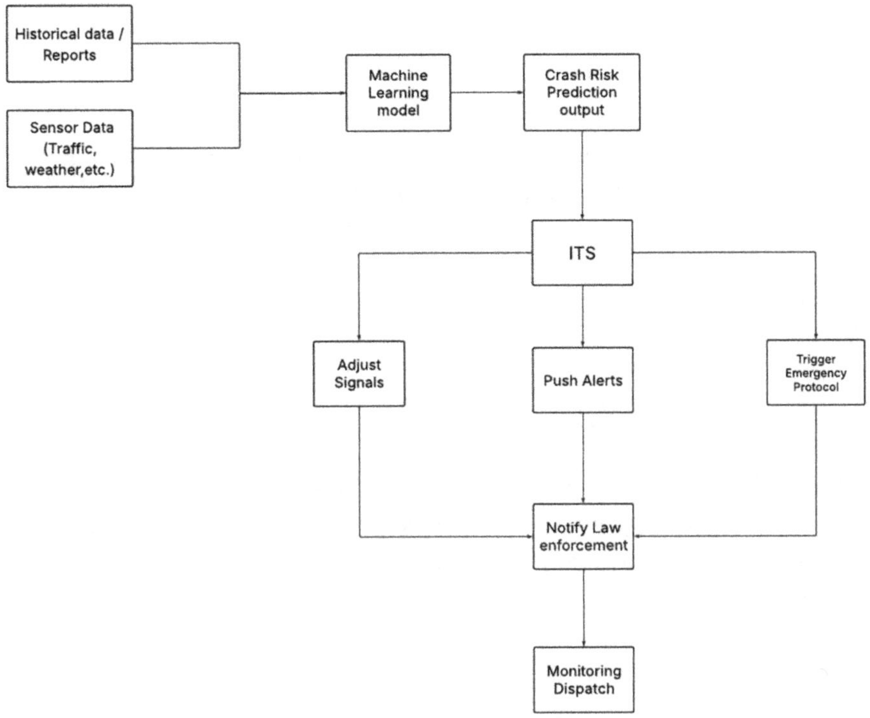

This flowchart in Figure 3. illustrates how ML-based real-time crash risk predictions are channeled through ITS for initiating instant on-ground action. Whether it's adjusting signal timings, sending alerts, or alerting law enforcement, this ML-to-Police pipeline assists in converting data into direct real-time protection particularly in the case of areas that have vulnerable road users.

2. ML Engine ITS Government

Insights produced by ML models such as hot spot crash locations, risk trends over time, and patterns with vulnerable users are not only utilised for real-time ITS responses but also aggregated into formal reports. These are sent to city or state-level governments to guide infrastructure planning, policy updates, and investment strategies, fostering long-term transport accessibility and safety enhancements.

Figure 4. ML to Government

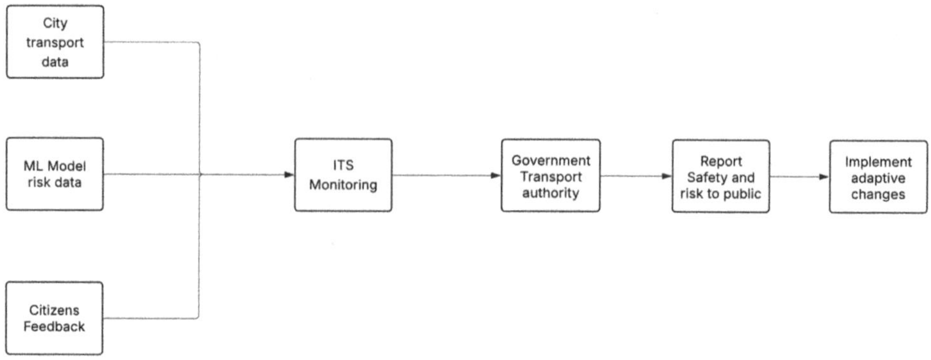

Figure 4 shows how risk insights from ML models, transport data, and user feedback flow via ITS to government bodies. These insights inform public reports, shape policies, and initiate changes such as safer infrastructure or enhanced access for vulnerable users.

3. Community ITS/ML Feedback

Citizens such as elderly and disabled users engage more with ITS using mobile applications or wearable technologies, providing feedback on street accessibility, safety concerns, or service needs. Their qualitative feedback is cycled back into the ML system to retrain and optimise prediction accuracy, developing a feedback loop where community experience informs wiser and more responsive transportation systems. Over time, this ongoing cycle assists the system in learning patterns associated with weak points or underreported incidents that may not be detected by traditional sensors alone. Feedback capabilities can come in the form of voice response, one-tap reporting, or visual indicators for users with differing capabilities. As this information builds up, traffic planners and local governments can see developing trends in accessibility gaps and allocate adaptive interventions in response that helps in building a city that is proactively transforming.

Figure 5. Public to ML

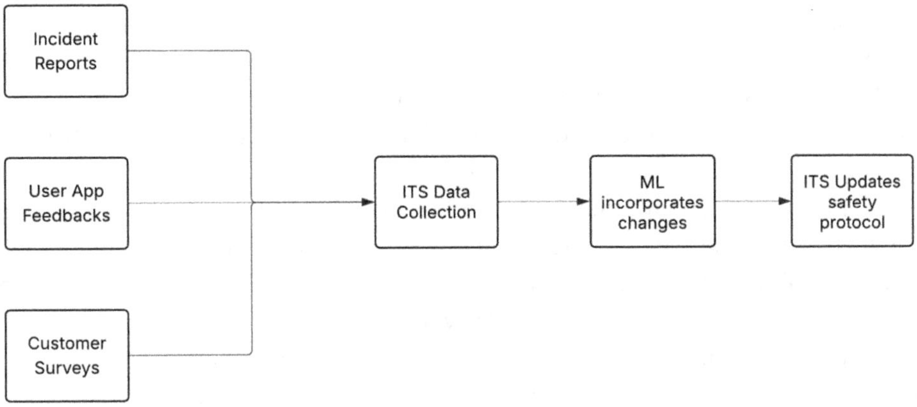

Figure 5 emphasizes on public input such as incident reports, app feedback, or surveys that gets picked up by the ITS. From there, it fuels the ML system, which adjusts safety protocol accordingly. It is a straightforward loop that keeps the system learning and responsive, particularly around things that impact the elderly and disabled, which sensors may otherwise overlook.

Community Feedback and Context-Aware Adaptation

While machine learning and ITS systems often rely on technical infrastructure and sensor data, a crucial non-technical dimension involves input directly from the communities they aim to protect particularly senior citizens and individuals with disabilities. Gathering feedback from these groups through surveys, community workshops, digital reporting tools, and participatory planning can guide smarter deployment of AI-enhanced traffic safety measures.

AI models can be improved not just by feeding in raw sensor data, but by integrating feedback that reflects lived experiences such as unsafe intersections, poorly lit sidewalks, or inaccessible crossings. Digital platforms can incorporate voice commands, large-text displays, or simplified input interfaces, allowing even those with sensory or mobility impairments to provide real-time reports.

Moreover, AI models can use this qualitative input to identify zones with higher concentrations of vulnerable users. When such zones are detected either from survey data or community behaviour patterns the system can proactively exaggerate safety responses: extending crossing times, adding audible cues, or even increasing law enforcement presence during peak hours.

Funding and Incentive Models for Inclusive ITS Adoption

Financing the integration of inclusive AI systems in transport infrastructure often poses a major barrier for municipalities. To overcome this, targeted funding models and incentives are necessary. Governments and international institutions should provide grants and subsidies to local agencies adopting ITS that prioritize accessibility and safety for vulnerable users.

Funding can be tied to measurable indicators of inclusion, for example, cities could receive incremental funding based on the deployment of adaptive crosswalks, installation of AI-based safety alerts in high-risk areas, or integration of real-time assistive navigation systems for the elderly and disabled.

Public-private partnerships should also be encouraged, especially in pilot-stage deployments. Companies that develop ML-based transport technologies could be offered tax benefits or recognition through smart city innovation awards when they implement or co-develop systems designed inclusively.

Long-Term Scalability and Maintenance of AI Systems

The success of AI in transport systems relies not just on launch, but on long-term scalability and adaptability. Urban environments evolve, and so must the ML models that monitor them. Systems should be regularly updated based on new data, changing demographics, emerging safety threats, and technological advances.

Cities should establish digital mobility councils or AI-infrastructure task forces responsible for overseeing continuous monitoring and maintenance of these systems. These teams can analyse usage trends, audit AI performance, and recommend updates that ensure models remain responsive to local mobility challenges.

Involving community stakeholders, such as aging citizen groups or disability coalitions, in these long-term reviews will also help ensure the AI remains grounded in real-world needs.

Collaboration Between Public and Private Sectors

The future of inclusive AI-driven transport systems depends on strong collaboration between governments, the tech industry, academia, and advocacy organizations. No single entity can solve urban mobility challenges alone.

Governments must create open regulatory environments that allow private firms to test innovative ideas while adhering to ethical and accessibility standards. Joint innovation labs between public transport authorities and AI firms can accelerate experimentation, reduce costs, and ensure that technology is developed with public benefit in mind.

Academic institutions and civil society groups should be brought in early to evaluate social impacts and improve public trust. Co-development models that blend technical expertise with lived experience will be key to designing truly inclusive, adaptable, and human-centered smart mobility ecosystems. The following section explains the methodology used in a case study to showcase how Machine Learning can be applied to improve traffic accident prediction.

Case Study: Applying ML in Transportation

Proposed Methodology

Figure 6. Proposed Research Methodology for the Case study implementation

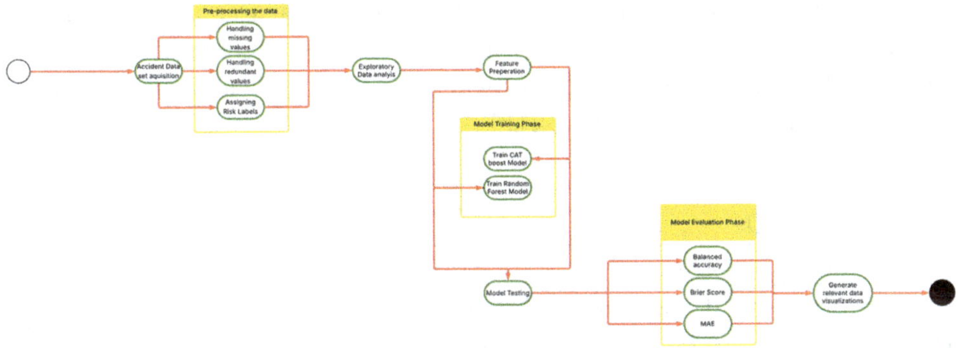

The case study methodology follows a structured machine learning workflow consisting of data acquisition, preprocessing, model training, evaluation, and result interpretation. The process is illustrated in Figure 6, outlining the major phases from raw dataset ingestion to final analysis and visualisation.

Initially, the dataset was preprocessed by dealing with missing and duplicate values to make it consistent and ready for modeling. The levels of accident risks were then attributed through K-Means clustering, grouping accidents as low, medium, and high risk. Because the data were imbalanced with a predominance of low-risk cases, random undersampling was used to balance the classes to facilitate unbiased learning. Exploratory Data Analysis (EDA) was performed to analyse patterns and check feature relevance. Categorical values were encoded in feature preparation prior to transitioning to model training.

Two models were used. CatBoost for overall accident forecasting because of its categorical feature efficiency, and Random Forest for street-level predictions because of its capability to manage difficult interactions. Both were trained on an 80:20 division.

Model performance was checked with Balanced Accuracy, Brier Score, and MAE, followed by visual results to understand trends and model behaviour.

Dataset Description

Accurate and reliable crash risk prediction relies significantly on the quality and comprehensiveness of the dataset used for model training. The dataset used in this study was obtained from Data.gov, a licensed and openly accessible source that allows unrestricted modifications and usage for study and research purposes. It includes details on vehicle/vehicle, vehicle/bicy- cle, and vehicle/pedestrian crashes in Tempe (Data.gov, nd). The dataset specifically focuses on attributes particularly processed through feature selection making it a suitable foundation for predicting crash risks in varying scenarios. This section provides a structured overview of the dataset's key attributes and modifications performed to enhance its predictive capability. The dataset consists of approximately 30,000 instances and includes a variety of features, described in the Table 1.

Table 1. Dataset Description

Attribute Name	Description
Street Name	Identifies the specific location where the crash occurred.
Weather Condition	Describes the environmental conditions such as clear, rainy, or foggy at the time of the crash.
Road Surface Condition	Indicates whether the road was dry, wet, or icy, etc.
Light Condition	Mentions the visibility conditions such as daylight, night- time, or streetlights.
Travel Direction	Represents the direction of the vehicle's movement.
Risk Attribute (Added column)	Categorizes the accident risk as low (0), medium (1), or high (2) based on predefined rules.

Exploratory Data Analysis

Understanding the dataset before training a model is crucial so as to make sure the model learns a series of meaningful patterns instead of the noise. EDA helps break down the structure of the data, revealing trends, relationships between features, themes and potential issues like missing values or imbalances. It plays a vital role in deciding what preprocessing steps needs to be taken in order to clean the dataset making it ready to be presented to the model. For this project particularly, EDA was carried out in a variety of types to examine how accident risks are distributed and how different factors like weather conditions, road surface states, and travel directions affect crash risk. This involved using histograms, correlation heatmaps and other visualisation methods which may be shown later on to understand feature relationships and highlight any imbalances in the dataset.

To better understand the dataset after balancing and assigning risk categories, data visualisation was used to illustrate how the risk levels are distributed post-processing. Imblearn library was imported for the use of its tools to balance the data set via random under sampling to ensure all the risk categories are equally represented. The visualisation below shows a bar graph representing the accident risk categories after applying random undersampling, ensuring that each risk level (low, medium, and high) is equally represented. The matplotlib is a visualisation library generally used to create and show various plots in the form of graphs.

Figure 7. Bar Graph Visualisation

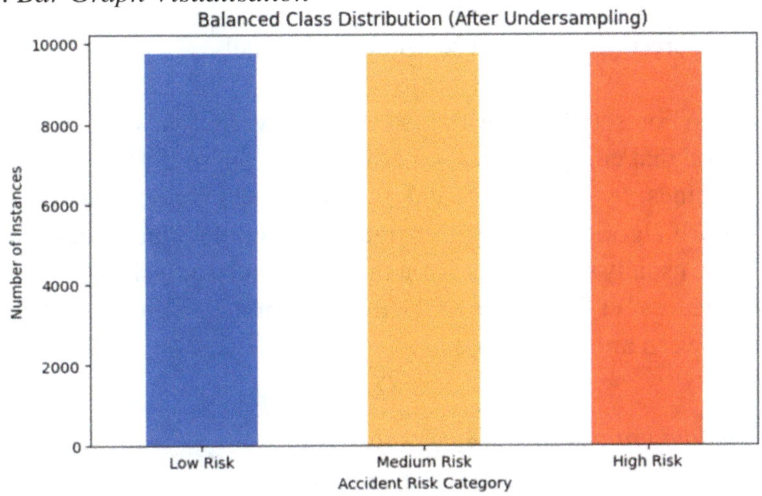

Machine Learning Techniques

Previous research has predominantly approached road accident prediction as a classification problem. These studies focus on predicting whether or not a traffic accident will occur without delving into the complex relationships between the factors contributing to these accidents. However, road accidents are influenced by various intertwined factors, such as weather, road conditions, and driver behaviour, which require more sophisticated modeling approaches. In this study, three machine learning models will be implemented to predict the likelihood of road accidents.

CATBoost (General Prediction Model)

CatBoost is a gradient boosting algorithm developed by Yandex that efficiently handles cat- egorical features without requiring manual encoding methods like one-hot encoding. It is particularly effective for binary classification tasks, such as predicting road traffic accidents, as it captures complex feature interactions while maintaining model interpretability. Additionally, numerical features can be normalized to further enhance performance (Alsulamy, 2024). Compared to traditional models like logistic regression, CatBoost has demonstrated greater accuracy and robustness across various fields, including traffic safety (Prokhorenkova et al., 2018). Its built-in ability to process categorical data directly reduces preprocessing time, making it computationally efficient. In this study, CatBoost serves as the baseline model to evaluate potential improvements offered by more advanced techniques such as Random Forest.

Random Forest (Street Specific Prediction Model)

The Random Forest (RF) algorithm, developed by Breiman (2001), is a machine learning method that enjoys great popularity in data science. This can be justified, among other things, by its fundamental building block, the decision tree. The operation of the RF algorithm is best illustrated by a single binary decision tree. By convention, one usually starts at the top at the "root" and works through the branches to one of the "leaves" at the bottom of the tree. The branches are called "nodes" and the lines in between are called "branches" (Schlenger, 2024).

Figure 8. Random Forest

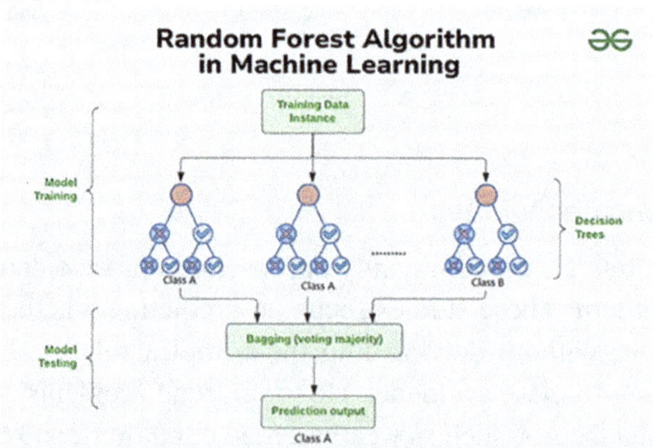

(GeeksforGeeks, 2024)

Evaluation Metrics

In order to compare the predictive accuracy of the machine learning models employed in this research, three most important metrics were used: Brier Score, Mean Absolute Error (MAE), and Balanced Accuracy. These metrics were used because they can measure various aspects of reliability in a model, ranging from probability calibration to numerical error of prediction to classification balance. The metrics, their purpose, and their formula for calculation are described below in Table 2.

Table 2. Evaluation Metrics

Metric	Description	Formula
Brier Score	Measures the accuracy of probabilistic predictions by computing the mean squared difference between predicted probabilities and actual outcomes. Lower values indicate better calibration.	$MAE = \frac{1}{n}\sum_{i=1}^{N}(f_i - o_i)^2$
Mean Absolute Error (MAE)	Calculates the average magnitude of prediction errors, giving a direct sense of how close predicted values are to actual outcomes.	$MAE = \frac{1}{n}\sum_{i=1}^{n}\lvert y_i - \hat{y}i \rvert$
Balanced Accuracy	Evaluates model performance across imbalanced datasets by averaging sensitivity and specificity. Helps ensure fair classification across all classes.	Balanced Accuracy= $\frac{1}{2}$ (Sensitivity+Specificity)

Experimental Setup

Building a predictive solution for a socially impactful problem like traffic crash risk required careful model selection. With the categorical nature and intensity of the dataset, it was enough to settle with two machine learning models that were capable of working with structured data effectively and giving useful outputs: CatBoost and Random Forest.

CatBoost was employed for overall accident risk forecasting based on conditions such as weather, road type, light conditions, and travel direction. Its native handling of categorical data without heavy preprocessing made it a perfect fit for this task and made the workflow more efficient.

Random Forest was used in street-specific prediction, where the names of streets were also part of the input feature. Known for its ability to detect localized patterns and perform well with structured, encoded data, Random Forest was a suitable choice for identifying accident-prone locations. There was a requirement of one-hot encoding in this particular variation.

CAT Boost Implementation

CatBoost was applied for overall accident risk prediction with emphasis on fundamental features like LightCondition, Weather, SurfaceCondition, and TravelDirection_One. CatBoost was selected due to its capability to naturally process categorical variables, minimizing preprocessing needs. As Kolli (2024) points out, CatBoost's ordered boosting and feature combination handling automatically make it very well qualified for structured classification tasks.

Some of the most important implementation steps involved:

Feature Selection:

Training was carried out on chosen categorical features, not including StreetName in order to preserve generalization.

Model Configuration: CatBoostClassifier was initialized with 100 iterations, a learning rate of 0.01, and a depth of 2.

Observations: CatBoost achieved an accuracy of approximately 0.97, suggesting strong learning, though further validation was required to rule out overfitting.

Deployment: The trained model was saved using Joblib for reuse.

Random Forest Implementation

In addition to general crash prediction, this study also explored street-specific risk assessment using a Random Forest model. This model incorporated all the above features plus StreetName so that it could pick up on local patterns and differences between various urban areas.

Random Forest was used because it can cope with high-dimensional input following encoding. It is robust to finding non-linear relationships and feature interactions. Its ensemble voting process that minimizes overfitting risk through aggregating predictions across many decision trees.

The implementation involved the following:

Score of 0.1508 with per-class scores of 0.1169 for Low risk, 0.1671 for Medium risk, and 0.1683 for High risk. These values demonstrate good calibration in the Low-Risk category with a slightly lower confidence agreement in Medium and High. Overall, the model generated well-calibrated probability estimates for One-hot encoding categorical variables: StreetName, LightCondition, Weather, SurfaceCondition, and TravelDirection_One.

Random Forest provided good performance, especially in classifying accident-risk streets according to environmental and directional criteria. The model's ability to learn from locality-encoded data enabled it to generate detailed, location-specific risk predictions, offering practical value for targeted urban traffic planning.

Evaluation results

Brier Score

The Brier Score metric was utilised to measure the calibration of probabilistic predictions for both CatBoost and Random Forest models. For CatBoost, the outcomes indicated near-perfect alignment between predicted probabilities and the true outcomes. Although this indicates great model confidence, this type of result could indicate overconfidence also known as overfitting, especially when dealing with smaller or less complex datasets. But additional testing and cross-validation also affirmed that the model was real performance, due to the sophisticated model design and the dataset structure. In comparison, the Random Forest model had a Brier risk-based decision-making.

Mean Absolute Error (MAE)

MAE was used to measure the average difference between predicted and actual risk values. CatBoost achieved a remarkably low MAE of 0.0229, highlighting its ability to generate precise predictions with minimal error. This supports the model's appropriateness for general accident risk categorization.

The Random Forest model also demonstrated strong performance with an MAE of 0.0446, indicating that its predictions remained closely aligned with actual accident risk labels. The two models performed consistently well in reducing the prediction error, with CatBoost possessing a minor advantage in accuracy.

Balanced Accuracy

To address the imbalanced nature of the dataset, Balanced Accuracy was computed for the Random Forest model. The score obtained of 0.9549 shows strong performance in all the accident risk classes, validating that the model performed fairly and without bias in predicting low, medium, and high-risk results. This measure ensured that Random Forest did not overfit the majority class and coped well with the class imbalance.

Data Visualisation and Comparisons

Visual analysis served as an essential step in connecting model predictions to real-world patterns within the dataset. By representing accident trends graphically, the visualisations provided clearer insights into high-risk areas and contributing factors, allowing for a more intuitive understanding of where and why accidents are most likely to occur. Visualisation was done to identify trends and patterns in the dataset that validate model predictions. One of the key visualisations involved the identification of the top five accident streets according to reported crash frequency. A horizontal bar graph indicated that Baseline Rd, Rural Rd, University Dr, Broadway Rd, and McClintock Dr ranked as having the most reported incidents.

Figure 9. Horizontal Bar Graph Visualisation

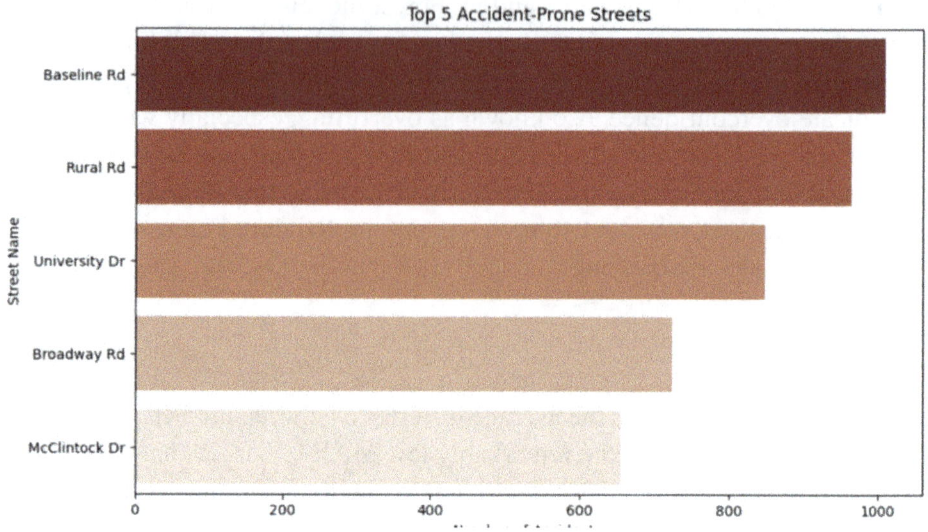

These observations draw attention to particular road sections that might need more scrutiny or specific safety measures. Such visualisations become highly important in linking model outputs with actual accident hotspots on the ground, allowing for more location-based and better-informed traffic management measures.

Conclusion of ML implementation

The implementation commenced with exploration of main accident-causing factors and went on to analyse and streamline a proper dataset for training. Feature selection and data preprocessing methods such as normalization and random undersampling were applied systematically to cleanse and prepare the data. The two models were then trained, tested, and validated using a stratified data split of 80:20, all with excellent scores in accuracy, Brier Score, MAE, and Balanced Accuracy. The implementation confirmed the reliability of the models and their applicability in real-world situations for urban planning and traffic safety measures.

This implementation not only proves the possibility of machine learning for transportation safety but also establishes the groundwork for further research to bring predictive AI and smart city infrastructure together. From data exploration to algorithm design and testing, the project was closely tied to its objectives in order to create a data informed framework that could be used to make real-time, risk-based traffic decisions.

FUTURE RESEARCH AND DIRECTIONS

Lack of Inclusive Dataset Development

Many existing datasets used for traffic prediction and urban mobility studies lack sufficient representation of vulnerable groups, especially senior citizens and people with disabilities. Future research should focus on developing inclusive datasets that capture a broader range of mobility behaviours, accessibility barriers, and real-world pedestrian conditions.

Crowdsourced mobility data, anonymised public transit usage records, and observational studies can be combined to generate datasets reflective of the daily challenges faced by vulnerable road users. Researchers should also explore data augmentation techniques and synthetic data generation to fill representation gaps while maintaining ethical standards and user privacy.

Multi-Modal Integration and Real-Time Adaptation

Studies should investigate how ML models can shift from purely predictive to fully adaptive responding to factors like sudden weather changes, fluctuating pedestrian densities, or emergency events. This level of responsiveness is particularly vital in ensuring timely interventions for vulnerable groups.

Ethical AI Governance and Policy Integration

As AI becomes more central to public infrastructure, particularly in mobility systems that affect people's safety and daily routines, the importance of strong ethical governance becomes increasingly urgent. Research must prioritise the development of frameworks that address the complex ethical challenges associated with ML applications in Intelligent Transportation Systems (ITS). These include algorithmic bias, data privacy violations, disproportionate surveillance, lack of transparency, and limited accountability for decisions made by autonomous systems.

Future studies should explore legal standards and ethical oversight mechanisms that go beyond compliance checklists. This includes creating AI impact assessment protocols, citizen review boards, and open auditing platforms that allow for third-party evaluation of mobility algorithms. It also calls for more research into explainability and interpretability of AI systems so that users especially those from disadvantaged groups can understand how and why decisions are made.

Municipal governments and national transport agencies must also develop policy tools that enable redress when systems fail and create a clear process for public feedback and accountability. Certification schemes, transparency labels, and ongoing ethical reviews should become standard components of AI deployments in public transport environments. As intelligent systems grow in influence, the urgency for embedding ethical responsibility in their governance grows equally pressing.

Addressing Model Generalizability and Transferability

One key challenge in applying machine learning to intelligent transportation systems is the generalizability of predictive models across different urban environments. A model trained on crash data from one region may underperform in another city due to differences in infrastructure, cultural behaviour, climate, and demographics. This limits the scalability and real-world utility of even the most advanced algorithms.

Future research must investigate strategies to enhance the adaptability and transferability of ML models. This could include the use of domain adaptation techniques, federated learning approaches that preserve local contextual data, or modular model architectures that can be customized regionally without complete retraining. Additionally, researchers should prioritize testing their models across a variety of contexts from highly urbanized metros to smaller towns and suburban environments to ensure broader applicability.

Understanding where and why certain models fail to generalize will also be essential in developing guidelines for future deployments. By making robustness and contextual flexibility central design priorities, researchers can ensure AI-driven transport safety solutions that are more effective and reliable regardless of geographic or demographic variation.

Research Gaps and Opportunities for Innovation

While the use of AI in transportation is advancing rapidly, numerous research gaps remain particularly in creating systems that serve all members of society equally. These gaps offer valuable opportunities for academic and policy-driven innovation.

Limitations in Datasets and Evaluation

A recurring issue in AI-based mobility research is the lack of high-quality, inclusive datasets. Most available datasets are region-specific, lack diversity in demographic representation, and often exclude contextual data that reflects the unique needs of senior or disabled users.

Underrepresentation in System Design

Despite growing awareness, people with disabilities and older adults remain underrepresented in the design, testing, and deployment phases of AI-driven transport systems. This gap not only affects system effectiveness but also deepens existing inequities in urban mobility.

Future research should prioritize co-design approaches that involve these users directly, ensuring their lived experiences shape the development of AI tools. This shift from user-centered to user-led design can significantly enhance inclusivity.

CONCLUSION

As urban environments become increasingly complex, the need for intelligent, adaptable, and inclusive transportation systems has never been greater. This chapter has examined how the integration of machine learning (ML) and AI-powered Intelligent Transportation Systems (ITS) can address critical challenges in mobility particularly for vulnerable road users such as senior citizens and individuals with disabilities. By leveraging data and automation, cities can build safer, more responsive, and more equitable transportation infrastructures. This chapter has been motivated by a need to enhance public safety through proactive, AI-enabled crash prediction models to inform interventions in real-time. The ultimate goal is to reduce accidents as well as improve safety of mobility among elderly citizens and the disabled.

REFERENCES

Abul Kalam Azad, T., Atkison, T., & Shahen Shah, A. F. M. 2024. A Review on Machine Learning in Intelligent Transportation Systems Applications. The Open Transportation Journal. [online] Available at: https://benthamopen.com/ABSTRACT/TOTJ-18-1

S. Alsulamy. 2024. Predicting construction delay risks in Saudi Arabian projects: A comparative analysis of CatBoost, XGBoost, and LGBM. Automation in Construction 152 (2024), 105072. https://doi.org/. autcon.2024.105072.DOI: 10.1016/j

Banerjee, K., Bali, V., Sharma, A., Aggarwal, D., Yadav, A. and Shukla, A., n.d. Traffic Accident Risk Prediction Using Machine Learning. IEEE.

Batrakova, L., & Gredasova, V. (2016). Road Safety and Traffic Psychology. *Procedia Engineering*, *150*, 1876–1881.

Chakraborty, M., Saha, S. and Sharmin, S., 2025. Quality-aware bus-driver scheduling for intelligent transportation system. Elsevier Transportation Research Part C: Emerging Technologies, [online] Available at: https://doi.org/DOI: 10.1016/j.trc.2024.104398

Department of Transport. (2019). *Road Traffic Accident Reporting Guide*. Department for Transport.

Elkateb, S., Métwalli, A., Shendy, A., & Abu-Elanien, A. E. B. (2024). *Machine learning and IoT–based predictive maintenance approach for industrial applications*. Alexandria University, Arab Academy for Science, Technology and Maritime Transport. DOI: 10.1016/j.aej.2023.12.065

Erickson, G. 2025. Uncovering Responsible AI's Biggest Challenge: Privacy and Fairness. [online] Available at: https://www.nimblegravity.com/blog/responsible-ai-privacy-fairness

GeeksforGeeks. 2025. CatBoost in Machine Learning. [online] Available at: https://www.geeksforgeeks.org/catboost-ml/

Infrastructure Australia. 2018. Future Cities: Planning for our growing population. [online] Available at: https://www.infrastructureaustralia.gov.au/

Koch, R. n.d. How AI in Traffic Management is Helping to Ease Traffic Congestion. [online] Available at: https://www.iotforall.com/how-ai-in-traffic-management-easing-congestion

Li, Y., Chen, M., Tang, Y., & Wu, Z. (2024). Impact of Road Environment and Driver Behaviour on Injury Severity. *Accident; Analysis and Prevention, 188*, 107–118.

Ministry of Transport (New Zealand). 2020. The Social Cost of Road Crashes and Injuries. [online] Available at: https://www.transport.govt.nz

National Safety Council. n.d. Night Driving Safety Facts. [online] Available at: https://www.nsc.org

Papageorgiou, G., Tsappi, E., & Wang, T. (2024). *Smart Urban Systems Planning for Active Mobility and Sustainability*. Elsevier Cities. [online], DOI: 10.1016/j.ifacol.2024.07.350

Prokhorenkova, L., Gusev, G., Vorobev, A., Dorogush, A. V., & Gulin, A. 2018. CatBoost: Unbiased Boosting with CategoricalFeatures.InAdvancesinNeuralInformationProcessingSystems(NeurIPS). https://arxiv.org/abs/ 1810.11363

Santhiya, R. and GeethaPriya, C., 2021. Machine Learning Techniques for Intelligent Transportation Systems—An Overview. 2021 12th International Conference on Computing Communication and Networking Technologies (ICCCNT), pp.1–7. DOI: DOI: 10.1109/ICCCNT51525.2021.9579970

Schlenger, J. 2024. Random Forest. 201–207. https://link.springer.com/chapter/ 10.1007/978-3-662-68313-2_24 C.M.C.Silva.2024.ADataScientist'sGuidetoBalancedAccuracy. https://blog.trainindata.com/a-data-scientists- guide-to-balanced-accuracy/

Suk, S., & Walter, A. (2018). Nighttime Visibility and Roadway Safety: A Literature Review. *Journal of Safety Research, 67*, 1–7.

Ushakov, D., Dudukalov, E., Shmatko, L., & Shatila, K. (2022). *Artificial Intelligence as a Factor of Public Transportation System Development*. Elsevier. [online], DOI: 10.1016/j.trpro.2022.06.276

Wang, S., Xiao, J., Liu, Y., Zhang, S., & Yan, G. (2025). *Real-time detection of intelligent transportation system based on 3D point cloud*. Elsevier Expert Systems with Applications. [online], DOI: 10.1016/j.inffus.2025.103213

World Health Organization. 2017. Managing Speed. [online] Available at: https://www.who.int/publications-detail/9789241511712

World Health Organization. 2021. Global Status Report on Road Safety. [online] Available at: https://www.who.int/publications/i/item/9789241565685

Yıldırım, M. Ş., Cavlak, M., Taştekin, B., Akçan, R., Tümer, A. R., & Balseven-Odabaşi, A. (2021). Road traffic injury-related disabilities in geriatric population. *Journal of Clinical Gerontology & Geriatrics*.

Zou, B., Li, J., He, S., & Zhang, Y. 2023. Weather Influence on Road Safety: A Data-Driven Analysis. Transportation Research Interdisciplinary Perspectives, 16, 100617. Data.gov. n.d. 1.08 Crash Data Report (Detail). https://catalog.data.gov/dataset/1-08-crash-data-report-detail- 498c3.

KEY TERMS AND DEFINITIONS

Artificial Intelligence (AI): A wide range of technology where machines stimulate human thinking across various different problems to find solutions.

Machine Learning (ML): A branch of AI where models are trained on data by analyzing and learning on patterns to make better predictions or do better actions without direct reprogramming.

Intelligent Transport System (ITS): Artificial Intelligence driven systems that support and optimise transport experience. Make real time decision using data, From Traffic signals to smart vehicles.

Exploratory Data Analysis (EDA): A data analysis process whereby you investigate more into the dataset characteristics to gain a deeper understanding of it.

Digital Mobility Council: A group that guides and monitors AI use in transport, ensuring it's ethical, efficient, and benefits society.

Inclusive ITS: Transport tech that uses AI to make systems fair and usable for everyone, including people with disabilities or other limitations.

CAT Boost: An open-source gradient boosting library that is inherently good with categorical data.

Random Forest: A ML model that builds multiple decision trees, then combines their predictions for better accuracy and stability.

LIDAR (light detection and ranging): LiDAR is a sensing technology that uses laser pulses to measure distances to objects. It generates precise 3D maps or point clouds of environments.

Data visualization: Visualisations of different forms based on various data analysis.

Public-Private Partnerships: Collabs between governments and tech companies to build AI-driven infrastructure, especially in smart mobility and public services.

Brier Score: The Brier Score measures the accuracy of probabilistic predictions. It is used when the model outputs a probability (between 0 and 1) for a binary classification.

Mean Absolute Error: Mean Absolute Error is the mean of the difference between actual and predicted values in absolute terms.

Chapter 6
Smartwatch-Based Semi-Supervised Fall Detection Using Anomaly Detection Techniques

Meshall Alshalaan
https://orcid.org/0009-0005-5356-7574
King Abdullah University of Science and Technology, Saudi Arabia

Fouzi Harrou
https://orcid.org/0000-0002-2138-319X
King Abdullah University of Science and Technology, Saudi Arabia

Ying Sun
King Abdullah University of Science and Technology, Saudi Arabia

ABSTRACT

Fall detection systems are crucial for seniors to mitigate significant health risks and severe fall-related injuries. Traditional supervised methods rely on extensive labeled datasets, which are challenging and time-consuming. Imbalanced datasets, where fall events are rare compared to daily activities, further complicate training. To bypass these challenges, we propose a semi-supervised fall detection approach using a One-Class Support Vector Machine (1SVM) with accelerometric data from smartwatches. 1SVM needs only fall-free data for training and effectively detects falls without labels. Specifically, we applied 1SVM to six features extracted from the accelerometric data, smoothed magnitude, moving window min-max difference, variance, maximum, and minimum. We evaluated this approach using publicly

DOI: 10.4018/979-8-3373-2033-5.ch006

available smartwatch data named the SmartFall dataset, demonstrating 1SVM's superior performance with an accuracy of 87%, outperforming SVM, k-nearest neighbors (KNN), and Naive Bayes.

1. INTRODUCTION

Falls represent a major public health concern, particularly for the elderly population, where they often result in serious consequences such as fractures, head injuries, reduced mobility, and long-term functional decline. According to the World Health Organization (WHO), falls are the second leading cause of unintentional injury deaths globally, with older adults being the most affected demographic. Beyond the immediate physical harm, falls can trigger a cascade of adverse outcomes, including loss of independence, increased fear of falling, social isolation, and higher healthcare utilization. These outcomes collectively reduce the quality of life and contribute to a higher risk of subsequent falls. As such, timely and accurate detection of falls is essential to enable rapid intervention, minimize complications, and support aging in place through proactive healthcare monitoring.

Despite significant advancements in fall detection using supervised machine learning, these approaches face several limitations when deployed in real-world settings. Supervised models rely heavily on large, labeled datasets that include representative examples of both normal activities and fall events. However, fall incidents are inherently rare and unpredictable, making it difficult to collect sufficient annotated fall data, particularly for diverse populations and contexts. Moreover, the variability in fall types, user behaviors, and sensor placements can lead to poor generalization and overfitting to specific training conditions. Labeling fall data also raises ethical and practical challenges, as inducing real falls for data collection poses safety risks. As a result, supervised models often fail to maintain high accuracy and robustness when deployed outside controlled environments, limiting their applicability in continuous, real-time monitoring scenarios.

Over the last decade, significant advancements have been made in fall detection technologies, driven by the development of various sensing modalities. Fall detection systems are typically categorized based on the type of sensors used: wearable sensors (e.g., gyroscopes, accelerometers, smartwatches), camera-based systems (e.g., RGB, depth, infrared), and environment-based sensors (e.g., acoustic and pressure sensors) (Zerrouki et al. 2021). Figure 1 illustrates this taxonomy. Wearable sensors, such as smartwatches, gyroscopes, smartphones, and belt-mounted devices, are among the most widely adopted due to their portability and direct motion capture (Pierleoni et al., 2015; Nooruddin et al., 2022; Newaz & Hanada, 2023). These devices commonly include inertial measurement units (IMUs) to track acceleration and angular velocity, enabling continuous monitoring of body movements (García-de-Villa et al., 2024). Camera-based systems, on the other hand, rely on visual data acquired from RGB cameras, depth sensors, or infrared cameras to detect abnormal posture changes or motion patterns (Gutiérrez et al., 2021; Tao et al., 2018; Mehta et al., 2021). While they offer rich spatial and contextual information, their use is generally confined to indoor spaces and raises privacy concerns (Wang et al., 2020).

Environment-based sensors provide a non-intrusive alternative by capturing fall-related environmental cues. These systems utilize acoustic sensors to capture impact sounds (Khan et al., 2015), floor or pressure sensors to detect sudden weight shifts (Popescu et al., 2008), presence devices to monitor occupancy and movement (Mahmud et al., 2025), and inactivity sensors to detect prolonged stillness that may indicate a fall (Igual et al., 2013). Among these, smartwatches have emerged as a practical and scalable platform for real-time fall detection in daily life. Their widespread adoption, embedded inertial sensors (e.g., accelerometers, gyroscopes), and seamless integration into daily routines make them ideal for unobtrusive health monitoring (Patel et al., 2012; Godfrey et al., 2018). Unlike dedicated medical devices, smartwatches are already worn by millions of users, making them an ideal platform for real-world health monitoring without additional hardware costs. Commercial smartwatches such as the Apple Watch, Fitbit, and Samsung Galaxy Watch now include fall detection, using accelerometers and gyroscopes to trigger emergency alerts after sudden impacts. While convenient and scalable, these proprietary black-box models lack transparency, personalization, and adaptability to atypical movement patterns. This limits inclusivity, as users with disabilities or mobility aids often face false positives or missed detections.

Figure 1. Overview of fall detection system categories based on sensing modalities.

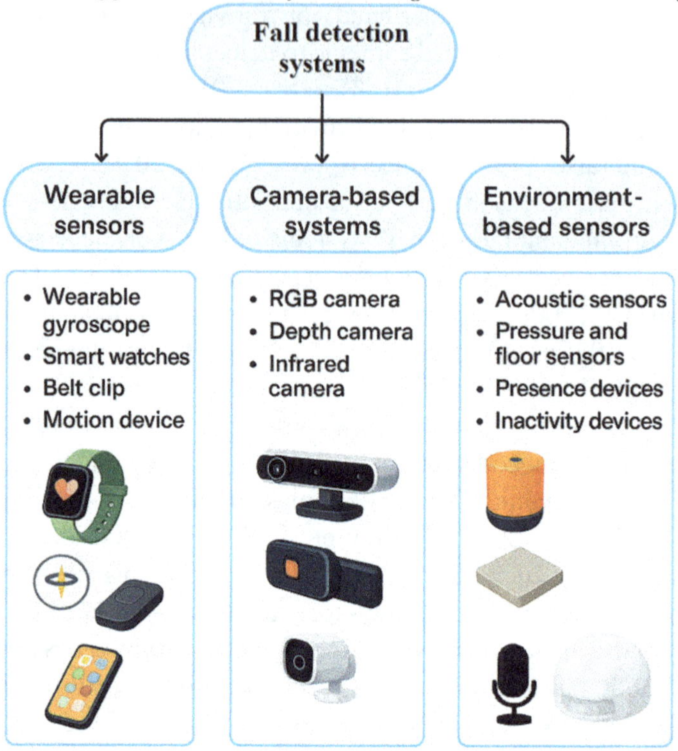

Although fall detection technologies are often designed for older adults, they must also accommodate individuals with disabilities, such as those with Parkinson's disease, stroke survivors, or prosthesis users, who face elevated fall risks due to atypical gait patterns, involuntary movements, or delayed motor responses. These atypical motion profiles often challenge conventional detection algorithms trained on standard movements. Wearable devices, particularly smartwatches equipped with inertial sensors, offer a promising platform for real-time monitoring due to their ubiquity, unobtrusiveness, and user familiarity. However, leveraging these devices effectively requires models that can adapt to the unique and evolving movement patterns of each user.

Over the past two decades, a wide range of machine learning (ML) and deep learning (DL) approaches have been developed to detect falls using wearable, vision-based, and environmental data. These methods differ in how they process sensor inputs, learn features, handle imbalanced data, and generalize across individuals. For example, Özdemir and Barshan (2014) developed a wearable fall detection system using motion sensors at six body locations. They evaluated k-nearest neighbor (k-NN), least squares method (LSM), support vector machines (SVM), Bayesian decision making (BDM), dynamic time warping (DTW), and artificial neural networks (ANN) on 2,520 trials from 14 subjects. Both k-NN and LSM achieved over 99% accuracy with low computational cost. (Hakim et al., 2017) proposed a smartphone-based fall detection system using built-in inertial measurement unit (IMU) sensors. A threshold-based algorithm was used to detect falls, combined with supervised machine learning to classify activities of daily living (ADLs). Four classifiers, SVM, decision tree, k-NN, and discriminant analysis, were evaluated on accelerometric data, with SVM achieving the highest accuracy of 99%. (Shrivastava & Pandey, 2021) proposed a stacking-based ensemble model using Naive Bayes, k-NN, J48, and Random Forest classifiers on features extracted from smartphone accelerometer data. This approach achieved high sensitivity (89%) and specificity (95%) compared to individual classifiers. (Mauldin et al., 2018) explored smartwatch-based fall detection and found that traditional classifiers like Naive Bayes and SVM had poor generalization with low recall rates (26% for SVM and 66% for NB). A deep learning model using four extracted features significantly improved the performance, achieving an accuracy of approximately 85%. (Casilari & Oviedo-Jiménez, 2015) proposed a dual-device system combining a smartphone and a smartwatch, each equipped with accelerometers and gyroscopes. Falls were confirmed only if detected by both devices. Testing on simulated falls and daily activities demonstrated that this dual-device approach effectively reduced false positives while maintaining high detection accuracy compared to single-device systems. (Khojasteh et al., 2018) explored threshold-based fall detection using on-wrist accelerometers, showing high accuracy but lacking robustness to fall variability. (Kwolek & Kepski, 2014) developed a low-cost, privacy-preserving fall detection system combining tri-axial accelerometer data with depth maps. A threshold triggers feature extraction, followed by SVM-based classification to reduce false alarms. (Theodoridis et al., 2017) proposed a low-cost fall detection method using only body-worn accelerometer data and Recurrent Neural Networks (RNNs). Data augmentation with random 3D rotations improved performance. Evaluated on the URFD dataset, the method achieved high accuracy with no false positives. (Liu et al., 2021) proposed a fall detection model using interpretable features, including body ratio, acceleration, and deflection, rather than raw pose keypoints. After oversampling to address data imbalance, KNN yielded the best results (F1: 1.00 for Normal, 0.85 for Fall, 0.96 for Lying), showing robustness to multi-person scenes and moderate occlusion.

Conventional supervised learning methods face significant limitations in fall detection due to the rarity and variability of falls and the ethical and logistical challenges associated with collecting labeled fall data (Mauldin et al., 2018; Bagala et al., 2012). In contrast, semi-supervised anomaly detection offers a more practical and scalable alternative by training models solely on abundant, passively collected normal activity data and identifying falls as deviations from learned patterns (Khan

& Hoey, 2017; Alam et al., 2022; Usmani et al., 2021). This approach enables learning personalized baselines without requiring extensive labeled fall events, making it particularly well-suited for real-world applications. Moreover, adaptive and privacy-preserving semi-supervised methods can enhance safety, reduce caregiver burden, and support independent living. In this context, we propose a cost-effective and accurate fall detection framework based on semi-supervised learning using accelerometric data from smartwatches. We employ a One-Class Support Vector Machine (1SVM) trained exclusively on normal (non-fall) activity to address the scarcity of labeled fall data and the inherent class imbalance in real-world deployments. The 1SVM is particularly effective for anomaly detection tasks where falls are treated as outliers relative to typical movement patterns. Six discriminative features are extracted from the smartwatch accelerometer signals: smoothed magnitude, moving window min–max difference, variance, maximum, and minimum. Evaluated on the publicly available SmartFall dataset, the proposed model achieves a detection accuracy of 87%, outperforming conventional supervised classifiers such as standard SVM, KNN, and Naive Bayes. These results demonstrate the effectiveness of our semi-supervised approach in achieving robust fall detection.

The remainder of the chapter is organized as follows: Section 2 reviews recent literature on fall detection methods. Section 3 introduces the proposed fall detection strategy based on the 1SVM. Section 4 describes the dataset, experimental setup, and evaluation results. Section 5 discusses the limitations, challenges of generalizability, and the importance of inclusive design in fall detection systems. Finally, Section 6 concludes the chapter with key insights and outlines potential future directions.

2. LITERATURE REVIEW

Fall detection has been widely investigated through various computational approaches. Several prior surveys (e.g., Li et al., 2025; Gaya-Morey et al., 2024; Rassekh & Snidaro, 2025; Kaur et al., 2025; Liu et al., 2023) reviewed fall detection systems. To facilitate comparison and highlight key developments, this section organizes existing methods into three main groups: (i) classical machine learning (ML) methods, (ii) deep learning (DL) approaches, and (iii) semi-supervised anomaly detection techniques. For each category, we review representative recent studies, highlighting their contributions, limitations, and relevance to real-world deployment scenarios.

2.1 Classical Machine Learning Methods

Classical machine learning-based fall detection relies on handcrafted features extracted from sensor signals, followed by supervised classifiers trained on labeled datasets containing examples of both fall and non-fall activities (Zerrouki et al., 2022). Over the last two decades, several studies have explored diverse classifiers and feature engineering strategies to improve detection accuracy and system robustness. (Zerrouki et al., 2016a) compared Naïve Bayes, k-Nearest Neighbors (kNN), Neural Networks (NN), and Support Vector Machines (SVM) for fall detection using vision-based features. The evaluation was conducted on the FDD and URFD datasets. SVM achieved the best overall performance. In another study, (Zerrouki et al., 2016b) proposed a hybrid approach combining exponentially weighted moving average (EWMA) monitoring of accelerometric data with SVM-based classification, achieving superior performance to NN, kNN, and Naïve Bayes by focusing classification only on detected fall windows. (Chelli & Pätzold, 2019) extracted time- and frequency-domain features from accelerometer and gyroscope data to classify daily activities and falls. Among the tested classifiers, ensemble bagged trees (EBT) and quadratic SVM (QSVM) achieved up to 97.7% overall accuracy and 100% fall detection without false alarms. (Hussain et al., 2019) developed a wearable sensor-based system for fall detection and pattern recognition. The system achieved 99.80% accuracy in fall detection using k-Nearest Neighbors (KNN) and 96.82% accuracy in activity recognition with Random Forest (RF). (Noh et al., 2021) used gait features from shoe-mounted inertial sensors and trained an XGBoost model to classify fall risk in older adults. Stride length, walking speed, and stance phase were identified as key predictors. (Subburam et al., 2024) evaluated several classifiers for fall detection, including SVM, Logistic Regression, Random Forest (RF), AdaBoost, and Gradient Boosting. Results showed that the Extra Random Forest (ERF) achieved the highest accuracy. (Rastogi & Singh, 2023) proposed an ensemble-based fall detection system combining SVM, KNN, Decision Tree, and Deep LSTM using a greedy majority voting algorithm, achieving 99.98% accuracy and outperforming individual models. Despite their simplicity and interpretability, classical ML methods often struggle with generalization to unseen users, sensor placements, and device variations. They also rely heavily on labeled fall data, which limits their adaptability in real-world deployments.

2.2 Deep Learning-Based Methods

Deep learning (DL) models automatically extract hierarchical features from raw data and effectively capture spatial–temporal dependencies, making them well-suited for fall detection tasks. These methods have been widely adopted across various sensing modalities, including wearable inertial sensors, video data, and wireless signals, demonstrating strong performance in detecting and predicting falls. For instance, (Hu et al., 2025) proposed a hybrid convolutional neural network (CNN)–long short-term memory (LSTM) model for involuntary fall detection using wrist-worn sensors. It was tested on data from 49 participants and outperformed standalone CNN and LSTM models in accuracy and reliability. (Hsu et al., 2023) explored fall risk prediction in elderly individuals using wearable sensor data and deep learning. They compared LSTM and CNN-based transfer learning models on a public dataset of daily activities, with CNN achieving 98% accuracy on a public dataset. The study confirms the effectiveness of deep learning for multi-task assessment using accelerometer and gyroscope data. (Bui et al., 2024) proposed a dual-mode fall detection system combining vision-based detection (enhanced YOLOv5s) and WiFi-based detection (CNN-LSTM with channel state information). The system achieved high accuracy and real-time performance, offering a non-intrusive solution for elderly monitoring under varying visibility conditions. (Yu et al., 2025) introduced a lightweight, real-time skeleton-based fall detection method combining Temporal Convolutional Networks (TCN) and Transformer Encoders (TE). Validated on UP-Fall and Le2i datasets, it achieved over 99% accuracy and demonstrated efficient edge deployment for elderly care. (Wang et al., 2024) proposed a fall prediction framework using wearable inertial sensors and a spatio-temporal graph neural network (ST-GNN) to model human pose dynamics. The method was validated on two public benchmark datasets and one proprietary dataset, where it achieved superior performance compared to state-of-the-art approaches. The study highlights the promise of ST-GNNs in accurately predicting fall risks in privacy-sensitive, mobile contexts using low-cost wearable sensors. (Şengül et al., 2022) developed a smartwatch-based fall detection system using accelerometer and gyroscope data. A Bi-directional LSTM (BiLSTM) model, trained with features extracted via Bicubic Hermite interpolation and rolling windows, achieved 99.59% and 97.35% accuracy in leave-one-activity-out and leave-one-subject-out settings, respectively, with perfect fall vs. non-fall classification. (Kiran et al., 2021) proposed a deep learning-based Human Action Recognition (HAR) framework using ResNet-50 with domain transfer learning. Features from the Global Average Pooling (GAP) and Fully Connected (FC) layers were fused via Canonical Correlation Analysis (CCA) and selected using Shannon entropy. The method achieved high accuracy (e.g., 100% on YouTube, 99.7% on UCF Sports) and improved both performance and computational efficiency. DL models often outperform classical approaches in terms of accuracy and flexibility but come at the cost of high computational requirements, limited interpretability, and large data demands.

2.3 Semi-Supervised Anomaly Detection Methods

Semi-supervised methods train solely on normal daily activities, enabling the detection of unseen falls while mitigating class imbalance. Recent studies adopt this approach by modeling normal activity and flagging falls as deviations. (Chen et al., 2021) proposed a semi-supervised fall risk assessment method using a stacked auto-encoder (SAE) trained on time–frequency representations of triaxial accelerometer data during the Timed Up and Go (TUG) test. The model achieved high predictive accuracy across all axes (up to 94.1%), showing potential for remote mobility assessment without expert supervision. (Yu et al., 2024) introduced Semi-PFD, a semi-supervised pre-impact fall detection model that leverages abundant ADL data while reducing reliance on labeled falls. Evaluated on KFall and SisFall datasets, Semi-PFD outperformed supervised models, achieving higher F1-scores even with limited fall data, and addressing overconfidence issues common in fully supervised settings. (Harrou et al., 2017) proposed a lightweight fall detection approach using posture descriptors and Principal Component Analysis (PCA). The system monitors ignored components via an Exponentially Weighted Moving Average (EWMA) chart to flag falls as statistical anomalies. Tests on URFD and FDD datasets showed improved sensitivity over classical PCA-based methods. (Zerrouki et al., 2016) developed a method combining Multivariate EWMA (MEWMA) monitoring of silhouette changes with SVM classification. The MEWMA–SVM pipeline reduced false positives from fall-like gestures and outperformed NN, naïve Bayes, and KNN on URFD and FDD datasets. (Tran et al., 2022) focused on near-fall detection using a smart video surveillance system. Skeleton-based velocity features extracted via Keypoint R-CNN were analyzed using One-Class SVM, Gaussian Mixture Model, and Isolation Forest (IF). The best performance was achieved with IF (AUC = 92%), highlighting its relevance for early intervention in mobility decline. These approaches are particularly promising for real-world deployment, especially for users with disabilities or rare fall types, as they do not require labeled fall data and can adapt to individual baselines.

Table 1 summarizes the core strengths and limitations of each category, underscoring the practical trade-offs that motivate our choice of a lightweight, semi-supervised anomaly detection framework for smartwatch-based fall detection.

Table 1. Comparison of Fall Detection Method Categories

Approach	Key Characteristics	Advantages	Limitations
Classical Machine Learning	Handcrafted features + supervised learning (e.g., SVM, k-NN, Decision Trees)	- Simple and interpretable - Low computational cost - Works well with curated datasets	- Requires labeled fall data - Poor generalization to new users - Sensitive to sensor placement
Deep Learning-Based Methods	Automatic feature extraction from raw signals (e.g., CNN, LSTM, BiLSTM, GNN, Transformers)	- High detection accuracy - Captures complex temporal & spatial patterns - Adaptable to multimodal inputs	- Data-hungry (needs labeled fall data) - High computational cost - Limited interpretability
Semi-Supervised Anomaly Detection	Trained only on normal activity; falls treated as anomalies (e.g., 1SVM, autoencoders, Isolation Forests)	- No need for fall labels - Personalized modeling - More realistic for real-world deployment	- May flag borderline non-fall anomalies - Performance depends on quality of "normal" training data

3. FALL DETECTION STRATEGY USING ONE-CLASS SVM

This section introduces a semi-supervised fall detection framework based on the 1SVM, trained solely on normal activity data to detect falls as anomalies. Section 3.1 defines the problem, 3.2 outlines the 1SVM algorithm, 3.3 describes feature extraction from smartwatch accelerometer data, and 3.4 presents the complete detection pipeline.

3.1 Problem Formulation

The fall detection problem addressed in this study can be formulated as an anomaly detection task over time-series sensor data acquired from a smartwatch. Let $X = \{x_1, x_2, ..., x\}$ be the set of input samples, where each sample $x = [x_1, x_2, ..., x] \in \mathbb{R}$ represents a feature vector extracted from the tri-axial accelerometer readings over a sliding window. The goal is to determine whether a given sample corresponds to a normal activity or an abnormal event (i.e., a fall).

In a traditional supervised classification setup, the output label $\hat{Y}$ would be defined as:

$$\hat{Y} = \begin{cases} 0, \text{ Normal activity} \\ 1, \text{ Fall} \end{cases}$$

However, due to the scarcity and variability of fall data, we adopt a semi-supervised formulation using a 1SVM. This approach relies solely on normal activity data for training. The 1SVM learns a decision boundary that encapsulates the distribution of normal activities, and any test sample falling outside this boundary is flagged as a potential anomaly. The decision function for 1SVM can be expressed as:

$$\hat{Y}_A = \begin{cases} +1, \text{if } x_i \text{ is similar to normal activity (inlier)} \\ -1, \text{ if } x_i \text{ is anomalous (potential fall)} \end{cases}$$

where $\hat{Y}_A$ denotes the anomaly score predicted by the 1SVM. The primary objective of this formulation is to learn a mapping function:

$$f{:}X \rightarrow \hat{Y}_A$$

that accurately distinguishes between normal and anomalous patterns using only fall-free data during training. This enables reliable fall detection without requiring extensive labeled datasets, making it suitable for real-world, on-device deployment in wearable systems.

3.2 Anomaly Detection with the One-Class SVM Algorithm

In the context of fall detection, anomaly detection techniques, particularly one-class classification methods, are effective when labeled fall data is scarce or unreliable. Among these, the 1SVM is a widely used kernel-based method designed to model the boundary of normal data and detect deviations as anomalies (Schölkopf et al., 2001; Harrou et al., 2019; Zerrouki et al., 2020; Hejazi & Singh, 2013). Its ability to operate in a semi-supervised setting makes it particularly suitable for wearable fall detection, where collecting diverse and ethically acceptable fall examples is often impractical.

The 1SVM is employed in this study to detect fall events by identifying anomalous motion patterns from smartwatch accelerometer data (Schölkopf et al., 2001). Unlike traditional SVMs that require both positive and negative labeled examples, 1SVM is particularly well-suited for fall detection because it can be trained solely on normal (non-fall) activity data, an abundant and safe-to-collect class. This makes it efficient for scenarios where collecting real fall data is ethically challenging or practically infeasible. A conceptual illustration of the 1SVM decision boundary and its use for identifying fall-related anomalies is shown in Figure 2.

Figure 2. A basic illustration of the One-Class SVM (1SVM) model. The model is trained on normal data (green points) to learn a decision boundary (hyperplane) separating the majority class from the origin. Points outside the learned region (red crosses) are considered outliers or potential fall events during detection.

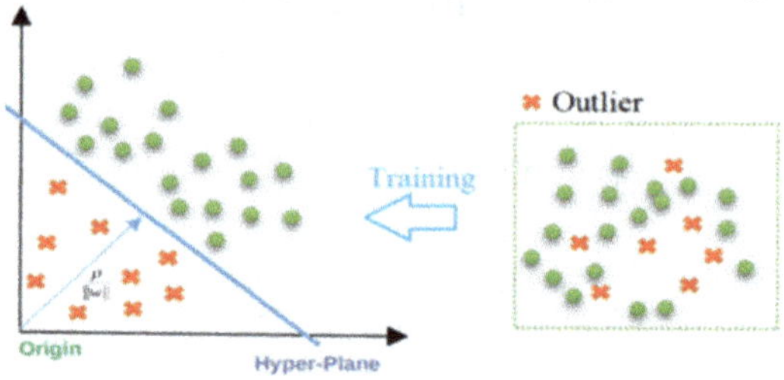

In this application, accelerometer signals from a smartwatch are segmented into fixed-length windows, and a set of statistical features is extracted from each window (see Section 2.3). These features form the input vectors for the 1SVM model, which learns a decision boundary that tightly encloses the "normal" feature space. Any test sample that deviates significantly from this space is flagged as a potential fall. The decision function in 1SVM distinguishes between normal and abnormal feature vectors based on their distance from the learned boundary. It is defined as:

$$F(x) = \text{sign}(w \bullet \phi(x)) - \rho) \tag{1}$$

Here, $\phi(x)$ is a kernel-based feature mapping function, **w** is the weight vector, and ρ is the bias term. If the function returns +1, the activity is considered normal; otherwise, −1 indicates an anomaly, potentially corresponding to a fall.

To compute this, the kernel function $K(x,x\ )$ measures similarity between feature vectors, allowing for non-linear separability in high-dimensional space. Common kernels such as the Gaussian radial basis function (RBF) are used to model the complex nature of human motion patterns.

During training, the parameters **w** and ρ are optimized by solving:

$$\min_{w,\rho}\left(\frac{1}{2}\left\|w\right\|^2 - \rho + \frac{1}{vl}\sum_{i=1}^{l}\varepsilon_i\right) \tag{2}$$

Subject to:

$$w \bullet \phi(x_i) \geq \rho - \varepsilon_i,\ \varepsilon_i \geq 0$$

Where:

1 is the number of training samples (normal activity),
ε_i are slack variables allowing margin violations,
$\nu \in (0, 1]$ controls the fraction of outliers and model complexity.

This formulation ensures that the model tightly fits the distribution of fall-free activities. At runtime, the trained model receives new feature vectors from the smartwatch. If a vector lies outside the learned normal boundary (i.e., classified as −1-), it is flagged as a potential fall event. To reduce false alarms from non-fall anomalies (e.g., abrupt but safe movements), post-processing filters such as temporal consistency or multi-window confirmation are applied. Thus, the 1SVM framework enables an efficient, label-free approach to fall detection using only normal daily activity data, making it robust and practical for real-world wearable applications.

3.3 Feature Extraction from Smartwatch Accelerometric Data

Accurate feature extraction is a critical step in transforming raw accelerometer signals into meaningful representations that capture the motion characteristics of normal and fall-related activities. In this study, tri-axial accelerometer data (a_x,a_y,a_z) are continuously collected from a smartwatch worn on the wrist. The raw data are first segmented using a fixed-length sliding window approach, with partial overlap to ensure temporal continuity and responsiveness.

From each windowed segment, six time-domain features are extracted to summarize the dynamic behavior of the movement. These features are selected for their ability to distinguish normal activities (e.g., walking, sitting, standing) from abrupt and irregular movements associated with falls. The computed features are:

- **Smoothed Magnitude**:

$$M_t = \sqrt{a_x^2 + a_y^2 + a_z^2}$$

A low-pass filtered version of the acceleration magnitude to suppress transient noise and capture general motion intensity.

- **Moving Window Min–Max Difference:** Let $W = \{a_1, a_2, ..., a_n\}$ be the accelerometer magnitude values in a sliding window. The min–max difference measures the range of variation within the window, capturing abrupt changes in acceleration typically observed during falls.

$$D_{\text{min-max}} = \max(W) - \min(W)$$

- **Variance:** The variance of the signal in the window is given by:

$$Var(W) = \frac{1}{n}\sum_{i=1}^{n}(a_i - \overline{a})^2$$

- **Mean:** The mean value of the accelerometer signal in the window is computed as:

$$\overline{a} = \frac{1}{n}\sum_{i=1}^{n}a_i$$

The mean helps characterize the overall acceleration level and provides a baseline for normalization. It represents the central tendency of the acceleration signals over the window, which helps normalize motion intensity across different users and activities.

All features are computed independently for each window and normalized to zero mean and unit variance before being input to the One-Class SVM model. This feature representation enables the model to learn a compact and generalizable boundary for fall-free motion patterns while being sensitive to abnormal fluctuations indicative of falls.

3.4 The Proposed One-Class SVM for Anomaly-Based Fall Detection

The proposed fall detection framework is built around a semi-supervised learning approach using the 1SVM, which is particularly effective in scenarios where fall instances are rare, diverse, and difficult to capture. By leveraging only normal (non-fall) data during training, the system learns a compact representation of daily activity patterns and identifies deviations from these patterns as potential falls. This eliminates the need for large, diverse, and ethically challenging labeled fall datasets.

As depicted in Figure 3, the detection process is divided into two key stages: training and testing. In the training stage, tri-axial accelerometer data are continuously recorded from a smartwatch worn on the wrist, with a sampling frequency of 31.25 Hz. The raw signal is segmented using a fixed-length sliding window with overlap to ensure temporal continuity and responsiveness. Each window is then processed to extract a set of handcrafted statistical features that summarize the motion characteristics of the wearer.

Figure 3. Flowchart of the proposed 1SVM-based fall detection system via smartwatch accelerometer data.

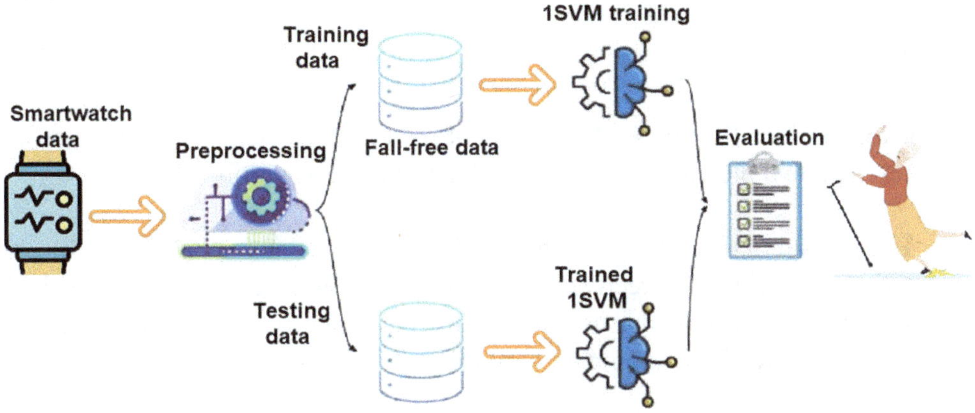

These features include the Euclidean norm of the accelerometer signal—computed as the magnitude of the acceleration vector and smoothed using a moving average filter to reduce noise artifacts. Additionally, the difference between the minimum and maximum values within the window is calculated to capture abrupt variations, which are typical of fall events. To further characterize the signal's behavior, basic statistical descriptors such as mean, variance, and standard deviation are also computed for each window. Together, these features form a compact and informative representation of the user's motion within each time frame.

To ensure consistency across different sessions and users, all feature vectors are normalized using z-score normalization, subtracting the mean and dividing by the standard deviation, prior to training. This step standardizes the scale of each feature, improving the generalization ability of the 1SVM model. The 1SVM is then trained using only the fall-free feature vectors to define a decision boundary that encloses the normal activity space. During the testing phase, the same preprocessing and feature extraction steps are applied to new accelerometer data, which may contain both fall and non-fall events. The trained 1SVM evaluates each windowed feature vector, and those falling outside the learned boundary are classified as anomalies, i.e., potential falls.

To rigorously assess the performance of the proposed 1SVM-based fall detection approach, three standard evaluation metrics were used: True Positive Rate (TPR), False Positive Rate (FPR), and Accuracy. These metrics provide a comprehensive view of the system's ability to detect falls while minimizing false alarms.

- True Positive Rate (TPR), also referred to as Recall or Sensitivity, measures the proportion of actual fall events that were correctly identified as falls by the model. A high TPR indicates that the system is effective in recognizing fall incidents. It is defined as:

$$TPR = \frac{TP}{TP + FN}$$

where: TP (True Positives): the number of correctly detected fall events, and FN (False Negatives): the number of actual fall events that were missed.

- False Positive Rate (FPR) quantifies the proportion of normal (non-fall) activities that were incorrectly classified as falls. Minimizing the FPR is critical in fall detection systems, as false alarms may lead to unnecessary interventions or reduced trust in the system. It is computed as:

$$FPR = \frac{FP}{FP + TN}$$

where: FP (False Positives): the number of non-fall events incorrectly identified as falls, and TN (True Negatives): the number of correctly identified non-fall events.

- Accuracy measures the overall correctness of the classifier by capturing both correct fall and non-fall predictions. It is defined as:

$$Accuracy = \frac{TP + TN}{TP + TN + FP + FN}$$

This metric is especially useful when the number of fall and non-fall samples is balanced. However, in highly imbalanced datasets, such as in fall detection scenarios where fall events are rare, accuracy should be interpreted with caution and supplemented with TPR and FPR. These metrics provide an objective basis for comparing the proposed 1SVM-based anomaly detection method against conventional classifiers. By analyzing the trade-off between TPR and FPR, the system's effectiveness in real-world deployment conditions can be better understood.

The overall procedure for implementing the proposed fall detection system is summarized in Algorithm 1. It outlines each step from raw smartwatch accelerometer data acquisition to final fall classification using a One-Class SVM model. The algorithm begins with signal segmentation and handcrafted feature extraction, followed by normalization to ensure feature consistency. In the training phase, the 1SVM model learns to represent the distribution of normal daily activities using only fall-free data. During inference, incoming feature vectors are evaluated against the learned boundary to detect deviations indicative of falls. Optional post-processing can be applied to suppress isolated false positives and enhance the reliability of the detection output. This structured process enables real-time, on-device fall monitoring in resource-constrained environments.

Algorithm 1: One-Class SVM-Based Fall Detection Using Smartwatch Accelerometric Data

Input: Raw tri-axial accelerometer data (a_x, a_y, a_z) from smartwatch
Output: Detected fall events

1. **Initialization:** Set window size *w*, overlap *o*, and 1SVM parameters *v*, kernel type.
2. **Data Acquisition:** Collect raw accelerometer data at 31.25 Hz from the smartwatch.
3. **Segmentation:** Apply a sliding window of length *w* with overlap *o* to segment the time-series signal.
4. **Feature Extraction (for each window):**
    - a. Compute Euclidean norm: $M_t = \sqrt{a_x^2 + a_y^2 + a_z^2}$
    - b. Smooth M_t using a moving average filter
    - c. Extract statistical features: mean, variance, standard deviation, min–max difference
    - d. Concatenate features into a feature vector x_t
5. **Normalization:** Apply z-score normalization to each feature vector.
6. **Training Phase:** Train the 1SVM model using only fall-free (normal) feature vectors.
7. **Testing Phase:**
    - a. Apply identical preprocessing and feature extraction to new test data
    - b. For each feature vector, compute decision function $F(x_t)$
    - - If $F(x_t) = +1$, classify as normal
    - - If $F(x_t) = -1$, classify as fall (anomaly)
8. **Post-Processing (optional):** Confirm a fall only if multiple consecutive anomalies are detected to reduce false positives.
9. **Output:** Return the final fall detection decision.

The next section reports on the empirical evaluation results obtained using the SmartFall dataset.

4. RESULTS AND DISCUSSION

4.1 Data description and analysis

The evaluation of the proposed fall detection system was conducted using the SmartFall dataset developed by (Mauldin et al., 2018), specifically designed for wrist-worn smart devices. The dataset consists of accelerometric data collected from seven healthy adult volunteers wearing a Microsoft Band 2 smartwatch on their left wrist. Participants were aged between 21 and 55 years, with heights ranging from 5 to 6.5 feet and weights from 100 to 230 pounds, ensuring inter-subject variability in body motion profiles. The subjects performed a structured protocol comprising both Activities of Daily Living (ADLs) and simulated falls. ADLs included jogging, sitting down, throwing objects, and waving hands, selected for their similarity to fall-like arm movements. These activities were automatically labeled as "NotFall". Simulated falls were executed in four directions: front, back, left, and right, onto a 12-inch-high mattress, with each type of fall repeated 10 times per subject to ensure consistency and diversity. Data collection was carried out at a sampling frequency of 31.25 Hz, chosen as a trade-off between signal fidelity and computational efficiency. Lower frequencies such as 4 Hz missed key dynamics of falls, while higher rates (e.g., 62.5 Hz) increased processing overhead without meaningful accuracy gains.

The SmartFall dataset provides fine-grained, time-series accelerometer recordings with real-time annotations. Labeling was assisted by a researcher who tagged fall instances during collection; additional post-processing was applied to ensure that the peak acceleration region of each fall was correctly labeled as "Fall," improving annotation quality. This dataset forms a representative benchmark for evaluating lightweight fall detection algorithms using wrist-mounted devices under constrained conditions where collecting real falls from elderly users is not feasible for ethical and safety reasons.

4.2 Preliminary Data Analysis

To gain insight into the characteristics of fall versus non-fall activities, we analyzed the distribution of raw tri-axial acceleration signals (a_x, a_y, and a_z) captured by the smartwatch. Figure 4 presents histograms comparing the value distributions of these components under two classes: Fall and No Fall.

Figure 4. Distribution of accelerometer components (a_x, a_y, and a_z) for fall and non-fall events in the SmartFall dataset.

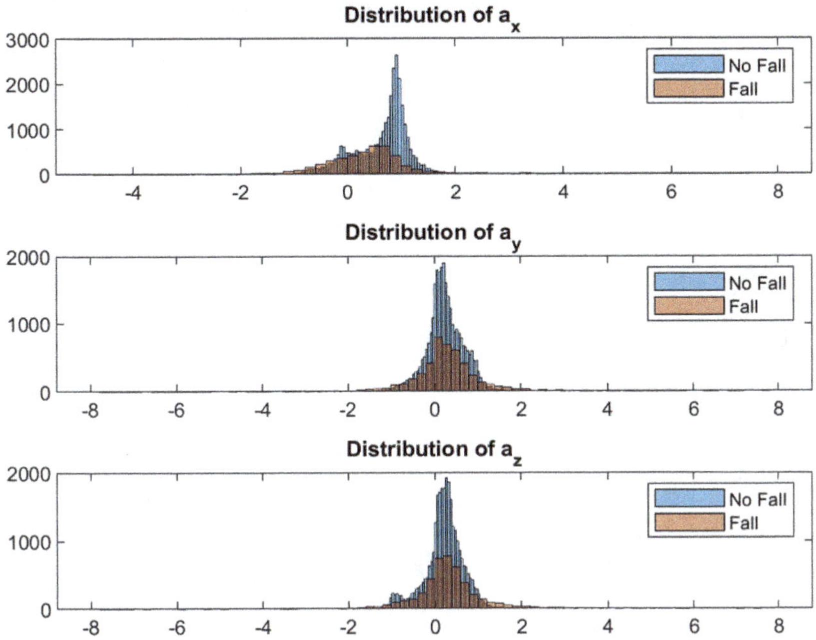

As shown in Figure 4, all three acceleration components (a_x, a_y, and a_z) exhibit distinct patterns under fall versus non-fall conditions. Fall events result in broader distributions and increased variance across all axes, with ax and az showing wider spreads and ay reflecting abrupt shifts, likely due to vertical or lateral impact. These disruptions introduce higher variability and heavier distribution tails, supporting the use of statistical features like variance, min–max difference, and smoothed magnitude in the proposed 1SVM-based anomaly detection framework.

In addition to individual components, the distribution of acceleration magnitude further highlights the contrast between fall and non-fall events. As shown in Figure 5, non-fall data are concentrated at low values, while fall events display a broader, heavier-tailed distribution, indicating more abrupt and intense motion. This supports the use of smoothed magnitude, maximum, and variance as effective features for distinguishing falls using simple time-domain analysis.

Figure 5. Distribution of acceleration magnitudes for fall and non-fall events in the SmartFall dataset.

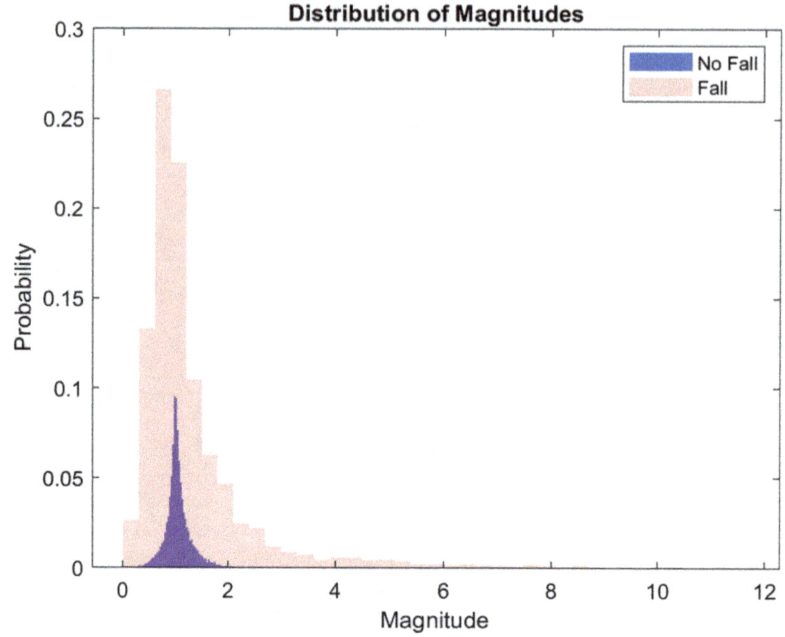

To explore temporal dynamics, we analyzed the autocorrelation of the three accelerometer components over a 200-sample lag window (Figure 6). Non-fall activities showed smoother, periodic patterns with slower decay, while fall signals exhibited sharper peaks and faster decay, indicating irregular, abrupt motion. These differences highlight the potential of temporal characteristics to aid fall detection and further justify the use of time-domain features like variance and min–max difference.

Figure 6. ACF of the three accelerometer components for fall (red) and non-fall (blue) segments in the SmartFall dataset.

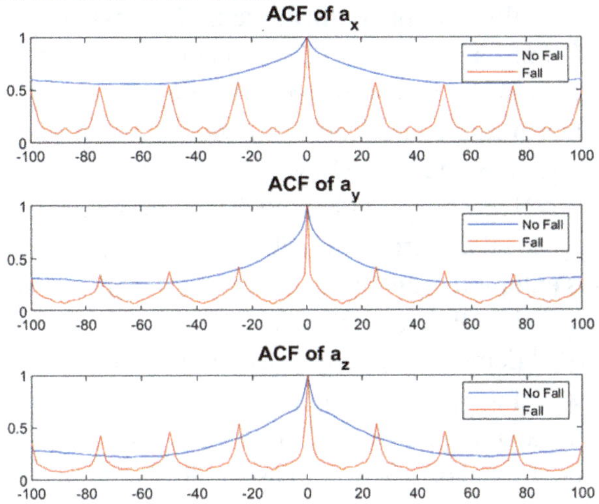

4.3 Fall detection results

To evaluate the effectiveness of the proposed fall detection method, six time-domain features were extracted from the smartwatch accelerometer signals: smoothed magnitude, moving window min–max difference, variance, maximum, and minimum. The 1SVM was then trained exclusively on fall-free samples using a radial basis function (RBF) kernel. The trained model was evaluated on testing data that included both fall and non-fall events. The performance metrics, TPR, FPR, and Accuracy, are reported in Table 2, and benchmarked against three baseline classifiers: k-nearest neighbors (kNN), Naive Bayes (NB), and standard SVM.

Table 2. Detection performance metrics on testing data.

Method	TPR	FPR	Accuracy
1SVM	74.00	0.10	88.00
kNN	51.03	6.79	87.64
NB	64.31	7.42	88.84
SVM	91.56	20.25	81.31

The 1SVM achieved a TPR of 74.00%, correctly detecting 74% of fall events. Notably, it maintained a very low FPR of 0.10, indicating minimal false alarms, and an overall accuracy of 88.00%. These results highlight the model's capacity to generalize well from normal activity patterns and to reliably identify fall-related anomalies with minimal noise. In contrast, the SVM classifier achieved the highest TPR at 91.56%, but its FPR of 20.25% rendered it impractical for real-world deployment due to excessive false positives. Although accurate in detecting falls, such a high false alarm rate could lead to frequent interruptions or alerts during regular activities. The kNN and Naive Bayes classifiers showed moderate detection performance, with kNN reaching a TPR of 51.03% and NB achieving 64.31%, both accompanied by higher false alarm rates (FPRs of 6.79% and 7.42%, respectively). While these models exhibit reasonable accuracy, their higher FPR undermines their suitability for a wearable fall detection system.

Overall, the 1SVM demonstrates a balanced trade-off between detection sensitivity and robustness to false positives, making it a compelling solution for real-time fall detection in wearable applications. However, while promising, there remains room for improvement, particularly in increasing TPR without compromising FPR, possibly through ensemble learning or hybrid anomaly detection strategies.

4.4 Comparison with Existing Methods

To further validate the effectiveness of the proposed 1SVM approach for fall detection, we conducted a comparative analysis using the same SmartFall dataset and benchmark results from the original study by (Mauldin et al., 2018). Table 3 presents the performance comparison based solely on smartwatch-derived accelerometric data under consistent experimental conditions. While the original study evaluated supervised models, including Support Vector Machine (SVM), Naive Bayes (NB), and a Gated Recurrent Unit-based Recurrent Neural Network (GRU-RNN), our approach adopts a semi-supervised learning paradigm, trained exclusively on fall-free data using six handcrafted time-domain features. Despite not using any labeled fall data, the 1SVM model achieved competitive accuracy and a significantly lower false positive rate, demonstrating the feasibility and robustness of anomaly-based fall detection using smartwatches in practical, real-world settings.

Table 3. Comparative performance between our approach and baseline methods on the SmartFall smartwatch dataset.

Method	TPR (Recall)	FPR	Accuracy	Supervision
1SVM (Ours)	74.00%	0.10%	88.00%	Semi-supervised (Normal only)
SVM [5]	86.00%	~20.25%	73.00%	Supervised
Naive Bayes [5]	92.00%	~7.42%	65.00%	Supervised
GRU-RNN [5]	100.00%	Not reported	85.00%	Supervised, Deep learning

Although the GRU-based model in the SmartFall paper achieves the highest TPR of 100%, it does not report false positive rates explicitly, and it comes with increased model complexity and training cost. Additionally, all supervised methods rely on fall-labeled data, which is often difficult, unethical, or impractical to obtain in real-world scenarios. In contrast, the proposed 1SVM model achieves a high accuracy of 88% while maintaining an exceptionally low FPR of 0.10%, which is critical in wearable healthcare systems to avoid false alarms. Despite a slightly lower TPR compared to supervised baselines, the 1SVM offers better robustness and deployability, making it more suitable for continuous monitoring in uncontrolled environments. These results demonstrate that semi-supervised anomaly detection techniques like 1SVM can serve as viable alternatives to traditional supervised models, especially when fall event labels are sparse or unavailable.

5. DISCUSSION: LIMITATIONS AND INCLUSIVITY IN FALL DETECTION

While the proposed semi-supervised fall detection framework demonstrates promising results on the SmartFall dataset, several limitations and broader considerations must be acknowledged to contextualize its applicability and alignment with the book's overarching theme of AI for enhanced quality of life.

5.1. Dataset Limitations and Generalizability

The SmartFall dataset used in this study includes accelerometric recordings of simulated falls and daily activities, primarily performed by young adult participants under controlled conditions. This introduces a limitation in terms of generalizability to real-world scenarios, particularly among older adults or individuals with disabilities who may exhibit distinct movement patterns. Real-world falls are often more variable in dynamics, environmental context, and user response, which simulated datasets may fail to fully capture. To address this, future work should validate the proposed approach using more diverse and ecologically valid datasets such as SisFall (Sucerquia et al., 2017), which includes recordings from elderly subjects; URFD (Kwolek & Kepski, 2015), which offers depth-based data with various fall postures; and UP-Fall (Martínez-Villaseñor et al., 2019), which contains multimodal recordings from multiple age groups. Incorporating such datasets would not only improve model robustness but also ensure fair evaluation across a wider range of users and conditions.

5.2. Broader Relevance to People with Disabilities

While fall detection research has focused on older adults, it is equally vital for individuals with disabilities who face increased fall risk. Individuals with physical, neurological, or cognitive impairments often exhibit atypical movement or balance issues that increase their fall risk. For example, individuals with Parkinson's disease often experience freezing of gait, instability, or motor fluctuations, leading to unpredictable and atypical falls unlike those seen in healthy elderly individuals. Similarly, stroke survivors may have hemiparesis or spasticity, resulting in asymmetric movements that are poorly represented in conventional fall datasets. People with conditions like cerebral palsy, multiple sclerosis, muscular dystrophy, or amputations often use assistive devices, adding further variability to their movement patterns. These populations face not only a higher incidence of falls but also increased risks of injury, hospitalization, and reduced independence. Most existing fall detection models are trained on data from individuals without disabilities or based on simulated falls by young adults in controlled settings. As a result, they may not generalize well to people with disabilities, leading to high false positive rates for atypical but normal movements, or false negatives when true falls deviate from standard patterns. This limits their real-world reliability and safety for these users.

The semi-supervised approach proposed in this chapter addresses these challenges by training solely on fall-free data to learn each individual's normal activity profile. Using a One-Class SVM, the model flags deviations as potential falls, making it well-suited to users with non-standard movement patterns and removing the need for labeled fall data, which is often scarce or ethically difficult to collect. Additionally, smartwatches, commonly used by people with disabilities for fitness, medication, and communication, provide a practical, non-stigmatizing, and cost-effective platform for deploying such personalized models. Beyond safety, inclusive fall detection systems can enhance independent living, self-confidence, and peace of mind for both users and caregivers. By enabling timely intervention and reducing the need for constant supervision, they help people with disabilities maintain autonomy and improve quality of life. Designing such systems with their needs in mind aligns with principles of universal design and digital health equity, ensuring that technological solutions are accessible, adaptable, and person-centered.

5.3. Commercial Systems and Practical Deployment

Commercial smartwatches such as the Apple Watch, Fitbit, and Samsung Galaxy Watch have played a major role in bringing fall detection to mainstream consumers. These devices use embedded inertial sensors, typically tri-axial accelerometers and gyroscopes, to detect rapid motion changes associated with falls. When a potential fall is detected, the watch may vibrate or emit an alert, allowing the user to cancel it if no help is needed. If there is no response, the system can automatically notify emergency contacts or services. This functionality makes fall detection passive, non-intrusive, and accessible, particularly for older adults or users seeking continuous monitoring without the stigma of traditional medical alert devices.

Despite their user-friendly design, commercial fall detection systems face critical limitations in transparency, adaptability, and clinical relevance. Their proprietary, black-box algorithms offer little insight into decision logic or tunable parameters, hindering validation and personalization. Typically trained on normative motion data from healthy individuals or simulations, these systems often fail to accommodate the diverse movement profiles of users with disabilities or chronic conditions. Consequently, reliability in non-standard populations remains limited. For instance, abrupt but non-fall-related movements in Parkinson's disease may trigger false alarms, while slow or asymmetric motions in stroke survivors may go undetected. Such shortcomings undermine user trust and system effectiveness. Moreover, these systems rarely support individualized baselines, contextual data integration, or clinical adaptation. Sensitivity tuning is limited, and concerns around data privacy persist, particularly when relying on cloud-based processing without user control.

Semi-supervised methods, such as the proposed One-Class SVM, offer a promising alternative by learning individual activity patterns from fall-free data, enabling more adaptive and potentially lower-error detection, especially for users with atypical movement. When deployed on smartwatches, these models have the potential to enable private, real-time monitoring and support broader clinical use, particularly for people with disabilities and high-risk older adults, as they can be trained using only fall-free data.

5.4. Toward Inclusive and Scalable Fall Detection

To fully realize the potential of AI-driven fall detection systems in real-world healthcare, future research must prioritize inclusivity, personalization, and robust validation. This includes testing across diverse user populations, real-life environments, and longitudinal conditions, as well as integrating additional data sources (e.g., gyroscope, heart rate, contextual sensors). Additionally, explainability and user trust are critical, particularly when deploying these systems in vulnerable populations. The proposed 1SVM-based framework offers a foundation for such adaptable and ethically grounded systems by focusing on fall-free data and treating falls as anomalies, a paradigm well-suited to deployment in smartwatches and edge devices.

In summary, addressing current limitations in data diversity, personalization, and transparency is essential for advancing fall detection systems. Inclusive, adaptive approaches, especially when integrated into wearable platforms, hold promise for extending reliable monitoring to broader and more vulnerable populations.

6. CONCLUSION

This chapter presented a semi-supervised fall detection approach based on One-Class SVM using smartwatch accelerometric data. Unlike traditional supervised methods, the proposed model is trained solely on fall-free data, making it suitable for real-world deployment where labeled fall events are scarce or impractical to collect. Statistical features such as smoothed magnitude, min–max difference, and variance were extracted from segmented time windows to capture motion characteristics. Experimental results on the SmartFall dataset demonstrated that the 1SVM model achieved a balanced trade-off between detection accuracy and false alarm rate, outperforming traditional classifiers like kNN and Naive Bayes in terms of robustness and practicality. While deep learning methods achieved higher sensitivity, the 1SVM offered the advantage of low complexity, interpretability, and minimal false positives. Overall, this study highlights the effectiveness of anomaly detection techniques for wearable fall detection and opens the door to future enhancements through temporal modeling or hybrid learning schemes.

Beyond algorithmic performance, this work has the potential to contribute to the broader goal of inclusive and accessible health monitoring. Its semi-supervised design could offer greater adaptability to atypical or disability-related movement patterns, making it a promising option for individuals with Parkinson's disease, stroke, or mobility impairments. Future work should focus on validating the approach using more diverse and representative datasets (e.g., SisFall, URFD, UP-Fall and investigating model personalization strategies to improve robustness and user-specific accuracy across real-world settings. Moreover, integrating multimodal sensing through sensor fusion, combining accelerometer data with gyroscope, barometer, heart rate or contextual signals, could enhance robustness and reduce ambiguity in borderline events.

As a future direction, functional data analysis methods, such as the Magnitude–Shape (MS) Plot, could be applied to fall detection by modeling sensor signals as functional trajectories. The MS-Plot captures both magnitude deviations (e.g., sudden accelerations) and shape deviations (e.g., atypical postural transitions) (Wang et al., 2026), offering a statistically principled and interpretable framework that can enhance detection accuracy and explainability. Another promising direction is federated learning, which enables collaborative model training across distributed smartwatches without exchanging raw sensor data (Douaidi et al., 2023). Each device can locally train a 1SVM on fall-free accelerometric signals, capturing user-specific movement patterns. Only model updates are shared with a central aggregator, preserving data privacy while improving global generalization. Federated learning is particularly suited for real-world deployment, offering scalability, personalization, and compliance with ethical data-sharing practices in health monitoring applications.

REFERENCES

Alam, E., Abu Sufian, P. D., & Leo, M. (2022). Vision-based human fall detection systems using deep learning: A review. *Computers in Biology and Medicine*, *146*, 105626. DOI: 10.1016/j.compbiomed.2022.105626 PMID: 35680453

Bagala, F., Becker, C., Cappello, A., Chiari, L., Aminian, K., Hausdorff, J. M., Zijlstra, W., & Klenk, J. (2012). Evaluation of accelerometer-based fall detection algorithms on real-world falls. *PLoS One*, *7*(5), e37062. DOI: 10.1371/journal.pone.0037062 PMID: 22615890

Bui, T., Liu, J., Cao, J., Wei, G., & Zeng, Q. (2024). Elderly fall detection in complex environment based on improved YOLOv5s and LSTM. *Applied Sciences (Basel, Switzerland)*, *14*(19), 9028. DOI: 10.3390/app14199028

Casilari, E., & Oviedo-Jiménez, M. A. (2015). Automatic fall detection system based on the combined use of a smartphone and a smartwatch. *PLoS One*, *10*(11), e0140929. DOI: 10.1371/journal.pone.0140929 PMID: 26560737

Chelli, A., & Pätzold, M. (2019). A machine learning approach for fall detection and daily living activity recognition. *IEEE Access : Practical Innovations, Open Solutions*, *7*, 38670–38687. DOI: 10.1109/ACCESS.2019.2906693

Chen, S. H., Lee, C. H., Jiang, B. C., & Sun, T. L. (2021). Using a Stacked Autoencoder for Mobility and Fall Risk Assessment via Time–Frequency Representations of the Timed Up and Go Test. *Frontiers in Physiology*, *12*, 668350. DOI: 10.3389/fphys.2021.668350 PMID: 34122139

Douaidi, L., Senouci, S. M., El Korbi, I., & Harrou, F. 2023, June. Predicting electric vehicle charging stations occupancy: a federated deep learning framework. In *2023 IEEE 97th Vehicular Technology Conference (VTC2023-Spring)* (pp. 1-5). IEEE. DOI: 10.1109/VTC2023-Spring57618.2023.10199832

García-de-Villa, S., Ruiz, L. R., Neira, G. G. V., Álvarez, M. N., Huertas-Hoyas, E., Del-Ama, A. J., Rodriguez-Sanchez, M. C., Seco, F., & Jiménez, A. R. (2024). Validation of an IMU-based gait analysis method for assessment of fall risk against traditional methods. *IEEE Journal of Biomedical and Health Informatics*. PMID: 39074006

Gaya-Morey, F. X., Manresa-Yee, C., & Buades-Rubio, J. M. (2024). Deep learning for computer vision based activity recognition and fall detection of the elderly: A systematic review. *Applied Intelligence*, *54*(19), 8982–9007. DOI: 10.1007/s10489-024-05645-1

Godfrey, A., Hetherington, V., Shum, H., Bonato, P., Lovell, N. H., & Stuart, S. (2018). From A to Z: Wearable technology explained. *Maturitas*, *113*, 40–47. DOI: 10.1016/j.maturitas.2018.04.012 PMID: 29903647

Gutiérrez, J., Rodríguez, V., & Martin, S. (2021). Comprehensive review of vision-based fall detection systems. *Sensors (Basel)*, *21*(3), 947. DOI: 10.3390/s21030947 PMID: 33535373

Hakim, A., Huq, M. S., Shanta, S., & Ibrahim, B. S. K. K. (2017). Smartphone based data mining for fall detection: Analysis and design. *Procedia Computer Science*, *105*, 46–51. DOI: 10.1016/j.procs.2017.01.188

Harrou, F., Dairi, A., Taghezouit, B., & Sun, Y. (2019). An unsupervised monitoring procedure for detecting anomalies in photovoltaic systems using a one-class support vector machine. *Solar Energy*, *179*, 48–58. DOI: 10.1016/j.solener.2018.12.045

Harrou, F., Zerrouki, N., Sun, Y., & Houacine, A. (2017). Vision-based fall detection system for improving safety of elderly people. *IEEE Instrumentation & Measurement Magazine*, *20*(6), 49–55. DOI: 10.1109/MIM.2017.8121952

Hejazi, M., & Singh, Y. P. (2013). One-class support vector machines approach to anomaly detection. *Applied Artificial Intelligence*, *27*(5), 351–366. DOI: 10.1080/08839514.2013.785791

Hsu, W. L., Liu, J. X., Yang, C. C., & Leu, J. S. (2023). A fall detection system based on FMCW radar range-Doppler image and bi-LSTM deep learning. *IEEE Sensors Journal*, *23*(18), 22031–22039. DOI: 10.1109/JSEN.2023.3300994

Hu, X., Yu, S., Zheng, J., Fang, Z., Zhao, Z., & Qu, X. (2025). A hybrid CNN-LSTM model for involuntary fall detection using wrist-worn sensors. *Advanced Engineering Informatics*, *65*, 103178. DOI: 10.1016/j.aei.2025.103178

Hussain, F., Hussain, F., Ehatisham-ul-Haq, M., & Azam, M. A. (2019). Activity-aware fall detection and recognition based on wearable sensors. *IEEE Sensors Journal*, *19*(12), 4528–4536. DOI: 10.1109/JSEN.2019.2898891

Igual, R., Medrano, C., & Plaza, I. (2013). Challenges, issues and trends in fall detection systems. *Biomedical Engineering Online*, *12*(1), 66. DOI: 10.1186/1475-925X-12-66 PMID: 23829390

Kaur, A. P., Nsugbe, E., Drahota, A., Oldfield, M., Mohagheghian, I., & Sporea, R. A. (2025). State-of-the-Art Fall Detection Techniques with Emphasis on Floor-Based Systems–A Review. *Biomedical Engineering Advances*, *9*, 100179. DOI: 10.1016/j.bea.2025.100179

Khan, M. S., Yu, M., Feng, P., Wang, L., & Chambers, J. (2015). An unsupervised acoustic fall detection system using source separation for sound interference suppression. *Signal Processing*, *110*, 199–210. DOI: 10.1016/j.sigpro.2014.08.021

Khan, S. S., & Hoey, J. (2017). Review of fall detection techniques: A data availability perspective. *Medical Engineering & Physics*, *39*, 12–22. DOI: 10.1016/j.medengphy.2016.10.014 PMID: 27889391

Khojasteh, S. B., Villar, J. R., Chira, C., González, V. M., & de la Cal, E. (2018). Improving Fall Detection Using an On-Wrist Wearable Accelerometer. *Sensors (Basel)*, *18*(5), 1350. DOI: 10.3390/s18051350 PMID: 29701721

Kiran, S., Khan, M. A., Javed, M. Y., Alhaisoni, M., Tariq, U., Nam, Y., Damaševičius, R., & Sharif, M. (2021). Multi-layered deep learning features fusion for human action recognition. *Computers, Materials & Continua*, *69*(3), 4061–4075. DOI: 10.32604/cmc.2021.017800

Kwolek, B., & Kepski, M. (2014). Human fall detection on embedded platform using depth maps and wireless accelerometer. *Computer Methods and Programs in Biomedicine*, *117*(3), 489–501. DOI: 10.1016/j.cmpb.2014.09.005 PMID: 25308505

Kwolek, B., & Kepski, M. (2015). Improving fall detection by the use of depth sensor and accelerometer. *Neurocomputing*, *168*, 637–645. DOI: 10.1016/j.neucom.2015.05.061

Li, Y., Liu, P., Fang, Y., Wu, X., Xie, Y., Xu, Z., Ren, H., & Jing, F. (2025). A Decade of Progress in Wearable Sensors for Fall Detection (2015–2024): A Network-Based Visualization Review. *Sensors (Basel)*, *25*(7), 2205. DOI: 10.3390/s25072205 PMID: 40218718

Liu, J., Li, X., Huang, S., Chao, R., Cao, Z., Wang, S., Wang, A., & Liu, L. (2023). A review of wearable sensors based fall-related recognition systems. *Engineering Applications of Artificial Intelligence*, *121*, 105993. DOI: 10.1016/j.engappai.2023.105993

Liu, Y. H., Hung, P. C., Iqbal, F., & Fung, B. C. (2021). Automatic fall risk detection based on imbalanced data. *IEEE Access : Practical Innovations, Open Solutions*, *9*, 163594–163611. DOI: 10.1109/ACCESS.2021.3133297

Mahmud, T., Kayastha, R., Kisi, K., Ngu, A. H., & Alamgeer, S. (2025). Evaluating the Effectiveness of Plantar Pressure Sensors for Fall Detection in Sloped Surfaces. *Electronics (Basel)*, *14*(15), 3003. DOI: 10.3390/electronics14153003

Martínez-Villaseñor, L., Ponce, H., Brieva, J., Moya-Albor, E., Núñez-Martínez, J., & Peñafort-Asturiano, C. (2019). UP-fall detection dataset: A multimodal approach. *Sensors (Basel)*, *19*(9), 1988. DOI: 10.3390/s19091988 PMID: 31035377

Mauldin, T. R., Canby, M. E., Metsis, V., Ngu, A. H., & Rivera, C. C. (2018). SmartFall: A smartwatch-based fall detection system using deep learning. *Sensors (Basel), 18*(10), 3363. DOI: 10.3390/s18103363 PMID: 30304768

Mehta, V., Dhall, A., Pal, S., & Khan, S. S. (2021, January). Motion and region aware adversarial learning for fall detection with thermal imaging. In *2020 25th international conference on pattern recognition (ICPR)* (pp. 6321-6328). IEEE. DOI: 10.1109/ICPR48806.2021.9412632

Newaz, N. T., & Hanada, E. (2023). The methods of fall detection: A literature review. *Sensors (Basel), 23*(11), 5212. DOI: 10.3390/s23115212 PMID: 37299939

Noh, B., Youm, C., Goh, E., Lee, M., Park, H., Jeon, H., & Kim, O. Y. (2021). XGBoost based machine learning approach to predict the risk of fall in older adults using gait outcomes. *Scientific Reports, 11*(1), 12183. DOI: 10.1038/s41598-021-91797-w PMID: 34108595

Nooruddin, S., Islam, M. M., Sharna, F. A., Alhetari, H., & Kabir, M. N. (2022). Sensor-based fall detection systems: A review. *Journal of Ambient Intelligence and Humanized Computing, 13*(5), 2735–2751. DOI: 10.1007/s12652-021-03248-z

Özdemir, A. T., & Barshan, B. (2014). Detecting falls with wearable sensors using machine learning techniques. *Sensors (Basel), 14*(6), 10691–10708. DOI: 10.3390/s140610691 PMID: 24945676

Patel, S., Park, H., Bonato, P., Chan, L., & Rodgers, M. (2012). A review of wearable sensors and systems with application in rehabilitation. *Journal of Neuroengineering and Rehabilitation, 9*(1), 1–17. DOI: 10.1186/1743-0003-9-21 PMID: 22520559

Pierleoni, P., Belli, A., Palma, L., Pellegrini, M., Pernini, L., & Valenti, S. (2015). A high reliability wearable device for elderly fall detection. *IEEE Sensors Journal, 15*(8), 4544–4553. DOI: 10.1109/JSEN.2015.2423562

Popescu, M., Li, Y., Skubic, M., & Rantz, M. (2008, August). An acoustic fall detector system that uses sound height information to reduce the false alarm rate. In *2008 30th Annual International Conference of the IEEE Engineering in Medicine and Biology Society* (pp. 4628-4631). IEEE. DOI: 10.1109/IEMBS.2008.4650244

Rassekh, E., & Snidaro, L. (2025). Survey on data fusion approaches for fall-detection. *Information Fusion, 114*, 102696. DOI: 10.1016/j.inffus.2024.102696

Rastogi, S., & Singh, J. (2023). Performance enhancement of vision based fall detection using ensemble of machine learning model. *Cluster Computing, 26*(6), 4119–4132. DOI: 10.1007/s10586-022-03818-6

Schölkopf, B., Platt, J. C., Shawe-Taylor, J., Smola, A. J., & Williamson, R. C. (2001). Estimating the support of a high-dimensional distribution. *Neural Computation, 13*(7), 1443–1471. DOI: 10.1162/089976601750264965 PMID: 11440593

Şengül, G., Karakaya, M., Misra, S., Abayomi-Alli, O. O., & Damaševičius, R. (2022). Deep learning based fall detection using smartwatches for healthcare applications. *Biomedical Signal Processing and Control, 71*, 103242. DOI: 10.1016/j.bspc.2021.103242

Shrivastava, R., & Pandey, M. (2021). Ensemble of multiple classifiers for accelerometer based human fall detection. In *Computer Networks and Inventive Communication Technologies: Proceedings of Third ICCNCT 2020* (pp. 865-874). Singapore: Springer Nature Singapore. DOI: 10.1007/978-981-15-9647-6_67

Subburam, R., Chandralekha, E., & Kandasamy, V. (2024). An elderly fall detection system using enhanced random forest in machine learning. *Engineering Proceedings, 59*(1), 172.

Sucerquia, A., López, J. D., & Vargas-Bonilla, J. F. (2017). SisFall: A fall and movement dataset. *Sensors (Basel), 17*(1), 198. DOI: 10.3390/s17010198 PMID: 28117691

Tao, L., Volonakis, T., Tan, B., Jing, Y., Chetty, K., & Smith, M. (2018). Home activity monitoring using low resolution infrared sensor. *arXiv preprint arXiv:1811.05416.*

Theodoridis, T., Solachidis, V., Vretos, N., & Daras, P. (2017, November). Human fall detection from acceleration measurements using a recurrent neural network. In *International conference on biomedical and health informatics* (pp. 145-149). Singapore: Springer Singapore.

Tran, K. C., Gassi, M., Nehme, P., Rousseau, J., Nguyen, T. K., & Meunier, J. (2022, November). *Comparison of anomaly detection algorithms for near-fall detection with video surveillance. In 2022 E-Health and Bioengineering Conference (EHB) (pp. 01-04).* IEEE.

Usmani, S., Saboor, A., Haris, M., Khan, M. A., & Park, H. (2021). Latest research trends in fall detection and prevention using machine learning: A systematic review. *Sensors (Basel), 21*(15), 5134. DOI: 10.3390/s21155134 PMID: 34372371

Wang, S., Li, X., Liao, G., Liu, J., Liao, C., Liu, M., Liao, J., & Liu, L. (2024). A spatio-temporal graph neural network for fall prediction with inertial sensors. *Knowledge-Based Systems, 293*, 111709. DOI: 10.1016/j.knosys.2024.111709

Wang, X., Ellul, J., & Azzopardi, G. (2020). Elderly fall detection systems: A literature survey. *Frontiers in Robotics and AI*, *7*, 71. DOI: 10.3389/frobt.2020.00071 PMID: 33501238

Wang, Z., Harrou, F., Sun, Y., & Genton, M. G. (2026). Exploring the magnitude-shape plot framework for anomaly detection in crowded video scenes. In *AI-Based Solutions for Engineering* (pp. 137–174). IGI Global Scientific Publishing.

Yu, X., Wan, J., An, G., Yin, X., & Xiong, S. (2024). A novel semi-supervised model for pre-impact fall detection with limited fall data. *Engineering Applications of Artificial Intelligence*, *132*, 108469. DOI: 10.1016/j.engappai.2024.108469

Yu, X., Wang, C., Wu, W., & Xiong, S. (2025). A real-time skeleton-based fall detection algorithm based on temporal convolutional networks and transformer encoder. *Pervasive and Mobile Computing*, *107*, 102016. DOI: 10.1016/j.pmcj.2025.102016

Zerrouki, N., Harrou, F., Houacine, A., & Sun, Y. (2016, November). Fall detection using supervised machine learning algorithms: A comparative study. In *2016 8th international conference on modelling, identification and control (ICMIC)* (pp. 665-670). IEEE. DOI: 10.1109/ICMIC.2016.7804195

Zerrouki, N., Harrou, F., Sun, Y., Ait Djafer, A. Z., & Amrane, H. (2022, September). A survey on recent advances in fall detection systems using machine learning formalisms. In *2022 7th International Conference on Frontiers of Signal Processing (ICFSP)* (pp. 35-39). IEEE. DOI: 10.1109/ICFSP55781.2022.9924708

Zerrouki, N., Harrou, F., Sun, Y., & Houacine, A. (2016). Accelerometer and camera-based strategy for improved human fall detection. *Journal of Medical Systems*, *40*(12), 284. DOI: 10.1007/s10916-016-0639-6 PMID: 27796842

Zerrouki, N., Harrou, F., Sun, Y., & Houacine, A. (2016). A data-driven monitoring technique for enhanced fall events detection. *IFAC-PapersOnLine*, *49*(5), 333–338. DOI: 10.1016/j.ifacol.2016.07.135

Zerrouki, Y., Harrou, F., Zerrouki, N., Dairi, A., & Sun, Y. (2020). Desertification detection using an improved variational autoencoder-based approach through ETM-landsat satellite data. *IEEE Journal of Selected Topics in Applied Earth Observations and Remote Sensing*, *14*, 202–213. DOI: 10.1109/JSTARS.2020.3042760

Chapter 7
Evolving Approaches to Static American Sign Language Fingerspelling Recognition

Ajay Menon
https://orcid.org/0009-0004-7476-7842
School of Mathematical and Computer Sciences, Heriot Watt University, Dubai, UAE

Mahmoud A. A. Mousa
https://orcid.org/0009-0007-2415-5655
School of Mathematical and Computer Sciences, Heriot Watt University, Dubai, UAE

ABSTRACT

This review synthesizes research on static American Sign Language (ASL) alphabet recognition from images, comparing traditional machine learning pipelines, convolutional neural network (CNN) transfer learning, and hybrid or transformer-based models. The analysis spans 2016 to 2025 studies that detail preprocessing, model design, and quantitative results on datasets such as the ASL Alphabet and Sign Language MNIST. Classical approaches using engineered features with classifiers such as Support Vector Machines (SVMs) or Random Forests perform well in controlled settings but rely on robust segmentation and handcrafted descriptors. Transfer learning on CNN backbones, including MobileNetV2, ResNet, EfficientNet, DenseNet, and the Visual Geometry Group (VGG) models, achieves near-perfect within-dataset accuracy; pure and modified Vision Transformers (ViTs)

DOI: 10.4018/979-8-3373-2033-5.ch007

and CNN–transformer hybrids also reach ceiling-level performance with favorable speed-to-accuracy tradeoffs. Most evaluations remain closed set and seldom report signer-independent splits, cross-dataset transfer, or deployment metrics.

INTRODUCTION

Hearing loss is a large and growing public health challenge with direct implications for communication access and equity. The World Health Organization (WHO) reports that more than 5% of the world's population, or about 430 million people, require rehabilitation for disabling hearing loss. By 2050, nearly 2.5 billion individuals are projected to be affected, including more than 700 million who will need rehabilitation. The annual global cost of unaddressed hearing loss approaches one trillion US dollars. In addition, over one billion young adults remain at risk due to unsafe listening practices (WHO, 2025). In parallel, disability affects an estimated 1.3 billion people worldwide, or roughly one in six, underscoring the systemic nature of access barriers in health, education, and employment (WHO, 2023b).

For deaf communities, timely access to information and services in sign language remains uneven despite international commitments to inclusion. The World Federation of the Deaf (WFD) reports that only about 41.5 percent of countries legally recognize their national sign languages, even as the global deaf population is often cited at roughly 70 million across more than 200 distinct sign languages (Dsane, 2024; WFD, 2025). Accessibility is integral to health information ecosystems and public communication, not peripheral accommodation, which places a premium on technologies that can bridge language and modality gaps at scale (WHO, 2023a). Within this context, automated recognition of signed alphabets offers a pragmatic entry point for communication aids, educational tools, and user interfaces, if models are accurate, efficient, and robust beyond laboratory conditions.

This review focuses on a small but important part of the landscape: static American Sign Language (ASL) alphabet recognition from images. The scope excludes temporal modeling of dynamic letters and continuous signing to examine, with greater depth, how current methods handle data curation and preprocessing, feature extraction, architecture choice, training protocols, and evaluation on static benchmarks. The aim is to synthesize what works, where, and at what computational cost, while making explicit the assumptions that underline near-ceiling results on curated datasets. The specific objectives are to compare traditional machine learning pipelines against transfer-learned convolutional neural network (CNN) models, hybrid CNN–transformer designs, and pure and modified transformer approaches; to align reported accuracies with dataset characteristics and splits; to identify gaps in signer diversity, cross-dataset validation, fairness, and deployment metrics; and to motivate a research agenda that shifts from incremental accuracy gains toward generalization, transparency, and real-world usability within static ASL applications.

METHODOLOGY OF REVIEW

This review followed the principles of systematic evidence synthesis as outlined in the Preferred Reporting Items for Systematic Reviews and Meta-Analyses (PRISMA). The time span of 2016 to 2025 was selected because it coincides with the rapid adoption of deep learning architectures for computer vision tasks, marking a methodological transition from handcrafted features to convolutional and transformer-based approaches. Literature prior to 2016 rarely employed modern deep models for sign recognition, whereas studies published after 2016 increasingly reported state-of-the-art architectures and benchmarks for static American Sign Language, establishing a coherent body of work for comparative analysis. The cut-off in 2025 ensures contemporaneity.

Peer-reviewed journal articles and reputable conference proceedings were identified through searches in databases such as IEEE Xplore, ACM Digital Library, SpringerLink, ScienceDirect, and MDPI, complemented by Google Scholar to capture additional relevant studies. Search strings combined keywords including "American Sign Language," "fingerspelling," "static," "alphabet," "CNN," "transfer learning," "transformer," and "gesture recognition." The initial set of records was screened at the title and abstract level, with duplicates removed and irrelevant items discarded. Full texts were then assessed for eligibility using explicit inclusion and exclusion criteria.

Studies were included if they reported static American Sign Language alphabet recognition from still images, provided details of preprocessing or feature extraction, specified the model architecture, and presented quantitative results with dataset size and class distribution. Exclusion criteria ruled out work on dynamic or continuous signing, temporal video models, non-ASL alphabets without ASL relevance, hardware or interface systems without a core recognition pipeline, and gesture datasets unrelated to ASL fingerspelling.

The final set of eligible studies was organized into three methodological categories, classical machine learning, convolutional (CNN) transfer learning, and hybrid or transformer-based models allowing like-for-like comparison across consistent dimensions of preprocessing, architecture, evaluation, and reported outcomes. This structured approach supports transparency in study selection and comparability of findings, consistent with PRISMA guidance.

BACKGROUND: PRINCIPLES OF STATIC ASL RECOGNITION

Alphabet Scope and Task Definition

Static ASL recognition focuses on images of handshapes that correspond to the 26 letters of the alphabet. In most benchmark datasets, the scope is narrowed to 24 letters, since the characters J and Z involve motion and therefore require temporal modeling rather than static classification. Their dynamic nature means that a purely image-based system cannot fully capture the trajectory or movement cues necessary for accurate recognition, which explains their exclusion in many studies. However, a few datasets and experimental setups incorporate static approximations of these dynamic letters by assigning a fixed representative posture. While this allows the entire alphabet to be addressed within a static framework, such representations are necessarily limited because they compress inherently temporal gestures into single frames. Beyond these issues, some datasets extend the recognition task to include control tokens such as space, delete, and nothing, yielding a total of 29 classes, while others add single-digit numerals (0–9), expanding the classification space to 36 categories. Across these variations, the common goal remains closed-set classification of handshapes under differing capture conditions, with the recognition scope shaped by whether or not dynamic letters are approximated in static form (Abu-Jamie & Abu-Naser, 2022; Cayamcela & Lim, 2019; Dabwan et al., 2024; Kumari & Anand, 2023).

Image Acquisition and Normalization

Pipelines begin with camera capture or utilize existing ASL datasets, then normalize inputs to reduce nuisance variation. Common steps include hand region localization or cropping, intensity and colour normalization, resizing to a fixed input (for example 28×28 for MNIST-style or 224×224 for CNN backbones), and optional background suppression. Robust systems aim for invariance to illumination, skin tone, scale, rotation, and viewpoint within a practical range (Cayamcela & Lim, 2019; Kumari & Anand, 2023; Pan et al., 2016; Qin & Wang, 2025; Tan, Lim, Lee, et al., 2023).

Representation of the Hand

Two broad strategies are used. Appearance-based methods operate directly on pixels and learn features end to end, as in transfer-learned CNNs and transformers. (Alsharif et al., 2023; Cayamcela & Lim, 2019; Dabwan et al., 2023; Lum et al., 2020; Tan, Lim, Chang, et al., 2023). Geometry based methods derive structured cues such as key points, contours, or shape descriptors, which can be more lightweight but may discard fine texture (Devi et al., 2023; Pan et al., 2016). Hybrid designs concatenate learned features with handcrafted descriptors to capture both local shape and global context (Killari, 2022; Kumari & Anand, 2023).

Learning Paradigms

Traditional machine learning applies classifiers like SVMs or Random Forests to extracted or engineered features after dimensionality reduction (Dayalan et al., 2025; Devi et al., 2023; Killari, 2022; Pan et al., 2016). Modern approaches skip the need of manual feature extraction or engineering and fine tune pretrained CNNs or transformers, replacing the final layer with a task specific head (Alsharif et al., 2023; Aly & Fathi, 2025; Cayamcela & Lim, 2019; Dabwan et al., 2024; Mousa et al., 2024; Dabwan et al., 2023; Lum et al., 2020; Tan, Lim, Lee, et al., 2023; Ismail & Mousa 2025). Attention modules can emphasize salient hand regions and suppress background patterns (Kumari & Anand, 2023; Qin & Wang, 2025; Tan, Lim, Chang, et al., 2023).

Training and Evaluation

Data augmentation, for example flips, rotations, and translations, improves generalization. Sound evaluation reports the class set, split protocol, and metrics such as accuracy, precision, recall, and F1. Signer-independent splits and cross-dataset tests provide stronger evidence of robustness than random holds.

Practical Considerations

Latency, memory, and energy budgets matter for on-device use. Fairness requires attention to demographic diversity, varied lighting and backgrounds, occlusion, and left-handed signing. These principles frame the comparative analyses in the following sections.

SURVEY OF METHODS

Traditional Machine Learning Algorithms

This subsection surveys three representative studies that exemplify classical computer vision pipelines for static fingerspelling recognition. These works were selected because they provide explicit pipelines involving preprocessing, handcrafted or geometric features, and non-deep classifiers, and because they represent some of the few contributions that focus specifically on static American Sign Language (ASL) alphabets. Very limited research in this area has relied on traditional machine learning, as most efforts since 2016 have shifted toward convolutional and transformer-based deep models. The following studies, therefore, serve as important benchmarks in demonstrating the strengths and shortcomings of classical approaches.

Pan et al. (2016) developed a real-time ASL alphabet recognition system for cluttered backgrounds, where segmentation quality is critical. Their pipeline selects stable video frames, applies adaptive skin-color modeling and morphological operations to extract hand masks, and computes composite features using SIFT, Hu moments, and Fourier descriptors. These features capture both local and global hand characteristics to reduce confusion among similar letters. Classification is performed hierarchically using PCA, LDA, and linear SVMs, with confusion-prone subsets isolated prior to making final decisions. Figure 1 illustrates the full pipeline.

Implemented using OpenCV and LibSVM for real-time performance, the method achieved 99.8% accuracy on a 7,800-image Chinese Sign Language dataset and 94% on the public ASL dataset by Barczak. Its strengths include robustness in complex backgrounds and a stacked PCA–LDA–SVM pipeline for handling confusable classes. However, it relies heavily on skin-based segmentation, which is sensitive to lighting and skin tone, and on handcrafted features that limit adaptability. The system was not tested in real-world settings, leaving usability unassessed.

Figure 1. Proposed Pipeline

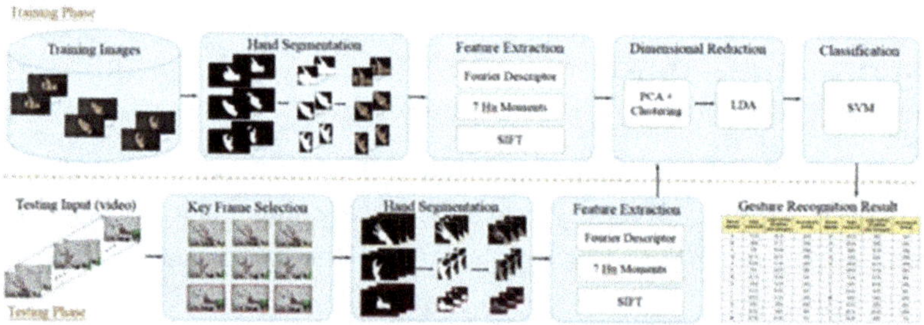

(Pan et al., 2016)

Devi et al. (2023) introduced a survey-style ASL recognition system combining a classical machine learning pipeline with a simple user interface. The system uses MediaPipe hand keypoints as features, capturing finger and palm geometry while discarding appearance, which improves robustness to lighting and background clutter. The workflow includes data loading, preprocessing, model training/testing, and interactive experimentation. Three classifiers—SVM, Random Forest, and k-NN—are compared using precision, recall, and F1 score, with model choice depending on the setting. Figure 2 illustrates the proposed pipeline.

Figure 2. Proposed Pipeline

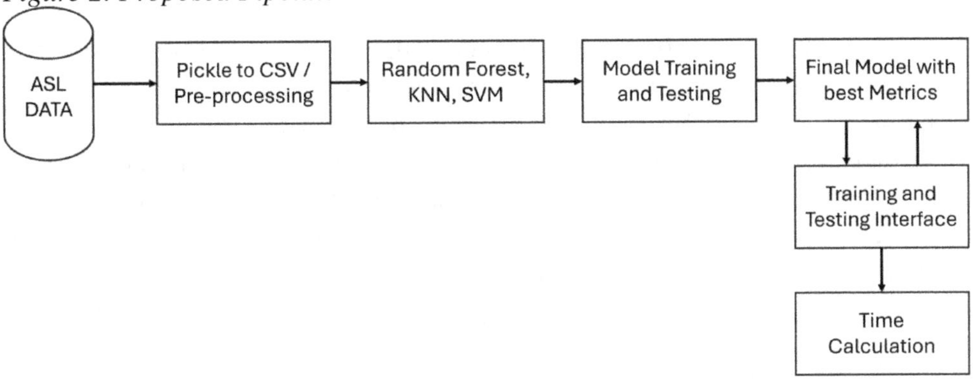

(Devi et al., 2023)

Consistent with its survey and tooling orientation rather than a dataset benchmarking focus, the paper does not commit to a single headline accuracy number in the material at hand (Devi et al., 2023). The advantages are clear for educational or prototyping contexts because the keypoint abstraction is easy to deploy and interpret and it decouples recognition from raw pixels, while the limitations stem from the same abstraction, since success depends on reliable keypoint detection and the loss of appearance cues can hamper discrimination among confusable handshapes or under occlusion and extreme hand poses. As with Pan et al. (2016), this system remains untested in practical deployment scenarios.

Dayalan et al. (2025) proposed a lightweight, real-time ASL fingerspelling system using live camera input. Their curated dataset includes approximately100 images per sign under uniform lighting and background. Preprocessing with OpenCV denoises and standardizes inputs, followed by manual landmark-style feature extraction to encode finger configurations. A Random Forest classifier is used for its efficiency and suitability for small, heterogeneous datasets. The pipeline flows from camera input to OpenCV preprocessing to Random Forest prediction. The system reports 98.8% accuracy, emphasizing ease of deployment and interpretability. However, its controlled data collection, handcrafted features, and lack of cross-dataset validation raise concerns about robustness in diverse real-world conditions.

Taken together, these three studies illustrate how traditional machine learning pipelines for static ASL recognition can achieve strong results under controlled conditions and modest data sizes, but also why they remain limited in scalability and robustness compared to deep learning alternatives which will be discussed in further sections. Table 1 summarizes the main contrasts in scope, features, model choices, datasets, and outcomes.

Critical Analysis

As shown in Table 1, the reviewed studies illustrate key trade-offs inherent in traditional ASL fingerspelling recognition pipelines. In scenarios with complex backgrounds, such as Pan et al. (2016), high recognition accuracy is achieved through precise segmentation and layered feature extraction, though generalization to external datasets remains limited. For low-latency applications on controlled datasets, Dayalan et al. (2025) demonstrate that compact feature representations combined with Random Forest classifiers can yield strong performance, albeit with uncertain robustness due to the absence of cross-dataset validation. In contrast, Devi et al. (2023) prioritize usability and interpretability by employing keypoint-based features and standard classifiers, offering a lightweight solution suitable for training and demonstration purposes, though with constrained accuracy compared to end-to-end deep learning approaches.

Table 1. Comparing Methodologies and Results of Studies Used Traditional Machine Learning Approaches

Study	Scope & Features	Model & Dataset	Classes & Performance	Noted limitations
Pan et al. (2016)	Real-time ASL alphabet recognition using SIFT, Hu moments, and Fourier descriptors in complex backgrounds	Hierarchical SVM on ASL Barczak public dataset	26 letters; 94% accuracy	Sensitive to lighting and skin tone; relies on handcrafted features
Devi et al. (2023)	ASL survey and training tool using MediaPipe hand keypoints	SVM, RF, k-NN on prototype (non-benchmark) dataset	36 (letters + digits); no definitive accuracy	Depends on keypoint reliability; lacks appearance cues
Dayalan et al. (2025)	Real-time ASL letters and numerals using OpenCV-based manual landmark cues under controlled conditions	Random Forest on curated dataset (~100 images/sign)	36 (letters + digits); 98.8% accuracy	Limited environmental diversity, no cross-dataset validation.

Despite the strengths demonstrated across the three studies, several critical limitations remain. None of the works conduct cross-dataset evaluations, signer-independent splits, or experiments in uncontrolled environments, leaving unresolved questions regarding robustness to variations in illumination, background clutter, camera hardware, and signer diversity. Additionally, performance reporting is often limited to aggregate metrics such as overall accuracy or precision, with insufficient attention to macro-averaged F1 scores, per-class confusion analysis, calibration error, or stress testing under adverse conditions. To improve the evidentiary rigor of future traditional pipelines, we recommend the adoption of standardized evaluation protocols that include cross-dataset transfer tests, signer-independent splits, mandatory reporting of macro F1 scores with per-class breakdowns and calibration metrics, and device-level assessments of latency, memory usage, and energy consumption on representative edge hardware. Furthermore, fairness audits across skin tones, lighting conditions, and capture devices should be incorporated to ensure equitable performance.

Key takeaways: Traditional pipelines demonstrate strong performance on curated datasets and offer advantages for lightweight deployment. However, their generalizability and readiness for real-world applications remain insufficiently evidenced. To advance their practical utility, future evaluations should incorporate standardized protocols, fairness-aware metrics, and deployment-oriented benchmarks.

The following section explores convolutional neural networks and transfer learning approaches, which have gained prominence since 2016. These methods reduce reliance on handcrafted segmentation and feature engineering by learning discriminative representations directly from raw pixel data, and have become the dominant paradigm for static ASL recognition within closed datasets.

CNNs and Transfer Learning Methods

This subsection reviews nine studies that employed convolutional neural networks and transfer learning techniques for ASL fingerspelling recognition. Unlike classical approaches that rely on handcrafted descriptors, these methods leverage ImageNet-pretrained backbones and incorporate attention mechanisms or short-term fusion blocks to learn discriminative features directly from pixel data. This shift has led to consistent improvements in within-dataset performance and marks a transition toward more scalable and data-driven recognition pipelines.

Cayamcela and Lim (2019)) applied transfer learning with AlexNet and GoogLeNet for real-time ASL alphabet recognition using a 78,000-image dataset across 26 classes. They replaced the original fully connected heads with a new 26-way classifier and fine-tuned the model at a small learning rate while freezing early layers. Images were resized (227×227 for AlexNet, 224×224 for GoogLeNet) and augmented with flips and ±30-pixel shifts. AlexNet achieved 99.39% accuracy and converged faster than GoogLeNet (95.52%). The study lacked cross-dataset and signer-diversity evaluation.

Lum et al. (2020) adapted MobileNetV2 for mobile-friendly ASL recognition using 87,000 RGB images across 29 classes. Inputs were resized to 224×224 and split 80/20 without augmentation. The model used ImageNet-pretrained MobileNetV2, followed by average pooling, a 1000-unit ReLU layer, 0.5 dropout, and a 29-class SoftMax output. The model achieved 98.67% accuracy and was optimized for on-device use.

Abu-Jamie and Abu-Naser (2022) fine-tuned VGG16 on the ASL Alphabet dataset, emphasizing evaluation protocols alongside accuracy. From ~87,000 images across 29 classes, they subsampled 43,500, resized to 64×64, and split 70/15/15 for training, validation, and testing. Due to variability across runs, they adopted k-fold validation and reported 100% test accuracy at epoch 20, supported by performance curves and a confusion matrix. While the protocol is clear and reproducible, the high accuracy may reflect overfitting or dataset simplicity, and the heavy backbone limits suitability for edge deployment.

Ma, Xu and Kim (2022) proposed a Two Stream Mixed CNN architecture that integrates short-term temporal cues by fusing features from two consecutive frames. As depicted in Figure 3, a fusion block combines and concatenates these features before passing them to a backbone network, enabling improved alphabet recognition from static image sequences.

Figure 3. Two Stream Mixed Convolutional Architecture

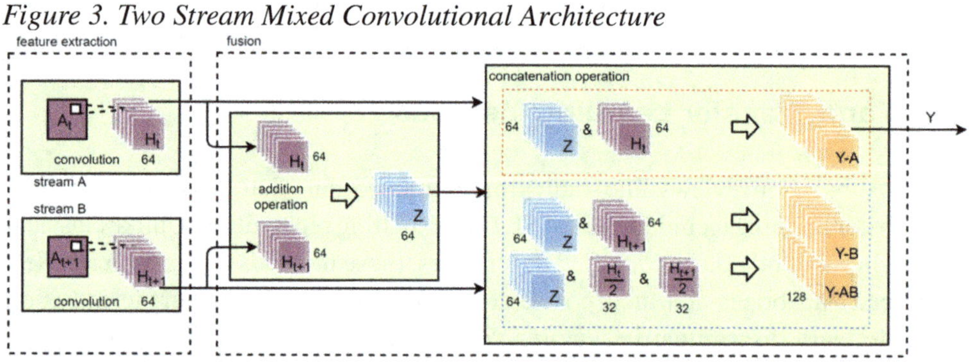

(Ma, Xu, & Kim, 2022)

Ma, Xu, and Kim (2022) evaluated Two Stream Mixed (TSM) architectures (as shown in Figure 4) using LeNet, AlexNet, ResNet18, and ResNet50 on the ASL Alphabet dataset (87,000 images, 29 classes). Preprocessing involved resizing camera images (250×250) to 229×229 for LeNet/AlexNet and 226×226 for ResNet18 and ResNet50, followed by grayscale normalization and augmentation (±10% translation, 10% scaling, and up to 45° rotation). The dataset was split 85/15 for training and validation. TSM-ResNet50 achieved the highest accuracy (97.57%). While effective, the two-frame design increased computational cost and required precise frame timing. Limitations included absence of cross-corpus validation, real-world testing, and unconstrained camera motion.

Figure 4. Proposed Methodology

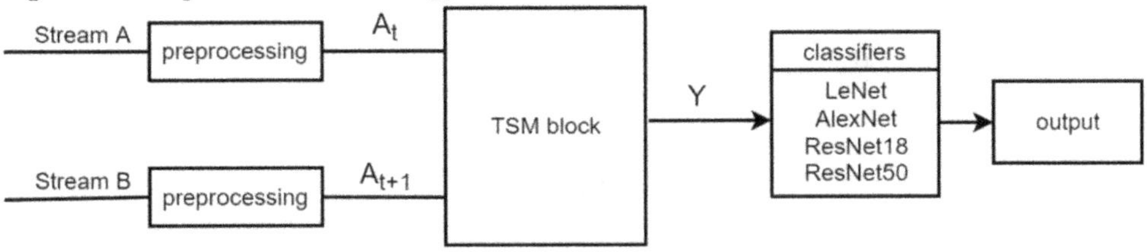

(Ma, Xu, & Kim, 2022)

Ma, Xu, Han, et al. (2022) proposed an ensemble transfer-learning framework for static ASL recognition using fine-tuned CNNs—LeNet, AlexNet, GoogLeNet, VGGNet, and ResNet—on the ASL Alphabet and ASLA datasets. Preprocessed inputs were grayscale-normalized, median-filtered, and resized (227×227 for LeNet/AlexNet, 224×224 for others). As shown in Figure 5, each model generated class probabilities, which were aggregated using an accuracy-based weighted voting rule. This rule assigned per-class weights to each CNN's output, optimized via two hyperparameters to balance classification accuracy and inference time. The final configuration outperformed SVM, Random Forest, AdaBoost, and soft voting baselines, achieving 98.83% and 98.79% accuracy on ASL Alphabet and ASLA, respectively. Strengths include backbone diversity and robust late fusion; limitations include within-dataset evaluation, lack of signer-independence, and increased pipeline complexity.

Figure 5. Proposed Framework

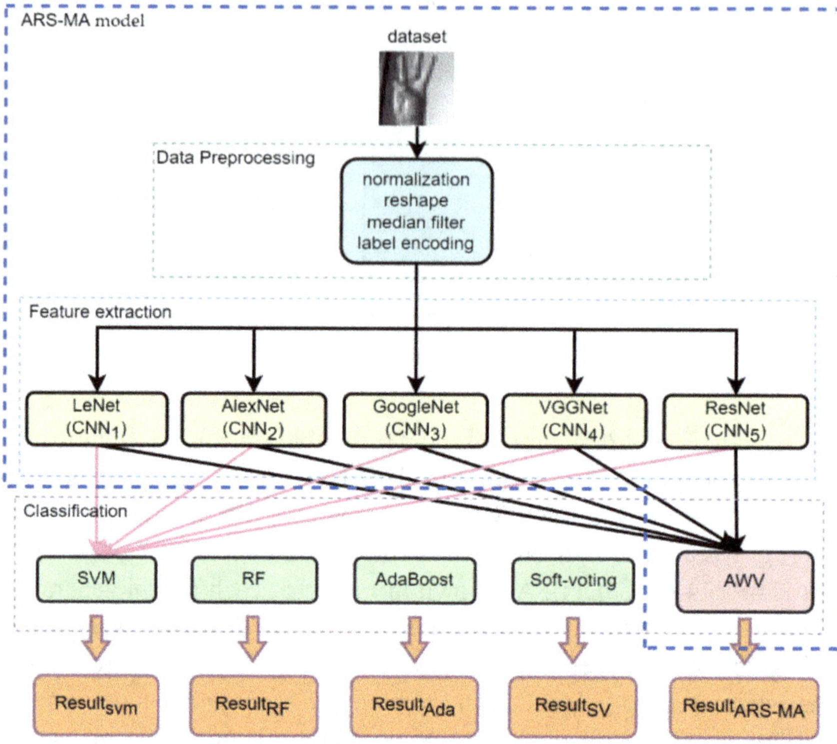

(Ma, Xu, Han, et al., 2022,)

Dabwan et al. (2023) evaluated VGG16 and VGG19 as baseline models for static ASL recognition using the Sign Language MNIST dataset, which comprises 28×28 grayscale images of 24 letters (excluding J and Z due to motion requirements). Inputs were normalized by a factor of 1/255 and split into standard training (27,455 images) and test (7,172 images) sets, approximating an 80/20 ratio. The authors fine-tuned the classification heads for 24-way recognition, reporting 97.5% accuracy for VGG16 and 96% for VGG19, along with precision, recall, and F1 scores. While the study offers a clear transfer-learning benchmark, it lacks cross-dataset validation and real-world testing, limiting its generalizability (Dabwan et al., 2023).

Kumari and Anand (2023) proposed a hybrid framework combining handcrafted and deep features for static ASL and ISL recognition. Inputs were resized to 128×128 and normalized; Histogram of Oriented Gradients (HOG) descriptors were computed using 8×8 cells and flattened into a vector. These features were concatenated with those extracted by a Convolutional Block Attention Module (CBAM)-enhanced CNN, designed to capture both fine-grained shape information and higher-level spatial context, as illustrated in Figure 6. The classifier comprised dense layers (300 and

150 units), L2 regularization, 0.5 dropout, and a SoftMax over 36 classes (digits 0–9 and all alphabets), illustrated in Figure 7. Evaluations on the Massey ASL and a static ISL dataset yielded 99.22% and 99.79% accuracy, respectively. The fusion of shape-driven and learned features improved fine-grained orientation recognition, though it increased feature dimensionality and computational cost. Additionally, the curated, static datasets limit conclusions about robustness in real-world conditions (Kumari & Anand, 2023).

Figure 6. Convolutional Block Attention Module Architecture

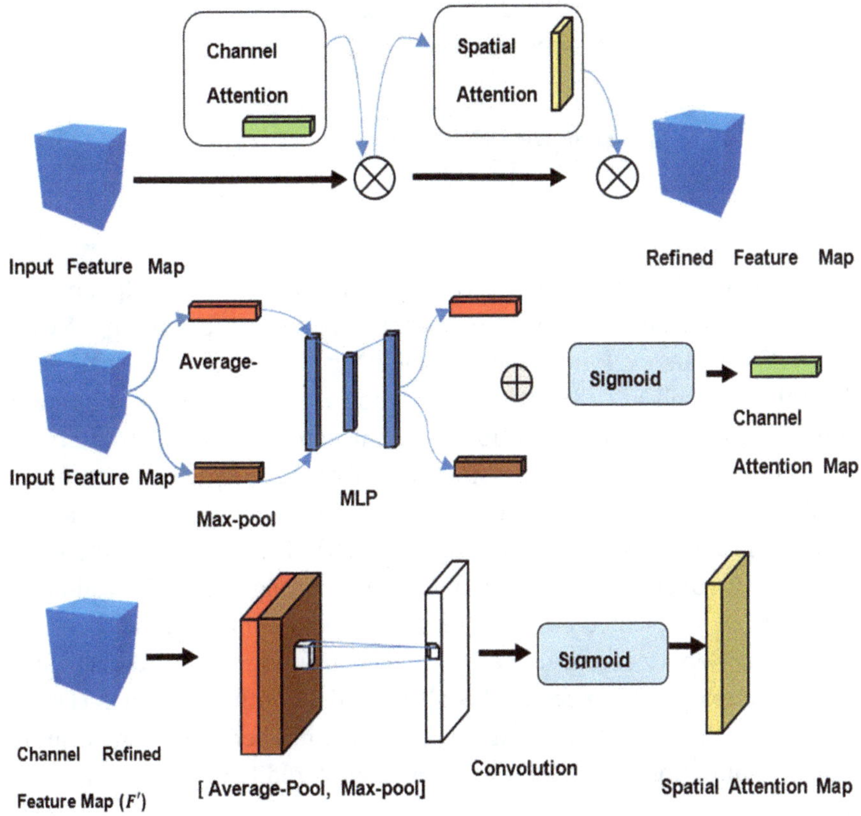

(Kumari & Anand, 2023)

Figure 7. Proposed Framework

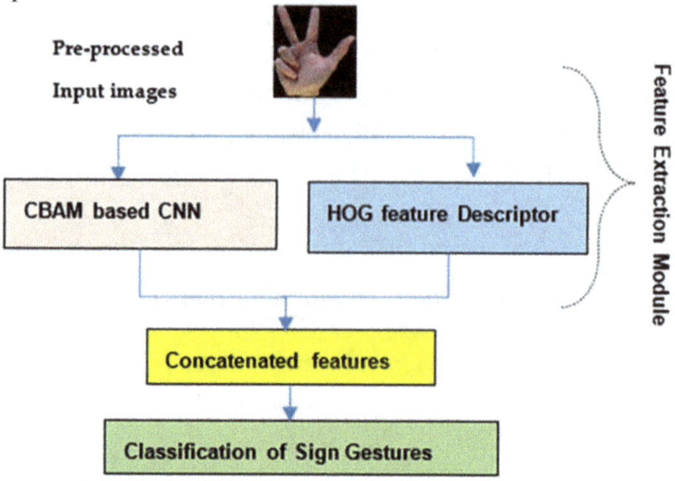

(Kumari & Anand, 2023)

Alsharif et al. (2023) compared five models on the ASL Alphabet dataset (>87,000 images, 29 classes) using consistent resizing and fine-tuning. ResNet-50 led with 99.98% accuracy, followed by EfficientNet (99.95%), ConvNeXt (99.51%), AlexNet (99.50%), and ViT (88.59%). The authors noted that resizing choices likely disadvantaged the transformer, cautioning against architectural over interpretation when input resolution and preprocessing differ from recommended settings.

In a follow-on study, Dabwan et al. (2024) proposed a DenseNet121 classifier for static ASL handshapes using a Sign Language MNIST-style split adapted for color inputs while still covering 24 letters with 27,455 training and 7,172 validation/test images. Inputs were rescaled by 1/255, and the model employed four dense blocks with a new head. Reported metrics were 97 percent training and 96 percent validation accuracy, accompanied by precision/recall/F1 and a confusion matrix (Dabwan et al., 2024). As with many static image evaluations, neither latency measurements, cross-dataset validation, nor generalization to cluttered backgrounds was directly assessed the study.

Extending toward real-time detection-oriented architectures, Elgohr et al. (2025) introduce a YOLOv11-based deep learning system designed for real-time recognition of American Sign Language (ASL), focusing on both alphabetic and transactional hand gestures. The proposed model employed a robust pipeline that included advanced data preprocessing and augmentation techniques, along with an optimized YOLOv11 architecture featuring enhanced components for feature extraction and classification. Training was refined using the AdamW optimizer and a composite loss function, resulting in high performance metrics – 95.4% precision, 94.8% recall, and 98.1% mean Average Precision (mAP) (Elgohr et al., 2025). The integration of GRAD-CAM and occlusion sensitivity further improved model interpretability.

Focusing on background robustness with minimal preprocessing, Qin and Wang (2025) proposed a dual channel star attention CNN that explicitly strengthens gesture features while suppressing background structure before fusion and classification over 24 static letters. Inputs were resized to 28 by 28 pixels and normalized to keep the pipeline lightweight. One channel focuses on enhancing the hand region through learned element wise weights, while the second channel attenuates background. A star attention mechanism aggregated and fused the two streams before the classifier. On an ASL finger spelling dataset the model achieved 99.81 percent accuracy, and the authors also reported strong results on an ISL benchmark (Qin & Wang, 2025). The design is promising for real time settings, although the low input resolution and static imagery may discard fine finger cues and the study does not present cross-dataset, signer-independent or real-world tests.

Finally, Hariharan et al. (2025) presented a modified deep residual CNN for static ASL that integrates an edge-aware segmentation stage with a streamlined ResNet-101 classifier. Images depicting 36 classes comprising digits 0 to 9 and letters A to Z are preprocessed with Gaussian filtering, contrast enhancement, histogram equalization, and averaging to denoise and standardize appearance, then segmented using a modified Canny Edge Detector that applied weighted least squares gradient estimation, non-maximum suppression, dual thresholds, and edge tracking to remove weak edges before classification. The classifier adapted ResNet-101 by reducing filters and residual blocks, inserting max pooling before convolutional blocks, and removing intermediate ReLU operations to lower complexity while retaining representational depth; the paper noted ImageNet pretraining as a basis for the architecture (Hariharan et al., 2025). Experiments on Kaggle ASL image set totalling 25,291 samples with an 80 to 20 train-to-test split reported 97% accuracy with a false positive rate of 0.05 percent, sensitivity of 0.90, specificity of 0.92, precision of 0.94, and F1 of 0.90, and comparisons indicated ResNet-101 outperforms ResNet-50 at 90% and ResNet-18 at 79% under the same pipeline (Hariharan et al., 2025). Training time was higher for the deeper model, but test time was similar across baselines, supporting the claimed accuracy to efficiency balance; strengths include explicit edge based segmentation coupled with a deep residual classifier that maintains performance while trimming parameters, whereas limitations included evaluation on a single curated dataset without signer-independent, cross-corpus or real-world tests, and reliance on a multi-step preprocessing chain that may be brittle under illumination change and background clutter.

Collectively, these studies documented the maturation of CNN-based and related architectures for static ASL alphabets, from early transfer-learned backbones to ensemble fusion, attention-augmented hybrids, dense-connectivity models, and detector-style pipelines. Most report excellent within-dataset accuracy on curated corpora, detailed preprocessing choices, and clear architectural descriptions that together chart the evolution of static ASL recognition during 2016–2025. Table 2 summarizes the main contrasts in scope, features, model choices, datasets, and outcomes.

Table 2. Comparing Methodologies and Results of Studies Using CNN-based Transfer Learning Approach

Study	Dataset and scope	Input and preprocessing	Backbone and head	Reported performance (Accuracy)	Notes and limitations
Cayamcela and Lim (2019)	Custom ASL; ~78,000 RGB; 26 classes	Resize: 227×227 (AlexNet), 224×224 (GoogLeNet); flips; ±30px translations	AlexNet, GoogLeNet; new 26-way softmax; frozen early layers	99.39% (AlexNet); 95.52% (GoogLeNet)	Transfer learning gains; only two backbones; no cross-dataset or signer diversity
Lum et al. (2020)	ASL Alphabet; ~87,000 RGB; 29 classes (letters + controls)	224×224; normalized; 80/20 split; no augmentation	MobileNetV2; avg pooling, dense 1000 (ReLU), dropout 0.5, softmax	98.67%	Mobile-friendly; single corpus; no latency or cross-dataset tests
Abu-Jamie and Abu-Naser (2022)	ASL Alphabet; 43,500 subsampled from ~87,000; static; 29 (letters + controls)	64×64 crops; 70/15/15 train/ validation/test; k-fold favored over single holdout	VGG16 fine-tuned	100% at epoch 20	Possible overfitting; heavy model; no cross-corpus testing
Ma, Xu and Kim (2022)	ASL Alphabet; 87,000; 29 classes; two-frame fusion	Original: 250×250; Resize: 229×229 (LeNet/AlexNet), 226×226 (ResNet); grayscale; rotation ≤45°, scale ±10%, translation ±10%	Two-Stream Mixed with LeNet, AlexNet, ResNet18/50	Best: 97.57% (TSM-ResNet50)	Higher compute; frame timing sensitive; no cross-corpus or motion testing
Ma, Xu, Han, et al. (2022)	ASL Alphabet: 29 classes, 200×200 RGB, 3,000/class; ASLA: 29 classes, 400×400 RGB, 7,000/ class;	Grayscale; median filter; resize: 227×227 (LeNet/ AlexNet), 224×224 (others)	Modified LeNet, AlexNet, GoogLeNet, VGG, ResNet; accuracy-weighted voting	98.83% (ASL); 98.79% (ASLA)	Ensemble boosts AUC; no signer-independence; added complexity

continued on following page

Table 2. Continued

Study	Dataset and scope	Input and preprocessing	Backbone and head	Reported performance (Accuracy)	Notes and limitations
Dabwan et al. (2023)	Sign Language MNIST; 28×28 grayscale; 24 classes (J and Z excluded)	Rescale 1/255	VGG16, VGG19; transfer-learned heads	97.5% (VGG16); 96% (VGG19)	Low-res grayscale; no RGB or real-world testing
Kumari and Anand (2023)	Massey ASL & static ISL; 36 classes (0–9 and A–Z)	128×128; normalized; HOG (8×8) + CBAM-CNN features	CBAM-CNN + HOG; dense 300/150; L2, dropout 0.5; softmax	99.22% (ASL); 99.79% (ISL)	Fusion improves orientation; higher compute; static datasets only; no cross-corpus testing
Alsharif et al. (2023)	ASL Alphabet; >87,000 images; 29 classes (letters + controls)	Resize to model input; ViT sensitive to size	AlexNet, ResNet-50, EfficientNet, ConvNeXt, ViT; fine-tuned	99.98% (ResNet-50); 99.95% (EfficientNet); 99.51% (ConvNeXt); 99.50% (AlexNet); 88.59% (ViT)	Strong CNNs; ViT underperforms due to input size; no cross-corpus testing
Dabwan et al. (2024)	Color MNIST-style; 27,455 train / 7,172 test; 24 classes (J and Z excluded)	Resize to network input; rescale 1/255	DenseNet121 with new classifier head	97% train; 96% validation	Static letters; no cross-corpus; RGB robustness untested
Elgohr et al. (2025)	ASL alphabet + transactional gestures; real-time; size not reported	Real-time frames; advanced preprocessing; resolution unspecified	YOLOv11; enhanced extractor; AdamW; composite loss; Grad-CAM	Precision 95.4%; Recall 94.8%; mAP 98.1	Detection focus; limited dataset info; no signer-independence; deployment complexity

continued on following page

Table 2. Continued

Study	Dataset and scope	Input and preprocessing	Backbone and head	Reported performance (Accuracy)	Notes and limitations
Qin and Wang (2025)	Kaggle ASL; 25,291 images; 36 classes (A–Z and 0–9)	Gaussian filter; contrast; histogram equalization; modified Canny	Streamlined ResNet-101; max pooling before conv blocks; some ReLUs removed; ImageNet-pretrained; softmax	97% accuracy; FPR 0.05; sensitivity 0.90; specificity 0.92; precision 0.94; F1 0.90; ResNet-101 > ResNet-50 (90%) > ResNet-18 (79%)	Higher training time; curated dataset; no signer-independent or cross-corpus evaluation; multi-step preprocessing may be brittle to illumination/background changes
Hariharan et al. (2025)	Custom ASL alphabet, balanced; ~78,000 RGB images (~3,000 per letter); 26 classes	Resize: 227×227 (AlexNet), 224×224 (GoogLeNet); flips; ±30px translations	AlexNet, GoogLeNet; new 26-way softmax head; early layers largely frozen; fine-tuned	99.39% (AlexNet); 95.52% (GoogLeNet)	Transfer learning gains; only two backbones; no cross-dataset or signer diversity

Critical Analysis

From Table 2, it is evident that transfer learning consistently yields near–state-of-the-art accuracy for static alphabetic recognition under controlled conditions (Cayamcela and Lim, 2019; Lum et al., 2020; Alsharif et al., 2023; Dabwan et al., 2024). AlexNet and MobileNetV2 offer fast convergence and efficient deployment for real-time scenarios on curated datasets, while deeper families such as ResNet and DenseNet sustain high accuracy with richer representational capacity. In this space, a modified deep residual approach that couples edge-aware segmentation with a streamlined ResNet-101 shows that explicit pre-segmentation can stabilize recognition in cluttered scenes while preserving test efficiency and outperforming shallower ResNet-50 and ResNet-18 despite higher training cost but similar inference time (Hariharan et al., 2025). Ensemble strategies that fuse heterogeneous CNNs with accuracy-based weighted voting demonstrate that late fusion can surpass single backbones while keeping inference practical, though they introduce a separate meta-classifier and fusion hyperparameters (Ma, Xu, Han, and Kim, 2022). Hybridization within the CNN family, either by concatenating HOG with attention-enriched features or by fusing two consecutive frames helps reduce confusions among visually similar letters at the price of added computation and pipeline complexity (Kumari and Anand, 2023; Ma, Xu, and Kim, 2022).

Despite these strengths, external validity remains underreported. Most works rely on within-dataset splits; cross-dataset transfer, signer-independent evaluation, and in-the-wild trials are seldom performed, leaving robustness to illumination changes, skin-tone variation, occlusion, left-handed signing, and background clutter uncertain. Deployment metrics are likewise sparse: few studies provide calibrated probabilities, macro-F1 with per-class breakdowns, confusion analyses beyond accuracy, or hardware-specific latency, memory, and energy profiles. Detection-oriented approaches such as YOLO variants report precision/recall and mAP, but dataset details and standardized comparators are often limited, complicating apples-to-apples assessment. To strengthen evidence, future CNN-based work should adopt standardized protocols that include signer-independent splits, at least one cross-dataset test, mandatory reporting of macro-F1, per-class errors, calibration metrics, and end-to-end latency on representative edge hardware, along with fairness-focused audits across lighting, skin tones, and capture devices.

Key takeaways: CNN transfer learning is reliable in closed settings; explicit pre-segmentation or late-fusion ensembles can reduce residual confusions; however, generalization and deployment readiness are under-evidenced. The next section turns to hybrids and transformer models, which aim to suppress background distractions and capture long-range dependencies with attention, potentially addressing some of these robustness gaps while introducing new trade-offs in complexity and compute.

Hybrids and Transformers

This subsection highlights architectures that extend beyond standard CNNs by integrating transformers or lightweight attention modules to enhance static gesture recognition.

Killari (2022) proposed a hybrid pipeline, shown in Figure 8, using LeNet-5 as a feature extractor for 28×28×1 grayscale images from the ASL MNIST dataset (24 static letters). The resulting 80-dimensional descriptors were classified using various models, including a single-hidden-layer neural network (120 units, softmax), decision tree, k-NN, and SVM. The neural network head achieved the highest accuracy (99.99%) under a 70/30 train–test split. The design is computationally efficient and suitable for low-resource settings. However, reliance on curated, low-resolution data without signer-independent evaluation limits generalizability (Killari, 2022). This lightweight hybrid serves as a reference for the transformer-based methods discussed next

Figure 8. Proposed Pipeline

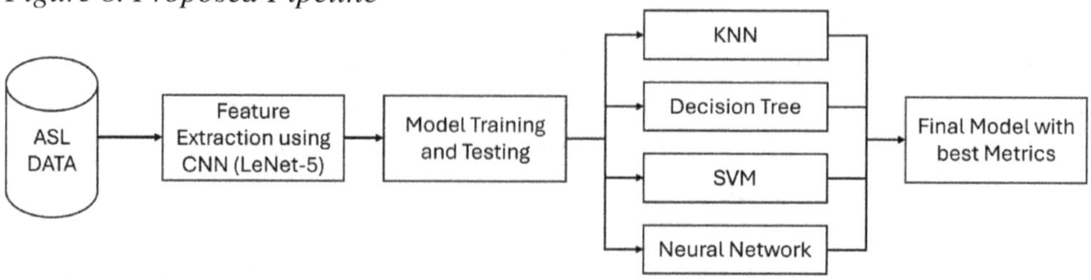

(Killari et al., 2022)

Building on that baseline, Tan, Lim, Chang, et al. (2023) and colleagues presented HGR ViT, a vision transformer pipeline tailored to static hand-gesture recognition that included the 24-class ASL alphabet, where J and Z were excluded because they require motion (Tan, Lim, Chang, et al., 2023). The method resized each image to 256×256, partitioned it into non-overlapping 32×32 patches, and mapped these patches to a token sequence with learned positional embeddings and a class token. This sequence was processed end-to-end by a standard transformer encoder, after which a linear classification head with softmax produced the final label. The authors fine-tuned an ImageNet-pretrained ViT-Base/32 using cross-entropy loss, keeping the pipeline deliberately free of handcrafted preprocessing so that attention maps could transparently reveal which regions drove the decision. Figure 9. depicts the framework proposed by Tan, Lim, Chang, et al. (2023).

On the 24-class static ASL dataset, the model attained 99.98 percent test accuracy under fivefold cross-validation, and attention maps concentrated over the hand region, supporting the claim that the transformer exploited pose-relevant structure rather than background artifacts. These characteristics set the stage for distilled and stacked variants that sought to retain global context while reducing computational footprint.

Figure 9. Proposed Framework

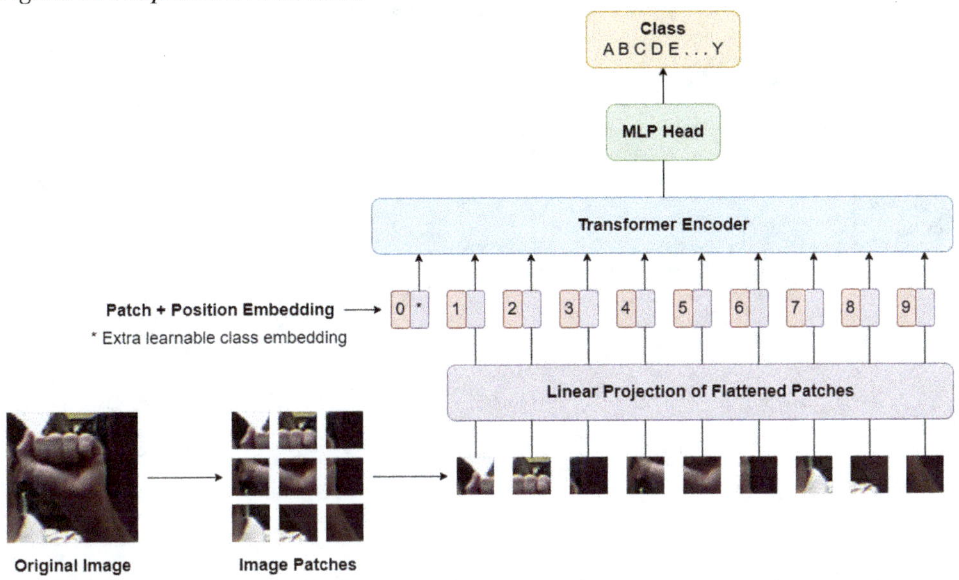

(Tan, Lim, Chang, et al., 2023)

Tan, Lim, Lee, et al. (2023) introduced SDViT, a stacked ensemble of distilled Vision Transformers for static hand gesture recognition. Inputs were resized to 256×256 and split into non-overlapping 32×32 patches. A ViT Base 32 pretrained on ImageNet21k+2012 was fine-tuned end-to-end using cross-entropy loss, early stopping, and adaptive learning rate scheduling. Distillation transferred soft targets from a larger teacher to four student ViTs (temperature 10, tuned mixing coefficient), which were combined via logistic regression stacking, as shown in Figure 10.

Figure 10. SDViT Architecture

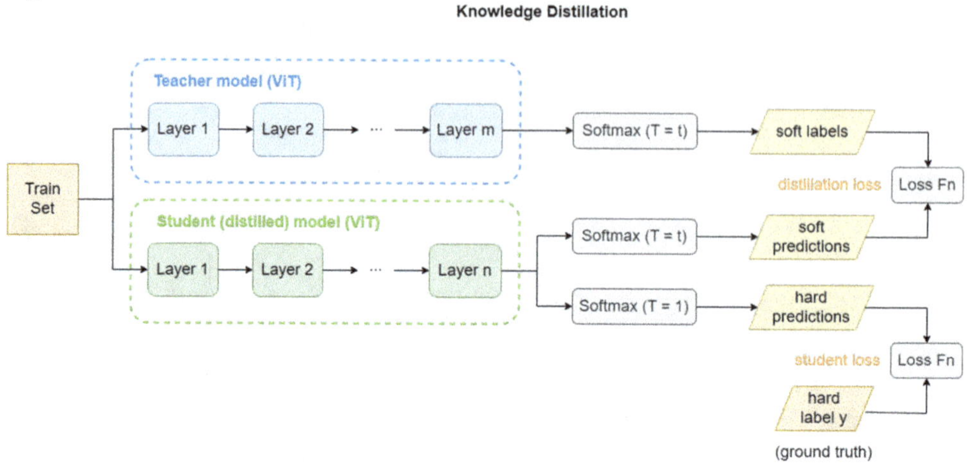

(Tan, Lim, Lee, et al., 2023)

Under fivefold cross-validation the system was evaluated on three benchmarks: an ASL set with 24 static letters totaling 65,774 images, an ASL with digits set of 36 classes with 2,515 images, and the NUS hand gesture set with 10 classes and 2,000 images; SDViT reports 100.00 percent on 24 class ASL, 99.60 percent on 36 class ASL with digits, and 100.00 percent on NUS, supported by confusion matrices and ablations comparing single ViT, distilled, and stacked variants (Tan, Lim, Lee, et al., 2023). Strengths include state-of-the-art accuracy from globally attentive features, parameter reductions via distillation, and robust gains from stacking, while limitations include reliance on large-scale pretraining, added deployment complexity from an ensemble, and continued focus on static curated datasets rather than signer-independent or in the wild evaluation.

To reconcile accuracy with efficiency and simplify deployment relative to stacked ensembles, Aly and Fathi (2025) proposed a hybrid transformer model that combined complementary convolutional streams with a lightweight vision transformer capturing longer-range dependencies without the cost of large ViT backbones (Aly and Fathi, 2025). The system operated on the ASL Alphabet dataset of approximately 87,000 RGB images across 29 classes, including letters and the tokens for space, delete, and nothing. Preprocessing included resizing to 64×64, normalization, and hand-region enhancement via adaptive thresholding, edge emphasis, and histogram equalization, followed by an 80/10/10 train–validation–test split. Two convolutional paths were optimized to capture complementary information, one with a global hand view and one with a hand-focused view; their feature maps were fused element-wise and passed to a lightweight transformer module that modeled global context before the final classifier (Aly & Fathi, 2025). Figure 11. depicts the model processing pipeline as proposed by Aly and Fathi (2025).

Figure 11. Model Processing Pipeline

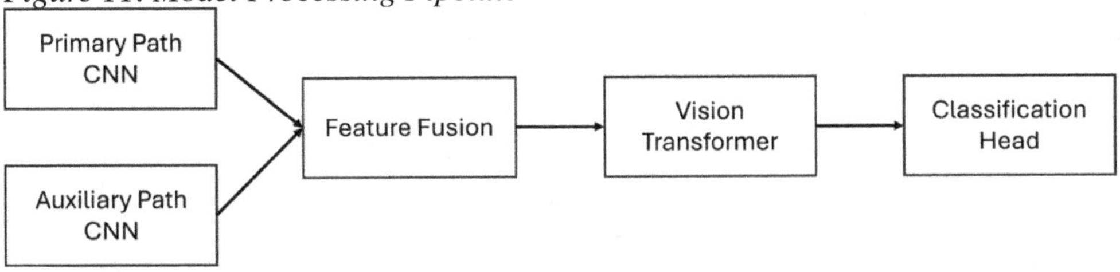

(Aly & Fathi, 2025)

Training incorporated strong data augmentation such as CutMix and added robustness-oriented strategies including contrastive learning and domain adaptation objectives. The resulting system reported 99.97 percent accuracy at roughly 110 frames per second with a computational budget of about 5.0 GFLOPs, indicating a favourable accuracy speed balance relative to heavier transformer variants (Aly & Fathi, 2025). The authors argued that the combination of explicit global and local cues with efficient attention underlies the performance gains; nevertheless, the approach used a relatively involved preprocessing chain, depending on the same dataset for both training and evaluation, and leaves generalization under cross-dataset or signer-independent conditions for future work.

Transformer-era and hybrid architectures span a range from lightweight CNN–classifier pipelines to full ViT models and stacked transformer ensembles, culminating in dual-path CNNs with compact attention modules. These studies demonstrate clear within-dataset gains while highlighting trade-offs in computational cost, model complexity, and design choices for static ASL recognition. Table 3 summarizes key differences in scope, features, models, datasets, and outcomes.

Table 3. Comparing Methodologies and Results of Studies Using Hybrid and Transformer Approaches

Study	Dataset and scope	Input and preprocessing	Architecture and feature pathway	Reported performance (accuracy)	Notes and limitations
Sajja et al., 2022	ASL MNIST; 27,455 grayscale; 24 classes	Resize to 28×28×1; LeNet-5 features (80D)	Single hidden layer NN (120 units, softmax) over LeNet features	99.99%	Low-res curated data; no dynamics; no signer-independence; no latency metrics
Tan et al., 2023 (HGRViT)	Static ASL; 24 classes (J, Z excluded)	RGB; resize to 256×256; 32×32 patches; positional embeddings, class token	ViT Base 32; fine-tuned; linear softmax head	99.98%	Heavy relative to compact CNNs, relies on large-scale pretraining; static data; no signer-independence
Tan et al., 2023 (SDViT)	Three benchmarks: ASL alphabet (24 letters, 65,774 images), ASL+digits (36 classes, 2,515 images), NUS hand-gesture (10 classes, 2,000 images); evaluated with 5-fold CV	RGB; resize to 256×256; 32×32 patches; positional embeddings, class token	Four distilled ViTs; global attention fused via logistic regression	100.00% (ASL); 99.60% (ASL+digits); 100.00% (NUS); Avg: 99.87%	Ensemble boosts accuracy; increases complexity; static curated datasets; no signer-independence or in-the-wild testing
Aly and Fathi, 2025	ASL Alphabet; ~87,000 RGB; 29 classes	Resize to 64×64; normalization; adaptive thresholding; edge detection; histogram equalization	Dual path CNN features fused element wise then refined by a lightweight ViT before classification	99.97%; ~110 FPS; ~5.0 GFLOPs	Complex preprocessing; same train/test split; static dataset; no signer-independence or in-the-wild testing

Critical Analysis

Studies shown in Table 3 collectively illustrate the spectrum of hybrid and transformer-era choices for static ASL recognition. A pure ViT approach, exemplified by HGR-ViT, achieves near-perfect accuracy with minimal domain-specific engineering and offers interpretable attention maps, yet it typically demands more compute and memory than mobile-oriented CNNs (Tan, Lim, Chang, et al., 2023). A complementary line explores knowledge distillation and stacking, as in SDViT, to retain global context while shrinking individual models and mitigating overfitting, though ensemble stacking increases deployment complexity and continues to rely on large-scale pretraining (Tan, Lim, Lee, et al., 2023). Hybridization proceeds along two paths. One retains a shallow CNN as a fixed feature extractor with a simple classical head, yielding an exceptionally light system that performs strongly on low-resolution grayscale data but is unlikely to sustain accuracy as capture conditions become more naturalistic (Killari, 2022). The other couples efficient convolutional streams with a slim transformer block and modern augmentation to capture both fine local structure and longer-range dependencies while staying within practical deployment footprints (Aly and Fathi, 2025). Despite these strengths, most reports remain confined to closed datasets: cross-dataset transfer, signer-independent splits, and real-world field trials are rarely conducted, and reporting often omits comprehensive robustness and fairness metrics such as macro-F1 with per-class breakdowns, calibration error, stress tests under occlusion and illumination change, and device-level latency, memory, and energy profiles.

To make progress, future hybrid and transformer work should adopt standardized protocols that include at least one cross-dataset evaluation and a signer-independent split; report macro-F1, per-class confusion, and calibration alongside accuracy; audit performance across skin tones, lighting, backgrounds, and capture devices; and provide end-to-end latency and energy on representative edge hardware. This will allow results to be compared fairly and will clarify the readiness of these architectures for deployment beyond laboratory settings. The next section turns from methodological contrasts to a consolidated discussion of results and reporting standards, followed by a brief "key takeaways" synthesis that highlights persistent gaps and emerging trends.

Key takeaways: Pure ViTs deliver ceiling-level accuracy with interpretability at higher computational cost; distilled and stacked transformers trade parameter count for added system complexity; hybrid CNN-attention models seek a sweet spot of accuracy and efficiency. Across all designs, standardized, fairness-aware, and deployment-oriented evaluation remains the primary unmet need.

GENERAL ANALYSIS

Results and Performance Landscape

According to the surveyed literature, near-perfect accuracy on static fingerspelling datasets is now routine when training and testing remain within the same curated distribution. Table 4 compares the overall approach and results of each study.

Table 4. Overall Comparison of Study Performance

Study	Dataset	Model/Approach	Reported Performance (accuracy)
Pan et al. (2016)	ASL Barczak; 26 classes	PCA → LDA → linear SVM	94%
Dayalan et al. (2025)	Static ASL; ~100 images/sign, uniform background and lighting; Letters and numerals classes	Random Forest on manual landmark features	98.8%
Cayamcela and Lim (2019)	Custom ASL; ~78,000 images; 26 classes	Transfer learning with new 26-way head, fine tuning at low learning rate	99.39% (AlexNet); 95.52% (GoogLeNet)
Dabwan et al. (2023)	MNIST; 28×28 grayscale; 24 classes (J and Z excluded)	Transfer-learned VGG16, VGG19	97.5% (VGG16); 96% (VGG19)
Dabwan et al. (2024)	Color MNIST-style; 24 classes	DenseNet121 with new classifier head	96%
Lum et al. (2020)	ASL Alphabet; ~87,000 RGB; 29 classes	MobileNetV2 with transfer learning and dropout 0.5	98.67%
Abu-Jamie and Abu-Naser (2022)	ASL Alphabet; ~87,000 RGB; 29 classes	VGG16 fine-tuned with preference for k-fold validation	100%
Ma, Xu and Kim (2022)	ASL Alphabet; ~87,000 RGB; 29 classes	Two-Stream Mixed fusion with LeNet, AlexNet, ResNet18, ResNet50	Best: 97.57% with TSM-ResNet50
Ma, Xu, Han, et al. (2022)	ASL Alphabet; ASLA; 29 classes	Ensemble of LeNet, AlexNet, GoogLeNet, VGGNet, ResNet + weighted voting	98.83% (ASL); 98.79% (ASLA)
Kumari and Anand (2023)	Massey ASL; 36 classes	CBAM-CNN + HOG + dense classifier	99.22%
Qin and Wang (2025)	ASL fingerspelling & ISL; 24 classes	Dual-channel star-attention CNN with feature fusion	99.81%

continued on following page

Table 4. Continued

Study	Dataset	Model/Approach	Reported Performance (accuracy)
Alsharif et al. (2023)	ASL Alphabet; ~87,000 RGB; 29 classes	Transfer learning across AlexNet, ResNet-50, EfficientNet, ConvNeXt, ViT	99.98% (ResNet-50); 99.95% (EfficientNet); 99.51% (ConvNeXt); 99.50% (AlexNet); 88.59% (ViT)
Hariharan et al. (2025)	Kaggle ASL; 25,291 images; 36 classes	Streamlined ResNet-101 with reduced filters and residual blocks, max pooling inserted before conv blocks, intermediate ReLUs removed; ImageNet pretraining; softmax classifier	97% (ResNet-101); 90% (ResNet-50); 79% (ResNet-18)
Killari (2022)	ASL MNIST; 27,455 grayscale; 24 classes	LeNet-5 + 1-hidden-layer NN	99.99%
Tan, Lim, Chang, et al. (2023)	Static ASL; 24 classes	ViT-Base 32; fine-tuned	99.98% (5-fold CV)
Tan, Lim, Lee, et al. (2023)	ASL (24 classes), ASL+digits (36 classes), NUS (10 classes)	Stacked distilled ViTs + logistic regression	100% (ASL); 99.60% (ASL+digits); 100% (NUS)
Aly and Fathi (2025)	ASL Alphabet; ~87,000 RGB; 29 classes	Dual-path CNN + lightweight ViT	99.97% accuracy; 110 FPS; ~5.0 GFLOPs

From Table 4, we can observe that traditional pipelines that rely on segmentation and handcrafted descriptors, such as hierarchical PCA, LDA, and SVM, still attain very high accuracy when backgrounds are controlled or segmentation is reliable, and Pan et al. provide a limited cross-corpus check by evaluating on Barczak's ASL images. The most consistent gains, however, come from transfer learning on convolutional backbones. On large RGB corpora like ASL Alphabet, MobileNetV2, ResNet-50, EfficientNet, and attention-augmented CNN variants commonly exceed 98 percent, with several reports approaching or exceeding 99.9 percent in closed settings. On Sign Language MNIST and related 28×28 grayscale benchmarks, VGG and DenseNet families also achieve exceptional scores, although the low resolution and static nature of these datasets constrain external validity. Vision Transformers show two patterns. A carefully tuned ViT with matched pretraining and input resolution, as in HGR-ViT, reaches near-ceiling accuracy with interpretable attention maps. In contrast, a generic ViT under mixed resizing and training protocols can lag well behind strong CNN baselines, as observed by Alsharif et al. Hybridization appears in two forms. One uses a shallow CNN as a fixed feature extractor with a classical head, which is extremely efficient and surprisingly accurate on MNIST-style data. The other couples efficient CNN streams with lightweight transformer blocks plus strong augmentation to produce favorable accuracy-to-throughput trade-offs, exemplified by Aly and Fathi's triple-digit frame rates with very high accuracy.

Robustness and Error Analysis

Evidence of robustness is uneven. A minority of studies report richer diagnostics such as sensitivity, specificity, macro-F1, ROC or AUC, or confusion matrices. Hariharan et al. provide sensitivity, specificity, precision, and F1 alongside accuracy, and several works include confusion matrices or attention visualizations. Most papers still emphasize overall accuracy, with limited signer-independent protocols, scarce cross-dataset transfer, and few stress tests for illumination, skin tone, occlusion, background clutter, and camera variation. Latency, memory, and energy are seldom measured on representative edge hardware, and probability calibration is rarely discussed. Table 5 summarizes robustness and deployment signals where they were explicitly reported.

Table 5. Robustness and Deployment Evidence at Glance.

Study	Consideration for robustness beyond accuracy	Cross-dataset or signer-independent	In-the-wild/ Field-Testing	Latency or throughput	Interpretability
Pan et al. 2016	Limited cross-corpus check; hierarchical error handling	Cross-dataset to Barczak images only	None reported	Not reported	Pipeline rationale; feature ablations implied
Cayamcela and Lim 2019	Basic augmentation	No	None reported	Not reported	None
Lum et al. 2020	Large dataset, no augmentation	No	None reported	Claimed mobile suitability; no measurements	None
Abu-Jamie and Abu-Naser 2022	k-fold preference; confusion matrix	No	None reported	Not reported	Confusion matrix
Ma, Xu, and Kim 2022 (TSM)	Augmentation; two-frame fusion ablations	No	None reported	Extra compute noted; no timing	None
Ma, Xu, Han, and Kim 2022 (ensemble)	ROC and AUC	No	None reported	Fusion complexity discussed; no timing	None

continued on following page

Table 5. Continued

Study	Consideration for robustness beyond accuracy	Cross-dataset or signer-independent	In-the-wild/ Field-Testing	Latency or throughput	Interpretability
Dabwan et al. 2023 (VGG)	Precision, recall, F1	No	None reported	Not reported	None
Dabwan et al. 2024 (DenseNet)	Precision, recall, F1; confusion matrix	No	None reported	Not reported	Confusion matrix
Kumari and Anand 2023	Orientation robustness argument	No	None reported	Not reported	None
Alsharif et al. 2023	Broad backbone comparison	No	None reported	Not reported	Discussion of ViT sensitivity to resizing
Qin and Wang 2025	Background suppression design	No	None reported	Not reported	Architectural attention mechanism
Hariharan et al. 2025	Sensitivity, specificity, precision, F1	No	None reported	Similar test time across backbones; training cost higher	None
Elgohr et al. 2025	Precision, recall, mAP	No	Demo style real time; no controlled field trial	Real-time intent; no device metrics	Grad-CAM and occlusion sensitivity
Killari 2022	Comparative heads on fixed features	No	None reported	Not reported	None
HGR-ViT 2023	Fivefold CV; attention maps	No	None reported	Not reported	Attention visualizations
SDViT 2023	Ablations on distillation and stacking	No	None reported	Ensemble complexity; no timing	Attention; stacking analysis
Aly and Fathi 2025	Strong augmentation; contrastive and domain-adaptation objectives	No	None reported	About 110 FPS and ~5.0 GFLOPs reported	Architectural rationale

Ethical and Deployment Challenges

Deployment-relevant questions receive limited, uneven coverage. Studies rarely audit performance across skin tones, age groups, left- and right-handed signing, or device diversity, which are central to fairness and accessibility. Privacy and consent practices for image capture and storage are seldom articulated. Human-factors aspects such as user fatigue, camera positioning, ambient lighting guidance, and error recovery in interactive systems are typically absent. For practitioners, a minimal deployment guide would include dataset governance and consent templates, instructions for on-device model execution and fallback logic, calibration and confidence thresholds, guidance for user prompts when predictions are uncertain, and clear reporting of latency, memory, and battery impact on representative mobile chipsets.

Scope Contrast: Static Alphabet Versus Continuous Signing

This chapter intentionally focuses on static ASL alphabets. Continuous signing introduces sequence modeling, coarticulation, temporal segmentation, signer rate variability, and a much larger label space that requires language modeling and alignment. The high scores achieved by static classifiers should not be interpreted as indicators of readiness for continuous, in-the-wild ASL understanding. Bridging the gap requires multimodal corpora with synchronized video and linguistic annotations, temporal models with alignment, and evaluation suites that reflect conversational variability.

Limitations and Open Challenges

The consolidated picture shows outstanding closed-set performance and maturing architectural diversity, but several gaps constrain real-world utility. Cross-dataset and signer-independent validation are rare, limiting claims of generalization. Robust audits are sporadic, and standardized reporting of macro-F1, per-class confusion, calibration error, and stress tests are uncommon. Few studies provide device-level latency, memory footprint, and energy measurements, and many rely on multi-step preprocessing that may be brittle under illumination shifts and cluttered scenes. For detection-style systems, dataset composition and comparators are often underspecified, making comparisons difficult.

FUTURE DIRECTIONS

This review has purposefully limited itself to static ASL alphabets, and the strongest near-perfect accuracies reported across many studies largely reflect closed-set training and testing under similar, curated conditions. A priority for future work is to replace convenience splits with signer-independent protocols, explicit cross-dataset transfer (for example, training on ASL Alphabet and testing on distinct collections captured in different environments), and rigorous stress testing against illumination changes, skin-tone diversity, background clutter, motion blur, occlusion, left-handed signing, and camera quality variation. Reporting should move beyond single accuracy numbers to calibrated confidence, per-class error analyses, and open-set behaviour in the presence of unknown or out-of-distribution hand poses. Fairness and accessibility need to be treated as first-order goals rather than afterthoughts, with demographic coverage assessed explicitly and failure modes documented. Reproducibility would benefit from standardized train, validation, and test partitions, consistent preprocessing definitions, and publicly released code with seeds and checkpoints so that results are verifiable and comparable.

Equally important is closing the gap between offline recognition and practical deployment. Models should be evaluated under strict latency, energy, and memory budgets on representative edge hardware, with systematic studies of compression, quantization, pruning, and distillation that preserve recognition fidelity while meeting real-time constraints. Privacy-preserving learning, including on-device and federated approaches, is directly relevant to camera-based applications and should be paired with transparent data governance. Robustness can be strengthened with domain adaptation, self-supervised or synthetic pretraining focused on hands and backgrounds typical of real use, and explicit uncertainty estimation that supports human-in-the-loop fallbacks. Although temporal modelling lies outside the scope of this review, bridging from static alphabets to practical interfaces will ultimately require careful integration of short-context cues, standardized human-factors evaluations, and end-to-end user studies that measure not only accuracy but also error recovery, responsiveness, and acceptability in everyday settings.

Actionable recommendations for researchers and practitioners: Future work should adopt a common protocol that includes at least one cross-dataset transfer test and a signer-independent split; mandatory reporting of macro-F1, per-class confusion, and calibration; stress tests for illumination, occlusion, background complexity, and left-handed signing; and device-level latency, memory, and energy on representative mobile hardware. Fairness and privacy should be addressed via stratified performance by skin tone and lighting, data-minimization practices, and explicit consent and governance. For deployment, provide a compact model card with robustness evidence and a reproducible reference implementation that includes preprocessing, quantization, and fallback behaviour.

CONCLUSION

Across static ASL recognition, modern transfer learning and hybrid designs reliably achieve very high accuracy on curated image corpora, with ResNet and EfficientNet families, MobileNetV2, ViT-based pipelines, and attention-augmented hybrids all reporting near-perfect results under within-dataset evaluation. Traditional pipelines that depend on segmentation and handcrafted descriptors can also perform strongly when backgrounds are controlled. The common recipe is clear: careful resizing and normalization, moderate augmentation, and fine-tuning of pretrained backbones yield consistent gains while keeping training practical.

At the same time, the evidence base remains narrow. Most studies evaluate on static, closed sets with similar capture conditions, limited signer diversity, and no true cross-dataset transfer. Dynamic letters are excluded by design in several benchmarks, and few works report signer-independent splits, latency and energy on edge hardware, or robustness to illumination, skin tone variation, occlusion, and clutter. Reported numbers therefore reflect best-case laboratory conditions rather than field readiness. Closing this gap will require standardized protocols, richer and more diverse datasets, transparent reporting beyond aggregate accuracy, and deployment-focused measurements that reflect real usage constraints. Within those bounds, the surveyed literature demonstrates that static ASL alphabet classification is effectively a solved problem in controlled settings, and the next advances will come from generalization, fairness, privacy, and usability rather than from incremental architecture tweaks alone.

REFERENCES

Abu-Jamie, T. N., & Abu-Naser, S. S. (2022). Classification of Sign-language Using VGG16. [IJAER]. *International Journal of Academic Engineering Research, 6*(6), 36–46.

Alsharif, B., Altaher, A. S., Altaher, A., Ilyas, M., & Alalwany, E. (2023). Deep Learning Technology to Recognize American Sign Language Alphabet. *Sensors (Basel), 23*(18), 7970. DOI: 10.3390/s23187970 PMID: 37766026

Aly, M., & Fathi, I. S. (2025). Recognizing American Sign Language gestures efficiently and accurately using a hybrid transformer model. *Scientific Reports, 15*(1), 20253. DOI: 10.1038/s41598-025-06344-8 PMID: 40550837

Cayamcela, M. E. M., & Lim, W. (2019). Fine-tuning a pre-trained convolutional neural network model to translate American sign language in real-time. *2019 International Conference on Computing, Networking and Communications (ICNC)*

Dabwan, B. A., Jadhav, M. E., Gadkari, A. S., Ali, Y. A., Almula, S. M., Ismil, O. A., & Mohammad, A. A. (2024). Hand gesture classification for individuals with disabilities using the DenseNet121 model. *2024 International Conference on Advancements in Power, Communication and Intelligent Systems (APCI)*

Dabwan, B. A., Olayah, F. A., Halawani, H. T., Mashraqi, A. M., Abdelrahman, Y. A., & Shamsan, A. F. (2023). Classification of Sign language Using VGG16 and VGG19. 2023 7th International Symposium on Innovative Approaches in Smart Technologies (ISAS)

Dayalan, K., Saman, D., Murugesan, H., & Prabhakaran, J. (2025). Sign language translation using random forest classifier. *AIP Conference Proceedings.*

Devi, V. A., Charulatha, T., & Dharishinie, P. (2023). A Survey on Sign Language Recognition and Training Module. ITM Web of Conferences

Dsane, D. N. A. A. B. (2024). Being understood: how to expand sign language access for the deaf community. Retrieved 19/08/2025 from https://blogs.worldbank.org/en/nasikiliza/how-to-expand-sign-language-access-for-the-deaf-community-

Elgohr, A., Elhadidy, M., El-Geneedy, M., Mohamed, S., & Mousa, M. (2025). Advancing Sign Language Recognition: A YOLO v.11-Based Deep Learning Framework for Alphabet and Transactional Hand Gesture Detection. *Proceedings of the AAAI Symposium Series, 6*, 209–217. DOI: 10.1609/aaaiss.v6i1.36055

Hariharan, U., Devarajan, D., Kumar, P. S., Rajkumar, K., Meena, M., & Akilan, T. (2025). Recognition of American sign language using modified deep residual CNN with modified canny edge segmentation. *Multimedia Tools and Applications*, *84*(31), 38093–38120. Advance online publication. DOI: 10.1007/s11042-025-20663-y

Ismail, M. I. M., & Mousa, M. A. (2025, August). Employing Computer Vision on a Smartphone to Help the Visually Impaired Cross the Road. In *Proceedings of the AAAI Symposium Series* (Vol. 6, No. 1, pp. 227-234). DOI: 10.1609/aaaiss.v6i1.36057

Killari, V. (2022). MACHINE LEARNING ALGORITHMS FOR ASL IMAGE RECOGNITION WITH LENET5 FEATURE EXTRACTION. *international journal of advanced research in computer science, 13*, 11–14. DOI: 10.26483/ijarcs.v13i3.6828

Kumari, D., & Anand, R. S. (2023). Fusion of Attention-Based Convolution Neural Network and HOG Features for Static Sign Language Recognition. *Applied Sciences (Basel, Switzerland)*, *13*(21), 11993. DOI: 10.3390/app132111993

Lum, K. Y., Goh, Y. H., & Lee, Y. B. (2020). American Sign Language Recognition Based on MobileNetV2. *Advances in Science, Technology and Engineering Systems Journal.*

Ma, Y., Xu, T., Han, S., & Kim, K. (2022). Ensemble Learning of Multiple Deep CNNs Using Accuracy-Based Weighted Voting for ASL Recognition. *Applied Sciences (Basel, Switzerland)*, *12*(22), 11766. DOI: 10.3390/app122211766

Ma, Y., Xu, T., & Kim, K. (2022). Two-Stream Mixed Convolutional Neural Network for American Sign Language Recognition. *Sensors (Basel)*, *22*(16), 5959. DOI: 10.3390/s22165959 PMID: 36015719

Mousa, M. A., Elgohr, A. T., & Khater, H. A. (2024). A novel hybrid deep neural network classifier for EEG emotional brain signals. *International Journal of Advanced Computer Science and Applications, 15*(6), 1045-1055. https://dx.doi.org/ DOI: 10.14569/IJACSA.2024.01506107

Pan, T.-Y., Lo, L.-Y., Yeh, C.-W., Li, J.-W., Liu, H.-T., & Hu, M.-C. (2016). Real-time sign language recognition in complex background scene based on a hierarchical clustering classification method. 2016 IEEE second international conference on multimedia big data (BigMM)

Qin, J., & Wang, M. (2025). Sign language recognition based on dual-channel star-attention convolutional neural network. *Scientific Reports*, *15*(1), 27685. DOI: 10.1038/s41598-025-13625-9

Tan, C. K., Lim, K. M., Chang, R. K. Y., Lee, C. P., & Alqahtani, A. (2023). HGR-ViT: Hand Gesture Recognition with Vision Transformer. *Sensors (Basel), 23*(12), 5555. DOI: 10.3390/s23125555 PMID: 37420722

Tan, C. K., Lim, K. M., Lee, C. P., Chang, R. K. Y., & Alqahtani, A. (2023). SDViT: Stacking of Distilled Vision Transformers for Hand Gesture Recognition. *Applied Sciences (Basel, Switzerland), 13*(22), 12204. DOI: 10.3390/app132212204

WFD. (2025). *The Legal Recognition of National Sign Languages*. Retrieved 19/08/2025 from https://wfdeaf.org/the-legal-recognition-of-national-sign-languages

WHO. (2023a). *The critical role of accessibility in health information*. https://www.who.int/europe/news-room/feature-stories/item/the-critical-role-of-accessibility-in-health-information

WHO. (2023b). *Disability*. Retrieved 19/08/2025 from https://www.who.int/news-room/fact-sheets/detail/disability-and-health

WHO. (2025). *Deafness and hearing loss*. Retrieved 19/08/2025 from https://www.who.int/news-room/fact-sheets/detail/deafness-and-hearing-loss

KEY TERMS AND DEFINITIONS

Accuracy Based Weighted Voting: A late fusion scheme that combines outputs from multiple classifiers by assigning weights based on their validation accuracy so that stronger models contribute more to the final decision.

Attention Mechanism: A module that learns to weight spatial or channel features so that the network emphasizes informative hand regions and deemphasizes distracting background patterns.

Confusion Matrix: A table that reports counts of predicted versus true classes, used to analyse which letters are commonly confused and to compute metrics such as precision, recall, and F1.

Cross-dataset Transfer: Testing a model trained on one dataset directly on a different dataset to assess robustness to changes in capture conditions, backgrounds, cameras, and demographics.

Data Augmentation: Synthetic transformations applied to training images, such as flips, rotations, translations, or color jitter, intended to improve generalization by exposing the model to plausible variations.

Fingerspelling: The use of handshapes that correspond to letters or numbers to spell words; in ASL studies it is often framed as a closed-set image classification problem over discrete classes.

Keypoint Based Features: Structured descriptors derived from hand landmarks detected by a pose model; they capture geometry while discarding appearance, enabling lightweight classifiers at the cost of fine texture cues.

MobileNetV2: A compact convolutional network that uses depth wise separable convolutions and inverted residual blocks to deliver high accuracy with low computation suitable for edge devices.

ResNet: A family of deep convolutional networks that employ skip connections to ease optimization of very deep models and to preserve gradient flow during training.

Segmentation: The process of isolating the hand region from the background using colour models, edges, or learned masks so that downstream features and classifiers focus on the relevant pixels.

Signer-independent Evaluation: An evaluation protocol where the people in the test set are not present in training, used to estimate how well a system generalizes to new users.

Static ASL Alphabet: A subset of ASL letters represented by still images of handshapes, typically 24 letters since J and Z require motion and are excluded from static benchmarks.

Transfer Learning: A training strategy that adapts a model pretrained on a large source dataset to a target task by replacing and fine tuning the final layers, which accelerates convergence and improves accuracy with limited labelled data.

Vision Transformer (ViT): An architecture that treats an image as a sequence of patches, applies self-attention to model long range dependencies, and predicts labels with a lightweight classification head.

Chapter 8
Deep Learning-Based Pakistan Sign Language Interpretation for Enhancing Communication for Individuals With Hearing Disabilities

Mehwish Raza
https://orcid.org/0000-0003-1778-6196
NED University of Engineering and Technology, Pakistan

Majida Kazmi
https://orcid.org/0000-0002-2767-3139
NED University of Engineering and Technology, Pakistan

Fauzia Yasir
https://orcid.org/0009-0004-2921-9046
NED University of Engineering and Technology, Pakistan

ABSTRACT

Sign language recognition is a critical area within computer vision and assistive technology, promoting inclusive communication for individuals with hearing impairments. While various international sign languages have been widely studied, Pakistan Sign Language (PSL) remains underexplored. This chapter, per the authors, presents

DOI: 10.4018/979-8-3373-2033-5.ch008

a real-time PSL recognition system using the YOLOv5 object detection framework. A custom dataset of 3,963 images, augmented to 9,522 using rotation, noise addition, and exposure adjustment, was developed using hand signs from students at the Ida Rieu School for the Blind and Deaf. The model achieved an accuracy of 94.67%, outperforming previous PSL systems in static sign classification. Comparative analysis shows improved generalization in real world conditions, particularly with complex backgrounds and partial occlusions. Unlike earlier approaches limited to controlled environments, this system demonstrates practical applicability in educational contexts. Future work includes optimizing for low-power edge deployment and dynamic sign recognition.

1. INTRODUCTION

Effective communication is central to human interaction, yet individuals with hearing impairments often face significant barriers in accessing this fundamental right. Sign languages serve as the primary mode of expression for the deaf community, employing visual-manual modalities to convey complex linguistic constructs. However, the lack of widespread knowledge of sign languages among the general population significantly limits the social inclusion and mobility of hearing-impaired individuals (ADCET, 2025). Globally, over 466 million individuals live with disabling hearing loss (a figure projected to rise to 900 million by 2050) (Mirza et al., 2022).

In Pakistan, where over 1.25 million people experience varying degrees of hearing loss (Pakistan Bureau of Statistics, 2021), Pakistan Sign Language (PSL) remains the principal form of communication within the deaf community. While PSL serves as the primary communication medium for this community, the general population's limited familiarity with PSL creates an isolation that extends far beyond simple conversation, affecting education, employment opportunities, healthcare access, and civic participation (Bae, 2023).

The emergence of artificial intelligence and deep learning technologies offers unprecedented opportunities to bridge this communication divide. Computer vision systems, particularly those employing Convolutional Neural Networks (CNNs) and object detection frameworks like YOLO (You Only Look Once) (Redmon & Farhadi, 2018) (Tyagi et al., 2023) have demonstrated remarkable success in visual recognition tasks. However, the majority of research in sign language recognition has focused on American Sign Language (ASL) and British Sign Language (BSL), very few studies have addressed PSL. Furthermore, the limited existing research on PSL often lacks real-world validation, which is crucial for practical deployment and long-term usability.

The novelty of this work lies in its comprehensive approach to PSL recognition. Unlike earlier studies that relied on controlled environments or non-native signers, our dataset was developed directly from native signers, ensuring natural fluency and linguistic accuracy. Data was collected in real-world conditions, capturing variations in lighting, backgrounds, and camera angles that better reflect deployment environments. To further strengthen the dataset, we adopted a hybrid strategy, combining authentic recordings with synthetic augmentation to increase diversity while preserving authenticity. Finally, the system was validated in practice at the Ida Rieu School for the Blind and Deaf, demonstrating its effectiveness in an inclusive educational setting.

The rest of the chapter is structured as follows: Section 2 presents a brief background, Section 3 reviews relevant literature in sign language recognition. Section 4 details the methodology, including dataset development, annotation, augmentation and model training. Section 5 presents the experimental setup, discusses the key results and presents a comparison of proposed work with existing studies. Finally, Sections 6 concludes the chapter.

2. BACKGROUND AND LITERATURE REVIEW

2.1 Background

Spoken languages use the “vocal-auditory” channel, meaning they are spoken with the mouth and heard by the ears. All writing systems are based on spoken language. In contrast, sign languages (SLs) use the “corporal-visual” channel, as they are expressed through body movements and are seen with the eyes. SLs are not uniform globally but vary across different deaf communities worldwide. They develop naturally when deaf people come together and need to communicate (Bragg et al. 2021). Each sign has a structure similar to that of the spoken words. For example, just as spoken languages form many words from a small number of sounds, sign languages form many signs from a small set of handshapes and movements. Therefore, signs are not just simple gestures; they are composed of small meaningful elements that work together. The fundamental components that form the basic structure of any sign language can be classified into two categories: manual and non-manual features, as illustrated in Figure 1. Manual features include hand shape, hand position, movement, and the orientation of the palm or fingers. Non-manual features include eye gaze, head movements, shoulder orientation, and facial expressions, including mouth movements. These features collectively form a unit known as gloss, which represents the closest equivalent to a word or a meaningful sign in sign language (Koller et al., 2021).

Figure 1. Fundamental components of SL: (a)Manual features (b)Nonmanual features

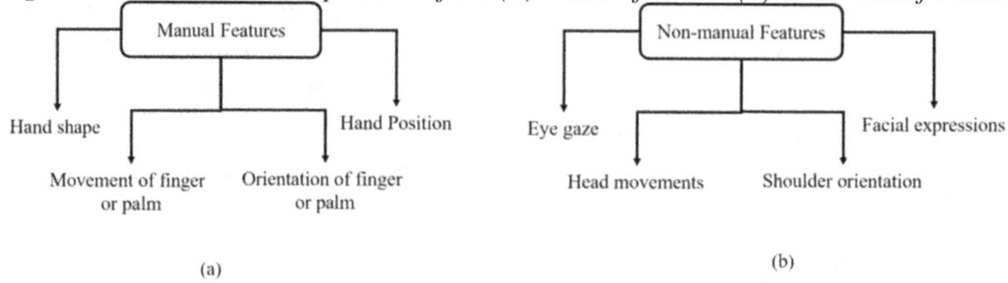

Both types of features are simultaneously used at the same time by signers to build sentences in an SL. Depending on the situation, a specific feature may be the most important factor in understanding gloss. It can change the meaning of a verb, provide information about time and place, and distinguish objects from people. For instance,

- In ASL, the sign for "give" uses the same hand movement, but the direction of the movement shows who is giving to whom, moving the hands from the signer toward another person means "I give to you," while moving from another location toward the signer means "you give to me."
- Similarly, facial expressions can completely change the meaning of a sign; the same hand movement with a questioning facial expression becomes a question, while with a normal expression it remains a statement.
- In PSL, eye gaze direction can indicate whether someone is talking about a person who is present or absent, and head nods can show agreement or emphasis.

PSL is the primary sign language used by the deaf community in Pakistan. Like other sign languages around the world, PSL has developed its own unique vocabulary and grammar rules that reflect Pakistani culture and society. PSL includes signs for religious concepts, family relationships, and social interactions that are specific to Pakistani culture. Research shows that PSL is used by approximately 200,000 people across Pakistan, making it an important communication tool for the deaf community (Rastgoo et al., 2021). The basic sentence structure of PSL follows a Subject-Object-Verb (SOV) pattern (Khan et al., n.d.), which is similar to Urdu but different from English.

- For example, where English would say "I eat rice," PSL signs it as I + RICE + EAT, this is called gloss, with the subject first, then the object, and finally the verb. This structure can be seen in other examples: "The boy reads a book" becomes BOY + BOOK + READ in PSL, and "She is going to school" becomes SHE + SCHOOL + GO.

- Questions in PSL are formed not by changing word order but by adding facial expressions such as raised eyebrows and forward head tilt. For instance, BOY + BOOK + READ with normal facial expression is a statement, while the same sign sequence with questioning facial expressions becomes a question.
- Negation is expressed through head shaking that accompanies the signs throughout the sentence, so I + RICE + EAT becomes negative when performed with continuous head shaking. Time expressions are typically placed at the beginning of sentences, such as YESTERDAY + I + SCHOOL + GO for "Yesterday I went to school" or TOMORROW + WE + MARKET + GO for "Tomorrow we will go to market."

Despite the structural richness and expressiveness of PSL, deaf individuals often face significant communication barriers in their daily lives, such as seeking help at service desks, filling out forms, or visiting healthcare facilities. In Pakistan, where most formal and public communication takes place in Urdu, the situation is even more complex. Deaf individuals who use PSL may struggle to communicate in environments where staff or services rely solely on spoken or written Urdu. For instance, at government offices like NADRA or utility centres, a deaf person may need to explain an issue or request assistance. In light of these persistent challenges, the development of a system capable of recognizing PSL gestures and translating them into written Urdu text is not just beneficial but it is a timely necessity to ensure inclusive and effective communication. Such a system would allow users to sign naturally in PSL while their gestures are interpreted and displayed in Urdu in real time, making communication more accessible, inclusive, and effective. This could significantly improve access to public services and formal communication channels for the deaf community in Pakistan. Moreover, it holds immense potential in educational contexts, enabling deaf students to connect PSL signs with written Urdu, thereby strengthening their literacy skills and overall academic performance.

Information Technology (IT) can play a transformative role in making this possible. With advancements in computer vision, machine learning, and natural language processing, IT provides the tools and frameworks needed to develop intelligent systems that can accurately interpret sign language in real time. Sign Language Recognition (SLR) is the process of automatically interpreting and understanding sign language gestures and movements using technology (Zhang & Jiang, 2024). Research in SLR can broadly be classified along two dimensions, on the basis of nature of sign and on the basis of technology approach, as shown in Figure 2.

The first dimension classifies SLR frameworks, by the type of signs they interpret. It refers to the nature of the signs, distinguishing between static signs, where gestures involve fixed hand poses and dynamic signs, which consist of continuous hand and body movements over time (Zhang & Jiang, 2024). Static sign recognition focusses on finger-spelling recognition. It primarily involves static signs, such as those used for alphabets and digits. These signs are characterized by fixed hand shapes and positions, while minor variations or slight movements may occur, their primary focus remains on the configuration and orientation of the hands rather than on motion. Fingerspelling involves spelling out words using individual signs for each letter or digit. These signs are mostly static, involving specific hand shapes and orientations. For example:

- A person signing the Urdu letter ' ' **(Bay)** by forming a specific hand shape held in a fixed position.
- Signing a phone number like **1-2-3** using distinct static signs for each digit.

Figure 2. SLR Classification

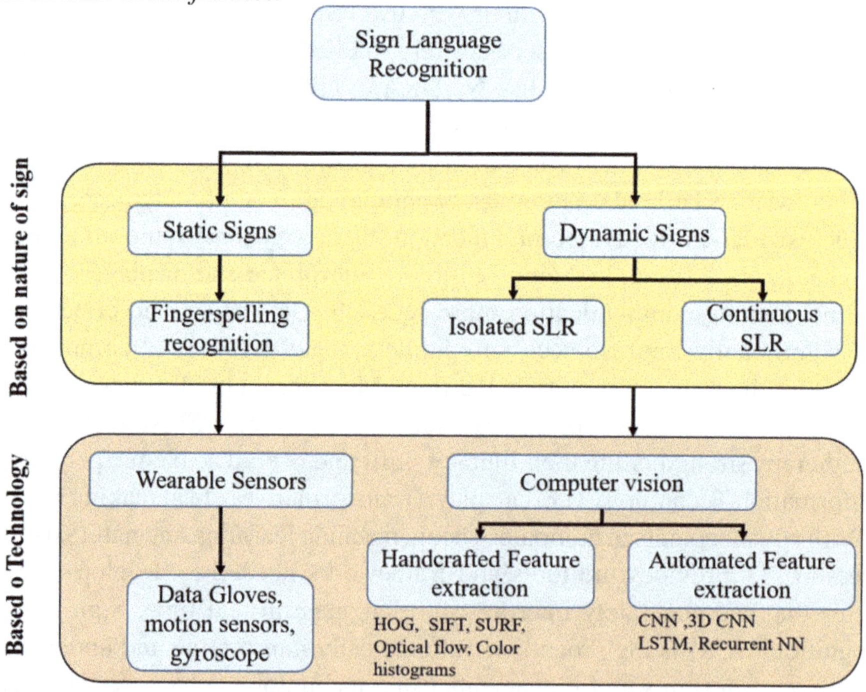

In contrast, dynamic sign recognition focusses on movement and sequence of signs. This category can be further classified into isolated and continuous recognition categories. Isolated sign recognition refers to the identification of individual signs performed separately, without any contextual linkage to preceding or succeeding signs. This task requires accurate detection of hand movements, facial expressions, and other non-manual cues specific to each gesture. These can be either static or involve motion but are not part of a sentence. For example:

- Signing the word **"WATER"** with a specific hand movement near the mouth.
- The sign for **"BOOK"**, involving a motion mimicking opening a book.
- Signing **"HELLO"** using a waving gesture.

On the other hand, continuous sign recognition aims to interpret full sentences or phrases expressed in sign language as in natural conversation. Unlike isolated recognition, it involves understanding the sequential and grammatical structure of multiple signs in real-time. This approach is essential for enabling natural, uninterrupted communication and for building systems capable of real-world sign language understanding. It includes understanding sign transitions, grammar, and temporal dependencies. For example:

- For a sentence like: "I am going to school", the PSL gloss will be like **I + SCHOOL + GO**, performed in one continuous motion.
- For a sentence like "He is not coming." The PSL gloss will be like **HE + COME + NOT**. Often signed with a strong head shake and a firm hand motion on "NOT," without pausing between the signs.

In addition to the nature of signs, the SLR frameworks can also be classified along the second dimension, based on the technological approach used. This dimension primarily includes two categories: wearable sensors-based methods and computer vision–based methods (Alyami et al., 2024). Notably, any method from the first dimension can be implemented using either of these technological approaches.

Wearable sensor-based methods use special equipment, such as data gloves, motion sensors, and depth cameras, to capture detailed information about hand and body movements (Amin et al., 2022). These methods can provide accurate measurements of hand positions and movements. While these methods can achieve high levels of accuracy in tracking manual gestures, their practical adoption remains limited due to several significant drawbacks. The main limitation of wearable sensor-based approach is the high cost of the equipment involved and the lack of accessibility of equipment, particularly in low-resource settings. Secondly, the wearable nature of the hardware can be uncomfortable, affecting the natural signing process (Zhang

& Jiang, 2024). Moreover, these systems require a complex setup and adjustment procedures that are difficult for regular users. Finally, most sensor-based systems can only capture hand (manual features) but miss important facial expressions and body language (non-manual features) that are essential for sign language understanding.

Due to these limitations of wearable sensor-based methods, researchers have moved toward computer vision-based methods. This approach uses regular cameras to capture video of signers and then use computer algorithms to analyse the visual information. Unlike wearable sensor-based methods, computer vision-based methods are non-intrusive, more accessible, and do not require specialized hardware. Most importantly, they have the potential to capture both manual features (such as hand shapes and movements) and non-manual features (such as facial expressions and head movements), which are essential for understanding sign language in a more accurate manner.

Building on this capability, computer vision based SLR systems are further enhanced through the application of machine learning and deep learning techniques. Two general approaches exist: handcrafted feature extraction and automatic feature extraction. In handcrafted approaches, domain-specific knowledge is used to manually design features, to capture important visual and motions cues such as hand shape descriptors and motion trajectories. Common handcrafted features include:

- **Histogram of Oriented Gradients (HOG)** – for capturing edge and shape information,
- **Scale-Invariant Feature Transform (SIFT)** – for identifying key points in images regardless of scale or rotation,
- **Speeded-Up Robust Features (SURF)** – similar to SIFT but optimized for speed,
- **Optical Flow** – for detecting and describing motion between frames,
- **Color histograms** or **skin color segmentation** – for isolating hands and facial regions.

Although handcrafted feature extraction methods have played significant role but these methods have certain limitations, such as they can be time-consuming and may not capture all the relevant information in the data. Additionally, these methods may struggle with handling complex and high-dimensional data, such as the spatiotemporal information present in sign language gestures. Moreover, these methods are often sensitive to variations in lighting, signer style, and background clutter, limiting their scalability (Zhang & Jiang, 2024).

In contrast, automatic feature extraction method, particularly those using deep learning models like CNNs and Recurrent Neural Networks (RNNs), offer a more scalable and adaptive solution. These models learn hierarchical patterns directly from data, eliminating the need for manual engineering and significantly improving robustness and generalization across different signers and environments. When integrated with natural language processing tools, these models can convert signs into text. These models can then be integrated with natural language processing pipelines to convert recognized signs into grammatically correct written text (Rastgoo et al., 2021).

Understanding the classification of SLRs, based on the nature of signs (static vs. dynamic) and technological approach (wearable sensor-based vs. computer vision-based) is important for designing systems that align with real-world needs. These classifications are not just theoretical distinctions; they directly inform the development of practical tools for deaf communication. The SLR tools not only enhance communication in public services but also opens up opportunities for application in other domains, particularly education. For instance, such technology can support deaf students in developing core literacy skills by helping them connect PSL gestures with corresponding Urdu alphabet characters. A PSL alphabet recognition system allows students to sign hand gestures representing individual Urdu letters, which are then recognized and displayed in real time, providing immediate visual feedback and reinforcing the learning process.

For example, if a student signs the PSL gesture for the letter ‘ ’ (Bay), the system recognizes it and displays ‘ ’ on the screen. This immediate visual feedback helps students practice recognizing letters, forming words, and even building simple sentences, thus bridging the gap between sign language and written Urdu.

Such a system can be:

- Deployed on tablets, laptops, or interactive whiteboards in classrooms.
- Integrated into language learning apps tailored for deaf children.
- Used by teachers who do not know PSL to facilitate effective instruction.

Overall, PSL recognition for Urdu alphabets can serve as a strong foundation for building more advanced recognition systems. Once a system can accurately identify individual letters, it can be expanded to recognize complete words and full sentences. This step-by-step development can lead to more powerful tools that support communication in a wide range of areas, not just in education but also in public services, workplaces, and daily life. In this way, alphabet-level PSL recognition becomes the starting point for creating a more inclusive and accessible digital environment for the deaf community in Pakistan.

2.2 Literature Review

Building on the foundational understanding of SLR classification and its practical relevance, particularly in the context of PSL, it is essential to explore the technological advancements that enable the development of such systems. Deep learning has emerged as a dominant approach due to its capacity to learn complex spatiotemporal patterns from raw visual data with minimal manual intervention, making it a critical component of modern SLR systems. These systems are primarily designed to detect and classify hand gestures, which are central to sign language communication. A review by (Zhang & Jiang, 2024) highlights the effectiveness of deep learning techniques in enhancing communication for the deaf community. More specifically vision-based models work better than sensor-based methods because they cost less and need simpler equipment (Zhang & Jiang, 2024). Given the strong potential of deep learning to handle both static and dynamic sign language data, the following section reviews recent research efforts in the field of SLR that leverage deep learning-based techniques.

Within deep learning-based SLR research, two broad approaches have emerged. The first approach involves training models from scratch, typically using custom CNN architectures tailored to specific datasets. These systems generally rely on a sequence of convolutional layers followed by pooling and fully connected layers to classify hand gestures. For example, Podder et al. (2023) developed a model for recognizing Arabic Sign Language by combining CNNs with a two-layer Long Short-Term Memory (LSTM) network to capture the time-based patterns in facial and hand movements. For classification, they introduced a modified version of a multi-layer perceptron (MLP). The model was trained on a custom dataset consisting of 50 sign classes, with input features extracted using the MediaPipe Holistic framework. Similarly, (Kothadiya et al., 2022) presented *DeepSign*, which combined CNN with recurrent networks such as LSTM and GRU to extract temporal dependencies from Indian Sign Language video sequences. The authors created a custom dataset with 11 commonly used signs captured under controlled background. The model achieves the accuracy of 97% but is limited to just 11 signs only. While such models can be tailored to specific tasks, they require large labelled datasets and often struggle to generalize when trained on limited or less diverse data which is a common limitation in sign language datasets, especially for less-resourced languages like PSL.

Because of these challenges, many studies have shifted towards using transfer learning with pretrained models, which can provide faster convergence, improved accuracy, and better generalization even with limited data. In transfer learning-based sign language recognition, detection models generally fall into two categories: two-stage and one-stage architectures. Two-stage models, such as R-CNN and Faster R-CNN, first generate region proposals and then classify them. While these models are known for their accuracy in static object detection, their multi-step process leads to longer inference times. This makes them less suitable for sign language recognition, which demands real-time response for effective communication. Therefore, we find no significant studies employing two-stage detection frameworks for SLR, particularly in the context of PSL.

On the other hand, one-stage detection models have shown tremendous improvements in SLR, especially those based on the YOLO framework. YOLO-based models integrate object localization and classification into a single forward pass, enabling faster detection with minimal compromise on accuracy. This quality makes them ideal for real-time gesture recognition. (Tyagi et al., 2023) conducted a comparative study on YOLOv5 and YOLOv8 for ASL detection. They found YOLOv5 to be more computationally efficient while still maintaining high accuracy, confirming its suitability for real-time systems, especially in resource-constrained settings. In a related direction, Khan et al. (2021) proposed a lightweight deep learning model for real-time human action recognition on constrained devices, highlighting strategies that are also applicable to sign language recognition in deployment-focused scenarios. Another work on ASL was presented by (Alsharif et al., 2024) where the author combined YOLOv8 for hand detection and MediaPipe for landmark tracking, trained on a diverse dataset of 29,820 images. In addition to ASL, YOLO methods have also been tested across different languages, like for example (Alaftekin et al., 2024) created a real-time Turkish sign language recognition system using improved YOLOv4 based on neural networks. Similarly, (Fan et al., n.d.) proposed a sign language recognition system for Chinese Sign Language, which takes a different direction from earlier studies that mainly focused on static gestures or recognizing individual alphabets. This study instead deals with the more challenging task of recognizing continuous sign language. In this study the author combined YOLOX with an attention mechanism to detect hands and head positions in sign videos and then used a BiLSTM model to recognize gesture sequences. This integration of a one-stage detector with a sequence model illustrates how SLR can evolve toward recognizing continuous sign language. However, despite the innovation, the model achieved a relatively low accuracy of 67.6%, highlighting the ongoing challenges in this area.

While a wide range of studies have explored SLR for ASL, BSL, and CSL, research dedicated to PSL remains limited. Among the few efforts, (Shah et al., 2021) proposed a vision-based method for static PSL alphabet recognition using handcrafted features and Multiple Kernel Learning with Support Vector Machine, achieving 91.98% accuracy. However, the model showed weak performance with certain features, such as speeded up robust features (SURF), which achieved only 15% accuracy. The authors also noted the need for a more diverse dataset and suggested exploring alternative robust features in future. Extending this line of research, (Mujeeb et al., 2023) developed a deep learning-based PSL recognition system trained on a custom dataset comprising 36 static hand gestures. The proposed architecture employed a six-layer convolutional neural network (CNN) and achieved a classification accuracy of 96%. While these results demonstrate the potential of CNN-based models for PSL recognition, the evaluation was conducted under highly controlled conditions, including a uniform black background. Such constraints limit the system's generalizability to real-world environments, where variations in background, lighting, camera angles, and signer characteristics (e.g., gender differences) are prevalent. Addressing these factors is essential for building robust and scalable PSL recognition systems suitable for practical deployment. In another related effort, (Nasim et al., 2024) developed an automated system aimed at supporting deaf and hard-of-hearing (DHH) individuals by translating English text into PSL gestures. The system uses natural language processing techniques such as tokenization and lemmatization, followed by machine translation methods to generate PSL lexical outputs. Although it does not perform gesture recognition, the system effectively converts English alphabets and words into PSL, achieving an accuracy of 89.58% for alphabet translation and 100% for word-level translation. This work highlights a different but important direction, facilitating communication access for DHH users, though it does not address the challenges of real-time PSL gesture detection.

Another promising study on PSL (Hamza & Wali, 2023) presented a deep learning-based recognition pipeline for PSL, integrating data augmentation techniques, specifically translation and rotation, to enhance the diversity and effectiveness of the training dataset. The proposed system was evaluated using a Convolutional 3D (C3D) model, which achieved an accuracy of 93.33%. The results demonstrated that applying augmentation significantly improves both accuracy and generalization. However, the dataset used in this study included only 80 sign words, with just two samples per word, one for training and one for testing. Furthermore, most of the signs were performed by the same individual, limiting the model's ability to generalize across different signers.

One more notable contribution on PSL is presented by (Mirza et al., 2022), who developed a vision-based recognition system for PSL alphabets utilizing the Bag-of-Words (BoW) model and SVM. The study constructed a dataset comprising 5,120 images for 36 signs, collected under controlled conditions from ten native PSL signers. Images were pre-processed, segmented, and SURF-based feature extraction was performed. These features were clustered using K-means++ to generate BoW representations, which were classified using SVM with fivefold cross-validation. The system achieved a classification accuracy of 97.80%, however the reliance on a highly controlled environment, uniform lighting, fixed camera angles, and plain white backgrounds, limits the model's ability to generalize to real-world settings.

Recent advances in the broader SLR field have shifted attention from static alphabets toward dynamic gestures and continuous signing, which more closely reflect natural communication. For example, (Ma et al., n.d.) proposed a Residual-LSTM framework enhanced with channel attention to capture spatiotemporal dependencies in sign video sequences, achieving ~91.2% accuracy on benchmark datasets and approaching the performance of advanced 3D ResNet models. Similarly, (Deng et al., 2025) introduced a Video Transformer Attention-based Network (VTAN) that prioritizes informative frames and hand regions, showcasing the growing role of attention mechanisms and transformer architectures in dynamic SLR. A further contribution is the Sign Language Transformer (SLT) by (Cihan Camgoz et al., 2020) which jointly performs continuous recognition and translation in a single model. By leveraging gloss-level representations, their approach achieved state-of-the-art performance on the RWTH-PHOENIX-Weather-2014T dataset, more than doubling translation accuracy compared to earlier methods. These studies highlight the importance of temporal modeling for advancing continuous sign recognition.

In parallel, researchers are increasingly focusing on multimodal approaches that integrate manual features (hand shapes, trajectories) with non-manual cues (facial expressions, gaze, and head pose). For instance, (Chen et al., 2024) proposed Sign-VTCL, a framework that fuses video, key points, and optical flow streams within a unified transformer-based model. This design enables the system to capture both linguistic detail (from hands and facial movements) and motion dynamics across frames, improving recognition of continuous sign sequences. Beyond these, researchers are also exploring the use of skeletal data combined with RGB video to extend multimodal sign recognition. For instance, the study (Hosain et al., 2019) combined skeleton-based features with RGB video across 51 ASL signs and 13,107 samples. The research study demonstrated the feasibility of leveraging depth sensors and 3D skeleton cues alongside vision for improved accessibility to digital assistants.

These multimodal directions underscore the need for PSL research to move beyond static hand configurations by incorporating richer manual and non-manual annotations and evaluating hybrid architectures in unconstrained environments.

Despite these advances, PSL-specific research remains limited and rarely tested in real-world contexts. Existing studies are constrained by small or highly controlled datasets, and importantly, YOLO-based approaches for PSL recognition remain unexplored, even though YOLO has proven highly effective for real-time sign detection in other languages. This lack of robust, field-tested PSL systems highlights a clear research gap in developing scalable and accessible solutions tailored to Pakistan's Deaf community.

To address these gaps, the proposed study presents real time PSL recognition system validated in real world settings. The core contributions of this work are as follows:

1. Development of a high-quality, manually annotated PSL dataset comprising 3,963 images representing 38 PSL alphabets.
2. Enhancement of dataset robustness through the application of both geometric and photometric data augmentation techniques, resulting in a threefold increase in dataset size and improved model generalization.
3. Implementation of an efficient deep learning-based PSL recognition system utilizing the YOLOv5 object detection model, optimized for high real-time accuracy of 94.6% and adaptability to resource-constrained environments.
4. Real-world validation and effectiveness assessment of the system through deployment in educational settings, specifically at the Ida Rieu School for the Blind and Deaf, demonstrating improved accessibility for hearing-impaired individuals.

Through these contributions, this work addresses the critical gap in inclusive communication technologies for Pakistan's deaf community, establishing a foundational framework for advancing AI-based PSL interpretation systems and paving the way for broader accessibility solutions in the region.

To address these gaps, the proposed study presents a real-time PSL recognition system validated in real-world settings. The novelty and core contributions of this work are as follows:

- **First linguistically valid PSL dataset** developed from **native signers** in **real-world conditions**, ensuring natural fluency, linguistic accuracy, and ecological validity.
- **Hybrid strategy of real data + synthetic augmentation**, expanding the dataset threefold (3,963 → 9,522 images) and enhancing model generalization.
- **Implementation of an efficient YOLOv5-based PSL recognition system**, optimized for real-time performance (94.6% accuracy) and deployment in real world environments.
- **Real-world validation in an educational setting** (Ida Rieu School for the Blind and Deaf), demonstrating practical effectiveness and accessibility for hearing-impaired individuals.

Through these contributions, this work establishes the first linguistically valid, real-world tested PSL recognition framework and sets a foundation for inclusive communication technologies and future PSL/SLR research.

3. METHODOLOGY

This section describes the step-by-step process used to develop and deploy the PSL recognition system. The methodology follows a systematic approach, starting from data collection to real-world testing in educational settings, as shown in Figure 3.

Figure 3. End to end workflow of the proposed PSL SLR framework

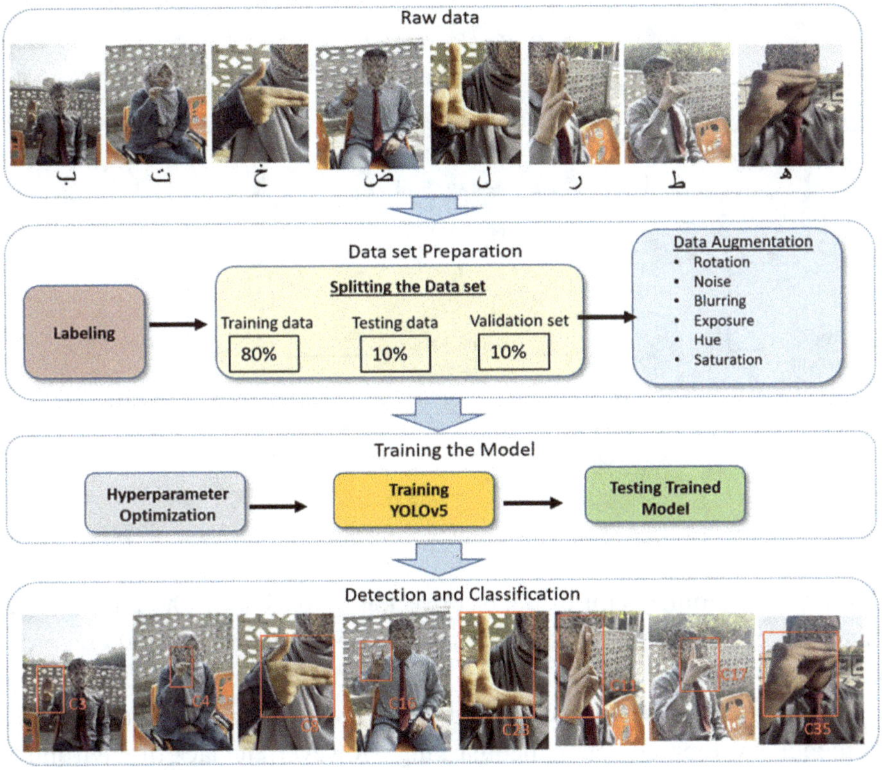

3.1 Dataset Development and Augmentation

An important factor in developing robust SLR systems is the diversity of the datasets used during training and evaluation. Diverse datasets are essential to ensure that SLR models can generalize effectively across the wide range of ways in which signs are performed, by individuals with different signing styles, across varying age groups, genders, and under diverse environmental conditions.

SLR dataset diversity can be characterized across three key dimensions, environmental conditions, data source type and signer's linguistic background, as shown in Figure 4.

Figure 4. Key dimensions contributing to the dataset diversity of Sign Language Recognition (SLR)

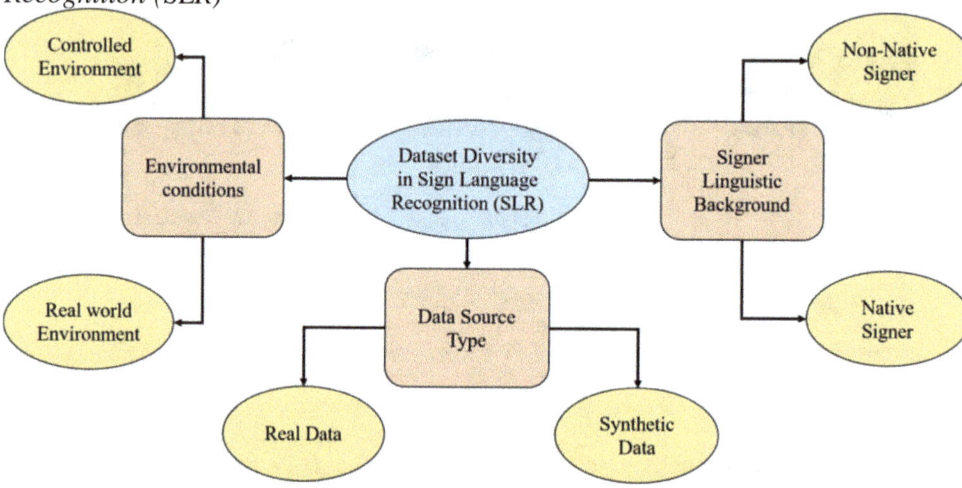

One important dimension of dataset diversity is based on the environment in which data is collected. Controlled environment datasets are typically recorded in laboratories or studios, where lighting, background, and camera angles are normally fixed. These datasets offer high-quality, noise-free samples that are ideal for initial model development and benchmarking. However, the lack of environmental variability in such datasets often results in models that are less effective when deployed in real-world settings, where lighting conditions fluctuate, backgrounds are non-uniform, and natural occlusions may occur.

In contrast, real-world datasets are collected in natural settings, such as classrooms, homes, or public spaces. These datasets capture the complexity of real-world settings, including diverse backgrounds, fluctuating lighting conditions, varying camera angles, spontaneous and unconstrained gestures. While they present greater challenges in terms of data annotation and pre-processing, models trained on real-world data are generally more robust and better suited for deployment in practical dynamic scenarios. A notable example of this approach is the Isharah dataset for Arabic Sign Language, which contains thousands of continuous sign samples recorded using smartphone cameras across varied real-world settings, intentionally capturing variations in lighting, angles, and background environments (Alyami et al., 2025).

This contrast between controlled and real-world data highlights the importance of using mixed-environment datasets to train systems meant for deployment in practical conditions.

Another critical dimension of dataset diversity is the linguistic background of the signers. There are two types of signers, native and non-native. Native signers are individuals who have acquired PSL as their first language from early childhood, produce data that is naturally fluent, consistent, and rich in the linguistic structures. This makes their contributions invaluable for training recognition systems that aim to reflect real-world usage accurately.

In contrast, data collected from non-native signers, who may have learned PSL later in life or use it less frequently, often lacks the linguistic authenticity and may introduce inconsistencies or unnatural signing patterns. Such inconsistency can degrade model performance and limit the system's ability to generalize. However, recruiting a large number of native signers can be challenging, especially for under-resourced languages like PSL.

To address the limitations of limited real-world and the challenges associated with recruiting native signers, researchers have increasingly explored synthetic data creation as an alternate solution. Synthetic dataset creation involves generating artificial sign language data using computational techniques rather than capturing it directly from human signers. In the context of SLR, this can be achieved through several methods, such as using 3D animated avatars to simulate sign gestures, pose estimation frameworks to manipulate joint coordinates for gesture replay, or Generative Adversarial Networks (GANs) to create realistic image sequences based on limited training samples.

Synthetic data offers several advantages. It enables the large-scale generation of diverse gesture samples, allowing researchers to simulate variations in sign types, signer appearances, lighting conditions, and backgrounds. This can help address class imbalance, expand underrepresented categories, and significantly reduce the labour and time involved in manual data collection.

However, despite these benefits, synthetic datasets present notable limitations. Artificially generated gestures often lack the subtle facial expressions and body movement that are critical to natural and expressive sign language communication. Additionally, models trained heavily or exclusively on synthetic data may struggle to generalize to real-world scenarios, particularly when synthetic samples fail to reflect realistic motion dynamics or environmental complexity. A further limitation of synthetic dataset is, it does not capture the diversity of real signers in terms of hand shape, skin tone, movement styles, and signer-specific articulation patterns.

A notable example of synthetic dataset creation is UAlpha40 dataset introduced by (Javaid et al., 2025). The dataset offers extensive coverage of the Urdu alphabets in PSL, including 40 PSL signs, collected from over 110 participants. The dataset employs diverse augmentation techniques such as gaussian noise, brightness, flip ratios, blurring and sharpening to increase dataset size. Despite its significance, the dataset is collected in a highly controlled environment, with uniform backgrounds, fixed lighting, and restricted signer poses. Moreover, the participant were non-native signers, reducing the linguistic accuracy of the signs. The dataset also relies heavily on synthetic augmentation to expand its size and variability, which, while useful, cannot fully replicate the natural articulation, motion dynamics, and signer-specific variations found in real-world communication.

In contrast to synthetic dataset creation, real data that is collected directly from human signers in natural or controlled environments, real data provides authentic representations of sign language. Such data captures authentic hand movements, facial expressions, and contextual tones essential for effective sign language recognition.

Each of these dataset types controlled/real-world, native/non-native, real/synthetic data has its own strengths and weaknesses. Controlled datasets are easy to annotate and ideal for algorithm development, but they lack real-world complexity. Real-world datasets provide valuable variability but are time-consuming and expensive to collect and annotate. Native signer data ensures linguistic consistency and accuracy but is often limited in scale, while synthetic data offers scalability but may lack realism.

Given these trade-offs, a hybrid approach that combines real-world data from native signers with synthetic data augmentation emerges as a promising solution for PSL SLR systems. Specifically, combining real-world data from native signers with synthetic data augmentation allows researchers to take advantage of both approaches. By building the dataset on authentic recordings from native users, capturing the natural fluency, grammar, and expressiveness of PSL, and complementing it with synthetically generated samples to fill gaps in signer diversity, environmental variation, or underrepresented classes, the resulting dataset becomes both linguistically valid and sufficiently diverse. This integrated approach significantly improves the model's ability to generalize across different signers, lighting conditions, camera perspectives, and regional sign variants, challenges that are often overlooked or underrepresented in existing PSL datasets.

In our work, we have adopted this hybrid strategy, collecting a core dataset from native PSL signers in natural environments and augmenting it with synthetic variations to simulate a wide range of real-world conditions. To the best of our knowledge, this is the first time a PSL dataset has been created using such a hybrid approach, combining native signer data collected in natural environments with synthetic augmentation to address class imbalance and environmental variability. This methodology not only addresses the scarcity of comprehensive PSL datasets but also ensures that our SLR system is both linguistically accurate and technically robust. By leveraging the strengths of both real and synthetic data, we aim to set a new standard for PSL recognition and contribute to more inclusive communication technologies for individuals with hearing disabilities in Pakistan.

Following this hybrid strategy of dataset creation (real world environment + native signer + synthetic augmentation), the dataset development process was carefully structured into two main phases: data collection and data pre-processing. Each phase was designed to ensure the resulting dataset met critical benchmarks of linguistic accuracy, environmental diversity, and technical quality, factors essential for training high-performance SLR systems tailored to the PSL context. To ensure high data quality, we defined inclusion and exclusion criteria for participant selection.

Inclusion Criteria:

- Only individuals with full knowledge of PSL were selected.
- Both male and female participants were included to avoid gender bias.
- Signers were selected from various age groups.
- Images were captured with consistent camera angles and varying lighting conditions.

Exclusion Criteria:

- Individuals lacking PSL proficiency were excluded.
- If minors were involved, parental consent was obtained.
- Participants with physical impairments that could affect signing were not included.

Participants were students from Ida Rieu School for the Blind and Deaf, representing grades 6 to 10. The signer group included 10 students, four female and six male students. Data acquisition was conducted using a digital camera, with careful consideration given to capturing variability across lighting, camera angles, and background complexity. This deliberate inclusion of visual variability aims to enhance the dataset's generalizability in real deployment settings.

The dataset comprises 38 PSL signs representing the Urdu alphabet with an average of 104 images per sign. A total of 3,963 images were collected across multiple sessions. Some samples from the dataset are illustrated in Figure 5, Figure 6, Figure 7, Figure 8 and Figure 9, showcasing the diversity in hand gestures, backgrounds, and participant characteristics captured during the data collection process.

Figure 5. PSL Dataset part 1

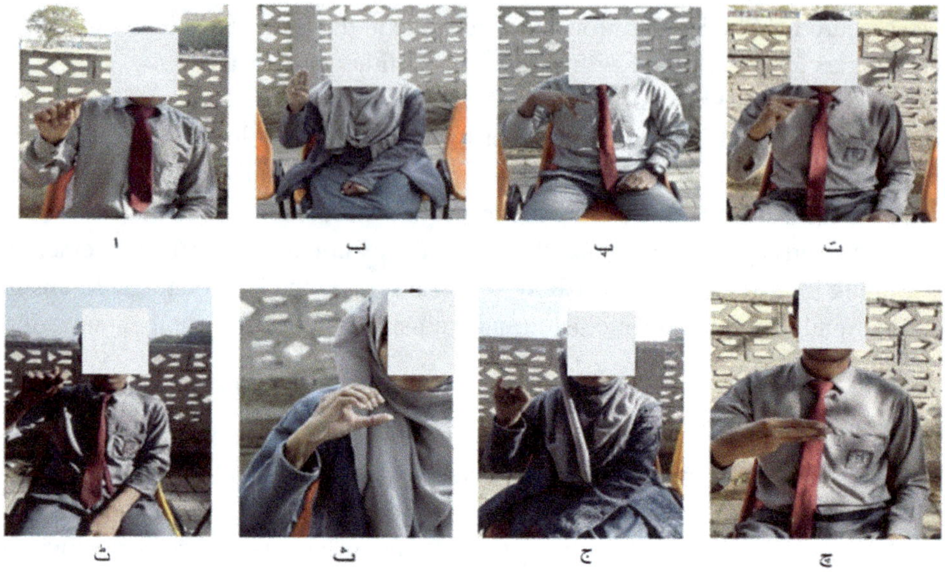

Figure 6. PSL Dataset part 2

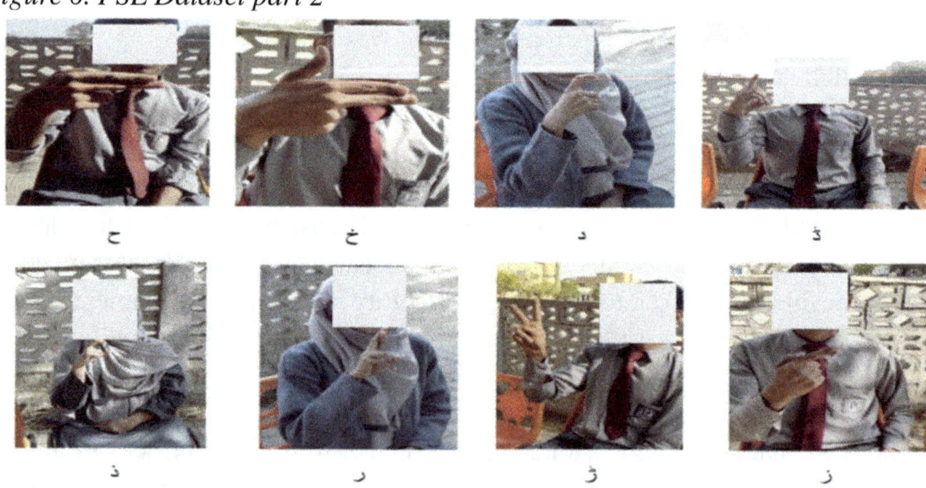

Figure 7. PSL Dataset part 3

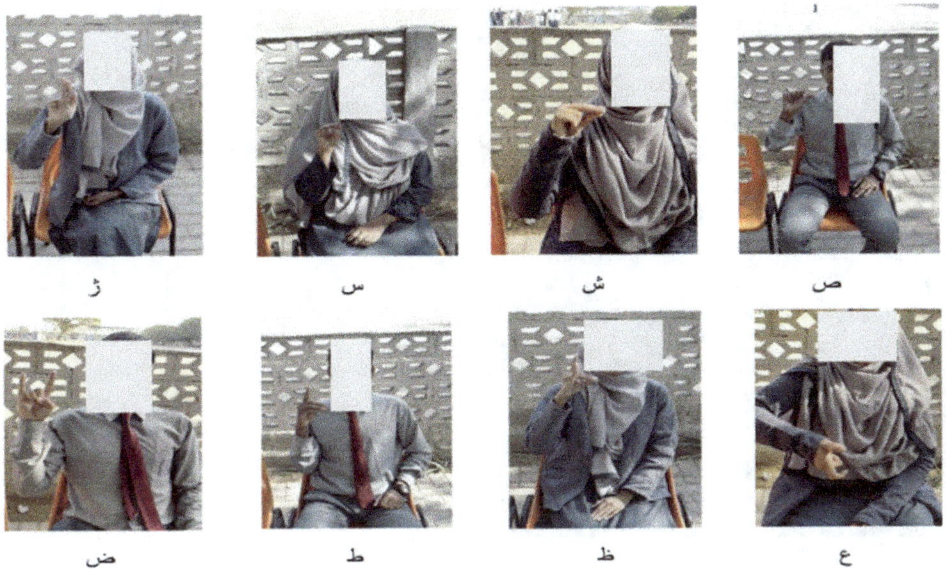

Figure 8. PSL Dataset part 4

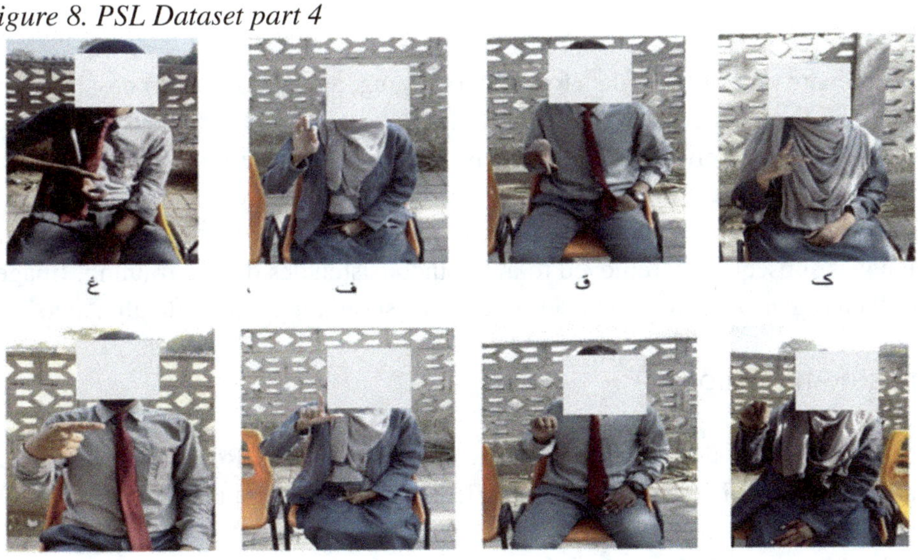

Figure 9. PSL Dataset part 5

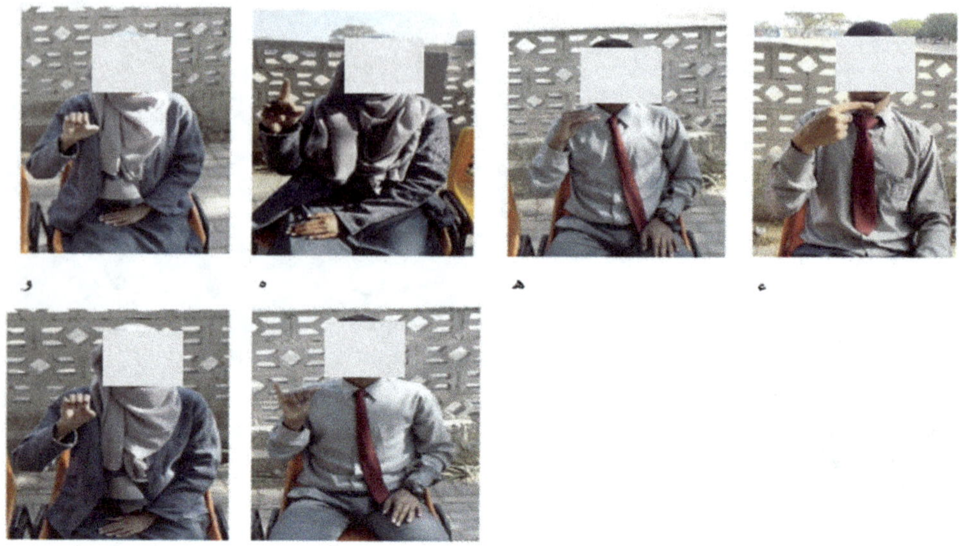

و ہ ھ ء

ی ے

Data Pre-processing

To prepare the collected data for model training, a series of pre-processing steps were applied to enhance consistency and reduce computational overhead. The images were resized uniformly to 640×640 pixels. To simplify processing, each image was converted to grayscale, thereby reducing the complexity of colour channels. Lastly, image orientations were standardized by correcting rotation using EXIF metadata, which was subsequently removed to avoid inconsistencies during training. Images were then organized into 38 classes, each corresponding to an Urdu alphabet.

Dataset Annotation

After preprocessing, annotation was conducted using Roboflow's platform, where all collected images were uploaded, and bounding boxes were manually drawn around the hand signs. Each image was labelled with its corresponding PSL alphabet class, and the annotated dataset was then exported in YOLO format, optimized for object detection tasks. To illustrate this process, sample annotated images are presented in Figure 10, showing bounding boxes accurately highlighting hand signs performed by different participants in varied real-world conditions. These examples reflect the diversity in participant appearance, gesture articulation, and lighting environments, all of which contribute to the dataset's robustness and the model's ability to generalize.

Figure 10. Sample annotated images from PSL showing bounding boxes drawn around hand signs by diverse participants

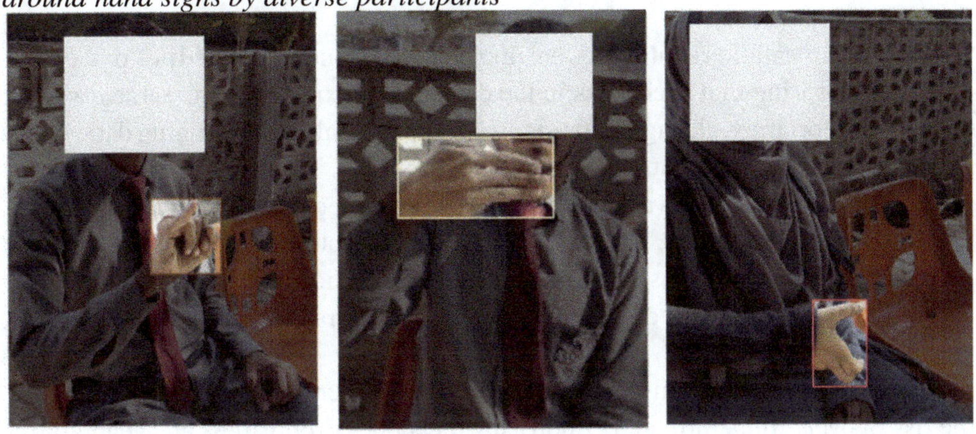

Data Augmentation

To further increase data diversity, we applied a variety of augmentation techniques. Data augmentation plays a crucial role in enhancing the diversity of the training dataset without the need to collect additional real-world samples. In this study, a set of carefully selected transformations was applied, as shown in Figure 11, to improve the generalization of the PSL recognition model, particularly in handling variations in hand shapes, lighting conditions, and backgrounds. These transformations were designed to reflect the kinds of visual noise and distortions often encountered in real-world settings, thereby making the model more robust.

The specific augmentation techniques used are as follows:

- **Rotation:** Each image was randomly rotated between $-13°$ and $+13°$, simulating natural variations in hand orientation during signing.
- **Noise Addition:** Salt-and-pepper noise was introduced to ~1.72% of image pixels, mimicking disruptions caused by camera sensors or noisy environments.
- **Blurring:** A Gaussian blur (σ = 0–0.5) was applied to reduce minor visual details and encourage the model to focus on essential shape and contour features.

- **Exposure Adjustment:** Image exposure was randomly altered between −10% and +10% to simulate both low-light indoor and bright outdoor conditions.
- **Saturation Adjustment:** Variations in saturation were introduced to help the model recognize signs under different levels of color richness and illumination.

These augmentation strategies were implemented using automated pre-processing pipelines, ensuring that each class in the dataset was exposed to the same transformations. Importantly, all augmentations were applied only to the training data, while validation and test sets contained only original images. This approach ensured that model performance was evaluated on unseen, unaltered samples, maintaining the validity of reported results. Furthermore, the augmentations were carefully chosen to mirror realistic variations, such as lighting changes, noise, and hand orientations, commonly encountered in deployment environments, rather than introducing artificial distortions.

Overall, augmentation not only expanded the dataset threefold but also reduced the risk of overfitting, ultimately improving the model's robustness and adaptability for real-world PSL recognition tasks.

Figure 11. Data augmentation techniques applied to PSL sign images. From left to right: original image, salt and pepper noise, random rotation, combined noise with rotation, and Gaussian blur

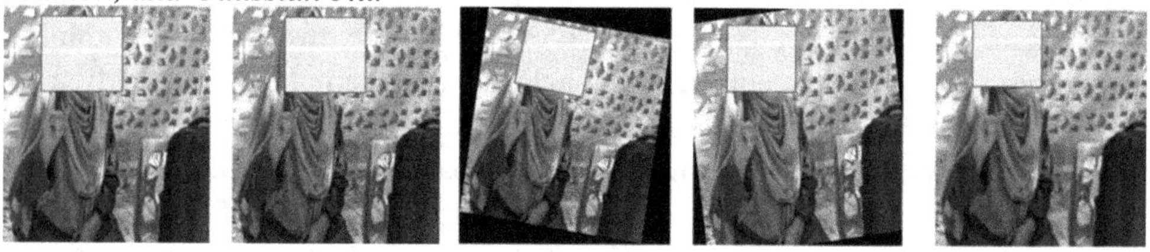

Final Dataset Composition

After applying pre-processing and augmentation, the dataset grew significantly. The dataset statistics at each stage are summarized in Table 1. This structured and well-balanced dataset provided a solid foundation for training the YOLOv5-based PSL recognition model, ensuring both quality and diversity necessary for robust performance.

Table 1. Dataset statistics by stages

Stage	Image Count
Before Augmentation	3,963
After Augmentation	9,522
Training Set	7618
Validation Set	952
Testing set	952

3.2 Model Architecture and Training

Following the development of a diverse and robust dataset, the next critical step was the selection of an appropriate deep learning model. The model selection was guided by the key design criteria including computational efficiency, deployment feasibility, generalizability, detection stability, and real-time performance.

A variety of state-of-the-art object detection models were evaluated based on key design criteria mentioned above. After evaluating several state-of-the-art object detection architectures, YOLOv5 was selected after evaluating multiple object detection models against key design criteria: detection stability, generalizability, computational efficiency, deployment feasibility, and real-time performance. Its multi-scale feature detection ensures robust gesture recognition across spatial resolutions. Generalization is enhanced through mosaic augmentation, adaptive anchors, and feature pyramid networks. YOLOv5 outperforms newer models in efficiency, making it ideal for resource-constrained devices. Its lightweight architecture allows seamless deployment on mobile and embedded systems, while fast inference speed supports real-time sign language recognition, essential for interactive and accessible communication in real-world educational and assistive settings.

To situate YOLOv5 within the broader landscape of detection models, we compared it with YOLOv8 (Ultralytics, 2024), EfficientDet(Tan et al., 2020), and RF-DETR (Roboflow, 2023) using benchmark results on the MS COCO dataset.

As shown in Table 2, YOLOv5n and YOLOv5s emerge as the most lightweight models, with significantly fewer parameters and faster inference speeds compared to YOLOv8, EfficientDet, and RF-DETR variants. This makes YOLOv5 highly suitable for real-time and resource-constrained PSL applications. However, YOLOv5 exhibits lower accuracy relative to EfficientDet and transformer-based detectors. These gaps can be addressed through augmentation pipelines, hyperparameter tuning, and optimization strategies, enabling YOLOv5 to remain competitive while retaining its strengths in speed and deployment feasibility.

Table 2. Comparison of YOLOv5 with other detection models on MS COCO

Model	**Accuracy (mAP 50:95)**	**Speed (ms)**	**Params (M)**
YOLOv5n	28	1.12	2.6
YOLOv5s	37.4	1.92	9.1
YOLOv8n	37.3	1.47	3.2
YOLOv8s	44.9	2.66	11.2
EfficientDET D0	53	12	3.9
EfficientDET D3	65.9	3.52	12
RF-DETR-N	48.4	2.32	30.5
RF-DETR-S	53	3.52	32.1

With these considerations, YOLOv5 was selected as the foundation for our PSL recognition system, ensuring that the model would not only perform well during offline evaluations but also support real-time deployment. The YOLOv5 architecture is composed of three interconnected modules: Backbone, Neck, and Head, which collaboratively process input images, extract meaningful features, and generate predictions in real time as shown in Figure 12.

Figure 12. YOLOv5 architecture

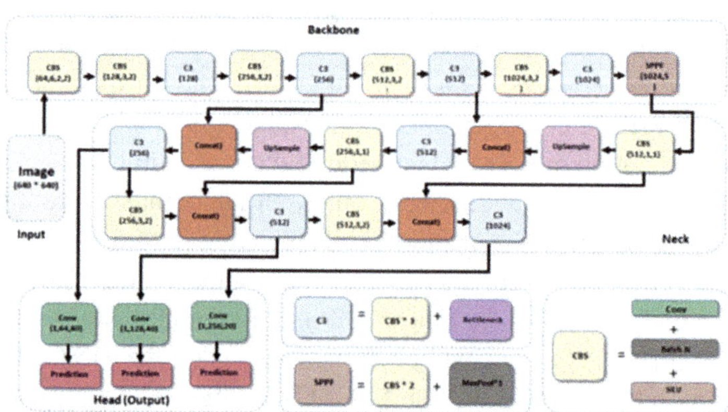

(Ultralytics)

Backbone: The backbone serves as the feature extractor. YOLOv5 utilizes the CSPDarknet53 architecture, which employs Cross Stage Partial connections to improve gradient flow and reduce computational cost. It consists of a series of convolutional layers combined with Batch Normalization and SiLU activation functions (CBS modules), along with C3 modules that capture spatial and semantic features.

The backbone concludes with a Spatial Pyramid Pooling - Fast (SPPF) block that efficiently captures multi-scale contextual information (Bochkovskiy et al., 2020).

Neck: The neck module aggregates and refines features from different scales to enhance detection robustness across object sizes. YOLOv5's neck combines Path Aggregation Network (PANet) and SPPF structures. It fuses feature maps at various resolutions using concatenation and up sampling operations, with additional C3 blocks for improved feature representation (Liu et al., 2018).

Head: The head generates the final detection outputs, including bounding box coordinates, object scores, and class probabilities. It predicts at three different scales, corresponding to small, medium, and large objects, enabling effective detection of varying hand sign sizes (Redmon & Farhadi, 2018).

This modular design achieves a strong balance between speed and accuracy, making YOLOv5 particularly suitable for real-time PSL recognition. YOLOv5 incorporates the Complete Intersection over Union (CIOU) loss function to enhance bounding box regression accuracy by considering overlap area, center distance, and aspect ratio alignment (Zheng et al., 2020).

The model was trained over multiple epochs using the following configuration:

- **Optimizer**: Stochastic Gradient Descent (SGD) with momentum
- **Learning Rate**: Initially set at 0.01 with decay applied
- **Loss Function**: Custom object detection loss combining bounding box regression and classification loss
- **Batch Size**: 16 images per iteration
- **Epochs**: 150, with early stopping based on validation accuracy

During training, the model's hyperparameters were adjusted through several trials to avoid overfitting and improve generalization. To improve generalization and reduce overfitting, the model employed data augmentation techniques in real time during training. This means that instead of applying augmentations beforehand and saving them as separate images, transformations such as rotation, noise, and exposure adjustments were applied dynamically to each image as it was loaded for training. This approach helped expose the model to a wider variety of inputs in each epoch, enhancing its ability to perform well in diverse, real-world scenarios. Figure 13 demonstrates a sample prediction, highlighting the model's ability to localize and classify hand signs with 95% confidence.

Figure 13. PSL recognition model prediction example showing input image(left) and the output image (right) with detected sign C2 at 95% confidence with bounding box localization

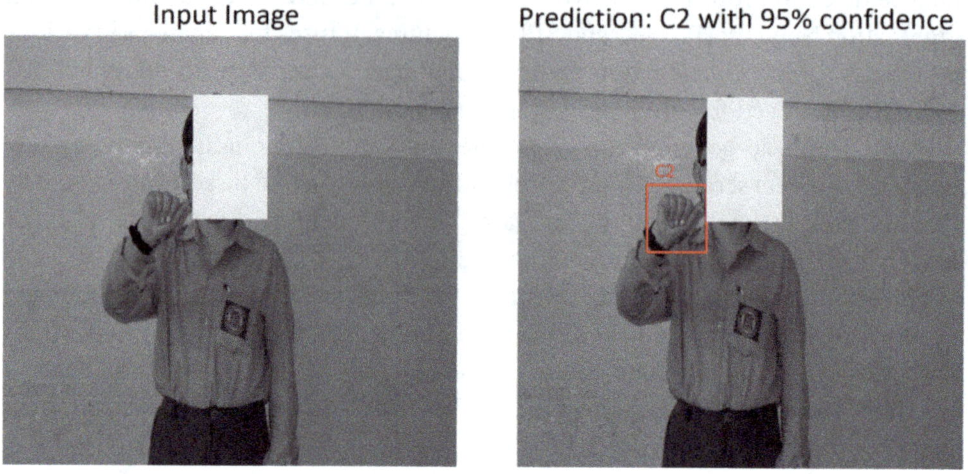

4. EXPERIMENTAL SETUP AND RESULTS

The PSL recognition model was developed and trained using the PyTorch framework, which provided the flexibility required for custom implementation and parameter tuning. Model training was performed on an NVIDIA Tesla T4 GPU to ensure efficient handling of large-scale training iterations and faster convergence.

This section presents a detailed evaluation of the proposed PSL recognition system, analyzing both headline metrics and deeper diagnostic studies including error analysis, ablation experiments, and statistical testing. These findings highlight the effectiveness of the YOLOv5-based architecture in accurately detecting and classifying PSL alphabet gestures, confirming its suitability for real-time sign language interpretation.

Figure 14. Training and validation performance of YOLOv5

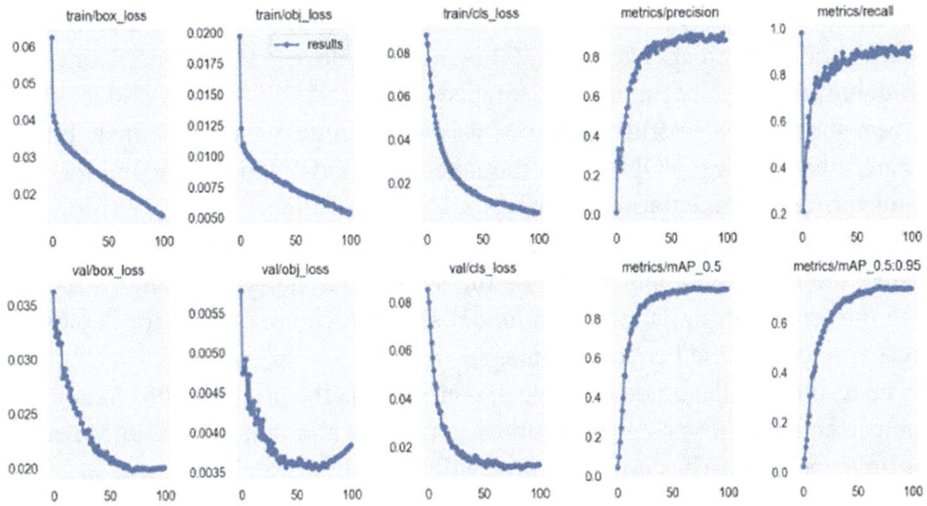

The training curves in Figure 14 illustrate the effectiveness of the loss functions used to optimize the model's performance. The *bounding box loss*, which measures how accurately the model locates hand signs within images, decreased from approximately 0.06 to 0.014, indicating better localization. The *object detection loss*, responsible for distinguishing hand signs from the background, dropped from 0.02 to 0.005, reflecting enhanced detection precision. Similarly, the *classification loss*, which evaluates the model's ability to correctly identify specific PSL alphabets, reduced from 0.08 to 0.008, showing notable improvement in classification accuracy throughout training. The *validation performance*, as shown in Figure 14, further supports the model's learning stability and generalization. The *validation box loss* decreased from 0.035 to 0.020, suggesting that the model maintained accurate hand sign localization on unseen data. Similarly, the *validation object loss* declined from 0.0048 to 0.0036, indicating consistent object detection across different samples. The *validation classification loss* also improved significantly, dropping from 0.08 to 0.015, which reflects the model's growing ability to correctly classify PSL alphabets during evaluation. Together, these trends confirm the model's robustness and its readiness for real-world application.

The training curves in Figure 14 show clear improvements in precision also along with the loss reduction. precision increased from 0.2 to 0.92, indicating that the model became significantly better at avoiding false positives, when it predicts a detection, while recall improved from 0.2 to 0.88, reflecting that the model's ability to find actual objects improved dramatically. To further quantify detection performance, the mean Average Precision (mAP) metrics provides an overall evaluation. The model achieved a mAP@0.5 of 0.94, indicating excellent overall detection performance, as this metric combines both precision and recall across different confidence thresholds, with 0.94 being very close to the perfect score of 1.0. Achieving such high accuracy on a linguistically valid PSL dataset collected from native signers in real-world conditions was a challenge, which was made possible by carefully selecting YOLOv5 as the detection model and optimizing the hyper parameters and augmentation strategy.

The performance evaluation also considered deployment-related metrics to validate the real-time applicability of the system. Along with accuracy, these include inference speed, latency, and model size, which are critical for deployment in resource-constrained environments.

The results, as illustrated in Table 3, confirm that the proposed PSL recognition system not only achieves high detection accuracy but also meets the requirements for real-time operation. The combination of 94% mAP, lightweight model size, and ~55 FPS inference speed demonstrates that the framework is suitable for deployment in both high-performance environments and resource-constrained edge devices, paving the way for portable and accessible PSL recognition solutions.

Table 3. Quantitative performance metrics of the proposed PSL recognition system

Metric	Result	Description
Precision	91.67%	Ability to avoid false positives
Recall	88.24%	Ability to detect actual signs correctly
mAP@0.5	94.67%	Overall detection accuracy combining precision and recall
F1-Score	89.92%	Harmonic mean of precision and recall
Model size	9.1 M parameters	Lightweight design suitable for deployment
Inference Speed	55 FPS	Real-time performance on NVIDIA Tesla T4 GPU

4.1 Error Analysis

Further evaluation was conducted using the confusion matrix shown in Figure 15, which illustrates the model's performance across all 38 PSL alphabet classes. The matrix reveals clear strengths and some systematic confusions:

- **Overall accuracy:** The high-intensity diagonal pattern confirms that most PSL signs were classified correctly, with many classes achieving over 90%

accuracy. This demonstrates the model's strong ability to discriminate across a diverse sign set.

- **Visually similar signs:** Misclassifications occurred primarily between signs that share close hand shape or orientation features. For instance, **(C4) and (C5)**, as well as **(C13) and (C14)**, were occasionally confused due to subtle finger positioning differences. Similarly, **(C12) and (C13)** showed overlaps, reflecting the challenge of distinguishing fine-grained visual cues.
- **Phonologically close signs:** Certain pairs like **(C6) and (C8)** were misclassified at times, which can be attributed to their similar base hand shape and minor differentiating strokes.
- **Background interference:** A few signs were misclassified as "background," particularly in cases of poor lighting or partial occlusion, suggesting sensitivity to environmental noise.

Overall, the confusion matrix confirms that the YOLOv5-based model demonstrates robust class-level performance with strong diagonal dominance. At the same time, it highlights challenging cases involving fine visual distinctions, pointing toward future improvements through targeted augmentation (e.g., hand rotation, illumination variation) and class-balanced dataset expansion.

Figure 15. Confusion matrix displaying classification performance across 38 PSL alphabets

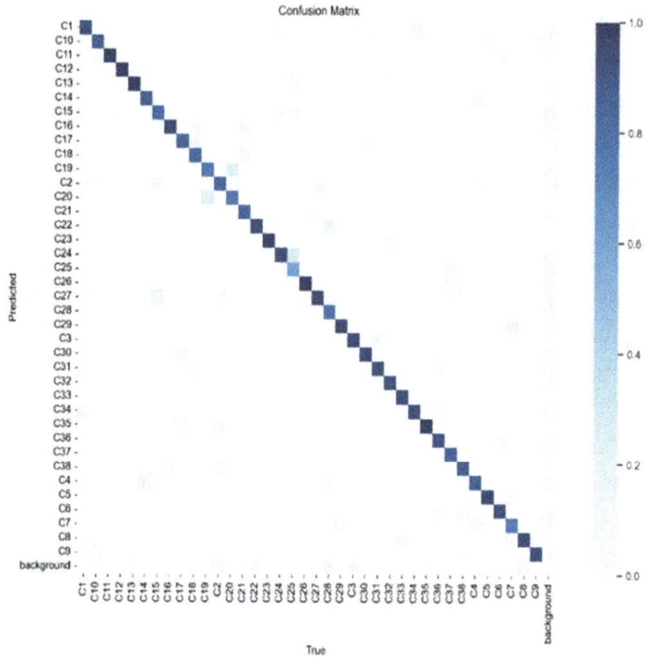

4.2 Ablation and Statistical Validation

To assess the contribution of data augmentation and to establish the statistical reliability of the observed improvements, an ablation study was performed, followed by formal statistical testing.

Table 4 summarizes the performance of the PSL recognition model trained with and without augmentation. The results demonstrate that augmentation yields consistent improvements across all metrics, most notably in accuracy (+4.3%) and F1-score (+5.1%), highlighting its critical role in enhancing generalization.

Table 4. Ablation study: performance with and without augmentation

Configuration	Accuracy	Precision	Recall	F1-Score
Without augmentation	90.4%	87.1%	82.6%	84.8%
With augmentation	94.7%	91.7%	88.2%	89.9%

To verify that these gains were not the result of random variation, a paired t-test was conducted.

Table 5 reports the observed accuracies across three independent runs of each configuration. The mean difference between augmentation and non-augmentation runs was 4.23%, with a standard deviation of 0.231. The paired t-test expressed as t, yielded $t(2)=6.27$, $p<0.05$ confirming that these gains are statistically significant and not attributable to random variation.

Table 5. Experimental runs used for paired t-test

Run	With Augmentation (%)	Without Augmentation (%)	Difference (d = X1 – X2)
1	94.8	90.2	4.6
2	94.3	90.6	3.7
3	94.5	90.3	4.2

Table 6. Comparison with existing studies on PSL recognition

Feature	Dataset	Dataset Type	Dataset diversity	Model	Accuracy	Real world Validation
(Mujeeb et al., 2023)	5,120 (images), 353 (videos)	PSL images and videos	Controlled environment, Non-native signers	CNN	96.17%	×
(Hamza & Wali, 2023)	160 (images)	PSL images	Controlled environment, Non-native signers	CNN	93%	×
(Shah et al., 2021)	6,633 (images)	PSL images	Controlled environment, Non-native signers	Multiple Kernel Learning (MKL)	91.98%	×
Our work, 2025	9,522 (images)	PSL images	Real world environment, native signers	YOLOv5	94.67%	✓

Table 6 highlights the key distinctions between our proposed work and previous studies. Our approach stands out by offering real-time recognition of the PSL alphabet using the YOLOv5 model, which is recognized for its high speed and accuracy in object detection. Unlike earlier studies, our dataset is both larger and more diverse, collected using native signers for better accuracy, comprising 9,522 images representing 38 PSL alphabet signs.

This diversity enhances the model's ability to generalize across different hand shapes and lighting conditions. Additionally, a significant contribution of our work is its real-world validation; the model was tested in an actual educational setting.

To the best of our knowledge, this is the first PSL recognition system to be field-tested in an educational environment with native signers, a contribution that advances prior PSL research beyond controlled laboratory settings. In contrast, many prior studies either used smaller datasets or lacked real-world testing, which may limit their practical usability. By integrating a robust dataset, real-time detection, and field validation, this study provides a more comprehensive and application-ready solution for PSL recognition.

5. LIMITATIONS AND FUTURE WORK

Despite achieving high accuracy and demonstrating real-world deployment, the proposed PSL recognition system has several limitations, each of which informs future research directions:

- **Hardware dependency**: The current system was deployed on a high-end GPU (NVIDIA Tesla T4), which has high power consumption and limits portability. *Future work will focus on optimizing the framework for deployment on edge devices such as Raspberry Pi or low-power embedded platforms to enable wider accessibility.*
- **Static recognition only**: The present framework focuses on static PSL alphabets and does not capture the richness of continuous signing. *Extending the system to dynamic, video-based recognition will better reflect natural communication.*
- **Lack of non-manual features**: Facial expressions, gaze, and head movements, crucial for natural sign language interpretation, were not included. *In future, multimodal approaches integrating both manual and non-manual cues will be explored.*
- **Dataset constraints**: Data was collected from a single institution without signer-independent or cross-dataset testing. *Broader data collection across institutions and the adoption of signer-independent protocols, cross-dataset, and cross-site validation will strengthen generalizability.*
- **Scalability**: Expanding to larger datasets and diverse populations may require greater computational efficiency. *Optimization strategies such as pruning, quantization, and distributed training will be investigated to maintain performance at scale.*

- **Short-term validation**: The system was evaluated in a single deployment phase without long-term monitoring. *Future studies will include longitudinal testing in classrooms and service centers to measure stability, user adaptation, and performance drift.*
- **Error handling**: The system currently provides only the most probable prediction. *Future versions will integrate confidence thresholds, top-k outputs, and interactive feedback loops to improve reliability in real-world use.*

6. CONCLUSION

This chapter presented the design, development, and evaluation of a deep learning-based system for recognizing PSL using static hand gestures representing Urdu alphabets. By employing the YOLOv5 object detection framework and constructing a custom dataset collected from hearing-impaired students, the model achieved high accuracy (94.67%) along with strong precision and recall. Through extensive data augmentation and careful annotation, the model demonstrated robustness to variations in lighting, hand shape, and environmental noise. The system's performance was validated through real-world deployment at the Ida Rieu School for the Blind and Deaf, where it successfully facilitated communication and interaction, highlighting its practical relevance and social value.

Beyond technical performance, user experience plays a central role in system acceptance. During deployment at the Ida Rieu School, students reported that the PSL-to-Urdu recognition system was both engaging and supportive for learning. Teachers observed that it facilitated classroom interaction, particularly for learners struggling with written Urdu. These early insights suggest strong potential for educational and assistive applications. Future deployments will include structured user experience (UX) evaluations with deaf users and instructors to assess usability, accessibility, and satisfaction, ensuring that the system meets the practical needs of its intended beneficiaries.

Despite these achievements, several challenges remain that can be addressed in future work. One key area is the extension of the system beyond static alphabets to dynamic gestures, which are essential for expressing full words and sentences in PSL. Another critical area is optimizing the model for deployment in low-power, edge computing environments, such as mobile devices and embedded systems commonly used in classrooms or public service centers. Reducing computational load and memory requirements without sacrificing accuracy will be essential to ensure reliable, real-time performance under power-constrained conditions. Techniques such as model pruning and quantization could be explored to make the system more suitable for widespread, energy-efficient deployment.

In conclusion, this research contributes a scalable, real-time PSL recognition solution built with local context and practical deployment in mind. It lays a foundational step toward inclusive communication technologies that address the needs of the deaf community in Pakistan, while offering a framework for similar initiatives in other underrepresented linguistic regions.

7. SUMMARY

This chapter presents a comprehensive exploration of a deep learning-based system developed to interpret Pakistan Sign Language (PSL), aiming to enhance communication accessibility for individuals with hearing disabilities in Pakistan. It addresses a critical technological and social gap by introducing a real-time recognition system capable of interpreting PSL alphabet signs with high accuracy using the YOLOv5 object detection model. The research is rooted in the broader context of challenges faced by the deaf community, where over 1.25 million people experience hearing impairment. Despite PSL being the primary communication mode for this community, it remains poorly understood by the general population, creating barriers to accessing education, employment, healthcare, and civic services.

The chapter highlights the linguistic and structural richness of PSL, which incorporates manual features such as hand shape, position, and movement, and non-manual features including facial expressions and head movements. This complexity enables expressive communication but poses challenges for systems attempting to interpret the language. While sign language recognition (SLR) research has progressed in languages like American Sign Language (ASL) and British Sign Language (BSL), PSL has received limited attention, particularly in developing practical, real-world systems. Most existing PSL models rely on small datasets and testing in controlled environments that fail to reflect the diverse, dynamic contexts in which PSL is used.

To bridge this gap, a custom PSL dataset comprising 3,963 images of hand signs was developed and expanded to 9,522 through augmentation techniques such as rotation, noise addition, and exposure adjustment. These images were collected from native signers—students at the Ida Rieu School for the Blind and Deaf, capturing a wide range of gestures, lighting conditions, and backgrounds. This dataset reflects real-world variability and includes linguistically accurate signs. The data was annotated using bounding boxes and labeled for YOLOv5 training, ensuring precise and effective input.

YOLOv5 was selected for its efficiency and accuracy in object detection. The model architecture includes a backbone for feature extraction, a neck for feature aggregation, and a head for prediction. Training was conducted using the PyTorch framework with optimization techniques such as stochastic gradient descent, data augmentation, and learning rate scheduling. The model achieved an accuracy of 94.67%, with a precision of 91.67%, recall of 88.24%, and F1-score of 89.92%. Loss curves from training and validation showed consistent improvements across detection, localization, and classification tasks.

A key contribution of this work is its validation in a real-world educational setting. The system was deployed at the Ida Rieu School, where it was used by students and instructors to facilitate communication. This testing demonstrated the model's ability to handle variations in signing style, environmental noise, and background complexity. Such validation distinguishes this work from prior studies limited to lab conditions and underscores its utility in educational and social settings. Deployment also showed the system's potential as a teaching aid, helping students connect PSL signs with written Urdu and enhance literacy.

The chapter outlines broader implications and future directions. A current limitation is that the system supports only static PSL signs, primarily fingerspelling of Urdu alphabets. To enable full communication, future work should incorporate dynamic sign recognition, which requires interpreting gestures in motion and understanding temporal relationships. This will involve advanced models such as recurrent neural networks or transformer-based architectures for processing video sequences. Optimizing the system for low-power devices like smartphones or tablets is also crucial for expanding accessibility, particularly in schools, public service centers, and rural areas. Techniques such as pruning, quantization, and knowledge distillation are proposed to support lightweight deployment.

In conclusion, this chapter delivers a substantive and practical contribution to assistive technology for the deaf community in Pakistan. It combines advancements in computer vision and deep learning with an understanding of PSL's linguistic structure, resulting in a system that is both technically sound and socially impactful. The development of a large, diverse annotated PSL dataset, the implementation of a real-time YOLOv5-based model, and successful deployment in a real-world educational setting collectively demonstrate the feasibility and value of AI-driven tools for underrepresented linguistic communities. This work provides a foundation for future PSL research and serves as a model for similar efforts in underserved regions.

ACKNOWLEDGMENT

We would like to extend our sincere thanks to the Ida Rieu Welfare Association for their collaboration and support during this project. We are also grateful to the students Mahad Sabih, Hasham Baig and Maaz Jawaid who actively participated in the data collection and early stages of model training.

REFERENCES

ADCET. (2025). *Deaf or hearing impaired.* Australian Disability Clearinghouse on Education and Training. https://www.adcet.edu.au/inclusive-teaching/specific-disabilities/deaf-hearing-impaired

Alaftekin, M., Pacal, I., & Cicek, K. (2024). Real-time sign language recognition based on YOLO algorithm. *Neural Computing & Applications*, *36*(14), 7609–7624. DOI: 10.1007/s00521-024-09503-6

Alsharif, B., Alalwany, E., & Ilyas, M. (2024). Transfer learning with YOLOV8 for real-time recognition system of American Sign Language Alphabet. *Franklin Open*, *8*, 100165. DOI: 10.1016/j.fraope.2024.100165

Alyami, S., Luqman, H., Al-Azani, S., Alowaifeer, M., Alharbi, Y., & Alonaizan, Y. (2025). *Isharah: A Large-Scale Multi-Scene Dataset for Continuous Sign Language Recognition* (No. arXiv:2506.03615). arXiv. https://doi.org//arXiv.2506.03615DOI: 10.48550

Alyami, S., Luqman, H., & Hammoudeh, M. (2024). Reviewing 25 years of continuous sign language recognition research: Advances, challenges, and prospects. *Information Processing & Management*, *61*(5), 103774. DOI: 10.1016/j.ipm.2024.103774

Amin, M. S., Rizvi, S. T. H., & Hossain, M. (2022). A Comparative Review on Applications of Different Sensors for Sign Language Recognition. *Journal of Imaging*, *8*(4), 98. DOI: 10.3390/jimaging8040098

Bae, S. (2023). A study on the difficulty of communication through sign language in non-English-speaking countries. *Open Journal of Social Sciences*, *11*(10), 494–506. DOI: 10.4236/jss.2023.1110028

Bochkovskiy, A., Wang, C.-Y., & Liao, H.-Y. M. (2020). *YOLOv4: Optimal speed and accuracy of object detection*. arXiv preprint arXiv:2004.10934. https://doi.org//arXiv.2004.10934DOI: 10.48550

Bragg, D., Koller, O., Bellard, M., Berke, L., Boudreault, P., Braffort, A., & Shillingsburg, T. (2021). Sign language recognition, generation, and translation: An interdisciplinary perspective. *Proceedings of the 21st International ACM SIGACCESS Conference on Computers and Accessibility*, 16-31.

Chen, H., Wang, J., Guo, Z., Li, J., Zhou, D., Wu, B., Guan, C., Chen, G., & Heng, P.-A. (2024). *SignVTCL: Multi-Modal Continuous Sign Language Recognition Enhanced by Visual-Textual Contrastive Learning* (No. arXiv:2401.11847). arXiv. https://doi.org//arXiv.2401.11847DOI: 10.48550

Chen, H., Wang, J., Guo, Z., Li, J., Zhou, D., Wu, B., Guan, C., Chen, G., & Heng, P.-A. (2024). *SignVTCL: Multi-Modal Continuous Sign Language Recognition Enhanced by Visual-Textual Contrastive Learning* (No. arXiv:2401.11847). arXiv. https://doi.org//arXiv.2401.11847DOI: 10.48550

Cihan Camgoz, N., Koller, O., Hadfield, S., & Bowden, R. (2020). Sign Language Transformers: Joint End-to-End Sign Language Recognition and Translation. *2020 IEEE/CVF Conference on Computer Vision and Pattern Recognition (CVPR)*, 10020–10030. DOI: 10.1109/CVPR42600.2020.01004

Cihan Camgoz, N., Koller, O., Hadfield, S., & Bowden, R. (2020). Sign Language Transformers: Joint End-to-End Sign Language Recognition and Translation. *2020 IEEE/CVF Conference on Computer Vision and Pattern Recognition (CVPR)*, 10020–10030. DOI: 10.1109/CVPR42600.2020.01004

Deng, Z., Liu, M., Li, L., Han, Q., & Min, W. (2025). VTAN: A Novel Video Transformer Attention-Based Network for Dynamic Sign Language Recognition. *Computers, Materials & Continua*, *82*(2), 2793–2812. DOI: 10.32604/cmc.2024.057456

Deng, Z., Liu, M., Li, L., Han, Q., & Min, W. (2025). VTAN: A Novel Video Transformer Attention-Based Network for Dynamic Sign Language Recognition. *Computers, Materials & Continua*, *82*(2), 2793–2812. DOI: 10.32604/cmc.2024.057456

Fan, D., Yi, M., Kang, W., Wang, Y., & Lv, C. (n.d.). OPEN Continuous sign language. *Scientific Reports*.

Hamza, H. M., & Wali, A. (2023). Pakistan sign language recognition: Leveraging deep learning models with limited dataset. *Machine Vision and Applications*, *34*(5), 71. DOI: 10.1007/s00138-023-01429-8

Hosain, A. A., Santhalingam, P. S., Pathak, P., Košecká, J., & Rangwala, H. (2019). Sign Language Recognition Analysis using Multimodal Data. *2019 IEEE International Conference on Data Science and Advanced Analytics (DSAA)*, 203–210. DOI: 10.1109/DSAA.2019.00035

Hosain, A. A., Santhalingam, P. S., Pathak, P., Košecká, J., & Rangwala, H. (2019). Sign Language Recognition Analysis using Multimodal Data. *2019 IEEE International Conference on Data Science and Advanced Analytics (DSAA)*, 203–210. DOI: 10.1109/DSAA.2019.00035

Javaid, S., Sajid, S., & Baloch, Y. K. (2025). UAlpha40: A comprehensive dataset of Urdu alphabet for Pakistan sign language. *Data in Brief*, *59*, 111342. DOI: 10.1016/j.dib.2025.111342

Khan, N. S., Abid, A., Abid, K., Farooq, U., Farooq, M. S., & Jameel, H. (n.d.). Speak Pakistan: Challenges in Developing Pakistan Sign Language using Information Technology. *South Asian Studies*.

Khan, W. U., Shah, N., Muntean, G.-M., Farman, H., Nasralla, M. M., Ullah, S., & Shabir, M. (2021). A lightweight deep learning model for real-time human action recognition on resource-constrained devices. *Soft Computing*, *25*(24), 15371–15385.

Kothadiya, D., Bhatt, C., Sapariya, K., Patel, K., Gil-González, A.-B., & Corchado, J. M. (2022). Deepsign: Sign Language Detection and Recognition Using Deep Learning. *Electronics (Basel)*, *11*(11), 1780. DOI: 10.3390/electronics11111780

Liu, S., Qi, L., Qin, H., Shi, J., & Jia, J. (2018). *Path aggregation network for instance segmentation*. In *Proceedings of the IEEE conference on computer vision and pattern recognition* (pp. 8759–8768). DOI: 10.1109/CVPR.2018.00913

Ma, D., Hirota, K., Dai, Y., & Jia, Z. (n.d.). *Dynamic Sign Language Recognition Based on Improved Residual-LSTM Network*.

Mirza, M. S., Munaf, S. M., Azim, F., Ali, S., & Khan, S. J. (2022). Vision-based Pakistani sign language recognition using bag-of-words and support vector machines. *Scientific Reports*, *12*(1), 21325. DOI: 10.1038/s41598-022-15864-6

Mujeeb, A. A., Khan, A. H., Khalid, S., Mirza, M. S., & Khan, S. J. (2023). A Deep Learning Approach to Pakistani Sign Language Recognition. *2023 20th International Bhurban Conference on Applied Sciences and Technology (IBCAST)*, 255–260. DOI: 10.1109/IBCAST59916.2023.10712904

Pakistan Bureau of Statistics. (2021). *Population and housing census: Persons with disabilities*. Government of Pakistan. https://www.pbs.gov.pk/

Podder, K. K., Islam, M. R., Hossain, M. I., & Akhand, M. A. H. (2023). Signer-independent Arabic Sign Language recognition system using deep learning model. *Sensors (Basel)*, *23*(16), 7156. DOI: 10.3390/s23167156

Rastgoo, R., Kiani, K., & Escalera, S. (2021). Sign language recognition: A deep survey. *Expert Systems with Applications*, *164*, 113794. DOI: 10.1016/j.eswa.2020.113794

Redmon, J., & Farhadi, A. (2018). YOLOv3: An incremental improvement. *arXiv preprint arXiv:1804.02767*. https://arxiv.org/abs/1804.02767

Roboflow. (2023). *RF-DETR: A robust transformer for object detection* [GitHub repository]. GitHub. Retrieved March 5, 2025, from https://github.com/roboflow/rf-detr

Shah, F., Shah, M. S., Akram, W., Manzoor, A., Mahmoud, R. O., & Abdelminaam, D. S. (2021). Sign Language Recognition Using Multiple Kernel Learning: A Case Study of Pakistan Sign Language. *IEEE Access : Practical Innovations, Open Solutions*, *9*, 67548–67558. DOI: 10.1109/ACCESS.2021.3077386

Tan, M., Pang, R., & Le, Q. V. (2020). *EfficientDet: Scalable and Efficient Object Detection* (No. arXiv:1911.09070). arXiv. /arXiv.1911.09070DOI: 10.1109/CVPR42600.2020.01079

Tyagi, S., Upadhyay, P., Fatima, H., Jain, S., & Sharma, A. K. (2023). *American Sign Language Detection using YOLOv5 and YOLOv8*. DOI: 10.21203/rs.3.rs-3126918/v1

Ultralytics. (2024). *YOLOv5 vs YOLOv8: Performance benchmarks*. Ultralytics Documentation. Retrieved March 5, 2025, from https://docs.ultralytics.com/compare/yolov5-vs-yolov8/#performance-benchmarks-yolov5-vs-yolov8

Ultralytics. (n.d.) *YOLOv5 architecture description*. https://docs.ultralytics.com/yolov5/tutorials/architecture_description/#1-model-structure

Zhang, Y., & Jiang, X. (2024). Recent Advances on Deep Learning for Sign Language Recognition. *Computer Modeling in Engineering & Sciences*, *139*(3), 2399–2450. DOI: 10.32604/cmes.2023.045731

Zheng, Z., Wang, P., Liu, W., Li, J., Ye, R., & Ren, D. (2020). Distance-IoU loss: Faster and better learning for bounding box regression. *Proceedings of the AAAI Conference on Artificial Intelligence*, *34*(07), 12993–13000. DOI: 10.1609/aaai.v34i07.6999

ADDITIONAL READING

Cooper, H., Holt, B., & Bowden, R. (2011). Sign language recognition. In T. B. Moeslund, A. Hilton, V. Krüger, & L. Sigal (Eds.), *Visual analysis of humans* (pp. 539–562). Springer London. DOI: 10.1007/978-0-85729-997-0_27

Revankar, G. D., & Kumar, S. S. (2025). American Sign Language Recognition Using Deep Learning Models. *Lecture Notes in Networks and Systems* (Vol. 1248, pp. 371–382). Springer. DOI: 10.1007/978-981-96-1758-6_31

KEY TERMS AND DEFINITIONS

Computer Vision: An area of artificial intelligence that enables machines to interpret and process visual information from the world, such as images or video frames, for tasks like detection, classification, and segmentation.

Dataset Diversity: The degree of variation within a dataset in terms of signer characteristics, environmental conditions, and gesture styles, which influences a model's ability to generalize to real-world scenarios.

Fingerspelling Recognition: The automatic identification of hand shapes corresponding to individual letters or numbers in a sign language alphabet, used for spelling names, places, or technical terms.

Generalizability: The ability of a machine learning model to perform well on new, unseen data that differs from the data it was trained on, reflecting its robustness in practical applications.

Native Signer: An individual who has acquired sign language as their first language from early childhood and uses it fluently and naturally in daily communication.

Pakistani Sign Language (PSL): The primary sign language used by the deaf and hard-of-hearing community in Pakistan, consisting of hand gestures, facial expressions, and body movements that convey meaning.

Sign Language Recognition (SLR): The process of automatically identifying and interpreting sign language gestures using computational models, often based on computer vision and machine learning techniques.

Synthetic Data Generation: The creation of artificial data using computational techniques, such as 3D avatars, pose estimation, or generative models, to augment or replace real-world data in machine learning applications.

Chapter 9
Security, Privacy, and Trust in Smart Systems for People With Visual Disabilities

Bülent Gürsel Emiroğlu
https://orcid.org/0000-0002-1656-6450
Kırıkkale University, Turkey

ABSTRACT

As smart systems become increasingly prevalent, ensuring their accessibility, security, privacy, and trustworthiness is paramount for individuals with visual disabilities. These users face unique interaction barriers. This chapter explores the intersection of smart technologies and these challenges, focusing on the heightened importance of security and privacy and their implications for user trust. It outlines essential design considerations for creating inclusive technologies, emphasizing multimodal feedback and compatibility with assistive tools. By highlighting case studies, best practices, and emerging trends, the chapter aims to provide valuable insights for researchers, practitioners, and policymakers dedicated to enhancing the quality of life for people with visual disabilities.

1. INTRODUCTION

The 21st century has witnessed a rapid and transformative evolution in technology, marked prominently by the advent and pervasive integration of smart systems into nearly every facet of daily life. These interconnected networks of devices, sensors, software, and artificial intelligence are reshaping how individuals interact with their

DOI: 10.4018/979-8-3373-2033-5.ch009

homes, workplaces, communities, and the world at large. From sophisticated smart home automation that controls lighting, climate, and security with voice commands, to wearable technologies that monitor health and provide real-time feedback, and intelligent mobile applications that offer navigation assistance and enhance communication, smart systems hold immense potential to improve efficiency, convenience, and overall quality of life for the general population (Smith & Johnson, 2022).

Disability studies literature consistently underscores the centrality of lived experiences in understanding disability (Shakespeare, 2017). Robust policy frameworks are essential to address these disparities, ensuring that technological advancements translate into tangible benefits for all disabled people, rather than exacerbating existing inequalities (Shakespeare, 2017). "Disability: The Basics" by T. Shakespeare (2017) provides a comprehensive and accessible introduction to the field of disability studies, exploring its fundamental concepts, historical evolution, and diverse theoretical models. The book critically examines key issues such as the social construction of disability, identity, human rights, and the ongoing struggle for inclusion and equality for disabled people. This perspective is crucial when examining socio-technical systems and accessibility frameworks in Human-Computer Interaction (HCI), as it moves beyond a purely medical model to recognize disability as a social construct shaped by environmental and systemic barriers (Ellis et al., 2020). Effective accessibility frameworks, therefore, must be grounded in the direct experiences of disabled people, ensuring that technologies are not only technically compliant but also genuinely usable and empowering (Anwar et al., 2022).

For individuals with visual disabilities, this technological paradigm shift carries a particularly profound significance. Historically, many aspects of daily living—such as navigating unfamiliar environments, managing household tasks, accessing written information, or engaging in spontaneous social interactions—have presented significant challenges, often requiring reliance on human assistance or specialized, sometimes cumbersome, assistive devices. Smart systems, when designed with accessibility in mind, offer unprecedented opportunities to dismantle these barriers, fostering greater independence, autonomy, and active participation in society. A smart navigation app providing real-time audio cues, a voice-controlled smart appliance simplifying kitchen tasks, or a wearable device offering non-visual environmental information can be truly life-changing tools, enabling visually impaired individuals to perform tasks and access information previously inaccessible to them independently (Fairchild & Stuerzlinger, 2020).

However, as these powerful and interconnected technologies become increasingly embedded in the fabric of daily routines, a complex interplay of concerns emerges, particularly regarding security, privacy, and the foundational element of user trust. Smart systems, by their very nature, are data-hungry, constantly collecting, processing, and transmitting information about users, their environments, and their behaviors. This ubiquitous data flow, while enabling personalized and intelligent services, simultaneously creates new vulnerabilities and risks (D'Silva & Kaur, 2020).

Individuals with visual disabilities often interact with smart environments using specific assistive technologies. Screen readers, which vocalize on-screen text and interface elements, and voice recognition systems, which allow control through spoken commands, are indispensable tools. While these technologies bridge critical accessibility gaps, their integration with smart systems can introduce unique security considerations (Fairchild & Stuerzlinger, 2020). For instance, a vulnerability in a voice assistant could potentially be exploited to gain unauthorized access to connected devices, or sensitive information vocalized by a screen reader might be inadvertently captured (D'Silva & Kaur, 2020).

A significant challenge highlighted in the literature is the economic accessibility of technologies for disabled people. Cost barriers and unequal access globally create substantial disparities, particularly in low-income regions (United Nations, 2007). These economic limitations are often compounded by intersectionality, where factors such as gender, socio-economic status, and geography exacerbate accessibility challenges. For instance, a disabled woman in a rural, low-income community may face significantly more hurdles in accessing assistive technologies or digital resources compared to a disabled man in an urban, high-income setting (Crenshaw, 1989; Mohanty, 2003). This layered disadvantage necessitates an intersectional approach to policy and design. "The Routledge Companion to Disability and Media" (2020), edited by Ellis, Goggin, Haller, and Curtis, offers a comprehensive exploration of the multifaceted intersections between disability and various forms of media. The volume delves into how disability is represented, produced, and consumed across different media platforms, examining the implications for disabled individuals and society at large. Karki et al. (2023) presents a "Smart Attendance Monitoring System" specifically designed for People with Disabilities (PwDs), utilizing face recognition technology to automate and streamline attendance tracking. The system aims to provide a more efficient and accessible method for monitoring attendance, addressing the unique needs and challenges faced by PwDs in various settings.

Furthermore, the extensive collection and processing of personal data by smart systems raise significant privacy concerns for all users, but these concerns can be amplified for visually impaired individuals. Understanding complex privacy policies, configuring granular data sharing settings, or even being aware of which data is being collected can be challenging without accessible interfaces and transparent communication (Gray & Cyan, 2022). The potential for misuse of collected data ranging from targeted advertising based on sensitive behavioral patterns to more malicious activities like stalking or identity theft can severely undermine a user's sense of safety and control (Chen et al., 2021).

These interwoven issues of security vulnerabilities and privacy risks directly impact the third critical element: trust. Trust is not merely a desirable feature; it is a fundamental prerequisite for the widespread acceptance and effective utilization of any technology, especially those deeply integrated into personal spaces and routines. For individuals who rely on smart systems for independence and safety, a lack of trust—whether stemming from fears of security breaches, concerns about data privacy, or simply the unreliability of inaccessible interfaces—can lead to hesitation, anxiety, and ultimately, the abandonment of potentially beneficial technologies (Gray & Cyan, 2022). If a visually impaired user cannot trust that their smart lock is secure, that their voice assistant isn't recording private conversations without consent, or that the navigation app will reliably guide them, the promise of increased independence evaporates, replaced by uncertainty and potential harm (Smith & Johnson, 2022).

The human dimension of disabled people's trust in smart systems and technologies is another critical area of inquiry. Trust, as a lived experience, is influenced by the reliability, usability, and perceived benefit of technologies, as well as the ethical considerations surrounding data privacy and algorithmic bias (Akhai, 2024b). Beyond individual trust, social and cultural barriers significantly impede the adoption and effective use of technologies by disabled people. These include a pervasive lack of training for users and support staff, insufficient institutional support for implementation, and societal stigmas that marginalize disabled individuals (Karki et al., 2023). Such barriers often stem from a broader lack of understanding and integration of disability perspectives within mainstream society and technological development. Anwar et al. (2022) introduces a conceptual framework for classifying the emotions of people with disabilities (PwDs) based on their utterances during online learning sessions. The aim is to leverage smart education technologies to better understand and respond to the emotional states of PwDs, thereby enhancing their online learning experience.

Disability scholarship and socio-legal perspectives provide a critical lens through which to analyze affordability, policy frameworks, and global inequalities. International instruments like the UN Convention on the Rights of Persons with Disabilities (United Nations, 2007) establish a legal and ethical imperative for inclusive technology and equitable access. This is a landmark international treaty designed to promote, protect, and ensure the full and equal enjoyment of all human rights and fundamental freedoms by all persons with disabilities. It establishes a comprehensive framework for their inclusion and participation in society, with the Optional Protocol allowing individuals to submit complaints regarding violations of the Convention. However, the gap between policy intent and practical implementation remains wide, particularly concerning the affordability of assistive technologies and the uneven distribution of resources globally.

Akhai (2024a) provides an overview of IoT-enabled air conditioners within smart home environments, highlighting their role in modern living. Expanding on this, Akhai and Wadhwa (2024a) delve into wireless networking solutions specifically for climate control and comfort in advanced air conditioning systems. The human element in such controlled environments is further explored by Akhai, Singh, and John (2016), who examine human performance in industrial design centers equipped with small unit air conditioning systems. In the realm of healthcare, several studies address the integration of digital and smart solutions. Mala et al. (2025) discuss digital health technologies for preventive cardiology, emphasizing their impact on improved healthcare delivery. Verma, Akhai, and Wadhwa (2024) investigate the application of smart materials in physiotherapy, exploring how sensor technology can revolutionize treatment. Akhai and Khang (2024) review innovations in medical manufacturing, specifically focusing on the transformative roles of 3D printing, robotics, and the Internet of Things, with a dedicated section on trust in smart systems. A significant theme across Akhai's recent work is Artificial Intelligence (AI) and the crucial aspect of trust and explainability. Akhai (2024c) addresses the future frontier of AI, moving "Towards Trustworthy and Reliable AI," while Akhai (2023) discusses the journey "From Black Boxes to Transparent Machines: The Quest for Explainable AI," highlighting the need for greater understanding of AI decision-making. Finally, Akhai and Kumar (2024) explore quantum resilience and distributed trust, underscoring the promise of blockchain and quantum computing in defense applications.

Achieving genuine technological inclusion for disabled people requires a holistic approach that integrates lived experiences, addresses economic and intersectional barriers, fosters trust, dismantles social and cultural obstacles, and is underpinned by strong socio-legal and policy frameworks that actively combat global inequalities. This chapter will therefore embark on a comprehensive exploration of the critical issues surrounding security, privacy, and trust within the context of smart systems specifically designed for or used by people with visual disabilities. It aims to provide a detailed overview of the unique challenges and significant opportunities presented by these technologies from this specific user perspective. By delving into the technical vulnerabilities, privacy implications, and the psychological and practical aspects of building trust, supported by illustrative case studies and discussions of best practices, this chapter seeks to offer valuable insights. The ultimate goal is to inform researchers, technology developers, practitioners, policymakers, and advocates about the critical considerations necessary for designing, deploying, and governing smart systems that are not only innovative and functional but also inherently secure, privacy-preserving, trustworthy, and truly inclusive, thereby genuinely enhancing the independence, safety, and quality of life for people with visual disabilities in an increasingly connected world.

2. UNDERSTANDING SMART SYSTEMS FOR INDIVIDUALS WITH VISUAL DISABILITIES

To fully appreciate the security, privacy, and trust implications, it is essential to first establish a clear understanding of what constitutes "smart systems" in this context and why their accessibility is of paramount importance for individuals with visual impairments.

2.1 Definition and Scope of Smart Systems

The term "smart systems" is broad and constantly evolving, but generally refers to interconnected ecosystems of physical devices, embedded sensors, software, network connectivity, and computational capabilities, often leveraging data analytics and artificial intelligence (AI) to perform tasks, make decisions, and interact with users and their environment in an intelligent or automated manner. These systems are characterized by their ability to collect data from their surroundings or user interactions, process that data, and respond or adapt based on predefined rules, learned patterns, or real-time conditions. The underlying principle is often to enhance efficiency, convenience, comfort, safety, or provide novel functionalities (Park & Kim, 2023).

Within the scope of daily life, particularly relevant to individuals with visual disabilities, smart systems manifest in various forms:

- **Smart Home Devices:** This category includes a wide array of appliances and systems designed to automate, monitor, or control aspects of a residential environment. Examples include smart lights (Philips Hue, LIFX), smart thermostats (Nest, Ecobee), smart locks (August, Yale Assure), smart security cameras and doorbells (Ring, Arlo), smart speakers and displays (Amazon Echo, Google Nest Hub), smart appliances (refrigerators, ovens), and smart plugs. These devices often communicate wirelessly (Wi-Fi, Bluetooth, Zigbee, Z-Wave) and can be controlled remotely via smartphone apps, voice commands through smart assistants, or automated based on schedules, sensor data, or user presence. For a visually impaired person, a smart thermostat controllable by voice eliminates the need to read a small display, or a smart light system allows turning lights on/off throughout the house without navigating in the dark (Smith & Johnson, 2022).
- **Wearable Technologies:** These are electronic devices worn on the body that collect and transmit data, often providing real-time feedback. Examples include smartwatches (Apple Watch, Fitbit), fitness trackers, and more specialized devices like smart glasses (though consumer adoption is still lim-

ited, devices like Envision Glasses or Microsoft HoloLens for enterprise demonstrate the concept). Wearables can monitor health metrics (heart rate, activity levels), provide notifications, and offer navigation assistance through vibrations or audio cues. For a visually impaired user, a smartwatch could provide discreet, non-visual alerts or basic navigation nudges. Future smart glasses hold potential for object recognition, text reading, and environmental description, offering a new layer of sensory information (Lee & Dey, 2020).

- **Mobile Applications:** While not physical devices themselves, "smart" mobile applications leverage smartphone capabilities (sensors, processing power, connectivity) and often cloud-based AI to provide intelligent services. This includes navigation apps (Google Maps, Apple Maps, specialized apps like BlindSquare or Lazarillo), object recognition apps (Seeing AI), currency readers, color identifiers, and apps that interact with smart home devices or wearables. These apps are crucial interfaces for visually impaired users, often relying heavily on screen reader compatibility and intuitive, non-visual interaction design. A smart navigation app, for instance, uses GPS, mapping data, and potentially camera input (via AI) to provide detailed audio instructions and descriptions of the surroundings (Oladimeji & Lee, 2021).

The underlying technologies enabling these systems are diverse and interconnected. Sensors (cameras, microphones, motion detectors, temperature sensors, GPS) collect raw data. Connectivity protocols (Wi-Fi, Bluetooth, cellular, Zigbee, Z-Wave) enable communication between devices and the cloud. Cloud computing provides storage and processing power for data analytics and AI algorithms. Artificial intelligence and machine learning enable systems to learn from data, recognize patterns (like faces or voices), understand natural language commands, and make predictive decisions. The user interface, while often visual (smartphone apps), increasingly includes voice interfaces (smart speakers, voice assistants on phones) and potentially tactile/haptic feedback (wearables) (Kulyk & Gajos, 2021).

2.2 Importance of Accessibility for Visually Impaired Individuals

Accessibility, in the context of technology, refers to the design and development of products, devices, services, or environments so that they can be used by people with the widest range of abilities and disabilities. For individuals with visual disabilities, accessibility is not merely a matter of convenience; it is a fundamental enabler of independence, participation, and equal opportunity in an increasingly digital and automated world. Without accessible technology, visually impaired individuals risk being excluded from essential services, information, and social interactions that the sighted population takes for granted (Kulyk & Gajos, 2021).

Smart systems, with their potential to automate tasks and provide information about the environment, hold particular promise for enhancing the independence of visually impaired individuals. When designed accessibly, they can significantly improve quality of life by providing:

- **Navigation Assistance:** Independent navigation is a significant challenge for many visually impaired people, especially in unfamiliar or complex environments. Traditional tools like white canes and guide dogs are invaluable but have limitations in providing detailed information about the broader environment, points of interest, or dynamic changes. Smart navigation apps and potentially future smart glasses can leverage GPS, mapping data, computer vision, and AI to provide real-time, detailed audio instructions, identify landmarks, describe intersections, alert users to obstacles, and even help locate specific shops or bus stops. This level of dynamic, granular information can dramatically increase confidence and autonomy in travel (Oladimeji & Lee, 2021).
- **Home Automation:** Managing a household involves numerous tasks that can be challenging without sight, such as adjusting lighting, controlling appliances, managing security systems, or identifying objects. Smart home technologies, when controlled via accessible voice interfaces or screen-reader-compatible apps, can empower visually impaired individuals to manage their living spaces independently. Turning lights on or off, adjusting the thermostat, locking doors, checking if the oven is on, or even identifying the contents of a pantry using a smart camera and AI – these tasks become achievable without sighted assistance, promoting a sense of control and reducing reliance on others (Kulyk & Gajos, 2021).
- **Information Access:** Accessing written information on product labels, documents, public signs, or digital screens is a daily hurdle. Mobile applications leveraging smartphone cameras and AI (like OCR - Optical Character Recognition) can read text aloud. Smart glasses could potentially do this hands-free. Smart assistants can provide quick access to information from the internet, weather updates, news headlines, and reminders through voice. This immediate, independent access to information is crucial for everything from managing finances to staying informed about current events (Mavroudis & Gritzalis, 2019).
- **Social Connectivity:** While not exclusively a smart system function, smart devices and accessible applications facilitate communication. Voice-controlled calling and messaging via smart speakers or phones, accessible

social media apps, and video assistance services (like Be My Eyes, which connects visually impaired users with sighted volunteers via video) leverage smart technology to reduce isolation and maintain social connections.

- **Task Management and Daily Living:** Smart systems can assist with a myriad of daily tasks. Smart scales can read weight aloud. Smart pill dispensers can provide audio reminders. Smart object identifiers can help sort laundry or identify groceries. These seemingly small conveniences collectively contribute to a significantly more independent and manageable daily life.

However, the potential benefits are contingent upon robust accessibility. If a smart device requires a sighted person for setup, its control app is incompatible with screen readers, its feedback is purely visual (e.g., a flashing LED), or its voice interface is unreliable, it becomes a source of frustration and exclusion rather than empowerment. Therefore, designing smart systems with accessibility for diverse visual needs from the outset is not an optional add-on but a fundamental requirement for realizing their transformative potential for this population. The challenges of security, privacy, and trust must be addressed within this crucial framework of accessibility (Oladimeji & Lee, 2021).

3. SECURITY CHALLENGES IN SMART SYSTEMS

Smart systems, by their very design, involve interconnected devices, data transmission, and often cloud-based processing. This interconnectedness, while enabling powerful functionalities, simultaneously introduces a complex attack surface that can be exploited by malicious actors. For individuals with visual disabilities, who may rely heavily on these systems for critical functions like safety, navigation, and communication, security vulnerabilities carry particularly severe implications, potentially leading to loss of autonomy, privacy violations, and increased dependency (Chen et al., 2021).

3.1 Vulnerabilities in Smart Devices

The security landscape of smart systems is fraught with vulnerabilities, often stemming from rapid development cycles, focus on features over security, and the diverse, sometimes resource-constrained nature of the devices themselves. Common security threats include:

- **Unauthorized Access:** This is a primary concern. Many smart devices are deployed with weak or default authentication mechanisms. Examples include:

Default Credentials: Devices shipped with easily guessable default usernames and passwords (e.g., admin/admin, 12345). If users do not change these, attackers can easily gain control.

Weak Password Policies: Systems that allow simple, short, or common passwords.

Lack of Authentication: Some devices or services may not require strong authentication for certain actions or data access.

Vulnerable APIs: Application Programming Interfaces (APIs) that allow devices or services to communicate may have security flaws that permit unauthorized access to data or control functions.

Physical Access Vulnerabilities: Some devices might store sensitive information or have configuration ports that are easily accessible physically, allowing attackers to bypass network security.

Brute-Force and Dictionary Attacks: Attackers systematically trying common passwords or combinations to gain entry.

- **Data Interception:** Data transmitted between smart devices, between a device and its mobile app, or between a device and the cloud can be intercepted if not properly encrypted.

Man-in-the-Middle (MITM) Attacks: An attacker positions themselves between two communicating parties (e.g., a smart bulb and the home Wi-Fi router) and intercepts, reads, or modifies the data being exchanged.

Unencrypted Communications: Data transmitted over local networks (Wi-Fi, Zigbee, Z-Wave) or the internet without strong encryption (like TLS/SSL) can be easily sniffed and read by anyone on the same network or along the data path.

Weak Encryption: Even if encryption is used, outdated or weak encryption algorithms can be cracked.

- **Malware Attacks:** Smart devices can be infected with malicious software. The Mirai botnet, which leveraged vulnerable IoT devices (like routers and cameras) to launch massive denial-of-service attacks, is a prominent example.

Exploiting Vulnerabilities: Malware can spread by exploiting known security flaws in device firmware or software.

Phishing/Social Engineering: While less direct for many smart devices, associated mobile apps or user accounts can be targeted via phishing, leading to compromised credentials that then grant access to devices.

Infected Updates: Attackers might compromise update servers to push malicious firmware updates to devices.

Types of Malware: Malware on smart devices can range from bots for DDoS attacks, ransomware (though less common on simple devices), spyware (e.g., turning on cameras/microphones), to malware designed to disrupt device functionality.

- **Denial of Service (DoS) Attacks:** Attackers flood a device or network with traffic, making it unavailable for legitimate users. While often used for broader network disruption, a DoS attack on a critical smart home device (like a smart lock or security system) could prevent a visually impaired user from accessing their home or receiving critical alerts.
- **Firmware Vulnerabilities:** The embedded software (firmware) that runs smart devices often contains bugs and security flaws that can be exploited. Unlike traditional computers, updating firmware on many smart devices can be difficult, inconsistent, or even impossible, leaving vulnerabilities unpatched.
- **Insecure Cloud Infrastructure:** Smart devices often rely on cloud services for processing, storage, and remote access. If the cloud infrastructure is compromised, vast amounts of user data and control capabilities can be exposed.
- **Lack of Security Updates:** Many manufacturers of low-cost smart devices fail to provide ongoing security updates after the initial purchase, leaving devices vulnerable to newly discovered threats.

3.2 Implications for Visually Impaired Users

The general security vulnerabilities in smart systems take on heightened significance and can have particularly severe consequences for individuals with visual disabilities due to their reliance on these technologies for independence and the challenges they may face in detecting or responding to security incidents.

- **Loss of Autonomy:** This is perhaps the most direct and impactful consequence. Unauthorized access to smart home systems can lead to a complete loss of control over one's living environment. An attacker could:

  i. Unlock doors, compromising physical safety.
  ii. Turn lights on/off erratically, causing confusion and potential hazards.
  iii. Adjust thermostats to uncomfortable or dangerous temperatures.
  iv. Disable security systems, leaving the home vulnerable.
  v. Control appliances like ovens or stoves, creating fire risks.
  vi. Manipulate assistive smart devices, rendering them useless or harmful.

For a visually impaired person, regaining control or even knowing that control has been lost is significantly harder. They cannot simply look at an interface to see if settings have changed or if a door is unlocked. Reliance on voice commands that suddenly fail, or unexpected changes in the environment, can be deeply disorienting and frightening, forcing them to depend on sighted assistance to diagnose and fix the problem. This directly undermines the independence the technology was meant to provide (Gray & Cyan, 2022).

- **Privacy Violations:** Data breaches and unauthorized access expose sensitive personal information, with potentially devastating outcomes:

Identity Theft: Compromised personal information (names, addresses, payment details linked to smart accounts) can be used for financial fraud.

Harassment and Stalking: Location data from smart devices or navigation apps can reveal routines and whereabouts. Unauthorized access to cameras and microphones can facilitate surveillance, leading to harassment, blackmail, or physical danger. For someone who is visually impaired, the inability to visually confirm if a camera is active or if a device is recording makes them particularly vulnerable to covert surveillance.

Exposure of Sensitive Data: Health data from wearables, details about daily routines, conversations captured by voice assistants, or even information about specific assistive needs could be exposed, leading to embarrassment, discrimination, or exploitation.

Financial Loss: Unauthorized purchases made through linked accounts or ransomware demanding payment to regain control of devices.

- **Increased Dependency:** When smart systems become unreliable or insecure, visually impaired users are often forced to rely more heavily on caregivers, family members, or technical support (which may not be accessible). Diagnosing a technical issue (is the smart lock broken, or has it been hacked?) is difficult without visual cues or accessible diagnostic tools. This increased reliance negates the very purpose of using smart technology for independence and can be a source of frustration and decreased confidence.
- **Physical Safety Risks:** Beyond unauthorized entry, security flaws can directly endanger physical safety. A compromised smart oven or stove could be turned on remotely. A hacked smart medical device could provide incorrect readings or dosages. A compromised smart car system (in the future) could pose severe risks.
- **Psychological Impact:** The constant worry about potential security breaches, the fear of being monitored, and the frustration of unreliable technology

can lead to significant stress, anxiety, and a decreased sense of security in one's own home and environment. This psychological burden is a major barrier to technology adoption and trust.

In summary, while security vulnerabilities are a risk for all users of smart systems, their consequences are often more profound and disabling for individuals with visual impairments. The inability to easily detect or respond to incidents, coupled with a higher reliance on these systems for basic independence, means that security failures can directly translate into a loss of autonomy, significant privacy breaches, and a forced return to dependency.

4. PRIVACY CONCERNS IN SMART SYSTEMS

Beyond security, the sheer volume and nature of data collected by smart systems give rise to significant privacy concerns (Chen et al., 2021). These concerns revolve around what data is collected, how it is processed, who it is shared with, and how it is protected from misuse. For individuals with visual disabilities, navigating and controlling their privacy in the smart ecosystem presents unique challenges, potentially leading to uninformed consent, data misuse, and a pervasive sense of surveillance.

4.1 Data Collection and Processing

Smart systems are inherently data-driven. Their ability to provide personalized services, automate tasks, and respond intelligently to their environment relies on continuous data collection and processing. The types of data collected are extensive and often deeply personal:

- **Personal Information:** This includes basic identifying information provided during setup, such as names, addresses, email addresses, phone numbers, and potentially demographic data. Account information, payment details, and login credentials are also stored.
- **Behavioral Data:** Smart systems track how users interact with them and how they behave in their environment. This includes:

Device Usage Patterns: When devices are used, for how long, and what functions are accessed (e.g., when lights are turned on/off, thermostat adjustments, door lock/unlock times).

Interaction History: Logs of voice commands given to smart assistants, queries made, and responses received.

Preferences: Settings configurations, preferred routines, entertainment choices.

App Usage Data: How associated mobile apps are used, features accessed, duration of use.

- **Location Data:** Many smart devices and associated apps collect precise or approximate location data:

GPS Data: From smartphones and wearables, providing detailed movement history.

Wi-Fi and Bluetooth Data: Used for indoor positioning or proximity detection.

IP Addresses: Provide approximate geographic location.

- **Environmental Data:** Sensors collect data about the physical environment. This includes temperature, humidity, light levels, motion detection, sound detection (including voice commands and background noise), and potentially video feeds from cameras. For example, a smart thermostat collects temperature data, a smart speaker collects audio data, and a smart camera collects video data.
- **Biometric Data:** Some smart devices, particularly wearables, may collect biometric data such as heart rate, sleep patterns, activity levels (steps taken, distance covered), and potentially more advanced metrics like blood oxygen levels or ECG data. Future devices might incorporate facial recognition or gait analysis.
- **Content Data:** For devices that process user-generated content, such as smart speakers transcribing voice commands or smart cameras analyzing video feeds, the content of these interactions is collected and often sent to the cloud for processing. This can include conversations, images, and other sensitive information.
- **Metadata:** Data about the data, such as timestamps of interactions, device identifiers, network information (IP address, Wi-Fi network name), and software versions.

This vast amount of data is processed for various purposes:

- **Providing Core Functionality:** Processing voice commands to control devices, analyzing sensor data to automate tasks, using location data for navigation.
- **Personalization:** Using behavioral data and preferences to tailor services, suggest routines, or provide customized responses.
- **Improving Services:** Aggregating anonymized or pseudonymized data to train AI models, improve voice recognition accuracy, or develop new features.

- **Troubleshooting and Support:** Using device data to diagnose issues and provide technical assistance.
- **Marketing and Advertising:** Analyzing user behavior and preferences for targeted advertising, either directly by the device manufacturer or by third parties with whom data is shared.

The sheer volume, variety, and velocity of this data collection, often occurring continuously in intimate spaces like homes, raise fundamental privacy questions. Users may not be fully aware of *what* data is being collected, *how* it is being processed, *where* it is being stored, *who* has access to it, and *for how long* it is retained. The complexity of data flows involving devices, mobile apps, cloud servers, and potentially third-party service providers makes it difficult for even technically savvy users to maintain control over their personal information (Gray & Cyan, 2022).

4.2 Privacy Risks for Visually Impaired Users

While privacy concerns in smart systems affect all users, individuals with visual disabilities face amplified risks and unique challenges in understanding and managing their privacy settings and data. Their reliance on non-visual interfaces and assistive technologies can inadvertently create new privacy vulnerabilities or make it harder to exercise privacy rights (Lazar & Greenidge, 2020).

- **Informed Consent:** Obtaining truly informed consent for data collection and processing is a significant challenge in the context of complex smart systems, and it is particularly difficult for visually impaired individuals.
- **Inaccessible Privacy Policies:** Privacy policies and terms of service are often lengthy, written in complex legal jargon, and presented in formats (e.g., small text, dense paragraphs, non-standard digital formats) that are inaccessible to screen readers or difficult to navigate without sight. Users may be forced to agree to terms they cannot fully read or understand simply to use a device or service essential for their independence.
- **Complex Opt-Out Mechanisms:** Managing privacy settings often involves navigating intricate menus within mobile apps or web interfaces. These interfaces may not be designed with accessibility in mind, making it challenging for screen reader users to identify options, understand their implications, and make informed choices about data sharing and collection. Opting out of certain data uses might be buried several layers deep in settings.
- **Lack of Real-Time Notification:** Users are often not clearly notified *in the moment* about what data is being collected (e.g., when a microphone is actively listening beyond the wake word, when a camera is recording, or when

location data is being transmitted). Visually impaired users lack the visual cues (like indicator lights) that might alert sighted users to data collection activities.

- **Data Misuse:** The collected data, if not properly secured or if shared inappropriately, can be misused in various ways, with potentially severe consequences for visually impaired users (Li & Ma, 2020).
- **Targeted Advertising and Discrimination:** Behavioral data, usage patterns, and even inferred information about a user's disability status could be used for highly targeted advertising or, more concerningly, for discriminatory practices (e.g., being shown different prices or being excluded from certain offers based on inferred characteristics).
- **Sharing with Third Parties:** Data collected by a smart device manufacturer might be shared with marketing partners, data brokers, or other third parties without explicit, informed consent. This can lead to unwanted solicitations or the aggregation of personal data across different platforms, creating a detailed profile of the individual.
- **Use in Legal Proceedings or Investigations:** Data from smart devices (e.g., voice recordings, location history, activity logs) could potentially be subpoenaed and used in legal cases, including civil or criminal proceedings. While this affects all users, the unique data generated by assistive interactions (e.g., specific commands related to a disability) could be particularly sensitive.
- **Exploitation of Disability-Specific Data:** Data related to the use of assistive features, frequency of certain commands, or patterns of interaction that reveal information about the user's visual impairment could be particularly valuable (and risky) if it falls into the wrong hands.
- **Surveillance:** The continuous monitoring capabilities of many smart systems can lead to a pervasive sense of being surveilled, impacting users' comfort, behavior, and trust.
- **Always-Listening Microphones:** Smart speakers and other devices with voice interfaces are designed to listen for a wake word, but the technical reality involves continuous audio processing. While manufacturers state recordings are only sent to the cloud after the wake word, the presence of always-on microphones in private spaces raises concerns, especially if there are vulnerabilities that could allow unauthorized activation or recording. Visually impaired users cannot see indicator lights that might signal recording (Lazar & Greenidge, 2020).
- **Smart Cameras:** Indoor and outdoor smart cameras provide security but also present significant privacy risks if accessed without authorization. An attacker gaining access could monitor activities within a home or observe who enters and leaves, posing a direct threat to safety and privacy.

- **Location Tracking:** Continuous location tracking via smart devices or apps, even if intended for navigation or safety features, creates a detailed record of a person's movements. This data is incredibly sensitive and vulnerable to misuse if not properly secured.
- **Behavioral Profiling:** Aggregating data from multiple smart devices can create a highly detailed profile of a person's daily routine, habits, social interactions (via voice analysis), and even health status (via wearables). This level of insight, while potentially used for personalization, is also a significant privacy risk if accessed or used inappropriately. For visually impaired individuals, whose routines might be more structured due to navigation needs, this profiling could be particularly revealing.
- **Challenges in Exercising Data Rights:** Regulations like GDPR and CCPA grant users rights regarding their data (e.g., the right to access, rectify, or erase personal data). However, exercising these rights often requires navigating complex online portals or submitting formal requests. These processes may not be designed accessibly, creating barriers for visually impaired individuals seeking to understand or control the data held about them.

The combination of extensive data collection, potential for misuse, and the specific challenges faced by visually impaired individuals in understanding and controlling their data creates a significant privacy gap. Addressing this requires not only robust technical safeguards but also a fundamental shift towards designing privacy-preserving and transparent systems with accessibility as a core principle, ensuring that visually impaired users can truly understand and manage their digital footprint (Mavroudis & Gritzalis, 2019).

5. TRUST IN SMART SYSTEMS

Trust is the cornerstone of any successful human-technology interaction, particularly when that technology is deeply integrated into personal spaces and critical daily functions. For individuals with visual disabilities, who may rely on smart systems for enhanced independence and safety, trust is not merely a matter of preference but a fundamental requirement for adoption and sustained use. A lack of trust can render even the most technologically advanced and potentially beneficial system unusable, leading to frustration, anxiety, and continued exclusion (Wang & Zhang, 2024).

5.1 The Role of Trust

Trust, in the context of smart systems for visually impaired users, is a complex construct influenced by multiple factors. It represents a user's belief that the system will consistently perform as expected, protect their interests (especially security and privacy), and ultimately contribute positively to their quality of life without introducing undue risks or dependencies (Zhao & Liu, 2021). Key components contributing to trust include:

- **Reliability and Performance:** Users must believe that the technology is dependable and functions correctly. For a visually impaired person, this means trusting that:
- A smart navigation app will provide accurate and timely directions and obstacle alerts.
- A voice command will be correctly interpreted and executed by a smart device.
- A smart lock will reliably lock and unlock the door when commanded.
- A smart medical device will provide accurate readings. Unreliable performance—such as voice commands failing, apps crashing, devices becoming unresponsive, or inaccurate information being provided—erodes trust quickly. For someone who cannot visually verify the system's state, reliability is even more critical.
- **Security Assurance:** Users must trust that the system is secure from unauthorized access, manipulation, and malicious attacks. This involves believing that:
- Their personal data and home environment are protected.
- Vulnerabilities are proactively addressed by the manufacturer.
- Their interactions are private and not being monitored without consent. Concerns about hacking, data breaches, or unauthorized surveillance directly undermine trust, leading users to feel vulnerable and unsafe when using the technology.
- **Privacy Protection:** Users must trust that their personal data is collected, processed, and used responsibly and transparently, and that they have control over it. This means trusting that:
- Data collection is minimized to what is necessary.
- Data is not shared with third parties without informed consent.
- Privacy policies are clear, understandable, and accessible.
- They have the ability to access, modify, or delete their data. A lack of transparency about data practices or perceived misuse of data can severely damage trust, as users feel their personal information is being exploited or mishandled.

- **Transparency:** Users need to understand how the system works, what data it collects, why it collects it, and what the potential risks are. Transparency in:
- **Functionality:** Clearly explaining what the device does and its limitations.
- **Data Practices:** Being upfront about data collection, processing, storage, and sharing.
- **Security Measures:** Explaining the security protocols in place and how users can enhance their own security.
- **Updates and Changes:** Communicating when updates are available and what changes they entail. Lack of transparency creates uncertainty and suspicion, making it difficult for users, especially those who cannot visually inspect interfaces or documentation, to build trust.
- **User Empowerment and Control:** Users need to feel that they are in control of the technology and their data, not controlled by it. This involves:
- Accessible and intuitive interfaces for managing settings.
- Granular control over data sharing and privacy options.
- Clear mechanisms for reporting issues and seeking support.
- The ability to easily disable features or disconnect devices if desired. Feeling powerless to manage a complex system or control one's own data is a major barrier to trust, particularly for individuals who value their independence.
- **Manufacturer and Service Provider Reputation:** Trust in the technology is often influenced by trust in the companies behind it. A company with a history of security breaches, privacy scandals, or poor customer support will struggle to earn the trust of users, especially vulnerable populations. Conversely, companies known for prioritizing security, privacy, and accessibility are more likely to be trusted.

For visually impaired users, the reliance on non-visual cues and the potential difficulty in independently verifying system states or navigating complex settings mean that the need for reliability, security, privacy, and transparency is even more acute. They must place a higher degree of *blind* trust in the system's design and the manufacturer's integrity. If that trust is broken, the consequences—loss of independence, privacy violations, safety risks—are particularly severe, and rebuilding trust can be a long and difficult process.

5.2 Building Trust in Smart Systems

Building and maintaining trust among visually impaired users requires a deliberate and sustained effort on the part of developers, manufacturers, service providers, and policymakers. It goes beyond simply adding accessibility features; it requires embedding trust considerations into the entire lifecycle of the technology, from conception and design to deployment, updates, and support.

- **User-Centric and Inclusive Design:** This is perhaps the most critical foundation for building trust.
- **Involve Users from the Outset:** Actively involving individuals with visual disabilities in the research, design, development, and testing phases is essential. Their insights are invaluable for identifying potential usability, accessibility, security, and privacy issues that might not be apparent to sighted developers. Co-design ensures that the technology truly meets their needs and preferences.
- **Prioritize Accessibility:** Design interfaces and interactions that are inherently accessible. This includes full compatibility with screen readers and voice control, providing clear audio feedback, using distinct non-visual cues (e.g., haptic feedback), and ensuring logical and easy-to-navigate structures in apps and settings. Accessibility builds trust by demonstrating respect for the user's needs and enabling independent interaction.
- **Predictable and Consistent Behavior:** Design systems that behave predictably and consistently. Unexpected actions or inconsistent responses are confusing and erode trust, especially for users who rely on auditory or tactile feedback.
- **Robust Security Measures:** Implementing and clearly communicating strong security protocols is fundamental to building trust in the system's safety.
- **Security by Design:** Security should be a core consideration from the very beginning of the design process, not an afterthought.
- **Strong Authentication:** Offer and encourage the use of strong, accessible authentication methods (e.g., accessible multi-factor authentication). Avoid relying solely on weak passwords.
- **Encryption:** Implement end-to-end encryption for sensitive data transmission whenever possible. Clearly communicate when and how data is encrypted.
- **Regular Security Audits and Penetration Testing:** Proactively identify and address vulnerabilities before they can be exploited.
- **Secure Update Mechanisms:** Ensure that firmware and software updates can be delivered securely and reliably to patch vulnerabilities. Make the update process accessible and clearly notify users when updates are available and recommended.
- **Clear Incident Response Plan:** Have a plan in place for responding to security breaches, including promptly notifying affected users and providing clear guidance on steps to take.

- **Enhancing Privacy Protections and Transparency:** Demonstrating a commitment to protecting user privacy is crucial for earning trust.
- **Data Minimization:** Collect only the data that is strictly necessary for the system to function and provide the requested services.
- **Purpose Limitation:** Clearly define the purposes for which data is collected and used, and do not use data for undisclosed purposes.
- **Accessible Privacy Policies:** Provide privacy policies and terms of service in accessible formats (e.g., screen-reader friendly web pages, audio summaries) and use clear, simple language. Consider providing layered information, starting with a concise summary and allowing users to delve into more detail if desired.
- **Granular and Accessible Privacy Controls:** Provide users with easy-to-find and easy-to-use controls over their data, allowing them to opt-in or opt-out of specific data collection or sharing practices. Ensure these controls are fully accessible via non-visual interfaces.
- **Just-in-Time Notifications:** Where appropriate, provide clear, non-visual notifications (e.g., distinct audio cues, haptic feedback) when sensitive data collection (like recording) is initiated.
- **Transparency Reports:** Consider publishing transparency reports detailing data requests from governments or other entities.
- **Transparent Communication:** Open and honest communication about the technology, its capabilities, its limitations, and its data practices is vital.
- **Clear and Accessible Documentation:** Provide user manuals, FAQs, and support materials in accessible formats.
- **Honest Marketing:** Avoid making exaggerated claims about security or privacy. Be realistic about potential risks.
- **Proactive Communication about Issues:** If a security vulnerability or privacy issue is discovered, communicate it promptly, clearly, and accessibly to affected users, explaining the risk and the steps being taken to mitigate it.
- **User Education and Support:** Empowering users with knowledge and providing accessible support builds confidence and trust.
- **Accessible Security and Privacy Education:** Provide accessible resources (audio guides, screen-reader friendly web content, webinars with audio descriptions) that educate users about common security threats, privacy risks, and best practices for protecting themselves when using smart systems.
- **Accessible Customer Support:** Ensure that customer support channels (phone, email, chat) are fully accessible to visually impaired users and that support staff are trained on accessibility issues and the specific needs of this user group.

- **Community Building:** Foster online communities or user groups where visually impaired users can share experiences, tips, and support regarding smart technologies.
- **Accountability:** Manufacturers and service providers must be accountable for the security and privacy of their systems. This includes adhering to relevant regulations, responding promptly to security reports, and taking responsibility when breaches or privacy violations occur. Demonstrating accountability builds confidence that the company is committed to user well-being.

Building trust is an ongoing process, not a one-time task. It requires continuous attention to security, privacy, and accessibility, coupled with open and respectful communication with users. For individuals with visual disabilities, who have historically faced barriers to technology access and may have valid reasons for skepticism, earning and maintaining their trust is paramount for the successful and ethical deployment of smart systems.

6. CASE STUDIES

Examining real-world examples provides valuable insights into the practical implications of security, privacy, and trust issues in smart systems for visually impaired users. These case studies, while sometimes hypothetical scenarios based on known vulnerabilities or challenges, illustrate the potential benefits and risks.

6.1 Case Study 1: Smart Home Technologies for Visually Impaired Users

Scenario: Sarah, who is blind, decides to install a smart home system to increase her independence. She gets a smart speaker (voice assistant), smart lights, a smart thermostat, and a smart lock for her front door. She relies heavily on voice commands to control these devices.

Potential Benefits: Sarah experiences significant improvements in daily life. She can turn lights on/off in different rooms without navigating in the dark, adjust the temperature comfortably, lock and unlock her door with voice commands when her hands are full, and check if the door is locked before going to bed. The voice assistant also helps her set timers for cooking, get weather updates, and make calls, further enhancing her autonomy.

Security Challenges

- **Vulnerable Smart Lock:** A vulnerability is discovered in the specific model of her smart lock that allows unauthorized remote unlocking if the attacker is on the same local network. Sarah, who cannot easily check the lock's status visually or navigate complex router settings to isolate the device, is unaware of this vulnerability. An attacker could potentially gain entry to her home.
- **Voice Assistant Spoofing:** Research demonstrates that voice assistants can potentially be tricked by synthesized voices or recordings, or even by ultrasonic commands inaudible to humans but detectable by microphones. An attacker near Sarah's house could potentially issue commands to her smart speaker to unlock her door or disable her security camera (if she had one), without her knowledge.
- **Network Intrusion:** If Sarah's home Wi-Fi network has a weak password, an attacker could gain access to her network and, from there, potentially access and control her connected smart devices, including lights, thermostat, and lock. Sarah might not notice unusual network activity without visual monitoring tools.

Privacy Concerns

- **Voice Command Data:** The smart speaker records voice commands and sends them to the cloud for processing. While intended for functionality, this data contains sensitive information about Sarah's routines, her interactions with visitors (if they speak commands), and potentially snippets of conversations if the wake word is accidentally triggered. If the manufacturer's cloud service is breached, this data could be exposed.
- **Activity Data:** The smart system logs when lights are turned on/off, when the thermostat is adjusted, and when the door is locked/unlocked. This creates a detailed log of Sarah's presence and activity within her home. This data, if accessed without authorization, could reveal when she is home or away, making her a potential target for burglary or other crimes.
- **Inaccessible Privacy Settings:** Sarah finds the smart system's mobile app difficult to navigate with a screen reader, making it hard for her to find and understand the privacy settings. She is unsure how to limit data collection or review what data is being stored.

Trust Implications:

- If Sarah experiences a security incident (e.g., her door unexpectedly unlocks) or learns about a privacy breach related to her smart speaker, her trust in the entire system will be severely damaged. She may feel unsafe in her own home, the very place the technology was supposed to make more secure and independent.
- The difficulty in managing settings and understanding data practices due to inaccessible interfaces erodes trust, making her feel powerless and vulnerable.
- Reliability issues, such as voice commands not being recognized consistently, also diminish trust in the system's ability to function as a dependable aid.

Study Findings (Hypothetical, based on common themes): A study exploring visually impaired users' experiences with smart homes might find that while participants initially express excitement about increased independence, they often harbor significant underlying concerns about security and privacy. Participants might report difficulty understanding how their data is used, challenges in configuring security settings, and a reliance on sighted family members to help manage the system, which can undermine the feeling of full independence. The study might conclude that manufacturers need to prioritize accessible security and privacy controls and provide clearer, non-visual indicators of system status and potential issues.

6.2 Case Study 2: Navigation Apps for the Visually Impaired

Scenario: David, who has low vision, uses a specialized navigation app on his smartphone to help him walk to familiar and unfamiliar destinations. The app uses GPS, mapping data, and sometimes crowdsourced information to provide detailed audio directions, identify intersections, alert him to upcoming turns, and point out landmarks or points of interest. He also uses a service like Aira via the app, which connects him to a live agent who can see his surroundings through his phone's camera and provide visual information.

Potential Benefits: The navigation app significantly enhances David's mobility and confidence. He can explore new routes, find specific addresses more easily, and navigate complex public spaces like train stations. The Aira service provides invaluable real-time assistance for tasks like reading signs, identifying bus numbers, or navigating busy areas.

Security Challenges:

- **Location Data Tracking:** The app continuously collects precise location data. If the app's servers are breached, or if the data is transmitted insecurely, an attacker could gain access to David's complete movement history, revealing his home address, workplace, places he visits regularly, and his daily routine. This poses a direct safety risk.
- **Account Compromise:** If David's account for the navigation service is compromised (e.g., via phishing), an attacker could potentially access his saved locations, trip history, and personal profile information.
- **Vulnerabilities in Live Assistance Services:** For services like Aira, the video feed from the user's phone is transmitted to a remote agent. While these services have security measures, a vulnerability in the app or the service's infrastructure could potentially allow unauthorized access to the live video feed or recorded sessions, leading to invasive surveillance.

Privacy Concerns:

- **Detailed Movement History:** The granularity of location data collected by navigation apps creates a highly detailed record of a user's life. This data can reveal sensitive information about their health (e.g., frequent visits to a hospital), social life, religious practices (visits to places of worship), and other personal aspects.
- **Data Sharing with Third Parties:** The navigation app provider might share aggregated or even pseudonymized location data with third parties (e.g., urban planners, advertisers). While often framed as beneficial, users may not be fully aware of this sharing or have the ability to opt-out.
- **Privacy of Live Assistance Sessions:** During a live assistance session, the agent (and potentially the service provider) has access to a real-time view of the user's environment and potentially conversations happening around them. While agents are typically bound by privacy policies, the potential for human error or malicious intent exists. Users need to trust that these sessions are handled with the utmost discretion and security.
- **Informed Consent for Data Use:** Understanding exactly how location data and video feed data are used, stored, and protected can be challenging due to complex privacy policies, which may be difficult to access and understand with assistive technologies.

Trust Implications:

- If David learns that his location history has been exposed or misused, his trust in the navigation app and service will be severely damaged. He may feel unsafe using it for independent travel, potentially limiting his mobility and independence.
- Concerns about the privacy of live assistance sessions could make him hesitant to use the service, even when he desperately needs visual information.
- Reliability issues, such as the app providing incorrect directions or losing GPS signal frequently, also erode trust in its ability to be a dependable guide.

Study Findings (Hypothetical): Research focusing on visually impaired users of navigation apps might highlight the tension between the immense value these apps provide for independence and the significant privacy concerns they raise. Participants might express anxiety about the constant tracking of their movements and the potential for this data to be misused. The study could emphasize the need for app developers to implement robust data security, provide clear and accessible privacy controls, and ensure transparent communication about data practices, particularly for sensitive location and video data.

6.3 Case Study 3: Smart Glasses for Enhanced Mobility and Information Access

Scenario: Maria, who is legally blind, begins using a pair of smart glasses equipped with a camera and AI capabilities. The glasses can identify objects, read text aloud from signs or documents, describe her surroundings, and potentially provide subtle navigation cues via audio or haptic feedback.

Potential Benefits: The smart glasses offer Maria a new level of real-time information about her environment. She can quickly identify objects in her path, read labels on products in a store, get descriptions of people's appearances, and read public signs independently. This significantly enhances her ability to interact with the world around her and reduces reliance on others for visual information.

Security Challenges:

- **Unauthorized Camera Access:** The most significant security risk is unauthorized access to the glasses' camera and microphone. If the device's security is compromised, an attacker could remotely activate the camera and microphone, gaining a real-time audio-visual feed of Maria's activities and surroundings without her knowledge. This is an extreme privacy violation and a major safety risk.

- **Data Storage and Transmission:** The glasses collect vast amounts of visual and audio data. If this data is stored insecurely on the device or transmitted without strong encryption to a companion app or cloud service, it is vulnerable to interception or theft.
- **Firmware Vulnerabilities:** Security flaws in the glasses' operating system or firmware could be exploited to gain control of the device, access data, or install malware.

Privacy Concerns:

- **Continuous Environmental Recording:** While the camera is intended to process information for the user, the potential for continuous recording of the environment and people within it raises significant privacy concerns, not just for the user but also for those around them. People interacting with Maria may not be aware that the glasses are processing visual information.
- **Biometric Data:** Future smart glasses might incorporate features like facial recognition for identifying known contacts. While beneficial, this involves collecting and processing biometric data, which is highly sensitive and requires stringent security and privacy protections.
- **Inferred Information:** The AI processing the visual and audio data can infer a great deal about Maria's life – where she is, who she is with, what she is doing, her emotional state (from voice analysis), and potentially even health information (e.g., signs of fatigue). This inferred data is highly personal.
- **Lack of Control for Others:** People in Maria's vicinity have no control over whether their image or voice is captured and processed by her smart glasses, raising privacy issues for the general public.

Trust Implications:

- Maria's trust in the smart glasses is contingent on her absolute belief that the camera and microphone cannot be accessed without her explicit knowledge and consent. Any credible report of a security vulnerability allowing remote access would be devastating to her trust and likely lead her to stop using the device, losing the significant independence it provides.
- Concerns about how the vast amount of visual and audio data is used, stored, and protected, and whether it is shared with third parties, directly impact her trust in the manufacturer and the technology.

- The social implications of using a device that constantly processes the environment also play a role in trust – Maria needs to trust that the technology is designed and used ethically, respecting the privacy of others.

Study Findings (Hypothetical): Research on early users of smart glasses for visual assistance might highlight the transformative potential for independence but also the profound privacy anxieties. Users might express discomfort with the idea of the device constantly processing their environment and worry about how the collected data is handled. The study could emphasize the critical need for manufacturers to implement state-of-the-art security for the camera and microphone, provide transparent and accessible controls over data collection and processing, and engage in public education about the technology's capabilities and privacy safeguards to build trust among both users and the general public.

These case studies underscore that while smart systems offer tremendous potential for enhancing the lives of individuals with visual disabilities, the inherent security and privacy risks are significant and can directly undermine the benefits by eroding trust. Addressing these issues is not a secondary concern but a fundamental requirement for ethical and effective technology development.

7. BEST PRACTICES FOR ENHANCING SECURITY, PRIVACY, AND TRUST

Addressing the challenges outlined in the previous sections requires a multifaceted approach involving technology design, organizational policies, regulatory frameworks, and user education. Implementing best practices across these areas is essential for building smart systems that are secure, privacy-preserving, and trustworthy for individuals with visual disabilities.

7.1 Implementing Strong Security Protocols

Security must be a foundational element of smart system design and deployment. Adhering to robust security protocols helps protect devices, data, and users from malicious attacks.

- **Security by Design and Default:** Security considerations should be integrated into every stage of the product lifecycle, from initial concept and design to development, testing, deployment, and end-of-life. Devices should ship with secure default settings rather than requiring users to configure security measures themselves.

- **Robust Authentication and Authorization:**
- **Strong Password Policies:** Enforce strong password requirements during setup and encourage users to change default credentials immediately.
- **Multi-Factor Authentication (MFA):** Offer and strongly recommend accessible MFA options (e.g., using a separate device for a code, accessible authenticator apps) to add an extra layer of security beyond just a password.
- **Principle of Least Privilege:** Devices and associated services should only have the minimum permissions necessary to perform their intended functions.
- **Encryption:**
- **End-to-End Encryption:** Implement end-to-end encryption for sensitive data transmission whenever technically feasible, ensuring that data is encrypted on the device and only decrypted by the intended recipient.
- **Encryption in Transit:** Use strong, up-to-date encryption protocols (like TLS 1.2 or higher) for all data transmitted over the internet or local networks.
- **Encryption at Rest:** Encrypt sensitive data stored on the device itself or in the cloud database.
- **Secure Communication Protocols:** Utilize secure and standardized communication protocols (e.g., HTTPS, secure MQTT) for device-to-device, device-to-app, and device-to-cloud communication.
- **Regular Security Updates and Patching:**
- **Over-the-Air (OTA) Updates:** Implement a secure and reliable mechanism for delivering firmware and software updates remotely.
- **Timely Patching:** Proactively monitor for vulnerabilities and release patches promptly.
- **Accessible Update Notifications:** Clearly notify users about available updates and the importance of installing them, using accessible communication methods.
- **Long-Term Support:** Commit to providing security updates for a reasonable lifespan of the device, not just for the first year or two.
- **Input Validation and Sanitization:** Implement rigorous input validation to prevent injection attacks and other vulnerabilities that exploit malformed data inputs.
- **Minimize Attack Surface:** Design devices and software with the smallest possible attack surface, disabling unnecessary ports, services, and functionalities.
- **Intrusion Detection and Monitoring:** Implement mechanisms to detect suspicious activity on devices or the network and alert users or administrators.
- **Secure API Design:** Design and implement APIs with security in mind, using authentication, authorization, and rate limiting.

- **Physical Security:** Consider physical security measures where appropriate, such as tamper-resistant hardware or secure boot processes.
- **Third-Party Component Security:** Vet the security of any third-party hardware or software components used in the smart system.
- **Responsible Disclosure Policy:** Establish a clear policy for security researchers to report vulnerabilities and commit to addressing them promptly.

7.2 Enhancing Privacy Protections

Prioritizing user privacy requires implementing technical measures and establishing clear, transparent policies that empower users to control their data.

- **Privacy by Design and Default:** Integrate privacy considerations into the design process from the beginning. Default settings should be the most privacy-preserving options.
- **Data Minimization:** Collect only the minimum amount of personal data necessary to provide the core functionality of the service. Avoid collecting data speculatively for potential future uses.
- **Purpose Specification and Limitation:** Clearly define the specific purposes for which data is collected at the time of collection. Do not use data for purposes incompatible with the specified ones without obtaining new, informed consent.
- **Anonymization and Pseudonymization:** Wherever possible, anonymize or pseudonymize data to reduce the risk of identifying individual users. Use strong anonymization techniques that prevent re-identification.
- **Data Retention Limits:** Establish clear policies for how long data is retained and securely delete data when it is no longer needed for the specified purpose.
- **Accessible Privacy Policies and Terms of Service:**
- Provide policies in multiple accessible formats (e.g., screen-reader friendly web pages, audio recordings, summarized versions).
- Use clear, concise, and easy-to-understand language, avoiding legal jargon where possible.
- Use visual design (for sighted users) and structural markup (for screen readers) that makes the policies easy to navigate and search.
- **Granular and Accessible Privacy Controls:** Provide users with fine-grained controls over their data and privacy settings. These controls should be easily discoverable and fully accessible via non-visual interfaces (voice commands, screen reader compatible menus). Users should be able to:
- Review what data is being collected.

- Opt-in or opt-out of specific data collection or sharing activities (beyond what is strictly necessary for core functionality).
- Access and download their personal data.
- Request correction or deletion of their data.
- Manage permissions granted to the device or associated apps (e.g., access to microphone, camera, location).
- **Transparent Data Flow Information:** Clearly communicate to users how their data flows through the system – where it is collected, where it is processed (on-device or in the cloud), where it is stored, and with whom it is shared.
- **Just-in-Time Privacy Notifications:** Provide clear, non-visual notifications (e.g., distinct audio cues, haptic feedback) when sensitive data collection, such as recording audio or video, is initiated. The user should be able to understand *why* the data is being collected at that moment.
- **Secure Data Storage:** Store collected data securely, both on the device and in the cloud, using encryption and access controls.
- **Third-Party Data Sharing Transparency and Control:** If data is shared with third parties, clearly disclose who these parties are, what data is shared, and for what purpose. Provide users with an accessible mechanism to consent to or opt-out of such sharing, unless required by law.
- **Regular Privacy Audits:** Conduct regular audits of data collection, processing, and storage practices to ensure compliance with policies and regulations.

7.3 Fostering Trust through User Engagement

Building trust is an ongoing process that requires active engagement with the user community, particularly visually impaired individuals. This involves more than just technical implementation; it requires a commitment to transparency, support, and empowering users.

- **Inclusive Design and Development Process:** As mentioned earlier, actively involve visually impaired individuals throughout the entire product lifecycle. This includes:
- **Consultation:** Seek input from individuals with diverse visual impairments and users of various assistive technologies during the requirements gathering and design phases.
- **Participatory Design:** Co-design features and interfaces with visually impaired users.

- **Accessibility Testing:** Conduct rigorous accessibility testing with actual users of screen readers, voice control, and other assistive technologies. Do not rely solely on automated testing tools.
- **Feedback Integration:** Establish clear channels for users to provide feedback on security, privacy, and accessibility issues and demonstrate that their feedback is valued and acted upon.
- **Transparent Communication about Security and Privacy:**
- **Clear and Accessible Explanations:** Explain security features, privacy settings, and data practices in plain language and accessible formats. Avoid technical jargon.
- **Proactive Security Notifications:** If a security vulnerability is discovered, communicate it promptly and clearly to affected users, explaining the risk, the impact, and the steps they should take (e.g., update firmware).
- **Data Breach Notification:** Have a clear and accessible plan for notifying users in the event of a data breach, explaining what data was compromised, the potential risks, and the steps the company is taking.
- **Accessible User Support and Education:**
- **Comprehensive and Accessible Documentation:** Provide user manuals, FAQs, troubleshooting guides, and security/privacy best practices in accessible formats (e.g., screen-reader friendly web pages, audio files, braille on request).
- **Accessible Customer Support Channels:** Ensure that customer support is available through channels accessible to visually impaired users (e.g., accessible phone lines, email support, accessible chat interfaces). Train support staff on accessibility and privacy issues relevant to visually impaired users.
- **Educational Resources:** Develop accessible educational materials (webinars with audio descriptions, audio tutorials, screen-reader friendly guides) that teach users about online safety, privacy management in smart systems, and how to use the device's security and privacy features effectively.
- **Empowering Users with Control:** Design interfaces that give users clear and easy control over critical settings, especially those related to security and privacy. Ensure that these controls are accessible via non-visual means.
- **Building a Community of Trust:** Foster a sense of community around the product or service where users feel comfortable sharing their experiences and getting support. Respond actively and empathetically to user concerns.
- **Demonstrating Accountability:** Be transparent about how security and privacy issues are handled. If a mistake is made, acknowledge it, explain what happened, and outline the steps being taken to prevent recurrence.

- **Compliance with Regulations and Standards:** Adhere to relevant data protection regulations (like GDPR, CCPA) and accessibility standards (like WCAG). Clearly communicate this compliance to users.
- **Ethical Considerations in AI Development:** If the smart system uses AI, ensure that the AI is developed and deployed ethically, with consideration for potential biases that could negatively impact visually impaired users, and with transparency about how AI is used and what data it processes.

By consistently implementing these best practices, developers and organizations can demonstrate a genuine commitment to the security, privacy, and well-being of their visually impaired users, thereby building the essential trust required for the successful and equitable adoption of smart systems.

8. FUTURE DIRECTIONS

The landscape of smart systems and assistive technologies is constantly evolving. Looking ahead, several key areas will shape the future of security, privacy, and trust for visually impaired users in this domain.

8.1 Advances in AI and Machine Learning

Artificial intelligence and machine learning are central to the functionality of many smart systems, enabling capabilities like voice recognition, image analysis, and predictive automation. Future advancements in AI hold significant potential to both enhance and challenge security and privacy for visually impaired users.

Potential Enhancements

- **Improved Anomaly Detection:** More sophisticated AI algorithms can potentially analyze user behavior patterns and device activity to detect anomalies that might indicate a security breach or unauthorized access in real-time. For example, an AI could flag unusual login attempts, unexpected device commands, or changes in data transmission patterns. This could provide a crucial, non-visual alert mechanism for visually impaired users.
- **Enhanced Biometric Authentication:** Advances in AI-powered facial recognition, voice recognition, or gait analysis could offer more secure and convenient authentication methods, provided they are developed with accessibility and privacy in mind and are not susceptible to spoofing.

- **Proactive Threat Identification:** AI could be used to analyze vast amounts of data from connected devices and networks to identify emerging threats and vulnerabilities before they are widely exploited.
- **Automated Privacy Management:** Future AI systems could potentially assist users, including those with visual impairments, in understanding and managing their privacy settings by summarizing complex policies, recommending privacy-preserving configurations based on usage patterns, and alerting them to potential privacy risks in new apps or devices.
- **Context-Aware Security:** AI could enable smart systems to adapt their security posture based on the user's context (e.g., stricter authentication when accessing sensitive data, relaxed authentication when performing routine tasks).

Potential Challenges and Risks

- **AI Bias:** If the data used to train AI models is not representative of visually impaired users or their interaction patterns, the AI could exhibit biases that lead to accessibility issues, security vulnerabilities (e.g., voice recognition failing for certain voices), or privacy risks.
- **Adversarial AI Attacks:** Attackers are developing techniques to trick AI systems (adversarial attacks). For example, subtle changes to audio commands or visual input could be designed to be misinterpreted by the AI, potentially leading to unauthorized actions or data breaches.
- **Increased Data Collection for AI Training:** Developing more sophisticated AI often requires vast amounts of data, potentially leading to increased pressure to collect more personal data from users, raising privacy concerns.
- **Lack of Explainability (Black Box Problem):** Some advanced AI models are complex "black boxes," making it difficult to understand exactly how they arrive at a decision or prediction. This lack of explainability can make it challenging to diagnose security or privacy issues related to the AI's behavior and can erode user trust.
- **Deepfakes and Synthetic Media:** Advances in generative AI could be used to create convincing deepfakes of a user's voice or appearance, which could potentially be used to bypass voice authentication systems or create malicious content.

The future integration of AI in smart systems for visually impaired users requires careful consideration of these potential benefits and risks. Development must prioritize ethical AI principles, transparency, explainability, and the proactive identification and mitigation of biases and adversarial vulnerabilities.

8.2 Development of Ethical Guidelines

As smart systems become more powerful and integrated, the need for clear ethical guidelines governing their design, deployment, and use becomes increasingly critical, particularly for vulnerable populations.

- **Specific Guidelines for Assistive Technologies:** Beyond general AI ethics, there is a need for specific ethical frameworks that address the unique considerations of smart systems used as assistive technologies. These guidelines should address:
- **Autonomy and Agency:** Ensuring that the technology enhances, rather than diminishes, user autonomy and control.
- **Equity and Non-Discrimination:** Preventing the technology from creating new forms of exclusion or discrimination based on disability.
- **Beneficence and Non-Maleficence:** Ensuring the technology provides genuine benefits and minimizes potential harm.
- **Privacy and Confidentiality:** Establishing stringent standards for the collection, use, and protection of sensitive data, especially health and behavioral data.
- **Transparency and Explainability:** Requiring clear communication about the system's capabilities, limitations, and data practices.
- **Multi-Stakeholder Collaboration:** The development of effective ethical guidelines requires collaboration among a wide range of stakeholders, including:
- **Technology Developers and Manufacturers:** Who are responsible for implementing ethical principles in design and development.
- **Policymakers and Regulators:** Who can establish legal frameworks and standards.
- **Visually Impaired Users and Advocacy Groups:** Whose lived experiences and perspectives are essential for identifying ethical challenges and priorities.
- **Researchers:** Who can study the societal impact of these technologies.
- **Ethicists and Legal Scholars:** Who can provide theoretical frameworks and legal expertise.
- **Addressing Power Imbalances:** Ethical guidelines must address the inherent power imbalance between technology providers and users, particularly when users are reliant on the technology for essential functions.
- **Accountability Mechanisms:** Guidelines should include mechanisms for accountability when ethical principles are violated, ensuring that companies can be held responsible for the harm caused by their systems.

- **Focus on Long-Term Impact:** Ethical considerations should extend beyond the initial deployment of the technology to consider its long-term societal impact and potential for unintended consequences.

The development and adoption of robust, disability-inclusive ethical guidelines are crucial for ensuring that smart systems are developed and used in a manner that respects the rights, dignity, and well-being of individuals with visual disabilities (Gray & Cyan, 2022).

8.3 Increased Awareness and Advocacy

Raising awareness among the general public, policymakers, and technology developers about the challenges and opportunities associated with smart systems for visually impaired individuals is essential for driving positive change.

- **Educating Developers and Designers:** Developers and designers need to be educated about the principles of universal design, accessibility standards (like WCAG), and the specific needs and interaction patterns of visually impaired users. This education should include hands-on experience with assistive technologies.
- **Advocacy for Inclusive Standards and Regulations:** Advocacy groups for people with visual disabilities play a critical role in pushing for the inclusion of accessibility, security, and privacy requirements in relevant technology standards and government regulations. This includes advocating for:
- Mandatory accessibility features in smart devices and their interfaces.
- Clear and accessible privacy policies.
- Requirements for robust security updates and long-term support.
- Data protection regulations that specifically address the unique risks faced by people with disabilities.
- **Public Awareness Campaigns:** Raising public awareness about the benefits of accessible smart technology and the importance of considering the needs of visually impaired users can help create market demand for inclusive products and encourage ethical development practices.
- **Highlighting Success Stories and Best Practices:** Sharing examples of smart systems that have successfully implemented strong security, privacy, and accessibility features can inspire other developers and demonstrate the feasibility and value of inclusive design.
- **Empowering Users through Education:** Providing visually impaired users with accessible information and training on how to choose, set up, and

securely use smart systems empowers them to make informed decisions and protect themselves.

- **Collaboration between Disability Organizations and Tech Companies:** Fostering ongoing dialogue and collaboration between disability advocacy organizations and technology companies can help bridge the gap between user needs and product development, leading to more inclusive and trustworthy technologies.

Increased awareness and sustained advocacy are vital for ensuring that the development and deployment of smart systems move beyond simply creating innovative gadgets to building a truly inclusive and safe connected world for everyone, including individuals with visual disabilities.

9. CONCLUSION

The integration of smart systems into the fabric of everyday life presents a landscape of both immense opportunity and significant challenge for individuals with visual disabilities. These technologies hold the potential to unlock unprecedented levels of independence, autonomy, and access to information and services, fundamentally improving quality of life. However, this transformative potential can only be fully realized if the critical issues of security, privacy, and trust are addressed proactively and comprehensively.

As this chapter has explored, visually impaired users face unique interaction barriers and amplified risks within the smart ecosystem. The inherent vulnerabilities in smart devices and the extensive collection of personal data pose significant threats, ranging from loss of control over one's environment and physical safety risks to pervasive privacy violations and the potential for discrimination or exploitation. For a population that relies on these systems for essential functions, the inability to easily detect or respond to security and privacy breaches, coupled with the challenges of navigating complex and often inaccessible interfaces, makes these risks particularly disabling (Mavroudis & Gritzalis, 2019).

The foundation of successful and ethical smart system deployment for visually impaired individuals lies in building and maintaining trust. Trust is not a given; it must be earned through a demonstrated commitment to reliability, security, privacy, transparency, and user empowerment. A lack of trust, stemming from fears of security breaches, concerns about data privacy, or frustration with inaccessible design, can severely limit the adoption of potentially beneficial technologies and negate their positive impact, perpetuating digital exclusion (Gray & Cyan, 2022).

Addressing these challenges requires a multi-pronged approach centered on best practices in design, development, and deployment. Implementing robust security protocols, such as security by design, strong authentication, and encryption, is essential to protect devices and data from unauthorized access and manipulation. Simultaneously, enhancing privacy protections through data minimization, transparent policies, accessible controls, and responsible data handling is crucial for respecting user autonomy and preventing misuse of sensitive information (Kulyk & Gajos, 2021).

Crucially, fostering trust requires active and genuine engagement with the visually impaired community. Inclusive design processes that involve users from the outset, coupled with accessible communication, comprehensive education on security and privacy, and responsive customer support, are vital for building confidence and ensuring that the technology meets real-world needs (Chen et al., 2021).

Looking to the future, advancements in AI and machine learning will continue to shape the capabilities of smart systems, presenting both opportunities for enhanced security and privacy features and new potential risks that require careful ethical consideration and proactive mitigation. The development of specific, disability-inclusive ethical guidelines and sustained advocacy efforts are essential to ensure that technological progress aligns with the rights and well-being of visually impaired individuals.

In conclusion, the journey towards a truly inclusive smart world for people with visual disabilities is not solely a technical challenge; it is an ethical and societal imperative. By prioritizing security, embedding privacy from the ground up, and actively working to build and maintain user trust through accessible and transparent practices, developers, organizations, and policymakers can create smart systems that genuinely enhance the independence, safety, and quality of life for this population, ensuring that they are empowered participants, not vulnerable bystanders, in our increasingly connected future. This chapter has aimed to provide a comprehensive overview of these critical considerations, serving as a resource for those dedicated to developing and deploying smart technologies that are not just innovative, but also equitable, safe, and trustworthy for all.

REFERENCES

Akhai, S. (2023). From Black Boxes to Transparent Machines: The Quest for Explainable AI. Social Science Research Network. DOI: 10.2139/ssrn.4390887

Akhai, S. (2024a). Smart Home Environment for Society: An Overview of IoT-Enabled Air Conditioners. In Modelling of Virtual Worlds Using the Internet of Things (Vol. 1, pp. 74-87). CRC Press.

Akhai, S. (2024b). Towards Trustworthy and Reliable AI The Next Frontier. In Explainable Artificial Intelligence (XAI) in Healthcare (Vol. 1, pp. 119-129). CRC Press, Taylor & Francis Group.

Akhai, S. (2024b). Towards Trustworthy and Reliable AI The Next Frontier. In Explainable Artificial Intelligence (XAI) in Healthcare (Vol. 1, pp. 119-129). CRC Press, Taylor & Francis Group.

Akhai, S., & Khang, A. (2024). Innovations in Medical Manufacturing: A Review of 3D Printing, Robotics, and Internet of Things (IoT). In The Quantum Evolution (Vol. 1, pp. 226-241). CRC Press.

Akhai, S., & Kumar, V. (2024). Quantum resilience and distributed trust: The promise of blockchain and quantum computing in defense. In Sustainable Security Practices Using Blockchain, Quantum and Post-Quantum Technologies for Real Time Applications (pp. 125-153). Springer Nature Singapore.

Akhai, S., Singh, V. P., & John, S. (2016). Human performance in industrial design centers with small unit air conditioning systems. *Journal of Advanced Research in Production Industrial Engineering*, *3*(2), 5–11.

Akhai, S., & Wadhwa, A. S. (2024). Wireless networking solutions for climate control and comfort in modern air conditioning systems. In *Intelligent Networks* (pp. 165–181). CRC Press. DOI: 10.1201/9781003541363-11

Anwar, A., Rehman, I. U., & Husamaldin, L. (2022, September). Smart education for people with disabilities (pwds): Conceptual framework for pwds emotions classification from student utterances (sus) during online learning. In 2022 IEEE International Smart Cities Conference (ISC2) (pp. 1-7). IEEE.

Chen, Y., Patel, R., & Lee, S. (2021). Building trust through inclusive design in assistive technologies. *International Journal of Inclusive Computing*, *12*(3), 150–165.

Crenshaw, K. (1989). Demarginalizing the intersection of race and sex: A black feminist critique of antidiscrimination doctrine, feminist theory and antiracist politics. *University of Chicago Legal Forum, 1989*(1), 139–167.

D'Silva, J., & Kaur, M. (2020). Privacy concerns in smart home environments: A review. *Journal of Cybersecurity and Privacy*, *2*(1), 1–18.

Ellis, K., Goggin, G., Haller, B. A., & Curtis, R. (Eds.). (2020). *The Routledge companion to disability and media* (p. 387). Routledge.

Fairchild, A., & Stuerzlinger, W. (2020). Designing smart home interfaces for visually impaired users. *Proceedings of the ACM on Interactive, Mobile, Wearable and Ubiquitous Technologies*, *4*(1), 1–22. PMID: 35846237

Gray, M., & Cyan, L. (2022). Ethical guidelines for assistive smart technologies: Inclusion and accountability. *Ethics in Technology*, *5*(2), 89–107.

Karki, N., Anwar, A., Rehman, I. U., Husamaldin, L., & Saadati, P. (2023, September). Smart Attendance Monitoring System Using Face Recognition for People with Disabilities (PwDs). In 2023 IEEE International Smart Cities Conference (ISC2) (pp. 1-7). IEEE.

Kulyk, O., & Gajos, K. Z. (2021). Enhancing accessibility and privacy in smart home devices for people with disabilities. *ACM Transactions on Accessible Computing*, *14*(4), 1–29.

Lazar, J., & Greenidge, K. D. (2020). Designing accessible voice interfaces for people with visual impairments. *Journal of Accessibility and Design for All*, *10*(1), 1–21.

Lee, S., & Dey, A. K. (2020). Using smart glasses to assist visually impaired people in indoor navigation. *IEEE Pervasive Computing*, *19*(3), 54–63.

Li, Y., & Ma, X. (2020). Privacy-preserving techniques for smart home IoT devices: A survey. *IEEE Internet of Things Journal*, *7*(7), 5986–6003.

Mala, S., Deep, U., Mala, E., & Akhai, S. (2025). Digital Health Technologies for Preventive Cardiology. In Impact of Digital Solutions for Improved Healthcare Delivery (pp. 379-400). IGI Global.

Mavroudis, V., & Gritzalis, S. (2019). Security and privacy challenges in smart homes for vulnerable users. *Computers & Security*, *85*, 1–14.

Mohanty, C. T. (2003). *Feminism without borders: Decolonizing theory, practicing solidarity*. Duke University Press.

Oladimeji, A., & Lee, S. (2021). Trust models for assistive smart systems: A systematic review. *Journal of Assistive Technologies*, *15*(4), 263–279.

Park, J., & Kim, S. (2023). AI-based privacy enhancement for assistive smart devices in home environments. *Sensors (Basel)*, *23*(4), 1789. PMID: 36850386

Shakespeare, T. (2017). *Disability: The basics*. Routledge. DOI: 10.4324/9781315624839

Smith, A., & Johnson, T. (2022). Accessibility and security considerations in smart home systems for visually impaired users. *Journal of Human-Computer Interaction*, *38*(5), 412–431.

. United Nations. General Assembly. (2007). Convention on the rights of persons with disabilities and optional protocol. UN.

Verma, R., Akhai, S., & Wadhwa, A. S. (2024). Use of smart materials in physiotherapy. In *Revolutionizing healthcare treatment with sensor technology* (pp. 300–319). IGI Global. DOI: 10.4018/979-8-3693-2762-3.ch019

Wang, L., & Zhang, Y. (2024). Trust and privacy in IoT-enabled assistive technologies: A user-centered approach. *IEEE Transactions on Human-Machine Systems*, *54*(1), 45–56.

Zhao, X., & Liu, H. (2021). Secure data sharing and privacy protection in smart healthcare and assistive devices. *IEEE Access : Practical Innovations, Open Solutions*, *9*, 123456–123468.

Chapter 10

Adaptive Materials for Transformative Rehabilitation

Rajni Verma
https://orcid.org/0000-0001-7904-0440
CGC University, Mohali, India

Mahapara Abbass
https://orcid.org/0000-0002-0838-2598
MMEC, Maharishi Markandeshwar University, Mullana, India

Amandeep Singh Wadhwa
https://orcid.org/0000-0002-7480-9254
University Institute of Engineering and Technology, Panjab University, Chandigarh, India

Shalom Akhai
https://orcid.org/0000-0002-7533-457X
MMEC, Maharishi Markandeshwar University, Mullana, India

ABSTRACT

This chapter examines how smart materials are driving a paradigm shift in disability rehabilitation, offering groundbreaking solutions to restore mobility, independence, and dignity. By leveraging responsive technologies like shape-memory alloys, electroactive polymers, and piezoelectric sensors, smart materials enable adaptive, personalized therapies that address the unique challenges faced by individuals with physical, sensory, or neurological disabilities. The chapter highlights real-world applications—from AI-powered prosthetics to self-adjusting exoskeletons—while

DOI: 10.4018/979-8-3373-2033-5.ch010

addressing barriers like cost and accessibility. It concludes with a vision for an inclusive future where smart materials erase limitations and redefine what's possible in rehabilitation.

1. INTRODUCTION: THE NEW ERA OF DISABILITY REHABILITATION

The field of disability rehabilitation is undergoing a extreme transformation, due to the advent of smart materials(Benouhiba et al., 2025). These innovative materials have the ability to sense, adapt, and respond in real time, revolutionizing rehabilitation approaches(Sali, Chai, & Ganesan, 2025). Traditional methods often fail to address the dynamic needs of individuals with disabilities, but smart materials are changing this narrative(Oro, 2025). For example, shape-memory alloys used in spinal braces can adjust their support as a patient progress, while electroactive polymers enable prosthetics to "learn" and adapt to grip patterns for amputees(Gherman et al., 2025). This technology is not just about creating better devices—it's about empowering individuals to reclaim their autonomy and live more independently.

- **Enhancing Adaptability -** One of the key features that make smart materials revolutionary is their responsiveness. These materials react to physiological cues such as temperature, pressure, and muscle activity, allowing prosthetics and orthotics to adjust themselves in real time based on the user's needs(Kantaros, Petrescu, &Ganetsos, 2025).For instance, a prosthetic limb made with smart materials can detect when the user is walking uphill and automatically adjust its stiffness to provide better support(Tabucol et al., 2025). This real-time adaptation is crucial for dynamic therapy, enabling individuals to participate in activities that were previously challenging or impossible(Zaydi, Maleh, &Khourdifi, 2025).
- **Personalization (Responsiveness): Tailoring Rehabilitation to Individual Needs -** Another major advantage of smart materials is their ability to provide personalized interventions. Traditional rehabilitation devices are often mass-produced with standard sizes and settings, which may not accommodate an individual's unique needs(Giansanti, 2025).Smart materials, however, can be customized to fit specific disabilities. For example, orthotic devices for children with cerebral palsy can have adjustable stiffness, allowing them to adapt as the child grows or as their condition evolves(Zawar et al., 2024). This level of personalization ensures that rehabilitation devices offer the most effective support possible, enhancing long-term outcomes(Abbas &Zlopasa, 2025).

- **Predictive and Preventive Care (AI Integration) -** The integration of smart materials with artificial intelligence (AI) amplifies their potential. AI-driven systems can analyze data from embedded sensors to predict and prevent complications(Ficili et al., 2025).For example, in individuals with multiple sclerosis, AI can anticipate muscle spasms and trigger preventive adjustments in a prosthetic or orthotic device, reducing discomfort and preventing injury. This predictive capability not only improves rehabilitation effectiveness but also enhances the user's overall quality of life (King & Colla, 2025; Zhang, 2025; Mala et al., 2025).).
- **Addressing Accessibility and Affordability -** The need for innovation in disability rehabilitation is more pressing than ever, with over 1 billion people worldwide living with disabilities(Bruce & Williams, 2025). Many lack access to advanced care, as traditional rehabilitation methods require extensive resources and specialized facilities that are often unavailable in low-income regions(Dereje et al., 2025). Smart materials bridge this gap by offering scalable, non-invasive solutions that integrate seamlessly into daily life. Advanced manufacturing techniques, such as 3D printing, enable the rapid and cost-effective production of customized prosthetics and orthotics(Shanmugam, 2025; Khang & Akhai, 2024). A prosthetic limb that traditionally costs thousands of dollars can now be produced for a fraction of the price, making assistive technologies more accessible to those who need them most(-Jamieson & Wijesundara, 2025; Akhai & Khang, 2024; Akhai & Wadhwa, 2024).
- **Reducing Abandonment Rates -** Another challenge with traditional rehabilitation devices is their high abandonment rate—studies indicate that 30% to 50% of users stop using prosthetics or orthotics due to poor fit or lack of functionality(Patricks et al., 2025).

Smart materials thus help solve this problem by being adaptable and responsive, ensuring that devices remain comfortable and effective over time.

1.1 What Makes Smart Materials Revolutionary?

Smart materials are transforming rehabilitation by introducing dynamic, adaptive, and personalized solutions(Sood, Lamba, & Singh, 2025). Unlike traditional materials, which are static and limited in functionality, smart materials can sense, respond, and adapt to changes in their environment or the user's condition(Enyan et al., 2025). This responsiveness is a game-changer for assistive technologies such as prosthetics, orthotics, and wearable rehabilitation devices(Waidi, 2025).One of their most remarkable features is the ability to react to physiological cues like temperature, pressure, or muscle activity(Kumar & Ranjan, 2025). For instance, artificial muscles made from smart materials mimic natural human movement without requiring heavy external components, making them ideal for wearable rehabilitation robots(Dewang et al., 2025; Akhai et al., 2025). These devices adjust in real time to the user's needs, enhancing mobility and functionality(Sharma et al., 2025). Personalization is another breakthrough. Rehabilitation devices made from smart materials can be tailored to individual needs. For example, orthotics for children with cerebral palsy can feature adjustable stiffness that adapts as the child grows or their condition evolves, ensuring long-term effectiveness and comfort(Gongor&Tutsoy, 2025).The integration of artificial intelligence (AI) further enhances smart materials. **Figure 1** hints the modern technologies application in healthcare. AI-driven sensors can predict and respond to issues before they arise. In individuals with multiple sclerosis, for example, AI can detect early signs of muscle spasms and adjust the device to prevent discomfort or injury. This predictive capability not only improves rehabilitation but also enhances overall quality of life(Chrysanthakopoulou&Koutsojannis, 2025).Additionally, smart materials enable continuous real-time monitoring during daily activities. Wearable devices track movements, posture, and other health metrics, providing valuable insights to clinicians(Mathunjwa et al., 2025). Motion sensors combined with wearable cameras can assess rehabilitation exercises with high accuracy, offering immediate feedback for posture correction and movement refinement(Han, Guffanti, &Brunete, 2025).

Figure 1. Modern technologies integration in healthcare.

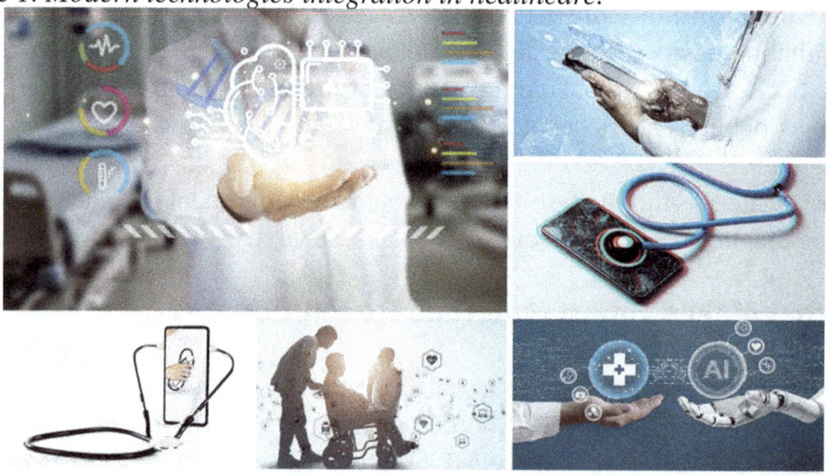

Key Advantages of Smart Materials in Rehabilitation include:

- **Responsiveness:** Adapts to real-time physiological changes for better support.
- **Personalization:** Custom-fits rehabilitation devices to individual needs.
- **AI Integration:** Predicts and prevents complications before they occur.
- **Continuous Monitoring:** Tracks user progress to refine therapy strategies.

In summary, smart materials revolutionize rehabilitation by delivering adaptive, personalized, and data-driven solutions. They integrate seamlessly into daily life, ensuring greater independence and a more effective rehabilitation experience(Y-ihun& Delgado, 2025).

1.2 The Imperative for Innovation in Disability Rehabilitation

Globally, over millions live with disabilities, yet many lack access to advanced rehabilitation due to high costs, limited facilities, and inadequate technology. This gap underscores the urgent need for affordable, scalable, and effective solutions, an area where smart materials have immense potential. Traditional assistive technologies face significant limitations. They are often expensive, rely on outdated manufacturing methods, and are frequently abandoned due to poor fit or discomfort(Rezaei, 2025). Smart materials address these challenges through adaptability, affordability, and enhanced usability(Karim et al., 2024). One of their most significant advantages is scalability. Advanced manufacturing techniques like 3D printing enable the rapid, cost-effective production of customized prosthetics and orthotics (Akhai 2023; Akhai 2024). A traditionally expensive prosthetic limb, for instance, can now be produced for a fraction of the cost using smart polymers(Borthakur, 2025). This breakthrough expands access to assistive technologies, particularly in low-income regions(Danemayer et al., 2023). Smart materials also enhance usability by evolving alongside the user's needs. Devices made from these materials can adjust their shape, stiffness, or functionality in response to changes in the user's condition or activity level(Pan et al., 2022). For example, shape-memory alloy spinal braces dynamically alter support levels based on whether the user is sitting or standing, ensuring long-term comfort and effectiveness (Muñoz Ruiz, 2024).Smart materials also enable remoterehabilitation, reducing the need for frequent clinic visitsas shown in **Figure 2**. Cloud-connected devices equipped with smart sensors can transmit real-time data to clinicians, allowing for adjustments without in-person consultations. This is particularly beneficial for users in remote areas or those with mobility challenges, ensuring consistent care without the logistical burden of travel(Ullah et al., 2023; Gao et al., 2021).Additionally, wearable rehabilitation devices incorporating AI and machine learning allow users to perform therapeutic exercises at home while receiving real-time feedback(Aziz et al., 2024). Soft wearable robots equipped with artificial muscles, for example, assist with movement therapy, providing ongoing support throughout daily activities(Gonzalez-Vazquez et al., 2023).

Figure 2. Remote monitoring of health via smart technologies and AI.

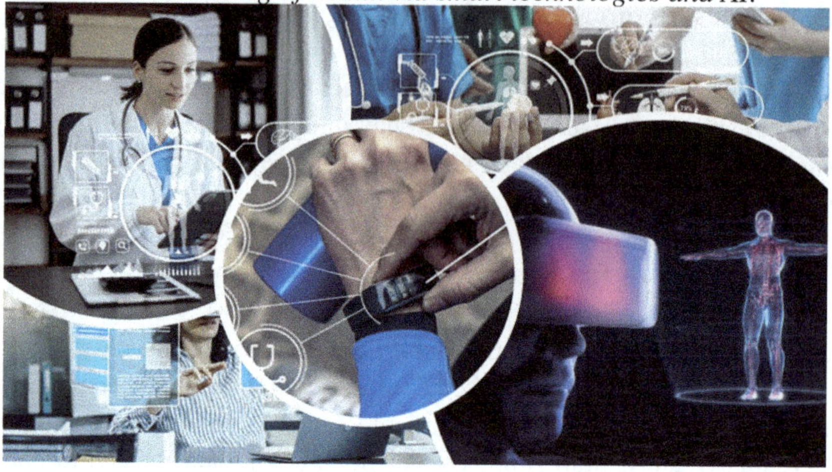

Emerging Technologies (VR & AR in Rehabilitation) - The integration of **virtual reality (VR) and augmented reality (AR)** with smart materials is further revolutionizing rehabilitation(Zhang et al., 2022):

- **VR** creates immersive environments where users can practice walking or object manipulation in a safe, controlled setting(Bagher et al., 2021).
- **AR** provides real-time visual cues for **posture correction and movement guidance** during therapy sessions(Theodorikakos, 2023).

Figure 3. Virtual reality applications for diagnose.

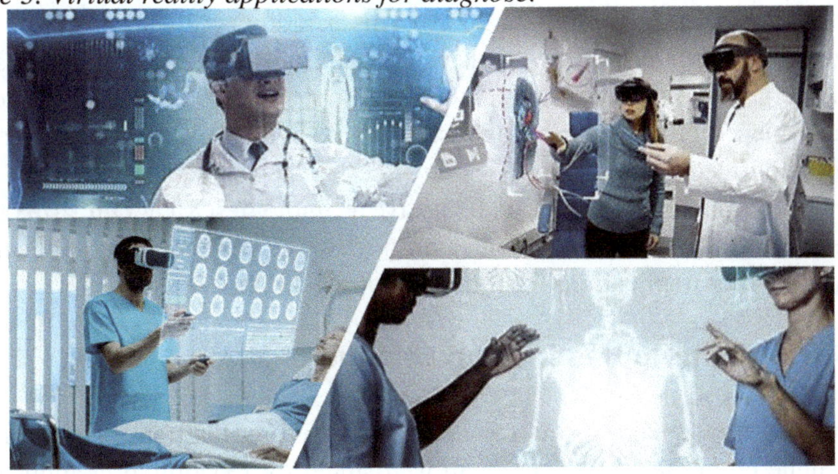

These technologies make rehabilitation more engaging and effective while fostering greater independence(Aderinto et al., 2023).Beyond individual users, smart materials are shaping the future of healthcare delivery. With aging populations and rising disability rates due to conditions like diabetes and stroke, healthcare systems face increasing pressure to provide efficient and cost-effective care(Coman et al., 2024). Smart materials enable decentralized rehabilitation, allowing individuals to manage their therapy independently at home, reducing healthcare burdens(Ahmad et al., 2022).

Overall, innovation in disability rehabilitation is no longer an option—it is an urgent necessity. Smart materials bridge critical gaps in accessibility, affordability, and effectiveness, providing adaptable solutions that empower individuals to reclaim autonomy(Rao & Nasir, 2024). By integrating advanced manufacturing, AI, and immersive technologies, we are shaping a future where everyone has access to high-quality rehabilitation, regardless of their circumstances as presented in **Figure 3**.

2. SMART MATERIALS: REDEFINING REHABILITATION PARADIGMS

The integration of smart materials in rehabilitation technologies is transforming the landscape of assistive healthcare(Zhang et al., 2024). Unlike traditional rehabilitation tools, which remain static in their functionality, smart materials introduce adaptive, responsive, and real-time adjusting systems that improve patient recovery and enhance the quality of life(Trovato et al., 2022). By responding to physiological and environmental cues, these materials enable rehabilitation devices to evolve alongside the user's progress, offering a personalized, efficient, and accessible approach to therapy(Kumar et al., 2023). This paradigm shift in rehabilitation is particularly significant for individuals with disabilities, post-surgical patients, and those undergoing long-term physical therapy(Lippi et al., 2023). With advances in materials science, bioengineering, and artificial intelligence (AI), smart materials are no longer confined to theoretical research—they are now actively shaping prosthetics, orthotics, wearable robotics, and assistive technologies(Xu & Qin, 2023). This chapter explores the core technologies driving this revolution, their applications, and their broader implications for the future of rehabilitation.

2.1 Core Technologies Driving Change

Several groundbreaking smart materials are driving this transformation, each with unique properties that make them well-suited for rehabilitation applications (Yang et al., 2024). These materials interact with external stimuli such as heat, pressure, electric fields, or biochemical signals, enabling assistive devices to provide dynamic, real-time support (Zarei et al., 2023). These technologies along with optimisations enhance the capabilities of engineered materials (Kumar, Wadhwa, Akhai, & Kaushik, 2024; Akhai, Srivastava, Sharma, & Bhatia, 2021; Akhai, Singh, & John, 2016; Kumar & Akhai, 2022; Kanda, Akhai, & Bansal, 2013). Some key smart materials and their transformative roles in rehabilitation are discussed below and detailed in **Table 1**:

- **Shape-Memory Alloys (SMAs):** Shape-memory alloys are metals that “remember” their original shape and can return to it when exposed to specific stimuli like heat (Behera & Behera, 2022). In rehabilitation, SMAs are used in spinal injury exoskeletons. These exoskeletons adjust their support dynamically as the user’s muscle strength improves during recovery(Urrea & Agramonte, 2023). For example, as a patient regains mobility, the exoskeleton reduces its stiffness, allowing for greater freedom of movement while still providing necessary support.
- **Electroactive Polymers (EAPs):** Electroactive polymers are flexible materials that change shape or size when an electric field is applied. They are widely used in bionic hands for amputees, where they mimic natural grip patterns through responsive finger actuators. This technology allows users to perform delicate tasks like holding a cup or typing on a keyboard with precision, making prosthetics feel more lifelike and functional (Ornaghi Jr et al., 2023).
- **Piezoelectric Sensors:** These sensors generate electrical signals when subjected to mechanical stress(Liu et al., 2022). In Parkinson’s tremor-monitoring wearables, piezoelectric sensors provide real-time data on tremor intensity

and frequency. This information helps optimize medication dosages and timing, ensuring better management of symptoms and improving the patient's daily functioning (Ukasi et al., 2024; singh and Akhai 2024).

- **Thermoresponsive Gels:** Thermoresponsive gels react to changes in temperature by altering their properties. In burn rehabilitation dressings, these gels release painkillers or anti-inflammatory drugs when they detect inflammation or elevated skin temperature. This targeted drug delivery reduces pain and accelerates healing while minimizing side effects associated with systemic medication (Al-Musawi et al., 2024; Singh and Akhai 2025; Akhai 2023).

These technologies demonstrate how smart materials can be tailored to address specific disabilities effectively, offering solutions that adapt to individual needs and conditions.

Table 1. Smart materials potential applications in rehabilitation and their impacts.

Smart Material	Description	Applications	Impact on Rehabilitation
Shape-Memory Alloys (SMAs)	Metals that "remember" their original shape and return to it when exposed to heat or electric current.	**Spinal Injury Exoskeletons**: Dynamically adjust support based on recovery progress, preventing muscle atrophy. **Adjustable Orthotic Braces**: Automatically modify stiffness for cerebral palsy or post-stroke patients, improving comfort and effectiveness.	**Personalization of Rehabilitation Devices**: Adapts in real time to the patient's physiology for better fit, comfort, and efficiency. **Enabling At-Home Rehabilitation**: Reduces need for clinical interventions, allowing continuous therapy at home.
Electroactive Polymers (EAPs)	Flexible materials that change shape or size under an electric field, mimicking muscle contractions.	**Next-Generation Bionic Hands**: Enable precise, lifelike movements in prosthetics. **Soft Robotic Rehabilitation Gloves**: Assist stroke patients in hand mobility exercises by reinforcing motor learning.	**AI-Driven Insights for Faster Recovery**: Enhances real-time therapy adjustments based on patient progress. **Cost-Effectiveness and Scalability**: Lightweight, flexible, and more affordable than traditional mechanical actuators.
Piezoelectric Sensors	Generate electric charge when subjected to mechanical stress, used for motion monitoring and real-time feedback.	**Parkinson's Tremor Monitoring**: Tracks tremor intensity, aiding medication adjustments. **Real-Time Gait Analysis**: Detects irregular walking patterns and provides haptic feedback for stroke patients.	**Personalization of Rehabilitation Devices**: Enables real-time monitoring and automatic therapy adjustments. **AI-Driven Insights for Faster Recovery**: Collects motion data for analysis, improving treatment precision.
Thermoresponsive Gels	Change properties based on temperature variations, useful in pain management and wound healing.	**Smart Burn Dressings**: Release drugs and adjust permeability based on skin temperature. **Heat-Responsive Compression Garments**: Provide pressure and heat therapy for pain relief.	**Enabling At-Home Rehabilitation**: Self-regulating materials provide automated pain relief and wound care without constant manual adjustments. **Cost-Effectiveness and Scalability**: Reduces dependency on frequent medical interventions, making therapy more accessible.

Overall, smart materials are ushering in a new era of rehabilitation, making assistive devices intelligent, adaptable, and personalized. From shape-memory exoskeletons to electroactive prosthetics, these technologies are breaking barriers in accessibility, efficiency, and effectiveness. As advancements in AI, bioengineering, and material science continue, smart materials will play an even greater role in shaping a future where rehabilitation is not just reactive—but proactive, predictive, and fully integrated into daily life(Dong et al., 2024; Sharma et al., 2023).

2.2 Bridging Gaps in Neurorehabilitation

Neurorehabilitation focuses on restoring function for individuals with neurological disorders or injuries such as strokes or spinal cord damage(Sharma et al., 2023). Smart materials play a pivotal role in bridging gaps in care by offering innovative solutions that enhance recovery outcomes(Farham & Baltazar, 2024).

- **Stroke Recovery** - Electroactive polymer-based gloves have emerged as a promising tool for stroke recovery. These gloves stimulate paralyzed hands using electrical impulses, encouraging muscle activation and improving motor control over time(Ghevondyan et al., 2025). Unlike traditional therapy methods that rely on manual exercises, these gloves provide consistent stimulation tailored to the user's progress, making rehabilitation more effective(Saldarriaga et al., 2024).
- **Spinal Cord Injuries** - For individuals with spinal cord injuries, exoskeletons equipped with shape-memory alloys offer adaptive support tailored to walking terrains such as stairs or flat ground(Zhou, 2024). These exoskeletons adjust their stiffness and flexibility based on the environment, enabling users to navigate diverse surfaces safely and confidently. This adaptability not only aids physical recovery but also empowers users to engage in daily activities independently(Enyan et al., 2025).

2.3 The Transformative Impact of Smart Materials

The integration of smart materials into rehabilitation devices has far-reaching implications for accessibility and efficiency:

- **Personalized Recovery** - Smart materials enable devices to adapt dynamically to individual needs, ensuring that rehabilitation is tailored to each user's condition and progress(Kantaros&Ganetsos, 2023). For instance, wearable robots with artificial muscles adjust their force output based on the user's activity level, providing optimal support during therapy sessions(Akbari et al., 2021).
- **Enhanced Accessibility** - Advanced manufacturing techniques like 3D printing make it possible to produce affordable prosthetics and orthotics using smart polymers. This reduces costs significantly compared to traditional

methods, making assistive technologies accessible to underserved populations worldwide(Pathak et al., 2023).

- **Real-Time Monitoring -** Wearable devices equipped with sensors provide continuous feedback during daily activities. For example, wearable cameras combined with motion sensors can classify rehabilitation exercises with high accuracy, offering immediate posture corrections during therapy(Huang et al., 2023).
- **Remote Rehabilitation -** Cloud-connected platforms allow clinicians to monitor patients remotely and make adjustments in real-time without requiring frequent clinic visits. This is particularly beneficial for individuals living in remote areas or those with mobility challenges(Dabla et al., 2021).

2.4 Future Directions

As smart materials continue to evolve, their applications in rehabilitation are expected to expand further:

- **Integration with Virtual Reality (VR) and Augmented Reality (AR):** VR environments can simulate real-world scenarios for practicing motor skills safely, while AR systems provide visual cues for correcting posture or movement during therapy(Cerritelli et al., 2021).
- **Nanotechnology:** Researchers are exploring nanomaterials for creating prosthetic limbs capable of mimicking sensory feedback like touch or temperature changes(Varaganti& Seo, 2024).
- **Soft Wearable Robots:** Artificial muscles made from smart materials are being developed for lightweight wearable robots that can assist users in performing therapeutic exercises at home(Pan et al., 2022).

In conclusion, smart materials are redefining rehabilitation paradigms by introducing intelligent systems that adapt dynamically to user needs while enhancing accessibility and personalization. Their transformative impact is paving the way for more inclusive and effective care models that empower individuals to reclaim autonomy and improve their quality of life.

3. REVOLUTIONARY APPLICATIONS IN DISABILITY CARE

The advancements in technology for disability care are groundbreaking and transformative. Innovations in mobility restoration, sensory and cognitive rehabilitation, and chronic pain management are enhancing the quality of life for individuals with disabilities(Jimbu et al., 2024). Smart prosthetics utilizing piezoelectric technology and AI-driven exoskeletons represent significant strides in mobility restoration(-Mikołajewska et al., 2025; Verma et al., 2024). Enhancements in sensory and cognitive rehabilitation are made possible with haptic feedback gloves and augmented reality combined with smart textiles, offering innovative solutions for individuals with sensory impairments(Irigoyen et al., 2024). Chronic pain and comorbidity management see advancements through drug-eluting smart patches and dynamic compression wear, which provide targeted therapies for various conditions(Gallagher et al., 2024). This text reviews these revolutionary applications and demonstrates the ways in which technology is aiding individuals who face physical disabilities. **Table 2** showcases innovative technologies transforming disability care, including advanced assistive technologies for mobility and rehabilitation, cutting-edge solutions in disability care and management, and revolutionary assistive devices.

Table 2. Advanced Assistive Technologies for Mobility and Rehabilitation.

Technology	*Functionality*	*Key Benefits*	*Applications*
Smart Prosthetics (Piezoelectric-powered damping)	Adjusts damping in real-time based on gait analysis.	Improves stability, reduces falls by 60%, and enhances natural movement.	Used by below-knee amputees for better mobility and balance.
AI-Driven Exoskeletons (MR Fluid-based adaptive support)	Stiffens dynamically based on movement needs, providing support during activities like stair climbing.	Enhances mobility, promotes independence, and reduces physical strain.	Assists spinal injury patients and individuals with limited lower-body strength.
Haptic Feedback Gloves (Piezoelectric materials for sensory rehabilitation)	Simulates touch and enhances sensory feedback for users with neuropathy or reduced sensation.	Restores tactile perception, improves grip control, and enables independent object handling.	Beneficial for diabetic neuropathy patients and individuals with sensory impairments.
Augmented Reality (AR) + Smart Textiles (Thermoresponsive sleeves for visually impaired users)	Uses temperature-sensitive materials to provide tactile navigation cues.	Enhances spatial awareness, improves navigation, and increases independence.	Supports visually impaired individuals in navigating environments safely.
Drug-Eluting Smart Patches (Automated medication release for cerebral palsy patients)	Releases medication at controlled intervals without manual intervention.	Ensures timely drug delivery, reduces spastic episodes, and improves treatment adherence.	Used in managing cerebral palsy and other conditions requiring consistent medication.
Dynamic Compression Wear (MR Fluid-based sleeves for lymphedema management)	Provides adaptive compression that adjusts based on the patient's real-time needs.	Reduces edema, improves circulation, and enhances patient comfort.	Helps lymphedema patients and individuals needing compression therapy.

3.1 Advanced Prosthetics, Exoskeletons, and Sensory Aids

- **Smart Prosthetics:** A piezoelectric-powered prosthetic reduces falls by 60% for below-knee amputees.
- **AI-Driven Exoskeletons:** Exoskeletons employ MR fluids to enhance mobility during stair climbing for spinal injury patients.
- **Haptic Feedback Gloves:** These gloves employ piezoelectric materials to bring tactile sensations to diabetic neuropathy patients.
- **Augmented Reality + Smart Textiles:**Thermoresponsive sleeves help visually impaired individuals navigate using tactile cues.
- **Drug-Eluting Smart Patches:** These patches deliver medication for cerebral palsy automatically, improving pain management.
- **Dynamic Compression Wear:** MR fluid-based sleeves help reduce edema in patients with lymphedema.

Thus, the overall Impact of such Innovations across multiple areas of disability care are leading to improved patient outcomes.

3.2 Advancements in Sensory Feedback and Rehabilitation

- **Impact on Mobility:** The integration of smart prosthetics represents a paradigm shift in mobility aids(Tan et al., 2022). The use of piezoelectric technology allows for a more natural gait by adjusting damping according to gait analysis. This not only provides comfort but significantly reduces falls, which is crucial for safety and independence among amputees(Bhat et al., 2023). The highlighted case study demonstrates a 60% reduction in falls, showing the effectiveness of this technology in real-world applications.
- **Exoskeleton Innovations:** AI-driven exoskeletons that utilize magnetorheological (MR) fluids provide adaptive support for users, enhancing their ability to navigate challenging environments, such as climbing stairs(Dostalova et al., 2022). This is especially beneficial for spinal injury patients, who otherwise might face mobility restrictions. By stiffening in response to movements, these exoskeletons offer vital support when needed, ultimately promoting autonomy(Siviy et al., 2023).
- **Sensory Feedback Advancements:** Haptic feedback gloves are a significant breakthrough for patients with diabetic neuropathy, a condition that often impairs sensation in the hands. The integration of piezoelectric materials allows these gloves to simulate touch, providing users with the ability to engage more fully with their environment(Nisky& Makin, 2024). This sensory res-

toration could improve the overall quality of life, making daily tasks feasible and less frustrating for those who previously struggled.

- **Augmenting Reality for Orientation:** Augmented Reality (AR) combined with smart textiles offers a unique approach to assist the visually impaired. The use of thermoresponsive sleeves, which provide tactile cues, represents an innovative method to improve navigation. By converting visual information into tactile signals, this technology paves the way for greater independence and confidence in mobility(Cerritelli et al., 2021; Varaganti& Seo, 2024)
- **Targeted Medication Delivery:** Drug-eluting smart patches present a frontier in chronic pain management by allowing for controlled, automated delivery of medications. For patients with cerebral palsy and other similar conditions, this technology ensures that medication is available when needed without the hassle of manual dosing, leading to better adherence and improved overall health management(Gallagher et al., 2024).
- **Weight Distribution and Edema Management:** Dynamic compression wear using MR fluids helps manage conditions like lymphedema by providing compressive support that adapitates to the body's need. This innovative solution reduces edema more effectively than traditional methods, contributing positively to the patient's comfort and mobility(Jiralerspong& Zhao, 2024). Advocates for smart textile technology suggest that such advances may also improve accessibility for individuals suffering from chronic pain-related conditions.
- **Comprehensive Impact on Disability Care:** Collectively, these revolutionary applications highlight the potential of technology to redefine disability care(Thacharodi et al., 2024). By addressing mobility, sensory processing, and chronic pain management, these innovations not only improve the functional capabilities of individuals with disabilities but also enhance their psychological wellbeing by promoting independence and enhancing quality of life(Thakur et al., 2024). The forward momentum of these technologies indicates an exciting future where disability care is increasingly effective and holistic.

In conclusion, the applications mentioned demonstrate the crucial impact that innovative technologies have on transforming disability care(Willingham et al., 2024). Each advancement not only caters to specific issues faced by individuals with disabilities but collectively indicates a promising trend towards inclusive health solutions that could redefine healthcare standards. Through personalized treatment and robust support systems facilitated by these technological advances, we can expect a significant enhancement in the lives of individuals living with disabilities.

4. ADVANTAGES VS. CHALLENGES IN REVOLUTIONARY ADOPTION

The adoption of revolutionary technologies in healthcare, particularly those designed to assist individuals with disabilities or chronic conditions, offers transformative benefits while presenting significant challenges(Rony et al., 2024). This section delves into the advantages and barriers associated with these innovations, focusing on precision, independence, cost-efficiency, high initial costs, durability, and ethical risks(Kocaaslan, 2024). **Table 3** provides a comprehensive analysis of revolutionary assistive technologies, their advantages and challenges, their potential solutions, and their impact on disability care. It also evaluates the functionality, impact, and implementation challenges of these technologies, and discusses opportunities, barriers, and adoption strategies for next-generation assistive devices.

4.1 Transformative Benefits

Revolutionary technologies offer transformative benefits such as precision in diagnosis and treatment, promoting independence for individuals with mobility challenges, and cost-efficiency over time(Singh & Nayyar, 2024). Piezoelectric sensors detect micro-tremors, allowing for personalized treatment plans(Azzi et al., 2025). Self-adjusting wheelchairs equipped with shape memory alloys enable users to navigate challenging environments autonomously(Yin et al., 2024). 3D-printed smart orthotics for children reduce costs and make advanced care more accessible, especially in low- and middle-income regions(Abbady et al., 2022).

4.1.1 Precision: Enhancing Early Detection and Intervention

One of the most profound advantages of revolutionary technologies is their ability to deliver unparalleled precision in diagnosis and treatment(El-Tanani et al., 2025). For instance, piezoelectric sensors have emerged as a game-changer in the management of Parkinson's disease. These sensors are capable of detecting micro-tremors—subtle, involuntary movements that often precede more pronounced symptoms of the disease. By identifying these early signs, healthcare providers can intervene sooner, potentially slowing the progression of the disease and improving the quality of life for patients. The precision of such technologies also allows for personalized treatment plans, tailoring interventions to the unique needs of each individual. This level of accuracy is particularly critical in neurodegenerative diseases, where early detection can significantly alter the disease trajectory.

4.1.2 Independence: Empowering Individuals with Mobility Challenges

Another transformative benefit of these technologies is the promotion of independence for individuals with mobility impairments. Self-adjusting wheelchairs equipped with shape memory alloys (SMAs) exemplify this advancement. SMAs are materials that can "remember" their original shape and return to it after deformation, enabling the wheelchair to adapt to uneven terrain autonomously(Pierzchlewicz et al., 2021). This innovation allows users to navigate challenging environments—such as gravel paths, steep inclines, or uneven sidewalks—without requiring external assistance. For individuals with limited mobility, this technology not only enhances their ability to move freely but also fosters a sense of autonomy and dignity. By reducing reliance on caregivers, these wheelchairs empower users to engage more fully in their communities and daily activities.

4.1.3 Cost-Efficiency Over Time: Reducing Long-Term Expenses

While the initial investment in revolutionary technologies can be substantial, they often prove cost-efficient in the long run. A prime example is the use of 3D-printed smart orthotics for children. Traditional orthotics can be expensive and require frequent replacements as children grow. In contrast, 3D-printed orthotics can be customized and rapidly produced, significantly reducing costs. Moreover, the adaptability of these devices ensures they remain effective even as a child's body changes, minimizing the need for repeated purchases. This cost-efficiency is particularly beneficial for families in low- and middle-income regions, where access to affordable healthcare solutions is often limited. Over time, the savings generated by such technologies can alleviate financial burdens and make advanced care more accessible.

4.2 Barriers to Overcome

High initial costs of innovative technologies like electroactive polymers (EAPs) and wearable devices for ALS patients pose barriers to widespread adoption(Sarker et al., 2025). These technologies are expensive and require scalable manufacturing processes and funding to subsidize underserved populations. To ensure durability, wearables must be ruggedized and tested rigorously. Ethical risks, such as algorithmic bias, must be addressed by prioritizing diversity, inclusivity, and involving disabled individuals in design and testing(Hanna et al., 2024).

4.2.1 High Initial Costs: A Barrier to Accessibility

Despite their long-term benefits, the high initial costs of revolutionary technologies pose a significant barrier to their widespread adoption. Prosthetics incorporating electroactive polymers (EAPs) illustrate this challenge. EAPs are materials that change shape or size in response to electrical stimuli, enabling prosthetics to mimic natural movements more closely(Jyothish & Mishra, 2024). However, the sophisticated materials and engineering required to produce these devices make them prohibitively expensive for many individuals, particularly in low-income regions. This disparity in access exacerbates existing inequalities, leaving those who could benefit most from such innovations unable to afford them. Addressing this issue requires concerted efforts to reduce production costs, develop scalable manufacturing processes, and establish funding mechanisms to subsidize these technologies for underserved populations.

4.2.2 Durability in Daily Use: Ensuring Reliability in Real-World Conditions

Another critical challenge is ensuring the durability of these technologies in real-world conditions. Wearable devices designed for patients with amyotrophic lateral sclerosis (ALS), for example, must withstand the rigors of daily use, including exposure to sweat, moisture, and physical wear and tear(Sheffield et al., 2025). Many current wearables are not adequately ruggedized, leading to frequent malfunctions or breakdowns that compromise their effectiveness(Al Khatib et al., 2024). For individuals with ALS, who rely on these devices for communication, mobility, and other essential functions, such failures can have severe consequences. To overcome this barrier, manufacturers must prioritize the development of robust, sweat-resistant designs that can endure the demands of daily life. This may involve the use of advanced materials, improved sealing techniques, and rigorous testing protocols to ensure reliability(Singh et al., 2024).

4.2.3 Ethical Risks: Addressing Algorithmic Bias in AI-Driven Devices

As artificial intelligence (AI) becomes increasingly integrated into healthcare technologies, ethical risks—particularly algorithmic bias—must be addressed(Hanna et al., 2024). AI-driven devices, such as those used for speech recognition or decision-making support, are trained on datasets that may not adequately represent diverse disability populations(Patel et al., 2025). This can result in biased algorithms that fail to perform equitably across different demographics. For example, a speech recognition system trained primarily on data from non-disabled individuals may struggle to accurately interpret the speech patterns of those with speech impairments. Such biases can exacerbate disparities in care and undermine the effectiveness of these technologies. To mitigate these risks, developers must prioritize diversity and inclusivity in their training datasets, implement rigorous testing for bias, and establish transparent accountability mechanisms. Additionally, involving individuals with disabilities in the design and testing phases can help ensure that these technologies meet the needs of all users.

Table 3. Comparative analysis of emerging assistive technologies.

Technology	Key Functionality	Advantages	Challenges	Potential Solutions
Piezoelectric Sensors for Early Diagnosis	Detects micro-tremors for conditions like Parkinson's, enabling early intervention.	High precision in detecting early disease symptoms, allowing for personalized treatment plans.	High cost and integration complexity in standard healthcare systems.	Research into low-cost alternatives; integration with wearable devices for broader accessibility.
Self-Adjusting Wheelchairs (Shape Memory Alloy-based)	Adapts to uneven terrains autonomously, promoting independent mobility.	Increases autonomy and reduces reliance on caregivers.	Requires frequent maintenance and may not be cost-effective for widespread use.	Developing energy-efficient, self-repairing materials; improving affordability through scalable production.
3D-Printed Smart Orthotics	Customizable orthotic solutions for growing children, reducing the need for frequent replacements.	Cost-effective in the long run; rapid production; improves accessibility in low-income regions.	High initial development costs; need for regulatory approvals before mass adoption.	Establishing open-source designs; government subsidies to reduce patient costs.
Electroactive Polymer (EAP)-Based Prosthetics	Mimics natural limb movement through electrical stimulation.	Provides lifelike motion and better adaptability than traditional prosthetics.	Expensive materials; requires significant power supply for prolonged usage.	Research on sustainable power sources (e.g., bioelectric energy); reducing material costs through mass production.
Wearable AI for ALS Patients	Assists with communication, movement tracking, and environmental interaction.	Enhances patient autonomy and communication efficiency.	Wearables lack durability; potential discomfort during prolonged use.	Development of sweat-resistant, durable materials; user-centered ergonomic design.

continued on following page

Table 3. Continued

Technology	Key Functionality	Advantages	Challenges	Potential Solutions
Augmented Reality (AR) Navigation for the Visually Impaired	Uses tactile cues and real-time feedback to assist with navigation.	Improves mobility and spatial awareness; provides real-time guidance.	High cost of AR integration; requires stable internet connectivity.	Lightweight AR wearables; offline functionality for better accessibility.
AI-Based Speech Recognition for Disabled Users	Enhances voice-assisted communication for individuals with speech impairments.	Enables independent interaction with digital systems.	AI bias in speech recognition; difficulty in processing atypical speech patterns.	Expanding diverse AI training datasets; user feedback integration for continuous improvements.

The adoption of revolutionary technologies in healthcare offers transformative benefits, including precision in diagnosis and treatment, enhanced independence for individuals with mobility challenges, and long-term cost-efficiency(Ahmad et al., 2022). However, significant barriers—such as high initial costs, durability concerns, and ethical risks—must be addressed to ensure these innovations are accessible, reliable, and equitable. Overcoming these challenges requires collaboration among researchers, manufacturers, policymakers, and the disability community to develop solutions that are both technologically advanced and socially responsible. By doing so, we can harness the full potential of these technologies to improve the lives of individuals with disabilities and chronic conditions, fostering a more inclusive and equitable future.

5. THE FUTURE: TOWARD INCLUSIVE, BOUNDARY-PUSHING REHABILITATION

The future of rehabilitation is poised to be transformative, driven by groundbreaking technological advancements, ethical imperatives, and collaborative frameworks. This section explores the emerging frontiers of rehabilitation, alongside the ethical and collaborative measures necessary to ensure inclusivity and accessibility for all.

5.1 Emerging Frontiers

The next wave of rehabilitation technologies will redefine the boundaries of human potential, offering solutions that are not only innovative but also deeply personalized and adaptive to diverse needs.

- **Brain-Material Interfaces:** The integration of piezoelectric skull implants with neural networks will enable direct brain-to-device communication, allowing individuals to control prosthetics with their thoughts(Garg et al., 2025). This technology promises unprecedented precision and fluidity in movement, bridging the gap between human intent and mechanical action. For example, a person with a spinal cord injury could operate a prosthetic limb as naturally as they would their biological one, restoring autonomy and functionality(Farina et al., 2023).
- **Self-Healing Materials:** Advances in material science will lead to the development of orthotics and prosthetics capable of repairing themselves in real time(Varaganti& Seo, 2024). Using polymers embedded with microcapsules of healing agents, these devices will autonomously mend cracks or damage caused by wear and tear(Dallaev, 2024). This innovation is particularly crucial for individuals with lifelong disabilities, ensuring their devices remain durable and functional over extended periods.
- **Climate-Adaptive Devices:** For healthier living human require a comfortable temperature (Akhai and Abbass 2025; Akhai 2024). Prosthetics and orthotics designed to adapt to extreme environmental conditions will become essential for populations in disaster zones or refugee camps(Kantaros et al., 2024). For instance, devices equipped with embedded sensors and thermal regulation systems will adjust to extreme heat or cold, ensuring comfort and functionality in challenging climates(Lokmic-Tomkins et al., 2023). This technology will be a lifeline for displaced individuals who rely on assistive devices to navigate their environments.

5.2 Ethical and Collaborative Imperatives

To ensure that these advancements benefit everyone, ethical considerations and inclusive collaboration must be at the forefront of innovation.

- **Co-Design with Disabled Communities:** End-users must be integral to the design and development process. For example, exoskeletons for individuals with quadriplegia should be prototyped and tested in collaboration with quadriplegic users to ensure they meet real-world needs. This participatory approach ensures that technologies are not only functional but also tailored to the lived experiences of those they aim to serve.
- **Global Accessibility Frameworks:** Governments and public health systems must prioritize the subsidization of smart materials and advanced assistive technologies. By making these solutions affordable and accessible, we can

bridge the gap between cutting-edge innovation and equitable distribution, particularly in low-resource settings.

- **Policy Advocacy:** Policymakers must mandate insurance coverage for adaptive technologies, such as AI-powered prosthetics and climate-adaptive devices. This ensures that financial barriers do not prevent individuals from accessing life-changing technologies. Advocacy efforts should also focus on creating international standards for the ethical development and deployment of rehabilitation technologies.

The future of rehabilitation is not just about technological breakthroughs but about creating a world where these innovations are accessible, inclusive, and ethical. By pushing the boundaries of science and engineering while centering the voices of disabled communities, we can build a future where everyone has the tools they need to thrive(MacLachlan et al., 2018; Correia et al., 2023). Even the latest technologies like IoT and artificial intelligence have a crucial role in shaping the future of modern advanced science (Akhai 2024)

6. DISCUSSION

Smart materials are not just technological innovations—they represent a fundamental shift in disability rehabilitation, transforming it from a process of recovery to one of empowerment. By integrating advanced material science with AI-driven intelligence, these materials create adaptive, personalized, and highly responsive rehabilitation solutions that improve mobility, therapy, and daily living. Technologies such as shape-memory alloys, electroactive polymers, and piezoelectric sensors enable assistive devices to respond in real time, making them more user-friendly and effective

Beyond functionality, the synergy between smart materials and AI enhances rehabilitation outcomes through predictive adjustments, remote monitoring, and AI-driven therapeutic exercises. This not only optimizes recovery but also reduces healthcare burdens by enabling home-based and decentralized rehabilitation models. Additionally, advancements in manufacturing, particularly 3D printing, have significantly reduced costs, making assistive technologies more accessible to underserved populations.However, despite their transformative potential, challenges remain. High initial costs, durability concerns, and ethical considerations, such as algorithmic bias in AI-driven rehabilitation, must be addressed to ensure equitable adoption. Inclusive design practices, rigorous testing, and policy interventions are necessary to bridge these gaps and ensure that smart rehabilitation technologies benefit all individuals, regardless of socioeconomic background.

Looking ahead, the future of rehabilitation lies in emerging innovations such as brain-material interfaces, self-healing materials, and climate-adaptive devices, which will further revolutionize disability care. By fostering collaboration among researchers, policymakers, and the disability community, we can drive ethical, inclusive, and sustainable advancements in rehabilitation technology.

To fully harness the potential of smart materials in disability rehabilitation, a collective effort is required. Key actions include:

1. **Investing in Open-Source Smart Material Platforms:** Encouraging collaboration among researchers, engineers, and designers will accelerate the development of affordable, accessible solutions and ensure technological breakthroughs reach those who need them most.
2. **Training Clinicians in Adaptive Technology Integration:** Equipping healthcare professionals with the skills to integrate smart materials into rehabilitation programs will enhance patient outcomes and bridge the gap between innovation and real-world application.
3. **Amplifying Stories of Impact:** Sharing the experiences of individuals who have regained independence through smart materials will inspire innovation, challenge societal perceptions of disability, and foster a culture of inclusivity.

The journey toward a more inclusive world is driven by innovation, collaboration, and empathy. By investing in smart materials, advancing inclusive policies, and centering the voices of individuals with disabilities, we can create a future where rehabilitation is not just about overcoming challenges, it's about unlocking limitless potential. The future of disability rehabilitation is not just about what we can create, it's about who we can empower.

7. CONCLUSION

- Smart materials are transforming disability rehabilitation from a recovery process to one of empowerment. They combine advanced material science with AI-driven intelligence to create adaptive, personalized, and highly responsive rehabilitation solutions. Technologies like shape-memory alloys, electroactive polymers, and piezoelectric sensors enable assistive devices to respond in real time, making them more user-friendly and effective. The synergy between smart materials and AI enhances rehabilitation outcomes through predictive adjustments, remote monitoring, and AI-driven therapeutic exercises, optimizing recovery and reducing healthcare burdens. Advancements in manufacturing, particularly 3D printing, have significantly reduced costs, making assistive technologies more accessible to underserved populations.

- However, challenges remain, such as high initial costs, durability concerns, and ethical considerations like algorithmic bias in AI-driven rehabilitation. Inclusive design practices, rigorous testing, and policy interventions are necessary to ensure equitable adoption of smart rehabilitation technologies. The future of rehabilitation lies in emerging innovations like brain-material interfaces, self-healing materials, and climate-adaptive devices.
- To fully harness the potential of smart materials in disability rehabilitation, a collective effort is required. Key actions include investing in open-source smart material platforms, training clinicians in adaptive technology integration, and amplifying stories of impact. The journey towards a more inclusive world is driven by innovation, collaboration, and empathy. By investing in smart materials, advancing inclusive policies, and centering the voices of individuals with disabilities, we can create a future where rehabilitation is not just about overcoming challenges but about unlocking limitless potential.

Chapter Summary

Table 4 summarizes the key points of each chapter, highlighting the transformative role of smart materials in disability rehabilitation, their applications, advantages, challenges, and future directions.

Table 4. Summary of chapter

Chapter Section	*Key Points*
1. Introduction: The New Era of Disability Rehabilitation	- Smart materials are revolutionizing disability rehabilitation by enabling real-time adaptation and responsiveness. - **Examples:** Shape-memory alloys in spinal braces, electroactive polymers in prosthetics. - **Benefits:** Enhanced adaptability, personalization, predictive care, and affordability. - **Challenges:** High abandonment rates of traditional devices due to poor fit or functionality.
1.1 What Makes Smart Materials Revolutionary?	- Smart materials sense, respond, and adapt to environmental or physiological changes. - **Applications:** Prosthetics, orthotics, wearable rehabilitation devices. - **Key advantages:** Responsiveness, personalization, AI integration, continuous monitoring. - **Example:** AI-driven sensors predict muscle spasms in multiple sclerosis patients.
1.2 The Imperative for Innovation in Disability Rehabilitation	- Over 1 billion people globally live with disabilities, many lacking access to advanced care. - Smart materials address limitations of traditional methods: high costs, poor fit, and discomfort. - Scalability through 3D printing reduces costs and improves accessibility. - Emerging technologies: Remote monitoring, VR/AR integration, and AI-driven rehabilitation.
2. Smart Materials: Redefining Rehabilitation Paradigms	- Smart materials introduce adaptive, responsive systems for personalized rehabilitation. - **Core technologies:** Shape-memory alloys, electroactive polymers, piezoelectric sensors, thermoresponsive gels. - **Applications:** Spinal injury exoskeletons, bionic hands, tremor monitoring, burn rehabilitation. - **Impact:** Personalized recovery, enhanced accessibility, real-time monitoring, remote rehabilitation.
2.1 Core Technologies Driving Change	- **Shape-Memory Alloys (SMAs):** Adjust support dynamically in spinal exoskeletons. - **Electroactive Polymers (EAPs):** Enable lifelike movements in prosthetics. - **Piezoelectric Sensors:** Monitor tremors in Parkinson's patients. - **Thermoresponsive Gels:** Deliver targeted drug release in burn dressings.
2.2 Bridging Gaps in Neurorehabilitation	- **Stroke Recovery:** Electroactive polymer gloves stimulate paralyzed hands. - **Spinal Cord Injuries:** Exoskeletons with SMAs adapt to walking terrains. - **Neurorehabilitation:** Smart materials enhance motor control and independence.

continued on following page

Table 4. Continued

Chapter Section	*Key Points*
2.3 The Transformative Impact of Smart Materials	- Personalized recovery through adaptive devices. - Enhanced accessibility via 3D printing and scalable manufacturing. - Real-time monitoring and remote rehabilitation reduce clinic visits. - Future directions: VR/AR integration, nanotechnology, soft wearable robots.
3. Revolutionary Applications in Disability Care	- **Smart Prosthetics:** Piezoelectric-powered damping improves stability. - **AI-Driven Exoskeletons:** MR fluid-based support enhances mobility. - **Haptic Feedback Gloves:** Restore tactile sensation for neuropathy patients. - **AR + Smart Textiles:** Thermoresponsive sleeves aid visually impaired navigation. - **Drug-Eluting Smart Patches:** Automate medication delivery for cerebral palsy. - **Dynamic Compression Wear:** MR fluid-based sleeves manage lymphedema.
4. Advantages vs. Challenges in Revolutionary Adoption	- **Advantages:** Precision in diagnosis, independence for mobility challenges, cost-efficiency over time. - **Challenges:** High initial costs, durability concerns, ethical risks like algorithmic bias. - **Solutions:** Scalable manufacturing, ruggedized designs, diverse AI training datasets.
5. The Future: Toward Inclusive, Boundary-Pushing Rehabilitation	- **Emerging Frontiers:** Brain-material interfaces, self-healing materials, climate-adaptive devices. - **Ethical Imperatives:** Co-design with disabled communities, global accessibility frameworks, policy advocacy. - **Collaborative Measures:** Inclusive innovation, equitable distribution, and ethical development.
6. Discussion	- Smart materials empower individuals by transforming rehabilitation into a personalized, adaptive process. - **Challenges:** High costs, durability, and ethical concerns must be addressed. - **Future innovations:** Brain-material interfaces, self-healing materials, and climate-adaptive devices. - **Call to action:** Invest in open-source platforms, train clinicians, and amplify impact stories.
7. Conclusions	- Smart materials combine material science and AI to create adaptive, personalized rehabilitation solutions. - Key technologies: Shape-memory alloys, electroactive polymers, piezoelectric sensors. - **Challenges:** High costs, durability, and algorithmic bias. - **Future:** Brain-material interfaces, self-healing materials, and inclusive policies. - **Goal:** Empower individuals with disabilities through innovation, collaboration, and empathy.

REFERENCES

Abbady, H. E., Klinkenberg, E. T., de Moel, L., Nicolai, N., van der Stelt, M., Verhulst, A. C., Maal, T. J. J., & Brouwers, L. (2022). 3D-printed prostheses in developing countries: A systematic review. *Prosthetics and Orthotics International, 46*(1), 19–30. DOI: 10.1097/PXR.0000000000000057 PMID: 34772868

Abbas, T., &Zlopasa, O. (2025). The Role of IoT and AI in Smart Prosthetics: Advancing Adaptive and Personalized Assistive Technologies.

Aderinto, N., Olatunji, G., Abdulbasit, M. O., Edun, M., Aboderin, G., & Egbunu, E. (2023). Exploring the efficacy of virtual reality-based rehabilitation in stroke: A narrative review of current evidence. *Annals of Medicine, 55*(2), 2285907. DOI: 10.1080/07853890.2023.2285907 PMID: 38010358

Ahmad, I., Asghar, Z., Kumar, T., Li, G., Manzoor, A., Mikhaylov, K., Shah, S. A., Höyhtyä, M., Reponen, J., Huusko, J., & Harjula, E. (2022). Emerging technologies for next generation remote health care and assisted living. *IEEE Access : Practical Innovations, Open Solutions, 10*, 56094–56132. DOI: 10.1109/ACCESS.2022.3177278

Akbari, A., Haghverd, F., & Behbahani, S. (2021). Robotic home-based rehabilitation systems design: From a literature review to a conceptual framework for community-based remote therapy during COVID-19 pandemic. *Frontiers in Robotics and AI, 8*, 612331. DOI: 10.3389/frobt.2021.612331 PMID: 34239898

Akhai, S. (2023). From Black Boxes to Transparent Machines: The Quest for Explainable AI. Available at: Social Science Research Network, DOI: 10.2139/ssrn.4390887

Akhai, S. (2023). Healthcare record management for healthcare 4.0 via blockchain: a review of current applications, opportunities, challenges, and future potential. In *Blockchain for Healthcare 4.0* (Vol. 1, pp. 211–223). CRC Press. DOI: 10.1201/9781003408246-11

Akhai, S. (2023). Navigating the Potential Applications and Challenges of Intelligent and Sustainable Manufacturing for a Greener Future. *Evergreen, 10*(4), 2237–2243. DOI: 10.5109/7160899

Akhai, S. (2024). A Review on Optimizations in µ-EDM Machining of the Biomedical Material Ti6Al4V Using the Taguchi Method: Recent Advances Since 2020. *Latest Trends in Engineering and Technology*, 395-402.

Akhai, S. (2024). Smart Home Environment for Society: An Overview of IoT-Enabled Air Conditioners. In *Modelling of Virtual Worlds Using the Internet of Things* (Vol. 1, pp. 74-87). CRC Press.

Akhai, S. (2024). The Impact of Artificial Intelligence on Healthcare: Opportunities and Challenges. *Journal of Advanced Research in Medical Science & Technology*, *11*(1&2), 1–6. DOI: 10.24321/2394.6539.202401

Akhai, S. (2024). Towards Trustworthy and Reliable AI The Next Frontier. In *Explainable Artificial Intelligence (XAI) in Healthcare* (Vol. 1, pp. 119-129). CRC Press, Taylor & Francis Group.

Akhai, S., & Abbass, M. (2025). Air Conditioning for Healthier Living. In Managing the Health Risks of Climate Change (pp. 135–154). IGI Global Scientific Publishing. DOI: 10.4018/979-8-3693-4183-4.ch006

Akhai, S., Abbass, M., Kaur, P., & Kaur, T. (2025). Digital Transformation Across Generations: Robotics and AI in Action. In *Impacts of Digital Technologies Across Generations* (pp. 23-40). IGI Global Scientific Publishing. DOI: 10.4018/979-8-3693-6366-9.ch002

Akhai, S., & Khang, A. (2024). Innovations in Medical Manufacturing: A Review of 3D Printing, Robotics, and Internet of Things (IoT). In *The Quantum Evolution* (Vol. 1, pp. 226-241). CRC Press.

Akhai, S., Singh, V. P., & John, S. (2016). Human performance in industrial design centers with small unit air conditioning systems. *Journal of Advanced Research in Production Industrial Engineering*, *3*(2), 5–11.

Akhai, S., Srivastava, P., Sharma, V., & Bhatia, A. (2021, August). Investigating weld strength of AA8011-6062 alloys joined via friction-stir welding using the RSM approach. *Journal of Physics: Conference Series*, *1950*(1), 012016. DOI: 10.1088/1742-6596/1950/1/012016

Akhai, S., & Wadhwa, A. S. (2024). Recent Advances in Bio-Tribology From Joint Lubrication to Medical Implants: A Review. *Journal of Materials*, *2*(2), 125–135.

Al Khatib, I., Shamayleh, A., & Ndiaye, M. (2024, July). Healthcare and the internet of medical things: Applications, trends, key challenges, and proposed resolutions. *Informatics (MDPI)*, *11*(3), 47. DOI: 10.3390/informatics11030047

Al-Musawi, M. H., Turki, S. H., Al-Naymi, H. A. S., Al-salman, S. S., Boroujeni, V. V., Alizadeh, M., & Tavakoli, M. (2024). Localized delivery of healing stimulator medicines for enhanced wound treatment. *Journal of Drug Delivery Science and Technology*, *101*, 106212. DOI: 10.1016/j.jddst.2024.106212

Aziz, R., Jawed, F., Khan, S. A., & Sundus, H. (2024). Wearable IoT Devices in Rehabilitation: Enabling Personalized Precision Medicine. In *Medical Robotics and AI-Assisted Diagnostics for a High-Tech Healthcare Industry* (pp. 281-308). IGI global.

Azzi, Z., Al Sayegh, H., Metwally, O., & Eissa, M. (2025). Review of Nondestructive Testing (NDT) Techniques for Timber Structures. *Infrastructures*, *10*(2), 28. DOI: 10.3390/infrastructures10020028

Bagher, M. M., Sajjadi, P., Wallgrün, J. O., La Femina, P. C., & Klippel, A. (2021). Move the object or move the user: The role of interaction techniques on embodied learning in VR. *Frontiers in Virtual Reality*, *2*, 695312. DOI: 10.3389/frvir.2021.695312

Behera, A., & Behera, A. (2022). Shape-memory materials. *Advanced Materials: An Introduction to Modern Materials Science*, 1-42.

Benouhiba, A., Holzer, S., Konstantinidi, S., Civet, Y., & Perriard, Y. (2025). The elastic frontier: Dielectric elastomer actuators in healthcare technology. *Smart Materials and Structures*, *34*(3), 033001. DOI: 10.1088/1361-665X/adae6a

Bhat, A., Rao, V. S., & Jayalakshmi, N. S. (2023). Review of the Evolution of Magnetorheological Fluid-Based Rehabilitative Devices: From the Perspective of Modeling, Sensors and Control Strategies. *IEEE Access : Practical Innovations, Open Solutions*, *11*, 88759–88777. DOI: 10.1109/ACCESS.2023.3305674

Borthakur, P. P. (2025). The Role and Future Directions of 3D Printing in Custom Prosthetic Design. *Engineering Proceedings*, *81*(1), 10.

Bruce, A., & Williams, L. A. (2025). Access and Citizenship for Those With Disabilities: Digitally Enabled Education and AI as a Bridge to Innovative Inclusion. In *Digital Citizenship and the Future of AI Engagement, Ethics, and Privacy* (pp. 31-78). IGI Global Scientific Publishing.

Cerritelli, F., Chiera, M., Abbro, M., Megale, V., Esteves, J., Gallace, A., & Manzotti, A. (2021). The challenges and perspectives of the integration between virtual and augmented reality and manual therapies. *Frontiers in Neurology*, *12*, 700211. DOI: 10.3389/fneur.2021.700211 PMID: 34276550

Chrysanthakopoulou, D. C., & Koutsojannis, C. (2025). Machine Learning Algorithms Introduce Evoked Potentials As Alternative Biomarkers for the Expanded Disability Status Scale Prognosis of Multiple Sclerosis Patients. *Cureus*, *17*(3). Advance online publication. DOI: 10.7759/cureus.80335 PMID: 40206919

Coman, L. I., Ianculescu, M., Paraschiv, E. A., Alexandru, A., & Bădărău, I. A. (2024). Smart solutions for diet-related disease management: Connected care, remote health monitoring systems, and integrated insights for advanced evaluation. *Applied Sciences (Basel, Switzerland)*, *14*(6), 2351. DOI: 10.3390/app14062351

Correia, C., Reis, R. L., Pashkuleva, I., & Alves, N. M. (2023). Adhesive and self-healing materials for central nervous system repair. *Biomaterials Advances*, *151*, 213439. DOI: 10.1016/j.bioadv.2023.213439 PMID: 37146528

Dabla, P. K., Gruson, D., Gouget, B., Bernardini, S., & Homsak, E. (2021). Lessons learned from the COVID-19 pandemic: Emphasizing the emerging role and perspectives from artificial intelligence, mobile health, and digital laboratory medicine. *EJIFCC*, *32*(2), 224. PMID: 34421492

Dallaev, R. (2024). Advances in materials with self-healing properties: A brief review. *Materials (Basel)*, *17*(10), 2464. DOI: 10.3390/ma17102464 PMID: 38793530

Danemayer, J., Holloway, C., Cho, Y., Berthouze, N., Singh, A., Bhot, W., Dixon, O., Grobelnik, M., & Shawe-Taylor, J. (2023). Seeking information about assistive technology: Exploring current practices, challenges, and the need for smarter systems. *International Journal of Human-Computer Studies*, *177*, 103078. DOI: 10.1016/j.ijhcs.2023.103078

Dereje, D., Lamba, D., Abessa, T. G., Kenea, C., Ramari, C., Osama, M., Kossi, O., Boma, P. M., Panda, J., Kushnir, A., Mourad, J., Mapinduzi, J., Fourtassi, M., Daniels, K., Deutsch, J., & Bonnechère, B. (2025). Unlocking the potential of serious games for rehabilitation in low and middle-income countries: Addressing potential and current limitations. *Frontiers in Digital Health*, *7*, 1505717. DOI: 10.3389/fdgth.2025.1505717 PMID: 39957725

Dewang, Y., Sharma, V., Baliyan, V. K., Soundappan, T., & Singla, Y. K. (2025). Research Progress in Electroactive Polymers for Soft Robotics and Artificial Muscle Applications. *Polymers*, *17*(6), 746. DOI: 10.3390/polym17060746 PMID: 40292598

Dong, H., Lin, J., Tao, Y., Jia, Y., Sun, L., Li, W. J., & Sun, H. (2024). AI-enhanced biomedical micro/nanorobots in microfluidics. *Lab on a Chip*, *24*(5), 1419–1440. DOI: 10.1039/D3LC00909B PMID: 38174821

Dostalova, K., Tomasek, R., Kalova, M., Janura, M., Rosicky, J., Schnitzer, M., & Demel, J. (2022). Review of ankle rehabilitation devices for treatment of equinus contracture. *Expert Review of Medical Devices*, *19*(9), 721–731. DOI: 10.1080/17434440.2022.2136029 PMID: 36225151

El-Tanani, M., Satyam, S. M., Rabbani, S. A., El-Tanani, Y., Aljabali, A. A., Al Faouri, I., & Rehman, A. (2025). Revolutionizing Drug Delivery: The Impact of Advanced Materials Science and Technology on Precision Medicine. *Pharmaceutics*, *17*(3), 375. DOI: 10.3390/pharmaceutics17030375 PMID: 40143038

Enyan, M., Bing, Z., Amu-Darko, J. N. O., Issaka, E., Otoo, S. L., & Agyemang, M. F. (2025). Advances in smart materials soft actuators on mechanisms, fabrication, materials, and multifaceted applications: A review. *Journal of Thermoplastic Composite Materials*, *38*(1), 302–370. DOI: 10.1177/08927057241248028

Farham, B., & Baltazar, L. (2024). A review of smart materials in 4D printing for hygrothermal rehabilitation: Innovative insights for sustainable building stock management. *Sustainability (Basel)*, *16*(10), 4067. DOI: 10.3390/su16104067

Farina, D., Vujaklija, I., Brånemark, R., Bull, A. M., Dietl, H., Graimann, B., Hargrove, L. J., Hoffmann, K.-P., Huang, H., Ingvarsson, T., Janusson, H. B., Kristjánsson, K., Kuiken, T., Micera, S., Stieglitz, T., Sturma, A., Tyler, D., Weir, R. F., & Aszmann, O. C. (2023). Toward higher-performance bionic limbs for wider clinical use. *Nature Biomedical Engineering*, *7*(4), 473–485. DOI: 10.1038/s41551-021-00732-x PMID: 34059810

Ficili, I., Giacobbe, M., Tricomi, G., & Puliafito, A. (2025). From Sensors to Data Intelligence: Leveraging IoT, Cloud, and Edge Computing with AI. *Sensors (Basel)*, *25*(6), 1763. DOI: 10.3390/s25061763 PMID: 40292910

Gallagher, K. A., Mills, J. L., Armstrong, D. G., Conte, M. S., Kirsner, R. S., Minc, S. D., Plutzky, J., Southerland, K. W., & Tomic-Canic, M. (2024). Current status and principles for the treatment and prevention of diabetic foot ulcers in the cardiovascular patient population: A scientific statement from the American Heart Association. *Circulation*, *149*(4), e232–e253. DOI: 10.1161/CIR.0000000000001192 PMID: 38095068

Gao, A., Murphy, R. R., Chen, W., Dagnino, G., Fischer, P., Gutierrez, M. G., Kundrat, D., Nelson, B. J., Shamsudhin, N., Su, H., Xia, J., Zemmar, A., Zhang, D., Wang, C., & Yang, G. Z. (2021). Progress in robotics for combating infectious diseases. *Science Robotics*, *6*(52), eabf1462. DOI: 10.1126/scirobotics.abf1462 PMID: 34043552

Garg, I., Verma, M., Kumar, H., Maurya, R., Negi, T., & Jain, P. (2025). Bioelectronic Therapeutics: A Revolutionary Medical Practice in Health Care. *Bioelectricity*, *7*(1), 2–28. DOI: 10.1089/bioe.2024.0039 PMID: 40342937

Gherman, B., Zima, I., Vaida, C., Tucan, P., Pisla, A., Birlescu, I., Machado, J., & Pisla, D. (2025). Robotic Systems for Hand Rehabilitation—Past, Present and Future. *Technologies, 13*(1), 37. DOI: 10.3390/technologies13010037

Ghevondyan, M., Davtyan, M., & Aghayan, M. (2025). Dielectric elastomer actuators: Medical applications review. *Discover Materials, 5*(1), 43. DOI: 10.1007/s43939-025-00225-7

Giansanti, D. (2025). Advancements in Ocular Neuro-Prosthetics: Bridging Neuroscience and Information and Communication Technology for Vision Restoration. *Biology (Basel), 14*(2), 134. DOI: 10.3390/biology14020134 PMID: 40001902

Gongor, F., & Tutsoy, O. (2025). On the Remarkable Advancement of Assistive Robotics in Human-Robot Interaction-Based Health-Care Applications: An Exploratory Overview of the Literature. *International Journal of Human-Computer Interaction, 41*(2), 1502–1542. DOI: 10.1080/10447318.2024.2342101

Gonzalez-Vazquez, A., Garcia, L., Kilby, J., & McNair, P. (2023). Soft wearable rehabilitation robots with artificial muscles based on smart materials: A review. *Advanced Intelligent Systems, 5*(4), 2200159. DOI: 10.1002/aisy.202200159

Han, X., Guffanti, D., & Brunete, A. (2025). A Comprehensive Review of Vision-Based Sensor Systems for Human Gait Analysis. *Sensors (Basel), 25*(2), 498. DOI: 10.3390/s25020498 PMID: 39860869

Hanna, M., Pantanowitz, L., Jackson, B., Palmer, O., Visweswaran, S., Pantanowitz, J., & Rashidi, H. (2024). Ethical and Bias considerations in artificial intelligence (AI)/machine learning. *Modern Pathology*, •••, 100686. PMID: 39694331

Huang, X., Xue, Y., Ren, S., & Wang, F. (2023). Sensor-based wearable systems for monitoring human motion and posture: A review. *Sensors (Basel), 23*(22), 9047. DOI: 10.3390/s23229047 PMID: 38005436

Irigoyen, E., Larrea, M., & Graña, M. (2024). A Narrative Review of Haptic Technologies and Their Value for Training, Rehabilitation, and the Education of Persons with Special Needs. *Sensors (Basel), 24*(21), 6946. DOI: 10.3390/s24216946 PMID: 39517844

Jamieson, A. R., & Wijesundara, H. D. (2025). A review of adaptive equipment and technology for exercise and sports activities for people with disabilities. *Disability and Rehabilitation. Assistive Technology, 20*(1), 33–45. DOI: 10.1080/17483107.2024.2372323 PMID: 38962933

Jimbu, D., Cristea, A. E., Iliescu, D. M., Oprea, D., Iliescu, M. G., Caraban, B. M., & Bordei, P. (2024). 664 The importance of advanced technologies in functional rehabilitation of the hand. *Balneo and PRM Research Journal*, *15*(1).

Jiralerspong, T., & Zhao, H. (2024). Soft Robotic Devices for Mechanotherapy of the Upper and Lower Extremities. *Advanced Materials Technologies*, •••, 2401530.

Jyothish, K. J., & Mishra, S. (2024). A survey on robotic prosthetics: Neuroprosthetics, soft actuators, and control strategies. *ACM Computing Surveys*, *56*(8), 1–44. DOI: 10.1145/3648355

Kanda, R., Akhai, S., & Bansal, R. (2013). Analysis of MOST technique for elimination of idle time by synchronization of different lines. *International Journal of Research in Advent Technology*, *1*(4), 151–158.

Kantaros, A., & Ganetsos, T. (2023). From static to dynamic: Smart materials pioneering additive manufacturing in regenerative medicine. *International Journal of Molecular Sciences*, *24*(21), 15748. DOI: 10.3390/ijms242115748 PMID: 37958733

Kantaros, A., Petrescu, F. I. T., Brachos, K., Ganetsos, T., & Petrescu, N. (2024). Leveraging 3D Printing for Resilient Disaster Management in Smart Cities. *Smart Cities*, *7*(6), 3705–3726. DOI: 10.3390/smartcities7060143

Kantaros, A., Petrescu, F. I. T., & Ganetsos, T. (2025). From Stents to Smart Implants Employing Biomimetic Materials: The Impact of 4D Printing on Modern Healthcare. *Biomimetics*, *10*(2), 125. DOI: 10.3390/biomimetics10020125 PMID: 39997148

Karim, M. R., Siddiqui, M. I. H., Assaifan, A. K., Aijaz, M. O., & Alnaser, I. A. (2024). Nanotechnology and Prosthetic Devices: Integrating Biomedicine and Materials Science for Enhanced Performance and Adaptability. *Journal of Disability Research*, *3*(3), 20240019. DOI: 10.57197/JDR-2024-0019

Khang, A., & Akhai, S. (2024). Green intelligent and sustainable manufacturing: key advancements, benefits, challenges, and applications for transforming industry. *Machine Vision and Industrial Robotics in Manufacturing*, 405-417.

King, M. R., & Colla, S. (2025). Muscle Rehabilitation Techniques and Prevention of Injury. *Veterinary Clinics: Equine Practice*.

Kocaaslan, R. (2024). The current state and future of robotic surgery in Urology: A Comprehensive Review. *Interdisciplinary Medicine. Health and Bioscience Researches*, *2024*, 77.

Kumar, , HWadhwa, , A. SAkhai, , SKaushik, , A. (2024). Parametric analysis, modeling and optimization of the process parameters in electric discharge machining of aluminium metal matrix composite. *Engineering Research Express, 6*(2), 025542. DOI 10.1088/2631-8695/ad4ba9

Kumar, K., & Ranjan, C. (2025). *Smart Materials: Electro-Rheological Fluids, Piezoelectric Smart Materials, and Shape Memory Alloys*. Walter de Gruyter GmbH & Co KG.

Kumar, P., & Akhai, S. (2022). Effective energy management in smart buildings using VRV/VRF systems. In *Additive Manufacturing in Industry 4.0* (pp. 27-35). CRC Press. DOI: 10.1201/9781003360001-2

Kumar, S., Pandey, D., & Chandra, S. (2023). Revolutionizing biofeedback and beyond: a journey through the evolving landscape of biomechanics. *Biochemical and Cellular Archives, 23*(S1), 23. DOI: 10.51470/BCA.2023.23.S1.1625

Lippi, L., Turco, A., Moalli, S., Gallo, M., Curci, C., Maconi, A., de Sire, A., & Invernizzi, M. (2023). Role of prehabilitation and rehabilitation on functional recovery and quality of life in thyroid cancer patients: A comprehensive review. *Cancers (Basel), 15*(18), 4502. DOI: 10.3390/cancers15184502 PMID: 37760472

Liu, H., Hu, J., Zheng, Q., Feng, X., Zhan, F., Wang, X., Xu, G., & Hua, F. (2022). Piezo1 channels as force sensors in mechanical force-related chronic inflammation. *Frontiers in Immunology, 13*, 816149. DOI: 10.3389/fimmu.2022.816149 PMID: 35154133

Lokmic-Tomkins, Z., Bhandari, D., Bain, C., Borda, A., Kariotis, T. C., & Reser, D. (2023). Lessons learned from natural disasters around digital health technologies and delivering quality healthcare. *International Journal of Environmental Research and Public Health, 20*(5), 4542. DOI: 10.3390/ijerph20054542 PMID: 36901559

MacLachlan, M., Banes, D., Bell, D., Borg, J., Donnelly, B., Fembek, M., Ghosh, R., Gowran, R. J., Hannay, E., Hiscock, D., Hoogerwerf, E.-J., Howe, T., Kohler, F., Layton, N., Long, S., Mannan, H., Mji, G., Odera Ongolo, T., Perry, K., & Hooks, H. (2018). Assistive technology policy: A position paper from the first global research, innovation, and education on assistive technology (GREAT) summit. *Disability and Rehabilitation. Assistive Technology, 13*(5), 454–466. DOI: 10.1080/17483107.2018.1468496 PMID: 29790393

Mala, S., Deep, U., Mala, E., & Akhai, S. (2025). Digital Health Technologies for Preventive Cardiology. In *Impact of Digital Solutions for Improved Healthcare Delivery* (pp. 379–400). IGI Global.

Mathunjwa, B. M., Kor, R. Y. J., Ngarnkuekool, W., & Hsu, Y. L. (2025). A Comprehensive Review of Home Sleep Monitoring Technologies: Smartphone Apps, Smartwatches, and Smart Mattresses. *Sensors (Basel), 25*(6), 1771. DOI: 10.3390/s25061771 PMID: 40292882

Mikołajewska, E., Mikołajewski, D., Mikołajczyk, T., & Paczkowski, T. (2025). A Breakthrough in Producing Personalized Solutions for Rehabilitation and Physiotherapy Thanks to the Introduction of AI to Additive Manufacturing. *Applied Sciences (Basel, Switzerland), 15*(4), 2219. DOI: 10.3390/app15042219

Muñoz Ruiz, C. (2024). Shape Morphing Wearable For Regulating the Nervous System Through Breathing.

Nisky, I., & Makin, T. R. (2024). A neurocognitive pathway for engineering artificial touch. *Science Advances, 10*(51), eadq6290. DOI: 10.1126/sciadv.adq6290 PMID: 39693427

Ornaghi, H. L.Jr, Monticeli, F. M., & Agnol, L. D. (2023). A Review on Polymers for Biomedical Applications on Hard and Soft Tissues and Prosthetic Limbs. *Polymers, 15*(19), 4034. DOI: 10.3390/polym15194034 PMID: 37836083

Oro, B. (2025). Perspective Chapter: Designing for Dignity–The Role of Esthetic Empathy in Assistive Technologies.

Pan, M., Yuan, C., Liang, X., Dong, T., Liu, T., Zhang, J., Zou, J., Yang, H., & Bowen, C. (2022). Soft actuators and robotic devices for rehabilitation and assistance. *Advanced Intelligent Systems, 4*(4), 2100140. DOI: 10.1002/aisy.202100140

Patel, P., Pampaniya, S., Ghosh, A., Raj, R., Karuppaih, D., & Kandasamy, S. (2025). Enhancing Accessibility Through Machine Learning: A Review on Visual and Hearing Impairment Technologies. *IEEE Access : Practical Innovations, Open Solutions, 13*, 33286–33307. DOI: 10.1109/ACCESS.2025.3539081

Pathak, K., Saikia, R., Das, A., Das, D., Islam, M. A., Pramanik, P., Parasar, A., Borthakur, P. P., Sarmah, P., Saikia, M., & Borthakur, B. (2023). 3D printing in biomedicine: Advancing personalized care through additive manufacturing. *Exploration of Medicine, 4*(6), 1135–1167. DOI: 10.37349/emed.2023.00200

Patricks, V., Twiste, M., Granat, M., Curtin, S., & Worsley, P. (2025). Clinicians' Perspectives of Activity Monitoring Applications and Facilitators for Lower-Limb Prosthetic Service Provision. *Journal of Prosthetics and Orthotics, 37*(1), 42–52. DOI: 10.1097/JPO.0000000000000518

Pierzchlewicz, K., Kępa, I., Podogrodzki, J., &Kotulska, K. (2021). Spinal muscular atrophy: the use of functional motor scales in the era of disease-modifying treatment. *Child neurology open, 8*, 2329048X211008725.

Rao, E., & Nasir, M. A. R. B. (2024). *IMPACT OF AFFORDABILITY, ADAPTABILITY, AND AVAILABILITY IN ACHIEVING SUSTAINABILITY: A SYSTEM-DYNAMIC APPROACH* (Doctoral dissertation, College of Electrical & Mechanical Engineering (CEME), NUST).

Rezaei, N. (2025). *Promoting Activity in People with Dementia through Assistive Technologies: A Comprehensive Approach from Conceptual Design to System Development* (Doctoral dissertation, Technische Universität Wien).

Rony, M. K. K., Parvin, M. R., Wahiduzzaman, M., Akter, K., & Ullah, M. (2024). Challenges and advancements in the health-related quality of life of older people. *Advances in Public Health, 2024*(1), 8839631. DOI: 10.1155/2024/8839631

Saldarriaga, A., Gutierrez-Velasquez, E. I., & Colorado, H. A. (2024). Soft hand exoskeletons for rehabilitation: Approaches to design, manufacturing methods, and future prospects. *Robotics (Basel, Switzerland), 13*(3), 50. DOI: 10.3390/robotics13030050

Sali, S., Chai, R., & Ganesan, B. (2025). Recent trends and digital technology applications in lower limb injury rehabilitation. In *Digital Technology in Public Health and Rehabilitation Care* (pp. 99–124). Academic Press. DOI: 10.1016/B978-0-443-22270-2.00007-1

Sarker, A., Ul Islam, T., & Islam, M. R. (2025). A review on recent trends of bio-inspired soft robotics: Actuators, control methods, materials selection, sensors, challenges, and future prospects. *Advanced Intelligent Systems, 7*(3), 2400414. DOI: 10.1002/aisy.202400414

Shanmugam, P. S. T. (2025). 3D Printing in Prosthetic. *Compendium of 3D Bioprinting Technology*, 256.

Sharma, B., Davies, J., Nicotra, E., Ji, A., Zhu, K., Phan, P. T., Nguyen, C. C., Hoang, T. T., Wan, J., Pruscino, P., Phan, H.-P., Lovell, N. H., & Do, T. N. (2025). A Soft Robotic Textile-Actuated Anthropomorphic Artificial Shoulder Mechanism. *Advanced Intelligent Systems, 7*(4), 2400807. DOI: 10.1002/aisy.202400807

Sharma, K., Verma, S., Sharma, S., & Jat, M. (2023). Neurorehabilitation Techniques. *Chief Editor Prof. Rajesh Kumar*, 41.

Sheffield, Z., Paul, P., Krishnakumar, S., & Pan, D. (2025). Current Strategies and Future Directions of Wearable Biosensors for Measuring Stress Biochemical Markers for Neuropsychiatric Applications. *Advancement of Science*, *12*(5), 2411339. DOI: 10.1002/advs.202411339 PMID: 39688117

Singh, A. B., Khandelwal, C., &Dangayach, G. S. (2024). Revolutionizing healthcare materials: Innovations in processing, advancements, and challenges for enhanced medical device integration and performance. *Journal of Micromanufacturing*, 25165984241256234.

Singh, B., & Nayyar, A. (2024). Navigating deep learning models and health monitoring infrastructure financing in smart cities: Review from legal perceptions and future innovations. *Deep Learning in Engineering, Energy and Finance*, 80-114.

Singh, S., & Akhai, S. (2024, July). Electronics in precision control for mechanical engineering: A brief overview. In *AIP Conference Proceedings* (Vol. 3121, No. 1). AIP Publishing. DOI: 10.1063/5.0221464

Singh, S., & Akhai, S. (2025). Tracking Drug Authenticity and Expiry with Blockchain: A Comprehensive Overview. *Blockchain-Enabled Solutions for the Pharmaceutical Industry*, 175-188.

Siviy, C., Baker, L. M., Quinlivan, B. T., Porciuncula, F., Swaminathan, K., Awad, L. N., & Walsh, C. J. (2023). Opportunities and challenges in the development of exoskeletons for locomotor assistance. *Nature Biomedical Engineering*, *7*(4), 456–472. DOI: 10.1038/s41551-022-00984-1 PMID: 36550303

Sood, S. K., Lamba, Y. S., & Singh, A. K. (2025). Exploring the Shift from 3D Printing to 4D Printing: A Review. *IEEE Sensors Journal.*

Tabucol, J., Kooiman, V. G., Leopaldi, M., Leijendekkers, R., Selleri, G., Mellini, M., Verdonschot, N., Oddsson, M., Carloni, R., Zucchelli, A., & Brugo, T. M. (2025). The MyFlex-ζ Foot: A Variable Stiffness ESR Ankle-Foot Prosthesis. *IEEE Transactions on Neural Systems and Rehabilitation Engineering*, *33*, 653–663. DOI: 10.1109/TNSRE.2025.3534096 PMID: 40031158

Tan, Q., Wu, C., Li, L., Shao, W., & Luo, M. (2022). Nanomaterial-Based Prosthetic Limbs for Disability Mobility Assistance: A Review of Recent Advances. *Journal of Nanomaterials*, *2022*(1), 3425297. DOI: 10.1155/2022/3425297

Thacharodi, A., Singh, P., Meenatchi, R., Tawfeeq Ahmed, Z. H., Kumar, R. R., v, N., Kavish, S., Maqbool, M., & Hassan, S. (2024). Revolutionizing healthcare and medicine: The impact of modern technologies for a healthier future—A comprehensive review. *Health Care Science*, *3*(5), 329–349. DOI: 10.1002/hcs2.115 PMID: 39479277

Thakur, S., Kumar, A., Dijkstra, A., & Thakur, A. (2024). Occupational therapy-based rehabilitation of sciatic nerve pain. *Brain-X*, *2*(4), e70010. DOI: 10.1002/brx2.70010

Theodorikakos, S. (2023). *AR & VR application research for medical rehabilitation* (Master's thesis, Πανεπιστήμιο Πειραιώς).

Trovato, V., Sfameni, S., Rando, G., Rosace, G., Libertino, S., Ferri, A., & Plutino, M. R. (2022). A review of stimuli-responsive smart materials for wearable Technology in Healthcare: Retrospective, perspective, and prospective. *Molecules (Basel, Switzerland)*, *27*(17), 5709. DOI: 10.3390/molecules27175709 PMID: 36080476

Ukasi, S., Pongampai, S., Panigrahi, B. K., Panda, S., Hajra, S., Kim, H. J., Vittayakorn, N., & Charoonsuk, T. (2024). Continuous tremor monitoring in Parkinson's disease: A wristwatch-inspired triboelectric sensor approach. *iScience*, *27*(12), 111480. DOI: 10.1016/j.isci.2024.111480 PMID: 39720518

Ullah, M., Hamayun, S., Wahab, A., Khan, S. U., Rehman, M. U., Haq, Z. U., Rehman, K. U., Ullah, A., Mehreen, A., Awan, U. A., Qayum, M., & Naeem, M. (2023). Smart technologies used as smart tools in the management of cardiovascular disease and their future perspective. *Current Problems in Cardiology*, *48*(11), 101922. DOI: 10.1016/j.cpcardiol.2023.101922 PMID: 37437703

Urrea, C., & Agramonte, R. (2023). Improving Exoskeleton Functionality: Design and Comparative Evaluation of Control Techniques for Pneumatic Artificial Muscle Actuators in Lower Limb Rehabilitation and Work Tasks. *Processes (Basel, Switzerland)*, *11*(12), 3278. DOI: 10.3390/pr11123278

Varaganti, P., & Seo, S. (2024). Recent advances in biomimetics for the development of bio-inspired prosthetic limbs. *Biomimetics*, *9*(5), 273. DOI: 10.3390/biomimetics9050273 PMID: 38786483

Verma, R., Akhai, S., & Wadhwa, A. S. (2024). Use of smart materials in physiotherapy. In *Revolutionizing healthcare treatment with sensor technology* (pp. 300–319). IGI Global. DOI: 10.4018/979-8-3693-2762-3.ch019

Waidi, Y. O. (2025). Recent Advances in 4D-Printed Shape Memory Actuators. *Macromolecular Rapid Communications*, *46*(10), 2401141. DOI: 10.1002/marc.202401141 PMID: 40014667

Willingham, T. B., Stowell, J., Collier, G., & Backus, D. (2024). Leveraging emerging technologies to expand accessibility and improve precision in rehabilitation and exercise for people with disabilities. *International Journal of Environmental Research and Public Health, 21*(1), 79. DOI: 10.3390/ijerph21010079 PMID: 38248542

Xu, K., & Qin, S. (2023, May). An Interdisciplinary approach and advanced techniques for enhanced 3D-printed upper limb prosthetic socket design: A literature review. [). MDPI.]. *Actuators, 12*(6), 223. DOI: 10.3390/act12060223

Yang, H., Fang, H., Wang, C., Wang, Y., Qi, C., Zhang, Y., Zhou, Q., Huang, M., Wang, M., & Wu, M. (2024). 3D printing of customized functional devices for smart biomedical systems. *SmartMat, 5*(5), e1244. DOI: 10.1002/smm2.1244

Yihun, Y., & Delgado, P. (2025). Enhancing Personalized Rehabilitation: Integrating Assist-as-Needed System With Real-Time Feedback. *Journal of Engineering and Science in Medical Diagnostics and Therapy, 8*(3), 031002. DOI: 10.1115/1.4066387

Yin, S., Yao, D. R., Song, Y., Heng, W., Ma, X., Han, H., & Gao, W. (2024). Wearable and Implantable Soft Robots. *Chemical Reviews, 124*(20), 11585–11636. DOI: 10.1021/acs.chemrev.4c00513 PMID: 39392765

Zarei, M., Lee, G., Lee, S. G., & Cho, K. (2023). Advances in biodegradable electronic skin: Material progress and recent applications in sensing, robotics, and human–machine interfaces. *Advanced Materials, 35*(4), 2203193. DOI: 10.1002/adma.202203193 PMID: 35737931

Zawar, S., Udhani, R., & Sathe, S. (2024). Closing the Gap on Access to Assistive Technology. *Journal of Research in Medical and Interpathy Sciences, 2*(1), 31–34.

Zaydi, M., Maleh, Y., & Khourdifi, Y. (2025). A new framework for agile cybersecurity risk management: Integrating continuous adaptation and real-time threat intelligence (ACSRM-ICTI). In *Agile Security in the Digital Era* (pp. 19-47). CRC Press.

Zhang, R., Zhou, Y., Zhang, J., & Zhao, J. (2024). Cloud-integrated robotics: Transforming healthcare and rehabilitation for individuals with disabilities. *Proceedings of the Indian National Science Academy. Part A, Physical Sciences, 90*(3), 752–763. DOI: 10.1007/s43538-024-00264-3

Zhang, W. (2025). Enhancing Rehabilitation Assessment with Artificial Intelligence: A Comprehensive Investigation of Posture Quality Prediction Using Machine Learning. In *ITM Web of Conferences* (Vol. 70, p. 02025). EDP Sciences. DOI: 10.1051/itmconf/20257002025

Zhang, Z., Wen, F., Sun, Z., Guo, X., He, T., & Lee, C. (2022). Artificial intelligence-enabled sensing technologies in the 5G/internet of things era: From virtual reality/augmented reality to the digital twin. *Advanced Intelligent Systems*, *4*(7), 2100228. DOI: 10.1002/aisy.202100228

Zhou, Y. (2024). User experience of lower extremity exoskeletons and its improvement methodologies: A narrative review. *Proceedings of the Institution of Mechanical Engineers. Part H, Journal of Engineering in Medicine*, *238*(11-12), 1052–1068. DOI: 10.1177/09544119241291194 PMID: 39552186

KEY TERMS AND DEFINITIONS

3D Printing in Rehabilitation: Cost-effective manufacturing of personalized prosthetics and orthotics using additive technology.

Adaptive Prosthetics: Prosthetic limbs with real-time stiffness and grip adjustment for varied terrains and user needs.

AI-Driven Rehabilitation: Use of artificial intelligence to predict complications, personalize rehabilitation strategies, and improve therapy outcomes.

Augmented Reality (AR) Rehabilitation: Real-time movement correction using digital overlays during therapy.

Brain-Material Interfaces: Emerging systems enabling brain-controlled prosthetics through neural integration with smart materials.

Climate-Adaptive Devices: Prosthetics and orthotics that adapt to extreme heat or cold, ensuring comfort and reliability.

Drug-Eluting Smart Patches: Automated medication delivery patches that release drugs based on physiological signals.

Dynamic Compression Wear: Sleeves using magnetorheological fluids to adjust compression levels for lymphedema patients.

Electroactive Polymers (EAPs): Flexible materials that deform under electric fields, enabling prosthetic devices to mimic natural muscle movements.

Exoskeletons: Robotic wearables powered by smart materials to restore mobility in spinal injury and neuromuscular patients.

Haptic Feedback Gloves: Sensory gloves restoring touch sensation for patients with neuropathy or sensory loss.

Orthotics: Custom-fit external devices, increasingly using smart materials for dynamic support in conditions like cerebral palsy.

Piezoelectric Sensors: Sensors that generate electrical signals under stress, widely applied in tremor monitoring for Parkinson's disease and gait analysis.

Chapter 11 Advancing Skin Cancer Diagnosis Using Computer Vision to Aid the Visually Impaired

Ratish Palanisamy
https://orcid.org/0009-0009-3555-7435
Heriot-Watt University, UAE

Drishty Sobnath
https://orcid.org/0009-0001-9639-0079
Heriot-Watt University, UAE

Heba Elshimy
https://orcid.org/0000-0001-8465-8050
Heriot-Watt University, UAE

ABSTRACT

Skin cancer is one of the most common forms of cancer, with early detection being crucial for effective treatment. Individuals with visual impairment often struggle to monitor skin lesions independently, typically depending on caregivers or dermatologists for assistance. This study develops a skin cancer detection system using dermoscopic images from the HAM10000 dataset, evaluating four deep learning models to assist caregivers and dermatologists in providing faster analysis for the individuals who are visually impaired. The research employs segmentation masks to crop images during preprocessing, with data augmentation and transfer learning for optimizing performance. Among the models used, EfficientNetV2-L achieved the highest accuracy of 95.1% and a recall of 86.3% for malignant lesions in binary

DOI: 10.4018/979-8-3373-2033-5.ch011

classification, showing reliable classification of cancerous lesions. This system helps caregivers and dermatologists with a tool to efficiently monitor skin health for visually impaired individuals, reducing diagnostic delays and supporting faster decision making.

INTRODUCTION

Skin cancer is one of the most prevalent types of cancer worldwide, primarily caused by genetic and environmental factors, with prolonged exposure to ultraviolet (UV) radiation being a significant risk factor (Craythorne & Al-Niami, 2017). Skin lesions, which refer to areas of skin that differ from the surrounding skin, are common and often result from injuries or environmental exposure. Early detection is essential for better outcomes, but visually impaired individuals encounter distinct challenges in examining their own skin for suspicious lesions, often resulting in delayed diagnoses. The goal is to enable faster decision-making for dermatologists and caregivers in addressing skin cancer for the visually impaired individuals, improving their quality of life.

At least 2.2 billion people have vision impairment globally, with 1 billion cases being potentially preventable or are not addressed due to limited access to eye care services (World Health Organization, 2019). Additionally, according to recent statistics, over 331,722 new cases of skin cancer were reported in 2022, making it the 14th most common cancer among both men and women (World Cancer Research Fund, 2024). Visually impaired individuals often cannot visually inspect their skin for lesions, relying instead on caregivers or family members, which can result in inconsistent or delayed detection. Caregivers bear additional burdens, highlighting the need for tools that streamline this process.

Artificial Intelligence (AI) is transforming the healthcare industry by leveraging various machine learning techniques such as deep learning and computer vision. AI has been applied in healthcare to reduce costs, provide guidance during surgeries, support clinical trials, and improve patient care (Shaheen, 2021). Machine learning techniques, particularly convolutional neural networks (CNNs) and computer vision, play a significant role in analyzing skin cancer patterns. These technologies have been shown to outperform professional dermatologists in certain diagnostic scenarios, enhancing early detection accuracy and reducing healthcare workload. The use of machine learning in skin cancer detection leads to improved treatment outcomes and reduced mortality rates (Nahata & Singh, 2020).

While AI excels in general detection, a key gap lies in caregiver-focused applications for visually impaired individuals, where traditional methods like manual checks fall short. This chapter bridges this gap by evaluating deep learning models on the HAM10000 dataset, providing a deep learning-based skin cancer detection system for caregivers and dermatologists to aid in skin cancer detection for visually impaired individuals, enabling faster decision making. It also shows how combining CNN-based classification with segmentation masks can effectively classify cancerous lesions in dermatoscopic images. This chapter will also explore existing assistive technologies for visually impaired individuals, enabling early detection of potential skin cancer risks. Figure 1 shows the number of skin cancer cases globally in 2022.

Figure 1. Number of Skin Cancer cases globally in 2022

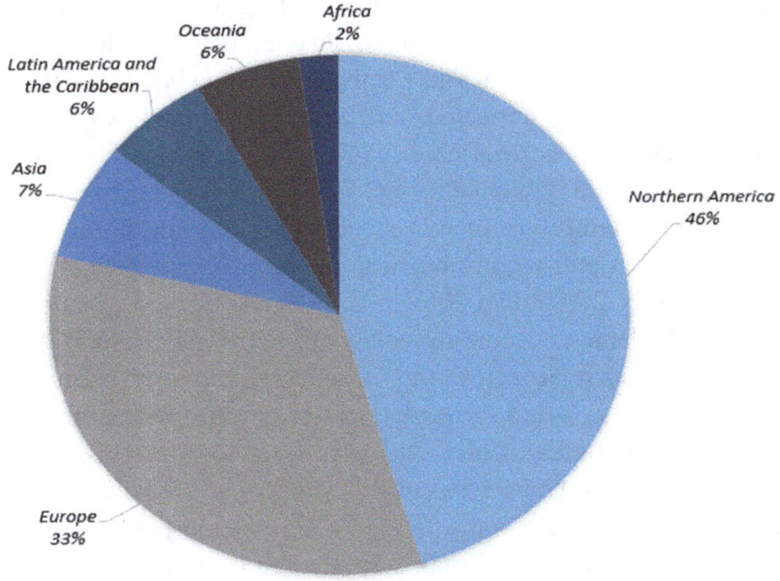

Note. Reprinted from Detection of Skin Cancer Based on Skin Lesion Images Using Deep Learning, by W. Gouda, N. U. Sama, G. Al-Waakid, M. Humayun, & N. Z. Jhanjhi, 2022, Healthcare, 10(7), Article 1183 (https://doi.org/10.3390/healthcare10071183). Licensed under CC BY 4.0.

The sections are organized as follows: Section 2 reviews the background on assistive technologies for the visually impaired and literature on deep learning for skin cancer diagnosis. Section 3 details the method and evaluation metrics. Section 4 shows the implementation of the study. Section 5 presents the evaluation and discusses the models performance. Section 6 provides the conclusion and recommendations for future research.

BACKGROUND

This section reviews foundational concepts, starting with skin cancer before linking to visual impairment challenges and assistive baselines, building towards AI's role in support for visually impaired individuals. It also reviews machine learning and image classification techniques in skin cancer detection.

Overview of Skin Cancer

Skin cancer generally occurs when abnormal cells grow in skin tissues, often due to UV exposure. Normally, new cells replace old ones, but UV light can disrupt this process, causing rapid cell growth. These cells can be either benign (non-cancerous) or malignant (cancerous). If untreated, skin cancer can spread, but early detection and treatment generally lead to a cure (Cleveland Clinic, 2021). Skin cancer is categorized into two main types: melanoma and non-melanoma. Melanoma is considered the most dangerous type of skin cancer, while non-melanoma skin cancers are less dangerous but still require medical attention. The incidence rate of new melanoma cases is 21.2 per 100,000 men and women per year (National Cancer Institute, 2018). Melanoma occurs in melanocytes, the cells responsible for skin pigmentation. It is often referred to as the "deadliest skin cancer" because it spreads easily and can appear as a dark, irregular spot or develop in existing moles. The ABCDE (Asymmetry, Border, Color, Diameter, Evolving) warning signs are used to detect melanoma early. Other types of skin cancer include basal cell carcinoma (BCC) and squamous cell carcinoma (SCC). BCC is the most common skin cancer, often occurring in individuals with fair skin, though it can affect other skin tones as well. BCC typically develops after prolonged sun exposure or indoor tanning and appears as a flesh-colored growth, pearl-like bump, or pinkish patch. SCC, the second most common type, manifests as a red, firm bump, scaly patch, or a sore that heals and reopens. SCC can grow deep into the skin, leading to significant damage and disfigurement. Another precancerous condition associated with skin cancer is actinic keratosis (AK). AK manifests as dry, scaly patches or spots on the skin and can develop into SCC. Early prevention and treatment of AK are essential to reduce the risk of progression to SCC (American Academy of Dermatology Association, 2024). Preventing skin cancer involves minimizing UV exposure from the sun, avoiding tanning beds, staying out of direct sunlight between 10 a.m. and 4 p.m., wearing protective clothing and hats, and applying SPF 30+ sunscreen every two hours (Bodemer, 2020). Skin cancer can become life-threatening when it spreads beyond the skin to organs and lymph nodes. However, early detection and treatment significantly improve the chances of successful prevention (Cleveland Clinic, 2021). Therefore, early detection is critical to prevent skin cancer from progressing into a more dangerous and life-threatening condition. For visually impaired individuals, this detection relies on caregivers and dermatologists, where AI systems can help in consistent monitoring.

Overview of Visual Impairment and Healthcare Access

Vision is an important human sense which is essential for learning, mobility, education, and employment. Visual impairment ranges from low vision to complete blindness, where vision cannot be corrected to normal levels through standard means such as glasses, contact lenses, or surgery (World Health Organization, 2023). The main causes include uncorrected refractive errors, cataracts, age-related macular degeneration, glaucoma, and diabetic retinopathy (World Health Organization, 2023). Individuals with vision impairment face a range of challenges that impact their ability to carry out daily activities such as managing the home, transportation, finances, shopping, and healthcare (Remillard et al., 2023). These difficulties not only arise from visual limitations like trouble reading fine print on medicines, navigating safely, or identifying objects, but also from the need to rely on caretakers or family members, inaccessible technology and websites which are not suitable for visually impaired individuals, and transportation barriers (Remillard et al., 2023). These issues faced by individuals with visual impairment can result in emotional stress which can reduce their confidence, and by environmental gaps and limited support services. Overall, vision impairment involves navigating a mix of personal, technological, and societal obstacles that gives less independence and access to everyday life activities.

The healthcare access barriers faced by visually impaired can be solved by multiple approaches. Traditional, non-AI-based assistive technologies remain as a foundation for supporting visually impaired individuals in healthcare settings. Screen readers and screen magnification software enable users to interact with electronic health records and digital health portals by converting text and graphical elements into speech (Giansanti & Pirrera, 2025). Additionally, traditional assistive technologies, such as white canes, Braille, and audiobooks, have supported visually impaired individuals for a long time (Naayini et al., 2025). While useful, these tools are limited when it comes to flexibility and personalization and are unable to adapt to diverse contexts. Basic consumer technology such as voice-activated assistants also can help in healthcare by enabling users to schedule appointments, set medication reminders, or query health-related information entirely through voice commands (Giansanti & Pirrera, 2025).

AI-Powered Assistive Technologies for Visually Impaired in Healthcare

Artificial intelligence (AI) has transformed assistive technologies for visually impaired individuals, particularly in healthcare settings. AI powered solutions take advantage of machine learning, computer vision, and natural language processing to enable greater independence and accessibility.

A significant advancement is the emergence of wearable AI devices capable of real-time object recognition, scene description, and reading both printed and digital text. For example, OrCam MyEye is a wearable device that uses computer vision to recognize faces, identify products, and read aloud from various text sources, helping visually impaired individuals interact with their environment and healthcare documents (Giansanti & Pirrera, 2025). Systems such as vision-based human activity recognition systems (HAR) are gaining attention as they allow for understanding of user behaviour in indoor settings. These systems can detect actions, movements, and potentially dangerous scenarios which increases both independence and safety. Such technology could alert users to obstacles, detect falls, or assist with tasks that require spatial awareness (Giansanti & Pirrera, 2025). Wearable devices such as Envision Glasses use camera-based vision with speech output to recognize text and faces, while the Sunu Band uses haptic feedback for detection of obstacles. These devices promote independence in daily living, but still face challenges related to high costs, short battery life, and reduced accessibility in low-income environments (Naayini et al., 2025).

A device known as AiSee is a wearable assistive device developed to help visually impaired individuals carry out everyday tasks more freely, especially for a setting like grocery stores (Boldu et al., 2020). It uses a wearable camera and uses large language models to identify objects and answer voice queries about them. AiSee helps solve common challenges such as identifying products, reading labels, and relying on caretakers or others for assistance. Instead of the need to hold a phone camera, the users just need to simply point in the direction of an object, and AiSee describes it out loud, helping them find difference between similar items and confirm details like product names (Boldu et al., 2020). Its design has also been developed in a way so it helps the visually impaired individuals feel more comfortable in public by being less noticeable than traditional tools. Few problems such as recognition errors and delayed responses also occurred occasionally.

A deep learning approach to address the challenges faced by visually impaired individuals in understanding visual content was proposed by Bipin & Abirami (2023), the approach involves using an image captioning system that functions by generating descriptive text explaining the image from input images which are provided. Bipin & Abirami (2023) proposed a model which uses a CNN model (Inception V3) as encoder with a Gated Recurrent Unit (GRU) for sequential text generation and it acts as the decoder, which is enhanced by an attention mechanism to focus on key image regions. Their system achieved a highest overall Bilingual Evaluation Understudy (BLEU) score of 34.89, with over 1,600 images receiving high or perfect scores. This architecture helps users who are visually impaired to receive clear, situation-based captions, supporting greater independence in daily activities such as reading labels or identifying objects. The caption accuracy outperformed by 10.59% compared to other approaches on the same dataset (Bipin & Abirami, 2023). Also, AI-powered systems use computer vision to translate visual information into accessible formats. Applications such as Microsoft's Seeing AI and Google Lookout identify objects, text, people, and scenes, while volunteer-based platforms like Be My Eyes provide real-time assistance through video connections (Naayini et al., 2025). While these tools enhance environmental awareness, they are limited by poor lighting or reliance on internet connectivity.

Natural Language Processing (NLP) has enabled visually impaired individuals to access and interact with digital content through screen readers like Job Access With Speech (JAWS) and Non-Visual Desktop Access (NVDA), which convert text into speech or Braille (Naayini et al., 2025). AI tools such as NaturalReader provide more realistic-sounding synthesis, and voice assistants such as Siri and Alexa allow for hands-free device control, task automation, and retrieving information. However, performance may be reduced in multi language contexts or when technical content is heavy (Naayini et al., 2025).

A review for AI-powered assistive technologies for the visually impaired individuals by Okolo et al. (2024) shows that most systems do not calculate object distance which seems to be a limitation, and deep learning frameworks like YOLO and SSD are popular due to their speed and efficiency. Many solutions aim to provide real-time assistance using audio feedback or sensor alerts (Okolo et al., 2024). AI-based assistive technologies show high accuracy but most still need improvements in estimating distance, adapting to different environments, and processing efficiency to fully support independent mobility for visually impaired individuals.

Machine Learning in Skin Cancer Detection

Early detection is vital for effective skin cancer treatment for visually impaired individuals. The gold standard for diagnosing skin cancer is by performing a biopsy, where a sample is taken from an abnormal lesion to check if it's cancerous. This process is generally very slow, painful, and costly. Computer-based methods make it possible to provide a faster, non-invasive, and more affordable approach. Non-invasive methods analyze skin lesions to identify melanoma and non-melanoma types. These are usually implemented through computer-aided skin cancer detection models, which include capturing an image, preprocessing it, segmenting areas of interest, extracting key features, and classifying the lesion (Dildar et al., 2021). Machine learning has made remarkable strides in the medical field, particularly in skin cancer detection, where it supports dermatologists through early detection or screening, automated image analysis and for decision support. In particular, deep learning and convolutional neural networks (CNNs) are considered powerful tools for skin cancer detection through image analysis. By training on large datasets, CNNs can recognize complex patterns, differentiate benign from malignant lesions, and achieve dermatologist-level accuracy. Techniques like image classification, feature extraction, and segmentation allow CNNs to study clinical and histopathological images. However, machine learning still requires large, unique datasets, interpretability, and strong privacy measures for optimal performance. Doctors acceptance is also crucial, as machine learning aims to support, not replace, medical professionals, ensuring improved diagnostic accuracy and early detection. As the technology evolves, incorporating patient and doctor feedback will be essential for broader clinical trust (Das et al., 2021). Therefore, machine learning (ML) and deep learning (DL) algorithms are being extensively used in cancer detection, both achieving varying levels of accuracy depending on the datasets provided. Researchers are primarily focused on developing and improving advanced ML and DL models to enhance diagnostic accuracy and adapt to different types of data. Future research should emphasize developing intelligent prediction models that enable early cancer detection without direct medical intervention (Selvaraj & Aruna, 2023). The cancer and non-cancer lesion detection process can be divided into several steps: inputting the image, preprocessing it, segmenting the image, extracting features, and classifying the image, which results in identifying whether the lesion is cancerous or non-cancerous. This process aids caregivers and dermatologists in monitoring visually impaired individuals by classifying lesions efficiently. These steps are illustrated in Figure 2.

Figure 2. Skin Cancer Detection Pipeline

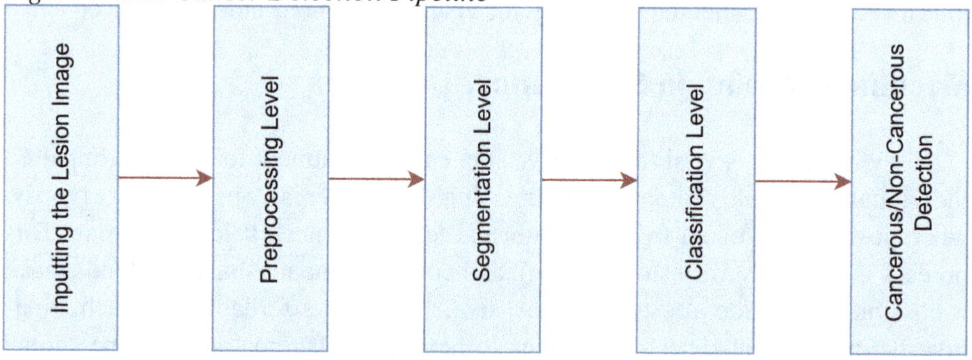

Image preprocessing is a vital initial step in computer vision tasks, especially in detecting skin cancer using dermoscopic lesion images. Image scaling enhances image quality by eliminating irrelevant areas and emphasizing key features, making the images more suitable for analysis. The main techniques researchers use include image scaling, color space transformation, illumination correction, contrast enhancement, artifact removal, noise removal, and hair removal (Oliveira et al., 2016). Overall, these preprocessing steps help give a more optimized image, resulting in better classification results. The methods used in preprocessing include several steps within them. They are mainly categorized as enhancement, restoration, and hair removal techniques. Image scaling is defined as changing the size of a digital image. In vector graphics, mathematical formulas show the path on how it is shaped and what color it is filled with; when resized, this is how they maintain their quality. On the other hand, raster graphics use arranged color pixels to display an image, and when resized, they create a new image with a different number of pixels. Image quality could be lost when pixels are reduced. Image scaling techniques are of great use since skin cancer images usually come in different shapes and sizes (Vocaturo et al., 2018).

Color space transformation mainly represents how the colors are arranged in an image. The color spaces generally used in image processing are RGB, HSI, CIE LAB, and CIE-XYZ. They are used to improve color information in an image, making skin cancer detection more efficient, and each color space has its own advantages. The RGB color space, consisting of red, green, and blue colors, is the most widely used as these colors are commonly present in images (Vocaturo et al., 2018). The illumination correction method doesn't involve many steps as it is based on the illumination of the image. Depending on whether it is dark or too bright, adjusting it accordingly will help locate the lesion better. Contrast enhancement plays an important role when it comes to enhancing the images and identifying key features in the lesion image. It uses brightness to show the difference between the object and its background. The main goal is to have everything in perfect contrast because if one area is highlighted more, other areas could lose their value. It is further divided into types: linear and nonlinear methods, with nonlinear methods being more frequently used in medical images. The linear technique mainly adjusts the image gray level values to stretch the histogram in upper and lower levels; it is often referred to as contrast stretching. Nonlinear methods include Histogram equalization (HE) and Adaptive Histogram equalization (AHE), and they work best when it comes to showing the important features in skin lesion images, making melanoma detection easier (Vocaturo et al., 2018).

Noise removal is considered an important step when preparing an image for analysis. Noise has different types, which include Gaussian noise, commonly present in the blue channel of cameras when taking skin lesion images; salt-and-pepper noise, which appears as white pixels in dark images and dark pixels in light images; Poisson noise, which appears grainy due to variations in electric charge and photon emission; and speckle noise, which is part of the granular type and often seen in radar images. These types of noise can affect image interpretation. Denoising techniques include methods such as spatial filtering and transfer domain filtering. For dermatoscopic images, mean filters are used for reducing Gaussian noise, median filters work best on salt-and-pepper noise, adaptive filters change according to pixel values and could be used for speckle noise, and statistical filters help with speckle noise. These filters greatly improve image quality during preprocessing (Vocaturo et al., 2018).

Artifacts consist of hair, shadows, reflections, water bubbles, skin markings, gel, and colored lesions. These artifacts, when present in images, can heavily affect the detection of skin cancer, resulting in incorrect classification. Hence, it is necessary that these artifacts are removed in image preprocessing (Oliveira et al., 2016; Vocaturo et al., 2018). Hair removal is necessary in dermatoscopic images, as hair can interfere with detecting small skin lesions. The methods used for hair removal include morphological operations, inpainting methods, top-hat transformations, the DullRazor tool (a software for hair removal), and fast hair segmentation. These methods ensure images are clear of hair artifacts, ensuring accurate skin cancer detection (Vocaturo et al., 2018).

Image Classification

This subsection will mainly talk about CNNs process and commonly used CNN architectures used in skin cancer detection. Then, it will also explore vision transformers used in skin cancer detection.

Convolutional Neural Networks (CNNs) for Skin Lesion Analysis

Convolutional Neural Networks (CNNs) are a part of neural networks and play a significant role in image processing and the computer vision domain. Researchers mainly focus on improving the structure of CNNs using optimized algorithms, which enhance their performance (Zhang et al., 2019). CNNs simplify the process of locating cancerous areas and identifying cancerous lesions, thereby reducing the workload of dermatologists and improving diagnostic accuracy. They are a more efficient type of artificial neural network, requiring fewer connections between their layers. The main layers of a CNN include convolutional, pooling, and fully connected layers (Nahata & Singh, 2020).

Convolutional Layer. CNNs are designed to process images by extracting only the key features that make them unique. They consist of convolutional layers, which play a vital role in feature extraction from images by using filters. These filters recognize edges, corners, and other characteristics of the skin lesion (Kumar et al., 2024; Nahata & Singh, 2020). While convolutional layers are excellent at identifying image features, increasing the number of layers results in a higher computational load. Activation functions such as ReLU, used in Kumar et al. (2024), can be applied to facilitate the learning of complex patterns.

Pooling Layer. The pooling layers in CNN help reduce the number of parameters while maintaining the key features, they also reduce the computational load overall. They consist of three types, Max pooling is the most commonly used as it helps reduce the computational load and perform dimensionality reduction tasks (Nahata & Singh, 2020).

Fully Connected Layer. Fully connected layers are also part of CNN, where the neurons are all connected to combine features from the previous layer. The last layers acts as the deciding factor whether the skin lesion is benign or malignant (Kumar et al., 2024).

CNN Architectures Used In Skin Cancer Detection

In the field of computer vision, different CNN architectures are used for creating algorithms.

VGG: VGG is known for its simplicity and effectiveness and is mainly part of the convolutional architecture. The commonly used models are VGG-16 and VGG-19. VGG-16 consists of convolutional layers, a max-pooling layer, fully connected layers, and the output layer. VGG-19 has also proven to be better than DenseNet in Barbadekar et al. (2023). It is exceptional at capturing fine image details and is valuable in the medical field. However, its downsides include requiring a lot of resources and having a heavy computational cost (Naqvi et al., 2023).

Inception V3: Inception V3 architecture uses various convolution filter sizes within each layer for processing features and capturing details across multiple resolutions (Gouda et al., 2022). Nahata & Singh (2020) have shown that when it comes to classifying skin lesions, it has achieved an average accuracy of 90%. Its ability to capture multiple resolutions allows it to classify both small and large lesions. Inception V3 has performed the best in Gouda et al. (2022) with an accuracy of 85.7% because of its ability to capture complex features. Inception V3 also outperforms models like VGG due to its flexibility in feature extraction, which makes it ideal for skin cancer detection compared to VGG's simple structure.

DenseNet: DenseNet is a CNN model whose architecture involves dense blocks that connect each layer to every other layer. Its design helps with efficiency and reduction of parameters (Naqvi et al., 2023). DenseNet is effective with small datasets and has feature reuse, which is beneficial in medical datasets where large datasets are not available. Barbadekar et al. (2023) has proven that DenseNet has an accuracy of 89.49%, whereas VGG-19 has an accuracy of 97.29% and has proven to be better than it in all aspects. Although DenseNet is known for its feature reuse, its dense connections increase memory requirements, which may be a problem in hardware-limited scenarios.

MobileNet: MobileNet is an architecture of CNN that is specifically designed for mobile applications. It doesn't have good accuracy compared to other models, its suitability for skin cancer detection on mobile devices is high (Nahata & Singh, 2020). While it doesn't perform as accurately as other models, its lightweight nature makes it possible for telemedicine and remote diagnosis, especially in areas with limited medical resources.

Residual Networks in Skin Cancer Detection

Residual Networks, introduced by He et al. (2015), helped deep learning by mitigating the vanishing gradient problem in very deep neural networks. It uses residual blocks and skip connections which enables the training of architectures with hundreds of layers and allows the model to learn hierarchical features with great effect. ResNet is commonly used in skin cancer detection due to its robustness, and it can adapt to complex datasets which have a wide variety of dermoscopic images and different classes associated with the images. ResNet has different types such as ResNet-50 and ResNet-101 which are used often as baselines or backbones in medical imaging analysis, thus showing their importance.

ResNet-50: ResNet50 has a huge impact on deep learning, especially in computer vision. It is a deep CNN model with a 50-layer Residual network and skip connections that bypass certain layers. This design mitigates issues related to the vanishing gradient, which allows for deeper networks and the capture of more information (Gouda et al., 2022). Prasher et al. (2023) used ResNet50 for skin cancer classification and applied transfer learning to achieve high accuracy, when pre-trained on ImageNet, ResNet50's transfer learning capabilities allow it to take advantage of the features from a big dataset, improving its performance on medical images. ResNet50 achieves considerable accuracy in skin cancer detection, although it performs slightly below InceptionV3 on the ISIC 2018 dataset in (Gouda et al., 2022). Compared with other ResNet models such as ResNet18 and ResNet34, ResNet50 have outperformed them by achieving 95.3% in skin cancer diagnosis (Alharith et al., 2024). In general, ResNet50 is ideal for complex medical images, but its deep depth can significantly increase computational load.

ResNet-101: ResNet-101 is a variant of ResNet that is 101 layers deep and is employed widely in skin cancer classification. Its architecture includes residual connections that remove the vanishing gradient problem, allowing the deeper networks to still maintain effective feature learning. ResNet-101 consists of 104 convolution layers in total, including 33 deep residual modules out of which 29 blocks directly taking outputs from previous layers through skip connections (Demir et al., n.d.). This guarantees efficient gradient flow and improved feature extraction. When compared to different models of ResNet in (Hossain et al., 2021), for detecting malignant and benign skin lesion, ResNet-101 achieved an accuracy of 89.09% just coming short of 0.55% compared ResNet-152 which was the highest. ResNet-101 has strong performance and, but it requires higher computational resources which could pose some challenges. Its ability to extract hierarchical feature from skin lesion images makes it a strong candidate despite the limitations.

EfficientNetV2 for Enhanced Classification

EfficientNetV2, introduced by Tan & Le (2021), shows strong advantage over the original EfficientNet family by optimizing both performance and training efficiency. It builds on the compound scaling principles of the original EfficientNet, but EfficientNetV2 includes FusedMBConv blocks, progressive learning, and adaptive regularization which helps it to achieve faster training and higher accuracy with just fewer parameters. These upgrades make EfficientNetV2 more appropriate for resource-constrained studies, such as skin cancer detection. In the vast scope medical image analysis, EfficientNetV2's ability to balance computational efficiency with high classification accuracy makes it a strong contender. EfficientNetV2 family consists of S, M, L for the small, medium and large versions of the model. Figure 3 shows the MBConv layer and Fused-MBConv layer in an EfficientNetV2 model.

Figure 3. MBConv and Fused-MBConv Layers in the EfficientNetV2 Architecture

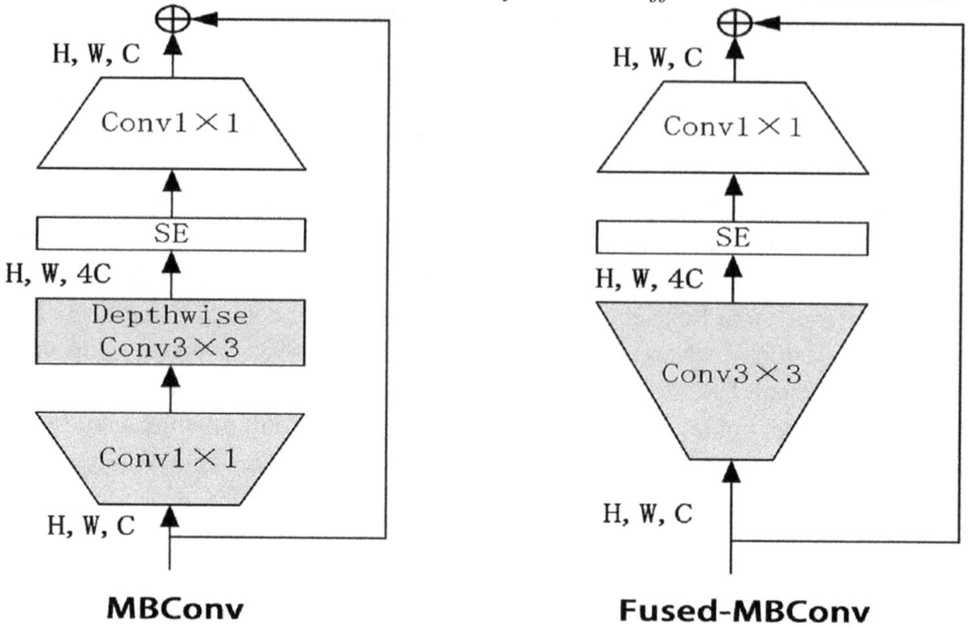

Note. Reprinted from EFFNet: A skin cancer classification model based on feature fusion and random forests, by X. Ma, J. Shan, F. Ning, W. Li, & H. Li, 2023, PLOS ONE, 18(10), e0293266 (https://doi.org/10.1371/journal.pone.0293266). Licensed under CC BY 4.0

EfficientNetV2-L: EfficientNetV2-L has around 120 million parameters, with it being one of the bigger models in the EfficientNetV2 family, it aims for high accuracy on complex tasks through its larger capacity. EfficientNetV2-L also uses MBConv and Fused-MBConv blocks that allows it for efficient feature extraction. EfficientNetV2-L has not only achieved higher accuracy than models like ViT-L/16 which is a vision transformer model, it has done it while training faster than it by 5x-11x (Tan & Le, 2021). EfficientNetV2-L was refined with transfer learning in Nasra (2024) for classification of benign or malignant skin lesions, it has performed extremely good by achieving 96% accuracy which is higher than other common CNN architectures. A novel ensemble was proposed by Rahman et al. (2025) combining EfficientNetV2-L with LightGBM (LGBM), but when EfficientNetV2-L was tested alone, it achieved higher than the EfficientNetV2-L model in Nasra (2024) by 1.47%.

ConvNeXt: A Modern CNN Architecture

ConvNeXt, introduced by Liu et al. (2022), shows a modern evolution of CNNs by taking design principles from transformer models while keeping the efficiency of traditional convolutional architectures. The ConvNeXt architecture has enhancements like larger kernels, inverted bottlenecks, and layer normalization, making it achieve performance competitive with or greater than transformers. ConvNeXt is a recent advancement that shows continuous innovation in CNN design for applications involving image classification. ConvNeXt family consists of T, S, B, L and XL for the tiny, small, base, large and extra large version of the model.

ConvNeXt-Tiny: The smallest variant in the ConvNeXt family is ConvNeXt-T, it has around 28 million parameters. Its improved architecture is inspired by ResNet, having depth-wise convolutions, increased kernel size (7x7), GELU activation, and layer normalization, which improves performance while maintaining computational efficiency especially for the tiny variant (Kablan & Ayas, 2024). A ConvNeXt ensemble model was proposed in Kablan & Ayas (2024) for skin cancer classification combining all ConvNeXt models and testing them separately also, ConvNeXt-T despite being the smallest achieved 96.9%, and was behind the large variant of ConvNeXt by a difference of 0.3% showing its efficient performance. ConvNeXt-T despite having less parameters compared to a model like Swin Transformer, it still achieves similar accuracy (Reddy et al., 2024).

Vision Transformers in Skin Lesion Classification

Vision Transformers (ViTs), introduced by Dosovitskiy et al. (2021), marks a change from the traditional convolutional neural networks (CNNs) by adapting to transformer architecture which was originally developed for natural language processing (NLP) to image classification tasks. While CNNs perform well at extracting hierarchical, localized features through convolutional filters, ViTs architecture takes advantage of self-attention to model long range dependencies across an image by dividing it into patches, applying patch embeddings, and processing them through transformer encoder layers with a classification head, which enables global feature capture for tasks like skin cancer detection (Dosovitskiy et al., 2021).

ViT-B/16: ViT-B/16 is the base variant of the Vision Transformer, where the B stands for base. It is characterized by a patch size of 16x16 pixels, 12 transformer encoder layers, and 12 attention heads per layer (Dahmani et al., 2024). ViT-B/16 when compared to ViT-B/32 in Dahmani et al. (2024) has outperformed it by getting an accuracy of 97% surpassing it by 2% in skin cancer classification, this is due to the fact that ViT-B/16 small patches result in larger sequence length allowing for finer feature extraction and improved classification performance. A pre-32trained ViT-B/16 is used in Elbedoui et al. (2024) along with EfficientNetV2-B0 and a CNN, when compared against each in classifying benign and malignant lesions, ViT-B/16 achieved higher accuracy than both the models, however, state-of-the-art CNN architectures such as VGG16 and ResNet18 showed better accuracy on the same dataset. ViT-B/16's ability to learn very detailed lesion characteristics through self-attention makes it a strong alternative to CNNs for skin cancer classification.

METHOD

In the system's architecture, images will be processed through a deep learning pipeline to detect skin cancer. Each image will first undergo preprocessing to improve quality and adjust image size, followed by using segmentation masks to crop images properly to isolate the lesion areas. The preprocessed skin lesions are then passed to a classification model using transfer learning to identify cancerous and non-cancerous types. This pipeline serves as a skin cancer detection tool for caregivers monitoring visually impaired individuals, enabling quick analysis. Figure 4 shows how the workflow of the model would look like.

Figure 4. System Methodology

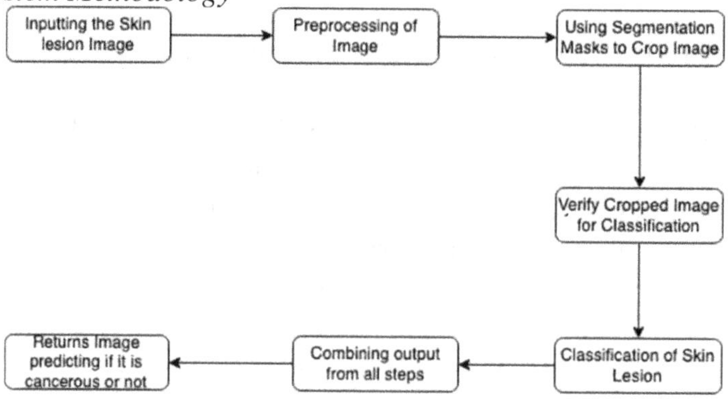

The process begins with inputting skin lesion images from the HAM10000 dataset. The images then go through preprocessing using segmentation masks to crop the image. When the images are preprocessed, data augmentation techniques are applied and then the image is normalized which is done programatically. After preprocessing and data augmentation, 4 deep learning models (ResNet-101, EfficientNetV2-L, ConvNeXt-T and ViT-B/16) using transfer learning will be used to classify whether the lesion is cancerous or non-cancerous. Optimization techniques such as AdamW is also used to improve performance of the model. The models will also perform multi-class classification of skin lesions.

Evaluation Metrics

Evaluation metrics are crucial to get the accuracy and effectiveness of skin cancer detection systems. These metrics provide a way to evaluate how well the model classifies lesions in skin images. The right evaluation of the model can help predict the system's helpfulness for the caregivers monitoring the visually impaired individuals. The metrics that are going to be used in evaluation of the models are Accuracy, Precision, Sensitivity/Recall and F1 score.

TP: True Positive (Skin lesion is actually cancerous and model predicts it correctly)
FP: False Positive (Skin lesion is non-cancerous but the model incorrectly predicts it as having cancer)
TN: True Negative (Skin lesion is actually non-cancerous and model correctly predicts it)
FN: False Negative (Skin lesion image is actually cancerous, but the model incorrectly predicts it as non-cancerous)

Accuracy

Accuracy is a metric that divides the number of accurate predictions by the total number of predictions.

$$Accuracy = \frac{TP + TN}{TP + TN + FP + FN}$$

Precision

Precision is defined as the proportion of true positives among all positive results predicted by the model.

$$Precision = \frac{TP}{TP + FP}$$

Sensitivity/Recall

The ability of the model to correctly identify actual positive cases is what sensitivity does.

$$Sensitivity = \frac{TP}{TP + FN}$$

F1 Score

The harmonic mean of precision and recall is the F1 score.

$$F1\ Score\ =\ 2\ \times \frac{Precision\ \times Sensitivity}{Precision + Sensitivity}$$

AUC (Area Under the Curve)

Area under the ROC curve measures the model's ability for differentiating between benign and malignant lesions.

AP (Average Precision)

Calculates Average precision across all recall levels, focusing on the positive class (malignant lesions) which is suitable for imbalanced datasets.

Macro-Average

For multi-class classification (7 classes), macro-averaged Precision, Sensitivity, and F1 Score are calculated by averaging the metric for each class which gives equal weight to all classes despite imbalances.

IMPLEMENTATION

Development Tools & Platform

The primary hardware platform for this study was a personal computer equipped with an NVIDIA RTX 3070 Ti GPU, an Intel Core i9-10850-K, and 32 GB of RAM. Nvidia CUDA (12.6) was used to enable GPU acceleration, significantly speeding up the training and inference processes for the deep learning models. This study is ran on a Windows 11 operating system, which provided a stable environment for development and compatibility with the chosen software tools.

Software and Libraries

This study used Python (version 3.13) as the main programming language because of its wide support for machine learning libraries and easy to use. Python was ideal for data preprocessing, model training and evaluation tasks. The development environment was set up using Anaconda to create isolated virtual environments which ensures compatibility of dependencies. All work, including preprocessing, training, and evaluation, was done in Jupyter Notebooks (.ipynb files). Several libraries were used in this study for skin lesion classification, as shown in Table 1. These tools were chosen for their efficiency in deep learning, computer vision, and data preprocessing tasks.

Table 1. Libraries Used for the Study

Library	Version	Purpose
PyTorch	2.6.0+cu126	Deep learning framework for model training and evaluation.
torchvision	0.21.0+cu126	Data loading, image transformations and access to pre-trained models (EfficientNetV2-L, ResNet-101, ConvNeXt-Tiny).
timm	1.0.15	Access to pre-trained Vision Transformer (ViT) model.
scikit-learn	1.5.1	Evaluation metrics (precision, recall, F1-score, confusion matrices).
NumPy	1.26.4	Numerical operations on image data for preprocessing
Pandas	2.2.2	Managing HAM10000 dataset metadata.
Matplotlib	3.9.3	Plotting graphs and visualizations.
Seaborn	0.13.2	Creating heatmaps and visualizations
OpenCV (cv2)	4.11.0.86	Image loading, resizing, and cropping using segmentation masks.

Dataset

HAM10000 Dataset Description

In this study, Human Against Machine with 10000 training images Tschandl (2018) (HAM10000) dataset is going to be used, containing 10,015 dermoscopic images representing various skin lesion types. Each image in the dataset is anonymized to ensure patient privacy and follows GDPR and other data protection regulations. Also, no personal information is associated with the images, making sure that the ethical guidelines are followed. These images include common and rare skin conditions, making it suitable for training deep learning models in skin cancer research. The total number of images in this dataset adds up to 10,015 images and contains seven classes of pigmented lesions which are: Actinic keratoses, Basal cell carcinoma, benign keratosis-like lesions (solar lentigines / seborrheic keratoses and lichen-planus like keratoses), dermatofibroma, melanoma, melanocytic nevi and vascular lesions (angiomas, angiokeratomas, pyogenic granulomas and hemorrhage, vasc). Out of these lesions, the benign ones are 'bkl', 'df', 'nv' and 'vasc', these are non-cancerous. The malignant lesions, which are cancerous, are 'akiec','mel' and 'bcc'. Figure 5 shows the seven types of skin lesion that exist in the dataset. The HAM10000 dataset includes images around 600x450 pixels. Each image is also associated with the metadata stored in the metadata file, which provides details such as the lesion's class label, patient demographics (e.g., age, sex), and where the lesion is located on the body. Additionally, it also contains segmentation masks for all images for the HAM10000 dataset (Tschandl et al., 2020). A significant challenge with the HAM10000 dataset is its class imbalance. The class distribution is as follows, akiec (327), bcc (514), bkl (1,099), df (115), vasc (142), mel (1,113) and nv (6,705) being the majority class. This imbalance made it necessary to carry out careful preprocessing and training strategies to make sure the models could effectively learn to classify all classes, especially the medically critical cancerous classes (akiec, bcc, mel).

Figure 5. Images of the seven types of skin lesions present in the dataset

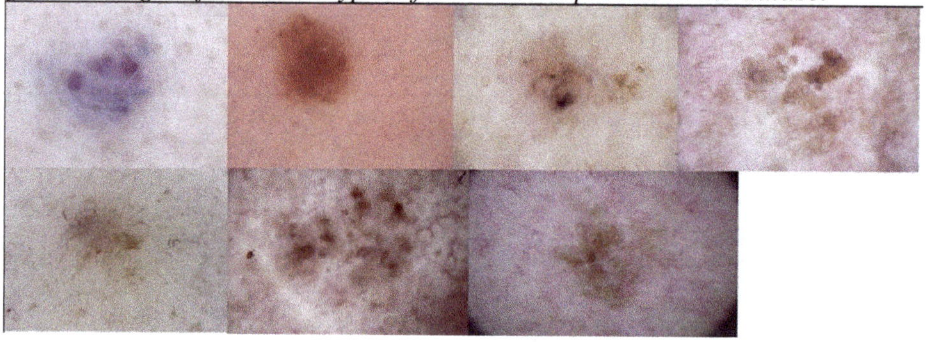

Data Preprocessing and Augmentation

To prepare the HAM10000 dataset for training deep learning models, various preprocessing and augmentation techniques were implemented. Preprocessing ensured that the images were in a suitable format for model input, while augmentation helped improve model ability to generalize by introducing variability in the training data. This topic details the preprocessing pipeline, including the use of segmentation masks and metadata for class organization, as well as the data augmentation techniques applied during training. The preprocessing consists of these three main steps:

- Cropping with Segmentation Masks: Used OpenCV (cv2) to crop images to the lesion area based on segmentation masks, focusing on the lesion.
- Resizing: Resized images to 224x224 pixels, the input size for models like ResNet-101 and ViT-B/16, using OpenCV.

- Used Pandas to load HAM10000 metadata and organize images into subfolders by class (e.g., akiec, bcc).

Data Augmentation Techniques

Data augmentation was applied programmatically during training to improve model generalization, particularly given the class imbalance in the HAM10000 dataset. Augmentation was performed using PyTorch's torchvision.transforms module and applied differently to the training and validation sets to ensure realistic evaluation. The transforms varied slightly depending on the model, with ViT-B/16 using an additional transformation to improve performance. Training Transforms for ResNet-101, EfficientNetV2-L, ConvNeXt-Tiny and ViT-B/16 were applied to the training data below:

- Training Transforms: Random horizontal flips (50% chance), random rotation (up to 15 degrees), color jitter (brightness, contrast, saturation), convert to tensor, and normalize it to ImageNet statistics (transforms.Normalize([0.485, 0.456, 0.406], [0.229, 0.224, 0.225]).
- Additional for ViT-B/16: Random resized crop (224x224, scale 0.8–1.0) and increased color jitter intensity, rest of the training transforms are the same.
- Validation/Test Transforms: Resize to 256x256, center crop to 224x224, convert to tensor, and normalizen, no augmentations were applied.

Dataset Splits

After preprocessing and organizing the HAM10000 dataset into class subfolders, the dataset was split into training, validation, and test sets to carry out model training and evaluation. The HAM10000 dataset (10,015 images) was split into training, validation, and test sets while having equal class distribution. A stratified approach was used with scikit-learn's train_test_split function, setting the stratify parameter to the class labels for the dataset's class imbalance. The splits were:

- Training Set: 70% (7,010 images)
- Validation Set: 15% (1,502 images)
- Test Set: 15% (1,503 images)

Model Implementations

The skin caner detection system to help the caregivers and dermatologists moitor the visually impaired individuals is done using four state-of-the-art deep learning models which were implemented using transfer learning: ResNet-101, EfficientNetV2- L, ConvNeXt-Tiny, and ViT-B/16. Each model was selected for its proven performance in image classification tasks, with structural modifications made to adapt to the HAM10000 dataset for skin cancer detection. This section provides an overview of each model's architecture, explains its suitability for classifying skin lesions as benign or malignant, structural adjustments applied during setup.

ResNet-101

ResNet-101 is a deep convolutional neural network with 101 layers, it was selected for its ability to capture detailed features for skin cancer detection. Its residual connections help avoid vanishing gradient issues, making it suitable for distinguishing between benign and malignant lesions. The model includes four stages of residual blocks, starting with a 7x7 convolution and max-pooling, and ending with global average pooling and a fully connected layer modified to output seven classes matching the HAM10000 dataset classes. Figure 6 shows the workflow of ResNet-101 in Skin Cancer detection.

Figure 6. WorkFlow of ResNet-101 in Skin Cancer detection

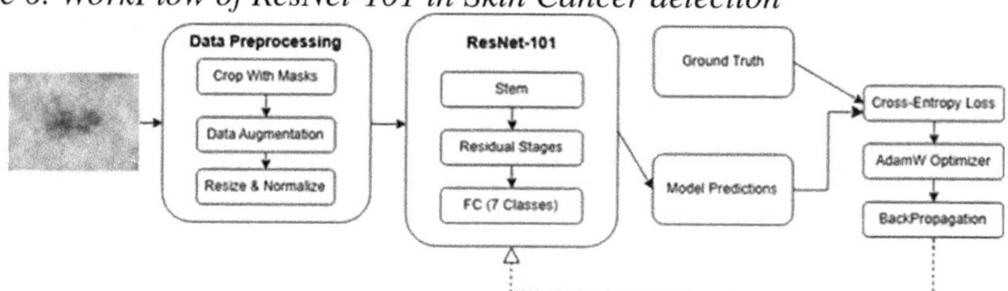

The model was implemented using PyTorch and torchvision with pre-trained ImageNet weights (maintainers and contributors, 2016). The final fully connected layer (model.fc) was replaced to output seven classes, and fine-tuning was applied by freezing layers up to layer2 and unfreezing layer3, layer4, and fc to learn specific features from the preprocessed image.

EfficientNetV2-L

EfficientNetV2-L is an advanced CNN and was chosen for its efficiency and high performance in skin cancer detection. Its balanced scaling of depth, width, and resolution makes it effective at capturing features of skin lesions, such as differences between benign and malignant types. The model includes seven stages with efficient blocks, starting with a 3x3 convolution stem, followed by global average pooling and a fully connected layer modified to output the seven classes. Figure 7 shows the workflow of EfficientNetV2-L in Skin Cancer detection.

Figure 7. WorkFlow of EfficientNetV2-L in Skin Cancer detection

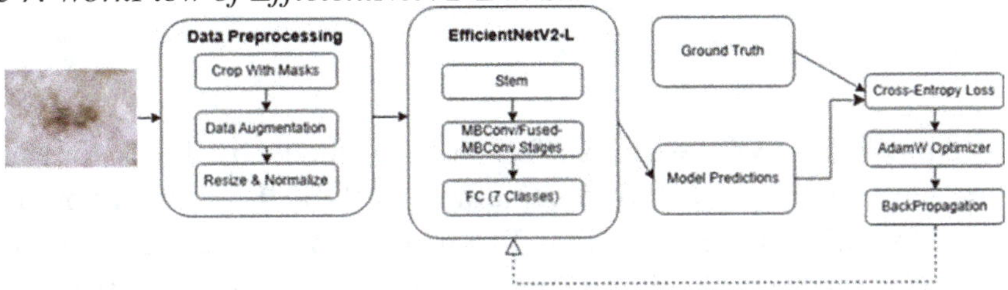

The model was implemented using PyTorch and torchvision with pre-trained ImageNet weights (maintainers and contributors, 2016). The final fully connected layer (model.classifier[1]) was replaced to output seven classes, and fine-tuning was applied by freezing earlier layers and unfreezing features.5, features.6, features.7, and classifier to learn specific features from the images.

ConvNeXt-Tiny

ConvNeXt-Tiny is a modern convolutional neural network, it was chosen for its ability to combine CNN and transformer strengths, its "Tiny" variant was selected for balancing performance and computational efficiency for skin cancer detection. Its hierarchical structure makes it effective at capturing features to differentiate benign from malignant lesions. The model includes four stages of ConvNeXt blocks, starting with a 4x4 convolution stem, followed by layer normalization, global average pooling, and a fully connected layer modified to output seven classes. Figure 8 shows the workflow of ConvNeXt-Tiny in Skin Cancer detection

Figure 8. WorkFlow of ConvNeXt-Tiny in Skin Cancer detection

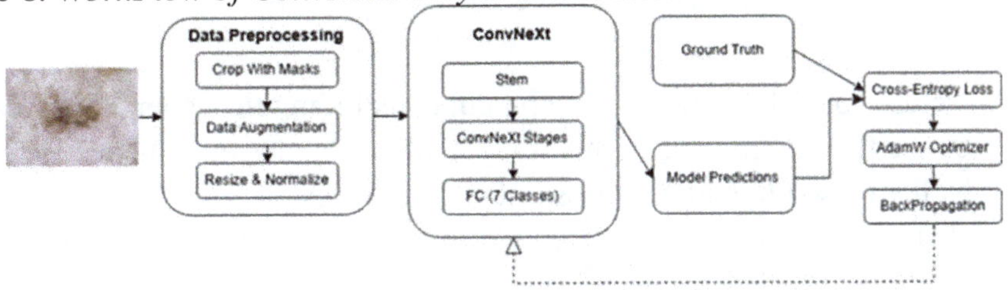

The model was implemented using PyTorch and torchvision with pre-trained ImageNet weights (maintainers and contributors, 2016). The final fully connected layer (model.classifier[2]) was replaced to output seven classes, and fine-tuning was applied by freezing earlier stages and unfreezing features.6, features.7, and classifier to learn specific features from 224x224 pixel images.

ViT-B/16

Vision transformer ViT-B/16, transformer-based model, is chosen for its ability to capture global features in dermoscopic images through self-attention, making it effective for skin cancer detection. The model divides 224x224 images into patches, embeds them with positional information, and processes them through 12 transformer layers with a CLS token. The output is passed to a fully connected layer modified to output seven classes. Figure 9 shows the workflow of ViT-B/16 in Skin Cancer detection.

Figure 9. WorkFlow of ViT-B/16 in Skin Cancer detection

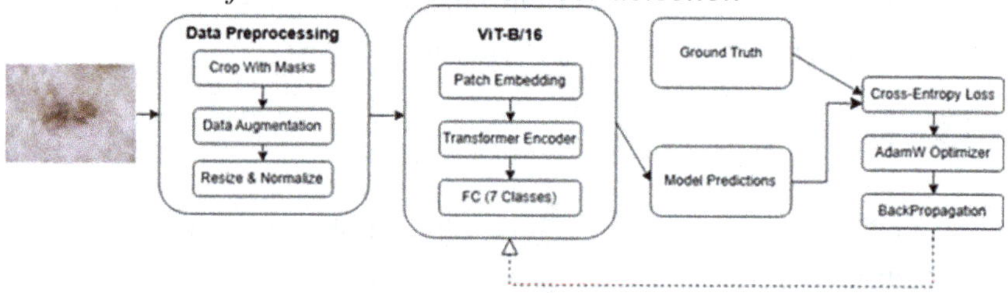

The model was implemented using PyTorch and the timm library with pre-trained ImageNet weights (Wightman, 2019). The final fully connected layer (model.head) was replaced to output seven classes, and fine-tuning was applied by freezing earlier layers and unfreezing the last four transformer blocks (blocks.8 to blocks.11) and head to learn specific features from the images.

Training

This section consists of the training pipeline, including the general optimization techniques used for the models in this study. It also includes model-specific adjustments which are used to address class imbalance issues.

Training Pipeline

The training pipeline for all models followed a standard supervised learning approach, implemented using PyTorch. Each model was trained on the HAM10000 training set, with validation performed on the validation set after each epoch to monitor performance and prevent overfitting. The training loop consisted of the following steps, (1) forward pass to calculate predictions, (2) computation of the loss using the Cross-Entropy Loss function, (3) backward pass to calcluate gradients, and (4) optimization step using the AdamW optimizer to update weights. During validation, the model was set to evaluation mode (model.eval()), and gradients were disabled (torch.no_grad()) to reduce memory usage and speed up the calculation process. The validation accuracy was calculated as the percentage of correctly classified samples, and the best model weights were saved based on the highest validation accuracy. Early stopping was applied for EfficientNetV2-L, ConvNeXt-Tiny, and ViT-B/16 to stop training if the validation accuracy did not improve for a specified number of epochs. The test set was used for final evaluation, where predictions were compared to ground truth labels to calculate evaluation metrics and a confusion matrix.

General Optimization Techniques

This section covers the optimization techniques used to train the models, for efficient convergence and strong performance on the HAM10000 dataset. Each technique is described below, followed by a summary of the hyperparameters for each model in Table 2.

AdamW Optimizer: All models used the AdamW optimizer, which improves regularization and convergence for finetuning pre-trained models by decoupling weight decay from the learning rate (Loshchilov & Hutter, n.d.) ResNet-101 and ConvNeXt-Tiny used a learning rate of 0.001, while EfficientNetV2- L and ViT-B/16 used 0.0001 to ensure stability.

ReduceLROnPlateau Scheduler: ResNet-101, EfficientNetV2-L, and ConvNeXt-Tiny used ReduceLROnPlateau scheduler to reduce the learning rate by 0.5 if validation loss did not improve for 5 epochs which helped the models converge better than other schedulers. ViT-B/16 relied on its lower learning rate and early stopping instead.

Cross Entropy Loss: All models used Cross-Entropy Loss, which measures the difference between predicted and true class probabilities for multi-class classification. Class weights were applied for ResNet-101, EfficientNetV2-L, and ConvNeXt-Tiny to address class imbalance. Label Smoothing EfficientNetV2-L used label smoothing (factor 0.1) to soften the target distribution, reducing overconfidence and improving generalization by preventing overfitting Szegedy et al. (2015), especially for visually similar classes.

Mixed Precision: Training EfficientNetV2-L used mixed precision training with PyTorch's torch.cuda.amp module to reduce memory usage on the GPU. This allowed for a larger batch size of 32, improving training efficiency. Mixed precision training uses a combination of 16-bit half precision and 32-bit full precision floating point operations to reduce memory usage and speed up model training while maintaining model accuracy.

Hyperparameters: Table 2 summarizes the hyperparameters for each model, including the optimizer, learning rate, weight decay, scheduler, and early stopping patience numbers.

Table 2. Hyperparameters Used for All Models

Model	Batch	Epochs	Optimizer	LR	WeightDecay	Scheduler	EarlyStopping
ResNet-101	64	50	AdamW	0.001	1e-4	ReduceLROnPlateau	None
EfficientNetV2-L	32	50	AdamW	0.0001	1e-5	ReduceLROnPlateau	10
ConvNeXt-Tiny	64	50	AdamW	0.001	1e-4	ReduceLROnPlateau	15
ViT-B/16	64	50	AdamW	0.0001	1e-4	None	15

Model-Specific Training Adjustments

To address the class imbalance in the HAM10000 dataset and improve performance on minority and medically important classes, model-specific adjustments were applied during training.

ResNet-101: Class imbalance was handled using two techniques. First, the Cross-Entropy Loss was weighted using inverse frequency weights, which assigns higher weights to minority classes (e.g., akiec, df). Second, a WeightedRandomSampler was used to oversample minority classes during training, with sampling weights derived from the same inverse frequency formula. This makes sure that the model saw more examples of underrepresented classes, improving its ability to generalize across all classes.

EfficientNetV2-L: Similar to ResNet-101, the Cross-Entropy Loss was weighted using inverse frequency weights. In addition to that, label smoothing was applied to the loss function to prevent overfitting. A WeightedRandomSampler was used with custom weights, mel (melanoma) and bkl (benign keratosis-like lesions) were oversampled with a weight of 2.0, while other classes had a weight of 1.0. This was used mainly because of the medical importance of melanoma and them performing worse compared to other classes.

ConvNeXt-Tiny: The Cross-Entropy Loss was weighted using square root inverse frequency weights, calculated as 1.0 / (count ** 0.5) and normalized to sum to 1. This approach reduced the dominance of majority classes such as nv while avoiding overly aggressive weighting of minority classes. A WeightedRandomSampler was used with custom weights, the base weights were 1.0 / count, with akiec and df multiplied by 1.5, and bkl and mel multiplied by 1.2. This balanced the focus on minority classes (akiec, df) and medically important classes (bkl, mel), improving the model's performance on these categories.

ViT-B/16: Unlike the other models, class weights were not applied to the Cross-Entropy Loss. It relied instead on a WeightedRandomSampler to handle class imbalance. The sampler used custom weights, mel and akiec were oversampled with a weight of 2.0, while other classes had a weight of 1.0. This focused training on melanoma and actinic keratosis, both of which are critical for skin cancer detection and are malignant lesions. No learning rate scheduler was used, as the lower learning rate (lr=0.0001) and early stopping (patience=15) were enough for ViT-B/16 to converge stably.

EVALUATION

This section evaluates performance of the four models (ResNet-101, EfficientNetV2-L, ConvNeXtTiny, ViT-B/16) on the HAM10000 dataset using transfer learning. The evaluation scenarios were divided as: (1) seven-class classification, where each class is treated individually, and (2) binary classification, where the classes were grouped into benign (bkl, df, nv, vasc) and malignant (akiec, bcc, mel) categories which is the study's primary goal. The metrics used for evaluation, accuracy, precision, recall, and F1-score were chosen to provide performance of the model, as detailed in Method section. In addition to that, ROC curves, precision-recall curves, and their respective summary metrics were calculated for the benign vs. malignant classification to evaluate the model's ability to separate benign and malignant categories across different thresholds. These metrics demonstrate the models strength in helping caregivers and dermatologists monitor visually impaired individuals with high reliability.

Results for Multi-Class Classification

The performance of each model on multi-class classification task is presented in the following tables and figure. Tables 3 to Table 6 detail the precision, recall, and F1-score for each class, along with the support which is the number of images for each class in the test set, macro-averaged metrics, and overall accuracy for each model. Figure 10 displays the confusion matrices for all models for classification performance across the seven classes.

Table 3 shows the multi-class classification metrics for ResNet-101, showing the model's performance on each of the seven classes. The table includes per-class precision, recall, and F1-score, and also the overall accuracy and macro averaged metrics.

Table 3. Multi-Class Classification Metrics for ResNet-101

Class	Precision	Recall	F1-Score	Support
akiec	0.79	0.69	0.74	49
bcc	0.91	0.92	0.92	77
bkl	0.87	0.81	0.84	165
df	0.81	0.76	0.79	17
mel	0.83	0.71	0.76	167
nv	0.93	0.97	0.95	1007
vasc	0.94	0.68	0.79	22
Macro Avg	0.87	0.79	0.83	1503
Accuracy	0.91			

Table 4 shows the multi-class classification metrics for EfficientNetV2-L, providing the model's performance across the seven classes. The metrics reflect the model's effectiveness in classifying both majority and minority classes, with macro-averaged values.

Table 4. Multi-Class Classification Metrics for EfficientNetV2-L

Class	Precision	Recall	F1-Score	Support
akiec	0.83	0.71	0.77	49
bcc	0.89	0.88	0.89	77
bkl	0.91	0.79	0.85	165
df	0.50	0.88	0.64	17
mel	0.83	0.83	0.83	167
nv	0.96	0.97	0.96	1007
vasc	0.96	1.00	0.98	22

continued on following page

Table 4. Continued

Class	Precision	Recall	F1-Score	Support
Macro Avg	0.84	0.87	0.85	1503
Accuracy	0.92			

Table 5 provides the multi-class classification metrics for ConvNeXt-Tiny, showing the model's performance on each class. The table shows the model's strengths and weaknesses with macro-averaged metrics.

Table 5. Multi-Class Classification Metrics for ConvNeXt-Tiny

Class	Precision	Recall	F1-Score	Support
akiec	0.73	0.49	0.59	49
bcc	0.83	0.84	0.84	77
bkl	0.78	0.76	0.77	165
df	1.00	0.76	0.87	17
mel	0.77	0.80	0.79	167
nv	0.95	0.96	0.95	1007
vasc	0.92	1.00	0.96	22
Macro Avg	0.85	0.80	0.82	1503
Accuracy	0.90			

Table 6 presents the multi-class classification metrics for ViT-B/16, showing how the model performed across the seven classes. The metrics shows the model's ability to classify skin lesions with macro-averaged values also.

Table 6. Multi-Class Classification Metrics for ViT-B/16

Class	Precision	Recall	F1-Score	Support
akiec	0.82	0.63	0.71	49
bcc	0.94	0.83	0.88	77
bkl	0.80	0.79	0.79	165
df	1.00	0.76	0.87	17
mel	0.76	0.81	0.79	167
nv	0.96	0.97	0.97	1007
vasc	0.91	0.95	0.93	22
Macro Avg	0.88	0.82	0.85	1503
Accuracy	0.91			

Figure 10. Multi-Class Confusion Matrices for All Models (ResNet-101, EfficientNetV2-L, ConvNeXt-Tiny, ViT-B/16)

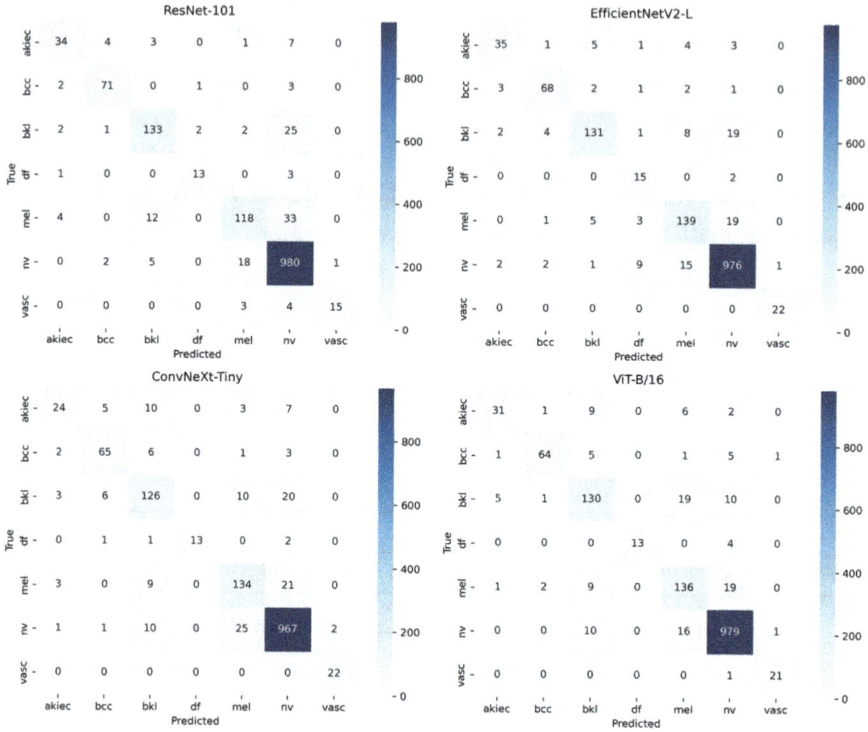

Analysis of Multi-Class Results

The multi-class classification results provides information into each model's ability to distinguish between the seven classes of skin lesions, which is challenging due to the class imbalance in the HAM10000 dataset. The analysis below examines the performance of each model, focusing on their strengths and weaknesses, particularly on minority classes (akiec, df, vasc) and majority classes (nv), and how these results may influence their performance.

ResNet-101: ResNet-101 achieved an overall accuracy of 0.91 and a macro-averaged F1-score of 0.83, indicating balanced performance across classes. It performed well on majority classes like nv (F1-score: 0.95) and malignant classes like bcc (F1-score: 0.92), but its recall for akiec (0.69) and vasc (0.68) was lower, it means it missed some occurrences of these classes. This will impact its ability to detect malignant lesions in the binary task, as akiec is a malignant class.

EfficientNetV2-L: EfficientNetV2-L had the highest overall accuracy (0.92) and a macroaveraged F1-score of 0.85, showing strong performance. It did excellent on nv (F1-score: 0.96) and vasc (F1-score: 0.98), with a perfect recall of 1.00 for vasc. However, its precision for df was low (0.50), but it had a high recall (0.88), which shows a higher rate of false positives for this class. Its balanced performance on malignant classes like mel (F1-score: 0.83) might make it perform well in the binary task classification.

ConvNeXt-Tiny: ConvNeXt-Tiny had the lowest overall accuracy (0.90) and a macro-averaged F1-score of 0.82. It struggled heavily with akiec (F1-score: 0.59, recall: 0.49), missing many occurences of this malignant class, which could lead to false negatives in the binary task. However, it performed well on nv (F1-score: 0.95) and vasc (F1-score: 0.96) and achieved a perfect precision for df (1.00), but its recall for df (0.76) shows some missed cases.

ViT-B/16: ViT-B/16 achieved an overall accuracy of 0.91 and a macro-averaged F1-score of 0.85, matching EfficientNetV2-L. It has the highest macro-averaged precision (0.88) which indicates fewer false positives. It performed well on nv (F1-score: 0.97) and bcc (F1-score: 0.88), but its recall for akiec (0.63) was relatively low, similar to ResNet-101. Its strong performance on mel (F1-score: 0.79) and vasc (F1-score: 0.93) shows it may be effective in the binary task.

The confusion matrices in Figure 10 further visualizes these findings. For example, ConvNeXtTiny's low recall for akiec is evident in its confusion matrix, where many akiec occurences were misclassified as other classes like mel or nv. EfficientNetV2-L's high recall for df resulted in some false positives, as seen in its confusion matrix, where df cases were correctly identified but other classes were misclassified as df sometimes. Overall, EfficientNetV2-L and ViT-B/16 appear to have the most balanced performance across classes, which may transfer to better results in the binary classification task, particularly in detecting malignant lesions.

Results for Benign vs. Malignant Classification

The performance of each model on the skin cancer classification task, where the seven classes were grouped into benign (bkl, df, nv, vasc) and malignant (akiec, bcc, mel) categories, is showed in Table 7 and Figure 11.

Table 7 summarizes the binary classification metrics for all models, focusing on their ability to distinguish between benign and malignant lesions. The table includes accuracy, as well as precision, recall, F1-score, AUC and AP values for both classes, allowing for a direct comparison of the model's performance in this critical task.

Table 7. Benign vs Malignant Classification Metrics for All Models

Model	Accuracy	Precision (Benign)	Recall (Benign)	F1-Score (Benign)	Precision (Malignant)	Recall (Malignant)	F1-Score (Malignant)	AUC	AP
ResNet-101	0.942	0.952	0.976	0.964	0.890	0.799	0.842	0.970	0.930
EfficientNetV2-L	0.951	0.967	0.973	0.970	0.885	0.863	0.874	0.940	0.910
ConvNeXt-Tiny	0.932	0.954	0.961	0.958	0.835	0.809	0.821	0.970	0.910
ViT-B/16	0.940	0.959	0.966	0.963	0.856	0.829	0.842	0.970	0.910

Figure 11 shows the confusion matrices for all models in the beingn and malignant classes, showing the true positives, false positives, true negatives, and false negatives for the benign and malignant classes. These matrices visualize each model's ability to correctly classify lesions especially for reducing false negatives for malignant cases.

Figure 11. Benign vs Malignant Confusion Matrices for All Models

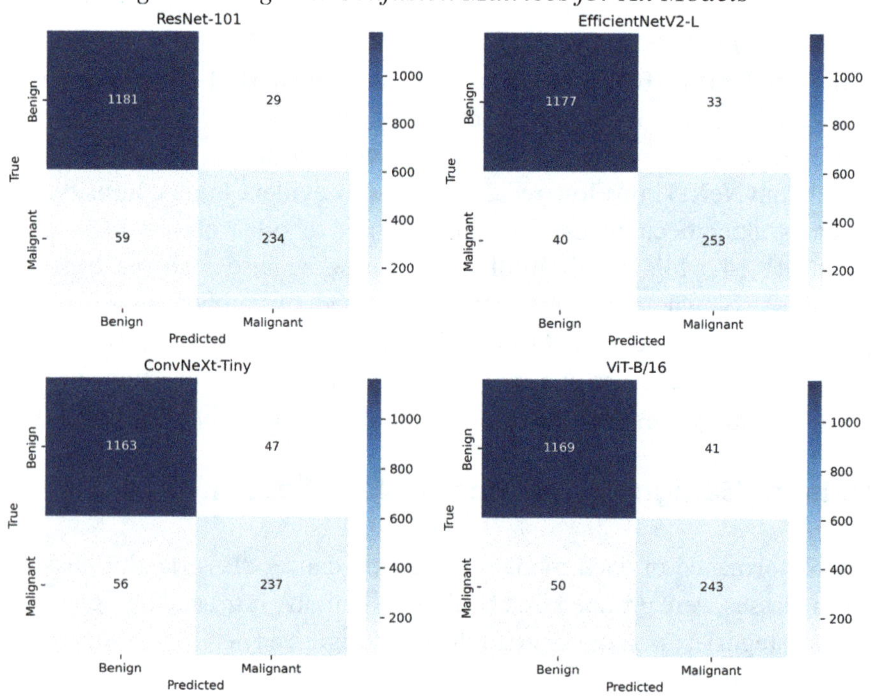

Figure 12 presents the ROC curves for all models, plotting the true positive rate (recall) against the false positive rate at various thresholds. The AUC values in Table 7 summarize the overall performance of each model between benign and malignant lesions.

Figure 12. ROC Curve for All Models

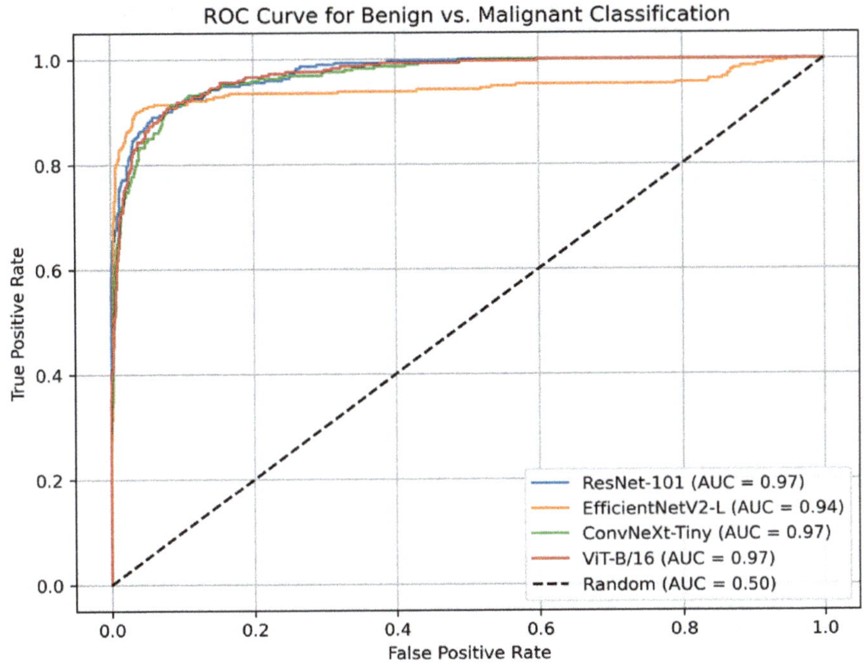

Figure 13 displays the precision-recall curves for all models, showing the trade-off between precision and recall for the malignant class.

Figure 13. Precision-Recall Curve for Benign vs. Malignant Classification

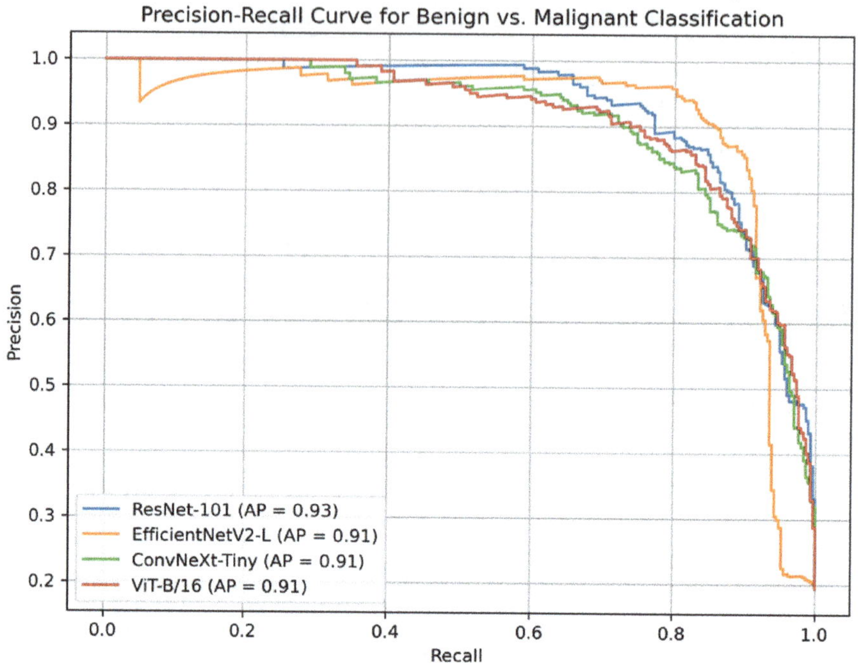

Analysis of Benign vs. Malignant Results

The Benign vs Malignant task focuses on distinguishing between benign (Non-Cancerous) and malignant (Cancerous) skin lesions, which is the primary objective of this study for skin cancer detection. The results in Table 7 and Figure 11 provide a clear comparison of the four model's performance. The analysis below evaluates each model's effectiveness.

ResNet-101: ResNet-101 achieved an accuracy of 0.942, with a strong F1-score for benign lesions (0.964) and decent F1-score for malignant lesions (0.842). It had the highest precision for malignant lesions (0.890) which shows fewer false positives when predicting malignancy. But its recall for malignant lesions (0.799) was the lowest among the models meaning that it missed some malignant cases. The confusion matrix in Figure 11 confirms this by showing higher number of false negatives for the malignant class compared to other models, which is a serious concern in a medical scenario where missing a malignant lesion could be dangerous. Its AUC (0.970) and AP (0.930) are the highest which is seen in Figure 12 and Figure 13 meaning that ResNet-101's predicted probabilities are well separated, but the default threshold of 0.5 is not optimal for maximizing recall for malignant lesions.

EfficientNetV2-L: EfficientNetV2-L performed better than the other models by achieving the highest accuracy (0.951), F1-score for benign lesions (0.970), F1-score for malignant lesions (0.874), and recall for malignant lesions (0.863). Its high recall for malignant lesions shows that it correctly identified most malignant cases, which is crucial for early detection of skin cancer. The confusion matrix in Figure 11 shows the fewest false negatives for the malignant class verifying its effectiveness. Additionally, its precision for benign lesions (0.967) was the highest, which shows a strong ability to avoid misclassifying benign lesions as malignant. But its AUC (0.940) and AP (0.910) are lower than the other models, as seen in Figure 12 and Figure 13. This inconsistency means that while EfficientNetV2-L performs best at the default threshold (0.5), its predicted probabilities for benign and malignant lesions may not be separated properly compared to other models.

ConvNeXt-Tiny: ConvNeXt-Tiny had the lowest accuracy (0.932) and F1-score for malignant lesions (0.821) among the models. Its recall for malignant lesions (0.809) was slightly better than ResNet-101 but still shows a significant number of missed malignant cases. The confusion matrix in Figure 11 reveals a higher number of false negatives for the malignant class, similar to ResNet-101, which could limit its reliability in a medical scenario. However, its precision for benign lesions (0.954) and F1-score for benign lesions (0.958) were strong, showing it performed well on the majority class. Its AUC (0.970) and AP (0.910) are good, matching ResNet-101 and ViT-B/16 in AUC, as seen in Figure 12 and Figure 13.

ViT-B/16: ViT-B/16 achieved an accuracy of 0.940, with an F1-score of 0.963 for benign lesions and 0.842 for malignant lesions, matching ResNet-101's F1-score for the malignant class. Its recall for malignant lesions (0.829) was higher than ResNet-101 and ConvNeXt-Tiny which indicates better detection of malignant cases. The confusion matrix in Figure 11 shows fewer false negatives for the malignant class compared to ResNet-101 and ConvNeXt-Tiny, which means it is more reliable for identifying malignant lesions. Its precision for benign lesions (0.959) was also strong, which suggests good balance in classifying both classes. The ROC and precision recall curves in Figure 12 and Figure 13 show an AUC of 0.970 and an AP of 0.910, showing a strong ability to separate the classes across thresholds.

Overall, EfficientNetV2-L showed the best performance at the default threshold, with the highest accuracy, recall for malignant lesions, and F1-scores for both classes. This also aligns with its strong performance in the multi-class classification task, where it showed balanced performance across all classes, including malignant ones like mel and akiec. However, it has lower AUC and AP compared to the other models. ResNet-101, ConvNeXt-Tiny, and ViT-B/16 all achieved a higher AUC, which means they had better overall separation of benign and malignant lesions across thresholds, but their lower recall for malignant lesions at the default threshold makes them less suitable for the chapter's goal of skin cancer detection to help the caregivers and dermatologists support the visually impaired individuals. The ability to minimize false negatives for malignant lesions makes EfficientNetV2-L the most suitable model for the study's goal of skin cancer detection.

Model Training Dynamics

This section analyzes the training and validation loss curves to understand how the models (ResNet-101, EfficientNetV2-L, ConvNeXt-Tiny, ViT-B/16) learned over 50 epochs using transfer learning. Figure 14 shows the loss curves, with solid lines for training loss and dashed lines for validation loss.

Figure 14. Training and Validation Loss Curves for all Models

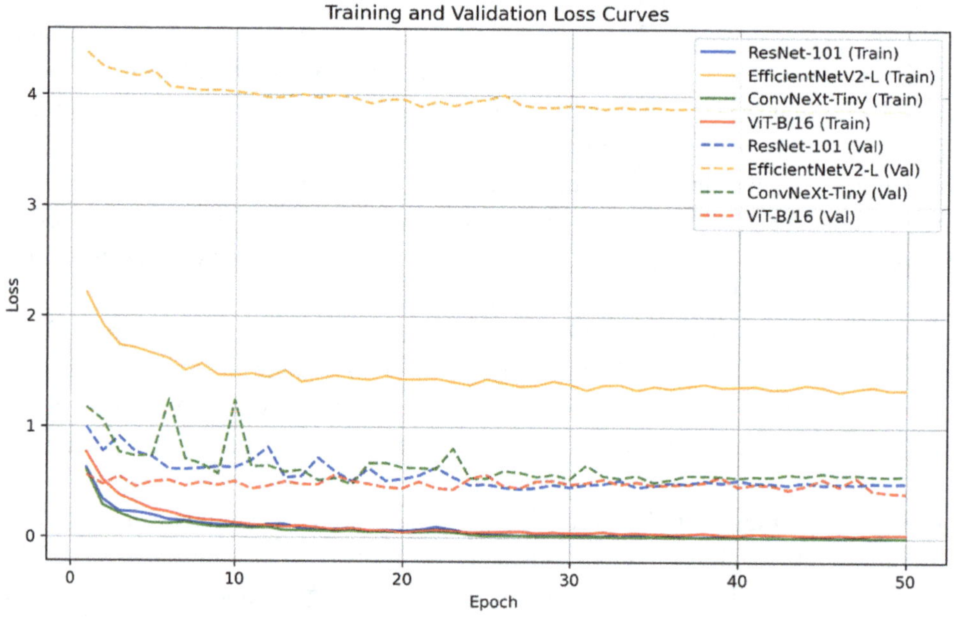

Figure 14 shows that all models training losses decrease steadily showing good learning on the training data, this due to the help by transfer learning from pre-trained ImageNet weights. ResNet-101, ConvNeXt-Tiny, and ViT-B/16 reach near 0 (0.0047, 0.0050, and 0.0341 by epoch 50), while EfficientNetV2-L's training loss drops from 2.2081 to 1.3446, but plateaus around 1.35. Validation losses reveal overfitting in all models, especially EfficientNetV2-L, with a large gap (1.3446 vs. 3.8724 at epoch 50). ResNet-101 and ConvNeXt-Tiny plateau around 0.5–0.6, while ViT-B/16 generalizes the best, reaching 0.4115. EfficientNetV2-L's overfitting explains its lower AUC (0.940), but its high accuracy (0.951) and recall (0.863) at the default threshold makes it the best model for skin cancer detection which is discussed in Results for Benign vs. Malignant Classification.

Web Interface

The system includes a web prototype, as proof-of-concept, to make skin cancer detection accessible for caregivers and dermatologists monitoring visually impaired individuals. The interface allows to upload dermoscopic images of skin lesions for analysis and once an image is uploaded, the system uses the saved model weights to make predictions based on the image uploaded. For example, a result might show "Benign" or "Malignant" with a confidence score. Figure 15 and Figure 16 shows the model predictions when a benign or malignant skin lesion image is uploaded.

Figure 15. Prediction on a Benign Skin Lesion Image

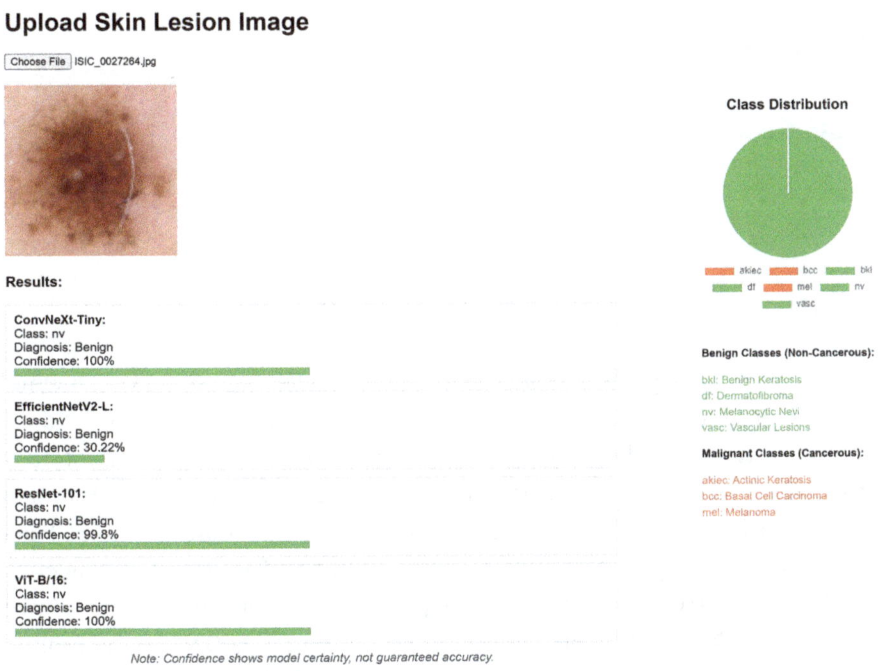

Figure 16. Prediction on a Malignant Skin Lesion Image

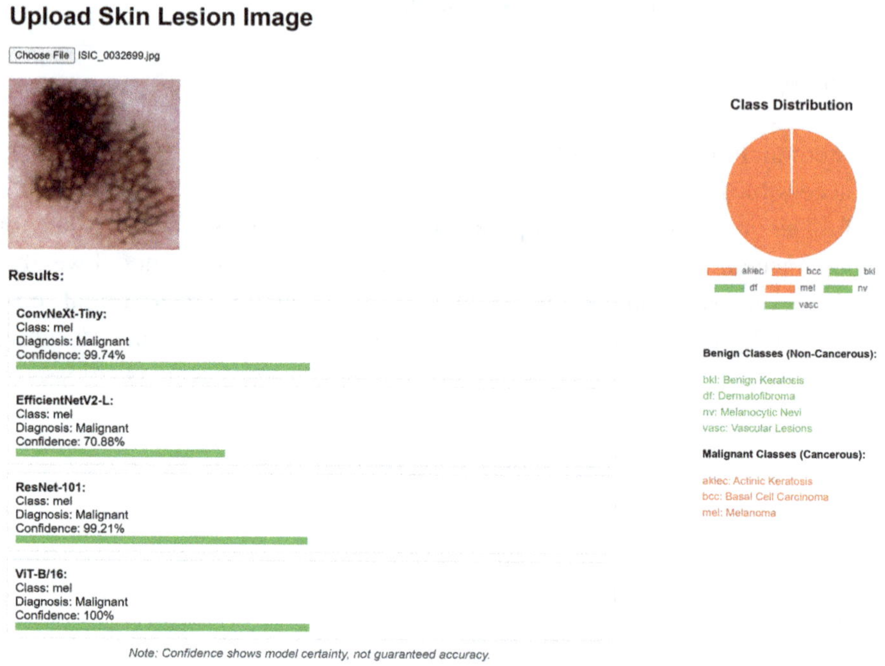
Upload Skin Lesion Image
Choose File ISIC_0032699.jpg
Results:
ConvNeXt-Tiny:
Class: mel
Diagnosis: Malignant
Confidence: 99.74%
EfficientNetV2-L:
Class: mel
Diagnosis: Malignant
Confidence: 70.88%
ResNet-101:
Class: mel
Diagnosis: Malignant
Confidence: 99.21%
ViT-B/16:
Class: mel
Diagnosis: Malignant
Confidence: 100%
Note: Confidence shows model certainty, not guaranteed accuracy.
Class Distribution
akiec bcc bkl df mel nv vasc
Benign Classes (Non-Cancerous):
bkl: Benign Keratosis
df: Dermatofibroma
nv: Melanocytic Nevi
vasc: Vascular Lesions
Malignant Classes (Cancerous):
akiec: Actinic Keratosis
bcc: Basal Cell Carcinoma
mel: Melanoma

Discussion

The results show strong performance of the skin cancer detection system which enables caregivers and dermatologists to monitor visually impaired individuals more effectively, reducing diagnostic delay. In the multi-class classification task, EfficientNetV2- L achieved balanced performance across seven lesion types. In the binary task, EfficientNetV2-L performed best with an accuracy of 0.951 and a recall of 0.863 for malignant lesions, making it the best for detecting cancerous lesions, while ResNet-101 performed decently with an accuracy of 0.942 but lower recall (0.799), and ConvNeXt-Tiny had the lowest accuracy at 0.932. The training dynamics show areas for improvement, where even though EfficientNetV2-L shows overfitting, it outperforms ViT-B/16, which generalizes better but has lower recall (0.829).

CONCLUSION

This section summarizes the chapter's achievements and also focusing on its limitations and suggesting future improvements.

Achievements

This study developed a skin cancer classification system using the HAM10000 dataset, focusing on helping caregivers and dermatologists in monitoring visually impaired individuals for skin cancer detection by evaluating four deep learning models (ResNet-101, EfficientNetV2-L, ConvNeXt-Tiny, ViT-B/16). Data preprocessing, data augmentation, resizing, and normalization, followed by training with AdamW optimizer, cross-entropy loss, and early stopping helped reduce overfitting. In the binary classification task, EfficientNetV2- L achieved the highest accuracy of 0.951 and a recall of 0.863 for malignant lesions with minimum false negatives critical for skin cancer detection. The multi-class task showed balanced performance across classes on all models, particularly for minority classes like akiec and mel, where data augmentation was used to address the dataset's imbalance. Overall, this aids caregivers and dermatologists in monitoring visually impaired individuals for better outcomes.

Limitations

Despite its achievements, this study faced several limitations and challenges. Even after using early stopping and weight decay, overfitting occurred which limited the model's accuracy, with EfficientNetV2-L's validation loss remaining high compared to its training loss, showing limited generalization. Additionally, advanced models such as NFNet-F1, CoAtNet could not be used for classification due to heavy memory usage on the GPU.

Further limitation arises from advanced augmentations like albumentations, MixUp and CutMix which could not be used for data augmentation since the GPU couldn't handle it, causing it to crash the kernel. Additionally, the models could only be trained for 50 epochs due to limited time, running the model for more epochs could have helped the models generalize better. Time constraints and limited GPU performance didn't allow for searching for more advanced hyperparameter tuning.

Future Work

Future enhancements could include improving generalization by exploring additional regularization techniques beyond weight decay, such as dropout, to further reduce overfitting. Implementing a segmentation model such as U-Net would provide better lesion boundaries leading to better accuracy. Additionally, using FocalLoss for addressing class imbalance issues, has the potential to tackle class imbalance issues more effectively. Further work would be including Explainable Artificial Intelligence (XAI) which focuses on making AI systems more understandable to humans and could enhance decision making support for doctors and caregivers without replacing their expertise. A future advancement could also include adding audio feedback and haptic interface to assist the visually impaired individuals and conduct usability studies with clinicians, caregivers, and visually impaired individuals to evaluate real-world feasibility. Further future work could include mitigating dataset biases by expanding to a larger dataset, which would have helped with better results and reliability in a medical scenario.

REFERENCES

Alharith, R., Ibrahim, A. O., Wahid, N., Ghazali, R., & Elsafi, A. (2024). Comparative Analysis of ResNet Models for Skin Cancer Diagnosis: Performance Evaluation and Insights. *Lecture Notes in Networks and Systems*, 370–378. DOI: 10.1007/978-3-031-66965-1_36

American Academy of Dermatology Association. (2024). *Types of skin cancer*. Www.aad.org. https://www.aad.org/public/diseases/skin-cancer/types/common

Barbadekar, A., Ashtekar, V., & Chaudhari, A. (2023). Skin Cancer Classification and Detection Using VGG-19 and DesNet. *2023 International Conference on Computational Intelligence, Networks and Security (ICCINS)*, 1–6. DOI: 10.1109/ICCINS58907.2023.10449996

Bipin, P. B., & Abirami, S. (2023). *Smart Assistant for Visually Impaired People using Deep Learning Algorithms*. 2023 International Conference on Sustainable Computing and Smart Systems (ICSCSS). https://ieeexplore.ieee.org/document/10169851

Bodemer, A. (2020). Skin-Cancer.pdf. https://www.va.gov/WHOLEHEALTHLIBRARY/docs/Skin-Cancer.pdf

Boldu, R., Matthies, D. J. C., Zhang, H., & Nanayakkara, S. (2020). AiSee. *Proceedings of the ACM on Interactive, Mobile, Wearable and Ubiquitous Technologies*, *4*(4), 1–25. DOI: 10.1145/3432196

Cleveland Clinic. (2021, November 19). *Skin Cancer Overview | Cleveland Clinic*. Cleveland Clinic. https://my.clevelandclinic.org/health/diseases/15818-skin-cancer

Craythorne, E., & Al-Niami, F. (2017). Skin cancer. *Medicine (Abingdon)*, *45*(7), 431–434. DOI: 10.1016/j.mpmed.2017.04.003

Dahmani, M. G., Tarhouni, M., & Zidi, S. (2024). Vision Transformers (ViT) for Enhanced Skin Cancer Classification. *2024 IEEE International Conference on Artificial Intelligence & Green Energy (ICAIGE)*, 1–6. DOI: 10.1109/ICAIGE62696.2024.10776698

Das, K., Cockerell, C. J., Patil, A., Pietkiewicz, P., Giulini, M., Grabbe, S., & Goldust, M. (2021). Machine Learning and Its Application in Skin Cancer. *International Journal of Environmental Research and Public Health*, *18*(24), 13409. DOI: 10.3390/ijerph182413409 PMID: 34949015

Demir, A., Yilmaz, F., & Köse, O. (n.d.). *Early Detection of Skin Cancer Using Deep Learning Architectures: Resnet-101 and Inception-v3*. https://biyoklinikder.org/TIPTEKNO19_Bildiriler/095.pdf

Dildar, M., Akram, S., Irfan, M., Khan, H. U., Ramzan, M., Mahmood, A. R., Alsaiari, S. A., Saeed, A. H. M., Alraddadi, M. O., & Mahnashi, M. H. (2021). Skin Cancer Detection: A Review Using Deep Learning Techniques. *International Journal of Environmental Research and Public Health*, *18*(10), 5479. DOI: 10.3390/ijerph18105479 PMID: 34065430

Dosovitskiy, A., Beyer, L., Kolesnikov, A., Weissenborn, D., Zhai, X., Unterthiner, T., Dehghani, M., Minderer, M., Heigold, G., Gelly, S., Uszkoreit, J., & Houlsby, N. (2021). *AN IMAGE IS WORTH 16X16 WORDS: TRANSFORMERS FOR IMAGE RECOGNITION AT SCALE*. https://arxiv.org/pdf/2010.11929

Elbedoui, K., Mzoughi, H., & Slima, M. B. (2024). Deep Learning Approaches for Dermoscopic Image-Based Skin Cancer Diagnosis. *2024 IEEE 7th International Conference on Advanced Technologies, Signal and Image Processing (ATSIP)*, 1–7. DOI: 10.1109/ATSIP62566.2024.10638968

Giansanti, D., & Pirrera, A. (2025). Integrating AI and Assistive Technologies in Healthcare: Insights from a Narrative Review of Reviews. *Health Care*, *13*(5), 556. DOI: 10.3390/healthcare13050556 PMID: 40077118

Gouda, W., Sama, N. U., Al-Waakid, G., Humayun, M., & Jhanjhi, N. Z. (2022). Detection of Skin Cancer Based on Skin Lesion Images Using Deep Learning. *Health Care*, *10*(7), 1183. DOI: 10.3390/healthcare10071183 PMID: 35885710

He, K., Zhang, X., Ren, S., & Sun, J. (2015). *Deep Residual Learning for Image Recognition*. https://arxiv.org/pdf/1512.03385

Hossain, M., Sadik, Kh., Rahman, Md. M., Ahmed, F., Hossain Bhuiyan, Md. N., & Khan, M. M. (2021, October 1). *Convolutional Neural Network Based Skin Cancer Detection (Malignant vs Benign)*. IEEE Xplore. DOI: 10.1109/IEMCON53756.2021.9623192

Kablan, E. B., & Ayas, S. (2024). Skin lesion classification from dermoscopy images using ensemble learning of ConvNeXt models. *Signal, Image and Video Processing*, *18*(8-9), 6353–6361. Advance online publication. DOI: 10.1007/s11760-024-03321-y

Kumar, A., Kumar, M., Bhardwaj, V. P., Kumar, S., & Selvarajan, S. (2024). A novel skin cancer detection model using modified finch deep CNN classifier model. *Scientific Reports*, *14*(1), 11235. Advance online publication. DOI: 10.1038/s41598-024-60954-2 PMID: 38755202

Liu, Z., Mao, H., Wu, C.-Y., Feichtenhofer, C., Darrell, T., & Xie, S. (2022, March 2). *A convnet for the 2020s*. arXiv.org. https://arxiv.org/abs/2201.03545 DOI: 10.1109/CVPR52688.2022.01167

Loshchilov, I., & Hutter, F. (n.d.). *DECOUPLED WEIGHT DECAY REGULARIZATION*. https://arxiv.org/pdf/1711.05101

Ma, X., Shan, J., Ning, F., Li, W., & Li, H. (2023). EFFNet: A skin cancer classification model based on feature fusion and random forests. *PLoS One*, *18*(10), e0293266–e0293266. DOI: 10.1371/journal.pone.0293266 PMID: 37871038

Naayini, P., Kumar, M. P., Bura, C., Jonnalagadda, A. K., & Kamatala, S. (2025). *AI-Powered Assistive Technologies for Visual Impairment*. ArXiv.org.

Nahata, H., & Singh, S. P. (2020). Deep Learning Solutions for Skin Cancer Detection and Diagnosis. *Learning and Analytics in Intelligent Systems*, 159–182. DOI: 10.1007/978-3-030-40850-3_8

Naqvi, M., Syed Qasim Gilani, Syed, T., Marques, O., & Kim, H.-C. (2023). Skin Cancer Detection Using Deep Learning—A Review. *Skin Cancer Detection Using Deep Learning—a Review, 13*(11), 1911–1911. DOI: 10.3390/diagnostics13111911

Nasra, P. (2024). Enhanced Melanoma Detection Using a Fine-Tuned EfficientNetV2-L Model on Dermoscopic Images. *2024 Second International Conference on Intelligent Cyber Physical Systems and Internet of Things (ICoICI)*, 1–7. DOI: 10.1109/ICoICI62503.2024.10696263

National Cancer Institute. (2018). *Melanoma of the Skin - Cancer Stat Facts*. SEER. https://seer.cancer.gov/statfacts/html/melan.html

Okolo, G. I., Althobaiti, T., & Ramzan, N. (2024). Assistive Systems for Visually Impaired Persons: Challenges and Opportunities for Navigation Assistance. *Sensors (Basel), 24*(11), 3572. DOI: 10.3390/s24113572 PMID: 38894363

Oliveira, R. B., Papa, J. P., Pereira, A. S., & Tavares, J. M. R. S. (2016). Computational methods for pigmented skin lesion classification in images: Review and future trends. *Neural Computing & Applications*, *29*(3), 613–636. DOI: 10.1007/s00521-016-2482-6

Prasher, S., Nelson, L., & Gomathi, S. (2023). Resnet 50 Based Classification Model for Skin Cancer Detection Using Dermatoscopic Images. *2023 3rd Asian Conference on Innovation in Technology (ASIANCON)*, 1–5. DOI: 10.1109/ASIANCON58793.2023.10270158

Rahman, M., Nobel, S. M. N., Meena, P. K., Meena, V. P., & Bahadur, J. (2025). Accelerated and Precise Skin Cancer Detection through an Enhanced Machine Learning Pipeline for Improved Diagnostic Accuracy. *Results in Engineering, 25*, 104168–104168. DOI: 10.1016/j.rineng.2025.104168

Reddy, C. K., Kumar, C. P., Gowtham, A. R. P. S., Maharaju, R., & Valupadasu, R. (2024). Cloud-Based Skin Cancer Classification: Training and Deploying a Model on AWS. *Lecture Notes in Networks and Systems*, 423–434. DOI: 10.1007/978-981-99-9521-9_32

Selvaraj, B., & Aruna, M. (2023). *A Review on Analyzing and Predicting the State of Cancer Disease using Machine Learning Algorithms*. DOI: 10.1109/ICIMIA60377.2023.10426268

Shaheen, M. Y. (2021). Applications of artificial intelligence (AI) in healthcare: A review. *ScienceOpen Preprints, 1*(1). DOI: 10.14293/S2199-1006.1.SOR-.PPVRY8K.v1

Szegedy, C., Vanhoucke, V., Ioffe, S., Shlens, J., & Wojna, Z. (2015, December 11). *Rethinking the inception architecture for computer vision*. arXiv.org. https://arxiv.org/abs/1512.00567

T. (2016). *TorchVision: PyTorch's Computer Vision library*. GitHub. https://github.com/pytorch/vision

Tan, M., & Le, Q. (2021). *EfficientNetV2: Smaller Models and Faster Training*. https://arxiv.org/pdf/2104.00298

Tschandl, P. (2018). The HAM10000 dataset, a large collection of multi-source dermatoscopic images of common pigmented skin lesions. *Harvard Dataverse*. https://doi.org/DOI: 10.7910/dvn/dbw86t

Tschandl, P., Rinner, C., Apalla, Z., Argenziano, G., Codella, N., Halpern, A., Janda, M., Lallas, A., Longo, C., Malvehy, J., Paoli, J., Puig, S., Rosendahl, C., Soyer, H. P., Zalaudek, I., & Kittler, H. (2020). Human–computer collaboration for skin cancer recognition. *Nature Medicine, 26*(8), 1229–1234. DOI: 10.1038/s41591-020-0942-0 PMID: 32572267

Vocaturo, E., Zumpano, E., & Veltri, P. (2018). *Image pre-processing in computer vision systems for melanoma detection*. Bioinformatics and Biomedicine., DOI: 10.1109/BIBM.2018.8621507

Wightman, R. (2019). *PyTorch Image Models* [Review of *PyTorch Image Models*]. GitHub. https://github.com/huggingface/pytorch-image-models

World Cancer Research Fund. (2024, October 4). *Skin cancer statistics | world cancer research fund.* World Cancer Research Fund. https://www.wcrf.org/preventing-cancer/cancer-statistics/skin-cancer-statistics/

World Health Organization. (2019, October 8). *World report on vision.* Www.who.int. https://www.who.int/publications/i/item/9789241516570

World Health Organization. (2023, August 10). *Blindness and vision impairment.* World Health Organization. https://www.who.int/news-room/fact-sheets/detail/blindness-and-visual-impairment

Zhang, N., Cai, Y.-X., Wang, Y.-Y., Tian, Y.-T., Wang, X.-L., & Badami, B. (2019). Skin Cancer Diagnosis Based on Optimized Convolutional Neural Network. *Artificial Intelligence in Medicine, 101756.* Advance online publication. DOI: 10.1016/j.artmed.2019.101756 PMID: 31980095

KEY TERMS AND DEFINITIONS

Assistive Technology: Devices or systems that assist individuals with disabilities in performing tasks which would otherwise be difficult.

Benign: A non-cancerous skin lesion that does not spread to other parts of the body.

Convolutional Neural Network (CNN): A type of deep learning architecture which is designed for image recognition that uses convolutional layers to extract visual features from skin lesion images for classification purposes.

Early Stopping: A regularization technique that stops training when validation performance does not improve for a set number of epochs which can prevent overfitting.

Epoch: An epoch in machine learning, especially in training deep learning models refers to one complete pass through the entire training dataset by the learning algorithm.

HAM10000 Dataset: A dermatological image dataset containing over 10,000 dermoscopic images of pigmented lesions, used for skin cancer classification.

Malignant: A cancerous skin lesion which can spread to other parts of the body.

Segmentation Mask: A mask of an image that shows the lesion boundaries precisely of the original image, used during preprocessing to crop and isolate skin lesions from surrounding skin.

Skin Lesion: An area of abnormal skin that differs in color, texture, or shape from surrounding areas of the skin, potentially indicating conditions such as skin cancer.

Transfer Learning: A strategy of initializing a model with weights which are pre-trained on a large dataset (e.g., ImageNet) and fine tuning it on a new dataset for better performance.

Visual Impairment: A condition ranging from low vision to complete blindness, which cannot be corrected by standard lenses or surgery and impacts mobility, communication, and access to healthcare services.

Chapter 12
Development of an IoT-Enabled Wearable Device for Monitoring Elbow Movements in Children With Cerebral Palsy Using MAS, AMS, and QUEST:
Improving Quality of Life of Cerebral Palsy Children

S. Thangam
https://orcid.org/0000-0003-2251-3651
Amrita School of Computing, Amrita Vishwa Vidyapeetham, Bengaluru, India

Ananya Ganapathi
https://orcid.org/0009-0002-2579-2545
Amrita School of Computing, Amrita Vishwa Vidyapeetham, Bengaluru, India

Deivanai Saravanan
https://orcid.org/0009-0005-5946-5421
Amrita School of Computing, Amrita Vishwa Vidyapeetham, Bengaluru, India

Sneha Thejassu Raghavan
https://orcid.org/0009-0006-2916-2929
Amrita School of Computing, Amrita Vishwa Vidyapeetham, Bengaluru, India

DOI: 10.4018/979-8-3373-2033-5.ch012

ABSTRACT

Cerebral palsy (CP) is a group of permanent movement disorders that significantly affect a child's ability to move and maintain balance and posture. Among the many challenges faced by children with CP, restricted joint movement, particularly in the elbows, severely impacts daily activities and motor development. The research proposes the design and development of an IoT-enabled wearable device aimed at assisting and monitoring elbow movements in children with cerebral palsy. The proposed solution integrates sensors such as accelerometers, muscle sensor, and flex sensors to capture real-time data on elbow flexion and extension. Tardieu, Modified Ashworth, Range of motion and Active movement scales are used for spasticity and movement assessment in order to provide thorough input. The sensor data is then transmitted to a cloud-based platform via WiFi. The proposed IoT solution provides real-time support for children with CP and offers a scalable platform for continuous improvement in therapeutic interventions.

INTRODUCTION

Cerebral palsy (CP) is one of the most prevalent motor disabilities affecting children worldwide, with around 2 to 3 children per 1,000 live births diagnosed with CP in India (Paul et al., 2022). It is estimated that over 25 lakh children in India are currently living with this condition. The disability is a neurological disorder caused by brain damage that primarily affects movement, posture, and coordination. Among the challenges faced by children with CP, restricted joint mobility, particularly in the elbows, significantly hampers their ability to perform essential daily tasks such as feeding, dressing, and writing. These impairments not only limit their independence but also affect their motor development and quality of life.

Traditional physical therapy approaches are commonly used to improve motor function. However, the methods often occur in controlled settings and lack continuous monitoring, which is crucial for the rehabilitation process. A review of interventions for children with CP shows that while physical therapy and motor learning approaches can be effective, their application is often constrained by the absence of real-time data monitoring and feedback (Novak et al., 2013). To address this gap, there is an increasing need for innovative technologies such as wearable devices that can offer continuous, real-time support to improve rehabilitation outcomes through sensors (Nascimento et al., 2020).

The research proposes the development of an IoT-enabled wearable device aimed at assisting and monitoring elbow movements in children with CP. The device incorporates advanced sensors such as accelerometers, muscle sensor, and flex sensors to collect real-time data on elbow flexion and extension during physical therapy. The data gathered by the sensors is securely transmitted via Wi-Fi to a cloud platform, where it can be analyzed to track progress and modify therapeutic interventions as needed. The system offers an advantage over traditional methods by enabling continuous, remote monitoring (Singh et al., 2020), thus providing more personalized and timely adjustments to therapy.

The wearable device also leverages modern networking protocols, such as MQTT, to ensure efficient and reliable communication between the device and the cloud. The proposed system combines cutting-edge sensor technology with cloud computing, allowing healthcare professionals to remotely monitor and adjust therapy plans. In doing so, it offers a scalable solution.

1 LITERATURE SURVEY

The study explains the use of assistive devices among young children with CP in Norway, analyzing data from 130 children to examine the types of devices used, frequency of use, and caregiver-reported benefits. It highlights that early intervention with assistive technologies, when integrated into daily routines, significantly improves quality of life by supporting mobility and self-care especially when tailored to the child's motor limitations (Moen & Østensjø, 2023).

Building on the importance of assistive technology, the study (Xiong et al., 2024) introduces a real-time monitoring system for CP rehabilitation that employs wearable devices to track physiological signals such as blood oxygen levels and heart rate. The system addresses the limitations of traditional rehabilitation methods by providing real-time feedback, enabling healthcare professionals to adjust rehabilitation intensity based on patient progress, leading to more effective and personalized therapy outcomes. In parallel, another paper (Cusimano et al., 2020) focuses on the development of an instrumented glove using digital manufacturing technologies for children under 5 years old, specifically targeting the "thumb in the palm syndrome." The glove offers a customized solution to assess thumb movement during therapy, addressing a significant gap in existing rehabilitation technologies for infants.

Continuing on these efforts, another study (Fadhlillah et al., 2020) presents an innovative system for continuous real-time monitoring of children with CP using IoT. By employing a sensor shield and micro-controller to collect data on heart rate and muscle contraction, the system transmits data to a cloud platform, allowing real-time analysis via an Android phone. The IoT-based system further supports the ongoing management of rehabilitation by providing immediate feedback, thus optimizing therapy and improving long-term outcomes for CP patients.

Various scales and tools are used to assess elbow movements. A few standardized scales are used to measure the movement of the elbow and general motor abilities. The Tardieu Scale is widely acknowledged for its high intra and inter-rater reliability as a reliable measure in evaluating muscle tone and spasticity of the elbow for children with CP. The Modified Tardieu Scale (MTS) has also been validated as having good reliability in the evaluation of spasticity among children with CP (Nourizadeh et al., 2024).

Apart from Tardieu scales, some of the widely practiced evaluations consist of Gross Motor Function Measure and Peabody Developmental Motor Scales. It basically evaluates the gross motor function

It is mainly based on the recording of the 4-point ordinal scale. On the other hand, PDMS explicitly evaluates the motor development and skills of a child. Both the tools are helpful in evaluating the functioning of the upper extremity, such as elbow movements (von Elling-Tammen et al., 2023).

Recent advancements have led to the development of instrumented assessment tools that provide objective measurements of elbow movements. The emphasis revolves around the use of motion capture systems and accelerometers for gaining accurate data on movement patterns (Rozaire et al., 2024). It is in instrumented measurements where quasi-quantitative information is afforded to the evaluation process concerning motor function, most especially in terms of bimanual tasks and basic activities.

Bimanual movements are crucial for daily activities, but children with cerebral palsy (CP) often have difficulty executing such functions due to motor impairment and disrupted coordination. Systematic review has found a range of instrumented assessment tools, including three-dimensional motion analysis and sensor-based technologies, which can be applied in clinical settings to assess these movements (Cacioppo et al., 2023).

Spasticity in cerebral palsy children would be best explained with reference to the elbow flexors in regulation of the threshold of tonic stretch reflex. Studies have shown that the measure of tonic stretch reflex threshold can be used as an effective marker for characterizing spasticity and the function of the motor system in such patients. This will give a sense of the muscular response to stretch and identify at what point spasticity becomes apparent in elbow flexors (Levin et al., 2024). With test-retest reliability and concurrent validity established for these measurements, their applicability in the clinical setting could become enhanced, offering a standardized method through which a change in treatment efficacy can be assured (Jobin & Levin, 2000). The spasticity measure will thus provide a valid source of data that can be used in tailoring specific rehabilitation strategies to enhance upper limb functions among the children diagnosed with CP.

A review of literature on the measurement systems referring to children with CP through movement in the upper limbs depicts an increasing interest in the utilization of instrumented tests in objective measures of the functionality of the upper limb. The review presented three-dimensional motion analysis systems that are commonly applied in monitoring spatiotemporal variables concerning movements in the upper limbs (Francisco-Martínez et al., 2021).

Instrumented assessments are important in the evaluation of function of the upper limb in children with cerebral palsy. There is a growing number of systematic reviews on these assessments and present them as increasingly significant in the clinical environment because of the basic necessities in quantifying the motor performance of a child, besides the accurate measurement of movement quality. Generally, such assessments involve the utilization of high-technology tools such as optoelectronic motion capture systems, which can form detailed kinematic parameters (Rozaire et al., 2024).

The Greek version of the FMS has established its reliability and validity as a tool for mobility assessment in children with CP, thus providing an environmentally valid classification system that physical therapists in Greece may apply with great confidence. Moreover, the scale has been validated to reflect accurately the capability of mobility the children with CP, thus becoming an excellent resource both in clinical and research practice. The Greek FMS is a step forward in assessing functional mobility and indeed helps to take a better approach regarding the planning of any therapy and monitoring of progress in pediatric rehabilitation for CP (Harvey, 2008; Skoutelis et al., 2022).

Multiple studies (Rathke et al., 2024; Wu et al., 2024) have explored the integration of the MQTT protocol for IoT applications, emphasizing its effectiveness in enabling real-time communication and data transmission. One study focused on an IoT-based gait kinetics monitoring system that used piezoresistive insole sensors to assess vertical ground reaction forces (vGRF) during walking. The system employed an ESP32 board to communicate via Wi-Fi through the MQTT framework, showing promising results for cost-effective gait disorder assessment .The use of this lightweight protocol also allowed the second system to maintain a 96.69% accuracy rate in facial recognition and rapid communication between devices, proving its reliability in critical care scenarios . These studies demonstrate MQTT's potential in creating robust, low-latency IoT solutions for both health monitoring and emergency assistance systems.

The research (Virupaxappa & Thangam, 2023) explores the ability of smartphone-connected inertial sensors and machine learning in offering accurate, real-time, and objective evaluations of dystonia severity outside clinical settings, which can improve regular monitoring and clinical management. Th methodology proposes an innovative solution in place of the traditional approach, as the time of clinical specialists is avoided while continuous, unbiased data are allowed to achieve better individualized planning of therapy.

Wearable technology, especially devices that have flex sensors, holds much promise for monitoring and even enhancing hand movements in neuropathological diseases (Thangam et al., 2024). Real-time data regarding finger movement captured by these devices could illustrate valuable insights into a patient's progress, and thus rehabilitation tracking and tailored treatments could be conducted. The IoT-enabled systems continuously monitor blood pressure, heart rate, and ECG, the data being stored securely in the cloud for accessing it remotely (Thangam et al., 2024). Smart gloves, provided with flex sensors and microcontrollers like Arduino, augment the interaction between the patient and the doctor as these gloves detect hand gestures and execute respective actions (such as turning on the light or fan) or send alerts to the caregivers in case of an emergency (Thangam et al., 2024). The approach assists in rehabilitation while offering a much more individualized and effective health care experience.

2 METHODOLOGY

2.1 Proposed Methodology System Architecture & Sequence Flow

The system works through a wearable device that constantly monitors the elbow movements of children with CP. This design uses an ESP32 core processing and communication module, several sensors, and cloud data storage for efficient and easy monitoring as shown in Figure 1. The three primary sensors enclosed within the wearable are flex sensors, muscle sensors, and an accelerometer capturing the real-time movement of the elbow. The data can track how well the child's elbow is moving, how much force is used, and how fast it was or how smooth. Health care providers can even use the data to understand the motor abilities of the child and review how therapy is helping the child. The device is for usage by children with cerebral palsy, which will follow the continuous tracking of their spasticity and possible therapeutic evaluation.

Figure 1. System Architecture Design

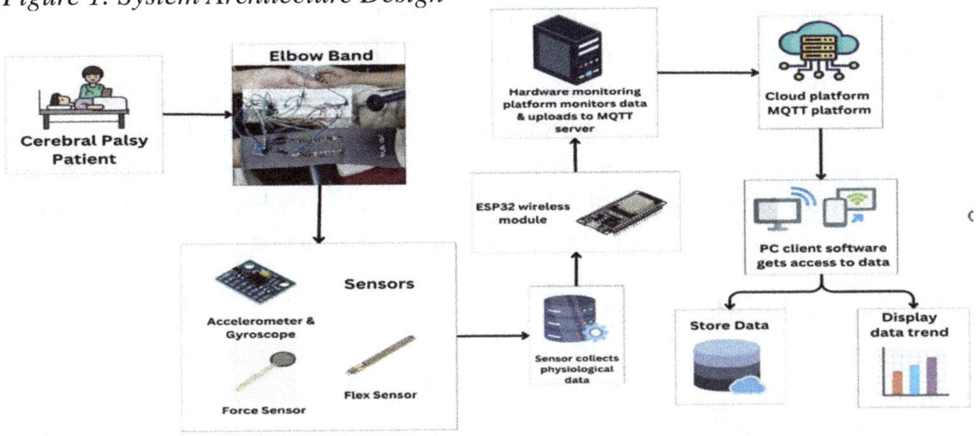

The proposed system presents a patient interface where a child wears an elbow band embedded with several sensors, including an accelerometer for tracking movement speed and orientation at the joint, a flex sensor to monitor joint angles, which could be used for analysis of range of motion, and a muscle sensor to measure resistance during a passive joint movement.

ESP32 is used as a data collection hub, which consists of a microcontroller that communicates as wireless as shown in Figure 2. The raw sensor data coming from the elbow band is received by the ESP32, processed, and then communicated through wireless to a hardware monitoring platform. The processed data is then uploaded to an MQTT server and accessed remotely with the security and scalability of the data.

Figure 2. Sequence of flow

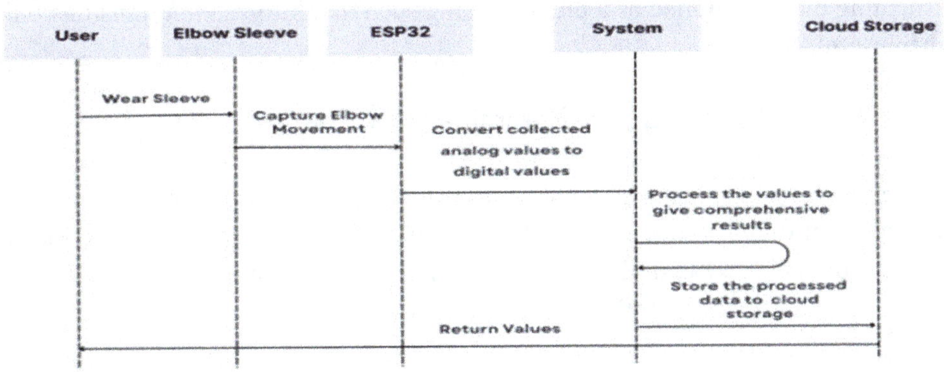

Once the data has been uploaded to the cloud platform, it's available for further analysis and storage. The cloud platform basically becomes a central repository, in which therapists and caregivers can view historical data, track trends in spasticity, and measure the effectiveness of their interventions in the course of time. Moreover, data is accessible through PC client software that picks information from the MQTT server. This software can graphically represent trends in data, meaning that one can visually report progress of the child for decision making when changing therapy. Flow of the execution of the proposed approach is as follows:

2.1.1 Patient Interface Setup

The child with cerebral palsy will be provided with the elbow band that carries all the sensors: accelerometer, flex sensor, and muscle sensor. The device is worn on the elbow to capture the necessary physiological metrics during passive and active movements.

2.1.2 Sensor Data Collection

The accelerometer measure the speed and angle of joint movements, thus discriminating between slow and fast stretches, which is essential in the evaluation of Tardieu Scale. The flex sensor measures the angle of the joints to measure the Range of Motion (ROM), which is useful in measuring the flexibility and mobility of the joints. The muscle sensor measures the resistance at which passive movements are performed and determines the "catch angle" or the point where increased resistance is detected, which is important for Modified Ashworth Scale (MAS) and Tardieu Scale measurements. It transmits this data to the ESP32 microcontroller. The ESP32 microcontroller stores the raw data from sensors. On the ESP32, filtering and data formatting may be applied as a preprocessing such that information transmits only when useful.

2.1.3 Data Processing and Preliminary Evaluation

It performs preliminary data processing at the ESP32 microcontroller, tracking the important values for the joint angle (ROM) and force at the catch angle to detect the level of spasticity and also move-ment speed for velocity response. Prepared data is then transmitted wirelessly.

2.1.4 MQTT wireless data transmission to cloud

Using its built-in Wi-Fi, the ESP32 transmits the processed data either to a hardware monitoring platform or directly to an MQTT server on a cloud platform. The MQTT protocol is used for effective and low-latency communication between the ESP32 and the cloud.

2.1.5 Cloud Data Storage and Long-term Tracking

The incoming data is safely stored into the cloud platform, providing a central storage space for both historical and real-time spasticity data. The stored data enables long-term tracking and analy-sis, allowing caregivers and therapists to monitor trends and progress over time.

2.1.6 Data Access through PC Client Software

Caregivers and therapists can access the data using PC client software that communicates with a cloud-based MQTT server. This client software allows accessing a specific data point or history records for further analysis purposes.

2.1.7 Visualization of Data Trends

The graphical user interface in the PC client soft-ware provides visualization for the trends in data on the metrics such as joint ROM, spasticity levels as measured by MAS scores, and catch angles over time. Visualiza-tion helps therapists monitor how the interventions are working overtime, observe how spasticity is changing, and makes it easy to make interventions more data-driven.

2.1.8 Therapeutic Feedback and Adjustments

Given all the data trends derived, caregivers and therapists are able to ascertain the speed of improvement made by the child, assess development in the motor function terms, or change therapy plans whenever deemed fit. This real-time feedback cycle ensures an adaptive, individually tailored care provision with a magnified overall therapeutic effect.

This sequence shown in Figure 2 leads to continuous assessment, supports the decision to adjust therapy based on the data, and eventually improves patient outcomes.

2.2 Scales used for the proposed solution

2.2.1 Joint Range of Motion (ROM)

The Joint Range of Motion (ROM) scale is a standardized method used to measure the degree of movement a joint can achieve, typically expressed in degrees. It quantifies the flexibility and mobility of a joint, allowing healthcare professionals to assess functional abilities and detect limitations caused by injury, illness, or developmental conditions. For example, a healthy elbow joint typically has a range from 0° (full extension) to about 140–150° (full flexion). The ROM scale is widely used in physiotherapy, sports medicine, and rehabilitation to monitor joint health, evaluate the effectiveness of treatments, and design personalized therapeutic interventions for conditions affecting joint mobility.

The most important metric used to measure the flexibility and mobility of the elbow joint in children with cerebral palsy is the Joint ROM. This involves using flex sensors and accelerometers that may capture actual data regarding real-time elbow flexion and extension. Flex sensors are gauges that determine the degree of movement in a joint by the change in resistance as the sensor bends, and this makes it possible to change the joint angle to degrees. This can be complemented with acceleration as acceleration during movement helps explain how fast and in what direction elbows are moving. Monitoring of the ROM continuously provides insight to the therapist as how over time the joints would gain mobility.

2.2.2 Active Movement Scale (AMS)

The Active Movement Scale (AMS) measures how actively a person can move his or her own joints by their own strength in muscles. This scale is different from the scale of passive movement, wherein the joint is moved for someone by a third person; active movements require control of the motion by the individual himself or herself. AMS is very useful to assess movement in children and also in people who have diseases that reduce muscle strength or coordination. It assists doctors and therapists to know the degree of movement control the patient has, weak points and enables them to track the progress of improvement or worsening during rehabilitation or therapy. The scoring of quality and range of these movements by AMS provides a clear picture of a person's functional abilities and guides the treatment plan.

AMS is one of the important measurement scales to be used in ascertaining the degree of active movement at the elbow joint. AMS uses accelerometers and flex sensors to evaluate the range and control of movements during active tasks at the elbow. The comparison of active movements to the passive assessment of Tardieu

Scale can allow therapists insights into muscle control and strength to adapt therapy approaches tailored toward improving voluntary motor skills.

2.2.3 Spasticity Measurement using Modified Ashworth Scale (MAS)

The Modified Ashworth Scale is a widely used method of measuring spasticity, which is the stiffness or tightness in muscles making movement difficult. Spasticity often occurs in conditions like cerebral palsy, where increased muscle tone can interfere with a child's ability to move freely. MAS works by assessing how much resistance is felt when passively moving a joint through its range of motion. The process helps in recognizing how great the spasticity actually is and which muscles are affected the most. Understanding spasticity is essential for the daily activities, mobility, and therapy goals because by measuring spasticity, therapists could design interventions that target reducing stiffness, improving movement and in general improve the quality of life for the child.

Muscle tone in children with cerebral palsy is well understood through the assessment of spasticity. One objective measure used for this purpose is the Modified Ashworth Scale, which uses muscle sensors to measure spasticity during passive elbow movement. The muscle sensors measure the amount of spasticity in the muscles, while the accelerometers measure how fast this resistance is increasing with each movement of the joint. This combination of sensor values can yield comprehensive measurements of spasticity that can easily be correlated to the qualitative judgments made during the Tardieu Scale. Objective data will therefore allow the therapist to base interventions clearly on specific child needs.

2.3 IoT enabled elbow device algorithm

The algorithm for the proposed solution consists of three primary phases: Data Collection and Data Processing and Data Transmission, designed to capture, process, and classify spasticity-related data to aid therapists in monitoring therapeutic progress.

2.3.1 Data Collection

The data collection process as given in Algorithm 1 starts when the microcontroller will establish a serial connection at a given baud, and after a small delay to ensure a stable start, it initiates an empty DataFrame for the purpose of storing sensor readings for later sessions. Every session, it will ask users or caregivers to move the elbow to specific angles-targeting active and passive movements. It records joint angles from the flex sensor, movement speed from the accelerometer, and resistance from the muscle sensor for 10 seconds. Structured data capture allows a richer information set to be collected pertaining to spasticity-related metrics. Recorded data is stored in the Data Frame; an Excel file is created, and the user is prompted to "Relax" before the next session.

Algorithm 1 Data Collection Process

```
Initialize and connect to the serial port at 9600 baud rate
Delay for 2 seconds
Initialize empty DataFrame for data collection
Display "Get ready!" and delay for 2 seconds
for each movement session from 1 to N do
Prompt user: "Prepare for assessment or perform elbow movement for session index"
Collect data for 10 seconds:
while data available and time < 10 seconds do
Read, decode, and split data into sensor values
if valid data for current session then
Append sensor values and timestamp to lists
end if
end while
Store lists in DataFrame and display "Relax."
Delay for 2 seconds
end for
Save DataFrame to an Excel file
Print "Data collection complete." =0
```

2.3.2 Data Processing and Analysis

In order to begin processing the collected data, cleaning is involved as seen from Algorithm 2 such as eliminating empty values, smoothing of sudden changes of based on some predefined thresholds and using valid data for any further analysis. For the metric specific evaluation of a particular reading during the analysis step, flex sensor data compute the ROM and classify as "Severe Impairment", "Moderate Impairment", and "Normal" based on the thresholds of angles. The resistance level is classified using the Modified Ashworth Scale (MAS) measured from muscle sensor data in spasticity. Active movement is measured by the Active Movement Scale (AMS) from accelerometer data, measuring the ability of voluntary movement. Furthermore, the Tardieu Scale metrics such as catch angle (R1) and rigidity angle (R2) are calculated from flex and muscle sensor data to measure spasticity levels.

The movement speed is further divided into two categories based on accelerometer thresholds, "Slow" and "Normal". The results are saved into a new Excel file for review by the therapist after processing.

Algorithm 2 Data Processing

```
Process data.
Read data and filter columns with "Flex," "Force," "Angle," "Accelerometer," etc.
Initialize a list to track previous valid sensor readings
for each row in the Excel file do
for each sensor value do
Handle empty values and convert to integer
if change exceeds predefined thresholds (for spastic
-ity, ROM, or angle changes) then
Use previous valid value
end if
Append current or previous value to list
end for
Write list to a new Excel file
end for=0
```

2.3.3 Data Transmission and Long-Term Analysis on the Cloud

The processed data is forwarded to a cloud-based system for storage. This platform can be used for longitudinal tracking, and through it, spasticity trends and treatment progress are monitored. The advanced models of machine learning can further be used for predicting changes in the future, hence enabling the refinement of the treatment plans in accordance with anticipated trends. All data is made accessible to caregivers and therapists through a simple dashboard, which aids in remote monitoring, providing real-time insights, and collaborative adjustments to the therapy plan. This integrated cloud system enables continuous, personalized rehabilitation tracking for improved patient outcomes.

Algorithm 3 Assessment of all the Scales and Movement Metrics

```
Assessment of scales:
Load processed data and define reference values for each relevant scale
for each muscle group or session in assessment do
```

```
Calculate passive movement response using flex sensor and angle data
if scale = "ROM" then
Calculate the elbow ROM based on flex sensor data
if ROM < 30 degrees then
Record "Severe Impairment"
else if ROM < 60 degrees then
Record "Moderate Impairment"
else
Record "Normal"
end if
else if scale = "MAS" then
Assess spasticity using muscle sensor data during passive movement
if resistance = 0 then
Record "No Spasticity"
else if resistance <= 2 then
Record "Mild Spasticity"
else if resistance <f= 4 then
Record "Moderate Spasticity"
else
Record "Severe Spasticity"
end if
else if scale = "AMS" then
Analyze active movement data from accelerometers
if active movement count < threshold then
Record "Limited Active Movement"
else
Record "Sufficient Active Movement"
end if
end if
end for
Print summary of classifications for each scale and muscle group
Save classification results to a new Excel file
Print "Assessment complete. Results saved." =0
```

3 IMPLEMENTATION DETAILS

3.1 Hardware requirement details

The patient interface of the device is an elbow band embedded with multiple sensors that collect all data relevant to spasticity and motor function. The hardware requirements for the wearable device is shown in Table.1.

Table 1. Hardware requirements for the IoT-enabled wearable device

Components	Specification	Quantity
Flex Sensors	5.6 CM Bend Sensor	5 units
Micro-controller	ESP32 with Wi-Fi capability	1 unit
Connecting Wires	Jumper Wires	Variable
Accelerometer	3-axis accelerometer, ADXL345	1 unit
Resistors	10k ohm	3 unit
Elbow Band	Adjustable for sensor attachment	1 unit
Muscle Sensor	Outputs analog signals (0–3.3V/5V)	1 unit
Battery	9 volts	2 units
EMG Electrodes	Ag/AgCl surface electrodes	3 units
Battery connectors	9V snap connector	3 units

The patient interface of the device is an elbow band embedded with multiple sensors that collect all data relevant to spasticity and motor function. The hardware requirements for the wearable device is shown in Table.1.

3.1.1 ESP32 Microcontroller

The ESP32 acts as the wearable's control unit. It takes data from a variety of sensors, namely the accelerometer, flex sensors, and muscle sensors, and processes the data in real time for instantaneous feedback. In addition, it transmits the data to a system hosted in cloud for storage and checks the data through its built-in Wi-Fi facility so as to assist the children throughout the day. Its small size ensures that it fits without bulking up inside the band, making it wearable-friendly.

3.1.2 Accelerometer (ADXL345)

The ADXL345 is important to watch how the arm is oriented and hence how it moves about. When placed on the band close to the elbow, it provides very important data on how the arm is located and moving in three-dimensional space. It ensures that the exercise in therapy is done correctly, helping in correction of movement and monitoring progress. The small size of the ADXL345 allows it to be easily accommodated in the wearable band.

3.1.3 Flex Sensors

The flex sensors are the main parts used to measure how much the elbow bends and straightens once they are fixed on both the inner and outer side of the elbow on the band. The sensors help figure out how much more movement the elbow has for them and keep track of the progress over time, which is very important for physical therapy. They are flexible and light, ideal for fitting into the band without losing comfort or ability to move.

3.1.4 Muscle Sensor

Muscle sensor (EMG) measures electrical activity from muscle contractions to assess spasticity and muscle performance. In an elbow wearable for children with cerebral palsy, it monitors biceps and triceps activity, providing real-time feedback to enhance therapy, complementing data from flex and muscle sensors for better spasticity evaluation and rehabilitation tracking.

3.2 Elbow Wearable Device Design

The proposed wearable technology is aimed at assisting the movement and elbow movement tracking in children suffering from cerebral palsy. The core of the device is the ESP32 processor, which powers the wearable core functionality. The ESP32 collects data from a variety of sensors embedded in the band and sends this data to a cloud platform for real-time monitoring and analysis. The accelerometer (ADXL345) measure the orientation and movement of the arm, which yields valuable insight into the range of motion for the elbow. Meanwhile, the flex sensors check the angle of bending or extension of the elbow joint, and a muscle sensor detects over-pressure during the movements to make sure the child is not under unhealthy conditions.

The data collected by the sensors are sent to a cloud-based platform using ESP32's Wi-Fi module. This enables caregivers and therapists to track the movements of the child in real-time. Networking protocols such as MQTT assure good communication between the device and the cloud, whilst secure encryption of sensitive patient data prevents data breaches.

The components are placed carefully as shown in Figure 3 and set up throughout the band to ensure a seamless user experience. The resulting product is a comfortable, efficient, and intelligent wearable band designed for children suffering from cerebral palsy to help them in enhancing the quality of their lives, specifically in motor function improvement.

Figure 3. Wearable elbow band

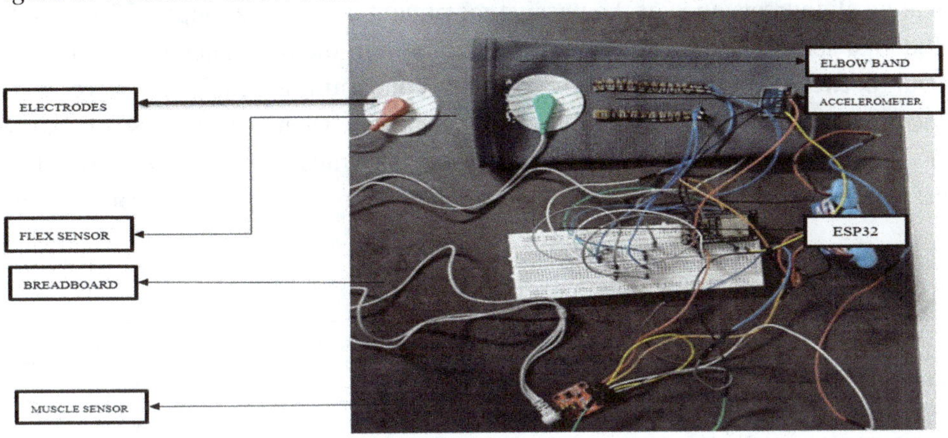

4 RESULT ANALYSIS

4.1 MQTT Connection

The MQTT connection was established using HiveMQ Cloud, utilizing secure communication over the TLS encryption. Using the provided credentials, the python script that included the code to listen to MQTT connected to the broker on cloud on port 8883; the connexion was confirmed by subscribing to the "elbowcn" topic and listening while returning a result code of 0.

Once subscribed the script could listen for incoming messages. When one came in, it would be encoded in base 64. The script would then decode the message and save the contents to a file where the sensor data with metrics is saved. This is actually what contained the transmitted sensor data in accurate and secure delivery. The output includes broker connection confirmation, topic subscription, and successful receipt and decoding of the transmitted file.

4.2 Scenario 1: Modified Ashworth Scale (MAS) Assessment

The MAS output as shown in Table 2 gives the categorization of spasticity as per the recorded force values with regard to muscle resistance. Normal resistance, no spasticity noted and observed with a force value below 200. Mild spasticity indicating slight resistance of the passive movement occurs in a range of 200 to 400. Moderate spasticity that shows a strong increase in the resistance by the muscles occurs between 400 and 600. Severe spasticity concerning a significant level of resistance with apparent mobility problems was recorded when force values were above 600. The classifications show the varying levels of muscle resistances throughout sessions thus giving important data to assess and monitor outcomes from therapy.

Table 2. Modified Ashworth Scale (MAS) Output

Timestamp	Muscle Sensor Value	MAS (Spasticity)
23:13:18.575	128	Severe Spasticity
23:13:19.587	61	Severe Spasticity
23:13:34.542	1619	Mild Spasticity
23:13:35.565	507	Mild Spasticity
23:13:39.542	4095	No Spasticity
23:13:40.558	77	Severe Spasticity

4.3 Scenario 2: Joint Range of Motion (ROM) Assessment

ROM data demonstrates two different patterns. For the first data collected, "Severe Impairment" is always reported because Flex1 and Flex2 values are less than 50 as shown in Figure 5 with considerable mobility restrictions along with muscle stiffness. For the second data collected, each session is labeled "Normal," and their Flex1 and Flex2 values are between 1800 and 2800 as depicted in Table 3, indicating normal joint movement. This actually calls for intervention during phases of "Severe Impairment", followed by regular monitoring at the "Normal" phases in order not to lapse into regression.

Table 3. Joint Range of Motion (ROM) Output

Timestamp	Flex1 Value	Flex2 Value	ROM (Impairment)
2024-11-22	2736	2537	Normal Impairment
2024-11-22	2288	2733	Normal Impairment
2024-11-22	2137	1963	Normal Impairment
2024-11-22	29	0	Severe Impairment
2024-11-22	49	82	Severe Impairment
2024-11-22	0	48	Severe Impairment

4.4 Scenario 3: Active Movement Scale (AMS) Assessment

Minimal movement is witnessed when the Accel X, Y, and Z readings are close to zero, leading to "Minimal Movement" classification in AMS as shown in Table 4. This means that an increased accelerometer reading would therefore be able to carry on "Limited Movement", for instance Accel X $\approx$ 5, Accel Y $\approx$ -11, Accel Z $\approx$ 9. Generally, there is "Full Movement" where readings are high, for instance, Accel X $\approx$ 20.045, Accel Y $\approx$ 16.397, and Accel Z $\approx$ 8.473. These could be a measure of the extent of voluntary control and muscle activation while moving.

Table 4. Active Movement Scale (AMS) Output

Timestamp	Accel X	Accel Y	Accel Z	AMS (Movement)
2024-11-22	0.000	0.000	0.000	Minimal Movement
2024-11-22	0.706	-2.079	5.413	Minimal Movement
2024-11-22	4.982	-5.688	-7.492	Limited Movement
2024-11-22	4.276	-9.218	-0.628	Limited Movement
2024-11-22	7.178	-11.219	2.707	Good Movement
2024-11-22	6.119	-2.197	9.022	Good Movement
2024-11-22	-14.004	20.045	-1.961	Full Movement
2024-11-22	-20.045	-20.084	2.667	Full Movement

Figure 4. Different scenarios of elbow bending (a) Elbow bending scenario with full movement b) Elbow bending with limited movement)

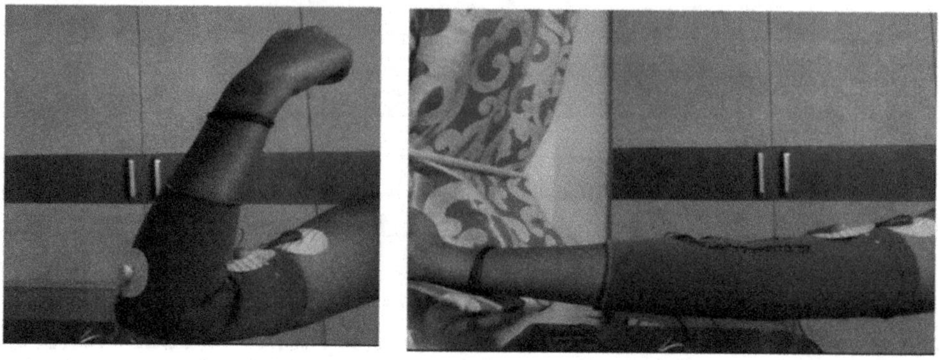

a) Elbow bending scenario with full movement b) Elbow bending with limited movement

5 CONCLUSION AND FUTURE SCOPE

The IoT-enabled wearable device for monitoring elbow movements in children with cerebral palsy marks a significant advancement in rehabilitation technology. The device uses sensors like accelerometers, muscle sensors and flex sensors using the different scales: Joint Range of Motion (ROM), Active Movement Scale (AMS) and Modified Ashworth Scale (MAS) while recording the most important aspects of ROM, movement speed, and resistance in the assessment of spasticity and motor function. The ESP32 microcontroller, MQTT protocol, and cloud computing is integrated to support secure and efficient data collection with remote monitoring that allows immediate feedback to healthcare providers for personalized therapy planning. The innovation bridges the gap between the traditional techniques of physical therapy, innovative technological solutions, and affordability with usability of devices toward better therapy outcomes.

Future work will involve including machine learning algorithms to these devices. Predictive analytics of therapy progress and outcomes may be enabled by embedding the latest machine learning algorithms. Finally, production costs should be reduced, and design shall be simplified for ease of manufacture and use to ensure the device is acceptable and used in a resource-limited setting.

REFERENCES

Cacioppo, M., Loos, A., Lempereur, M., & Brochard, S. (2023). Bimanual movements in children with cerebral palsy: A systematic review of instrumented assessments. *Journal of Neuroengineering and Rehabilitation*, *20*(1), 26. DOI: 10.1186/s12984-023-01150-7 PMID: 36849971

Cusimano, G., Longo, A., Uffreduzzi, A., Bravi, M., & Taffoni, F. (2020). "Design and development of an instrumented glove for hand rehabilitation in children suffering from cerebral palsy: a digital manufacturing approach," 2020 IEEE International Workshop on Metrology for Industry 4.0 IoT, Roma, Italy, pp. 521-525 DOI: 10.1109/MetroInd4.0IoT48571.2020.9138274

Fadhlillah, R., Susmartini, S., & Herdiman, L. (2020, February). Realtime health monitoring system design for children with cerebral palsy using internet of things. [). IOP Publishing.]. *Journal of Physics: Conference Series*, *1450*(1), 012119.

Francisco-Martínez, C., Prado-Olivarez, J., Padilla-Medina, J. A., Díaz-Carmona, J., Pérez-Pinal, F. J., Barranco-Gutiérrez, A. I., & Martínez-Nolasco, J. J. (2021). Upper Limb Movement Measurement Systems for Cerebral Palsy: A Systematic Literature Review. *Sensors (Basel)*, *21*(23), 7884. DOI: 10.3390/s21237884 PMID: 34883885

Harvey, A. R. (2008). *The functional mobility scale for children with cerebral palsy: reliability and validity*. University of Melbourne, School of Physiotherapy.

Jobin, A., & Levin, M. F. (2000). *Regulation of stretch reflex threshold in elbow flexors in children with cerebral palsy: a new measure of spasticity. Developmental Medicine &amp*. Child Neurology.

Levin, M. F., Piscitelli, D., & Khayat, J. (2024). Tonic stretch reflex threshold as a measure of disordered motor control and spasticity – A critical review. *Clinical Neurophysiology*, *165*, 138–150. DOI: 10.1016/j.clinph.2024.06.019

Moen, R. D., & Østensjø, S. (2023). Understanding the use and benefits of assistive devices among young children with cerebral palsy and their families in Norway: A cross-sectional population-based registry study. *Disability and Rehabilitation. Assistive Technology*, *19*(4), 1454–1462. DOI: 10.1080/17483107.2023.2198563 PMID: 37026592

Nascimento, L. M. S. D., Bonfati, L. V., Freitas, M. L. B., Mendes, J. J. A.Junior, Siqueira, H. V., & Stevan Jr, S. L. (2020). Sensors and systems for physical rehabilitation and health monitoring—A review. *Sensors (Basel)*, *20*(15), 4063. DOI: 10.3390/s20154063 PMID: 32707749

Nourizadeh, M., Shadgan, B., Abbasidezfouli, S., Juricic, M., & Mulpuri, K. (2024). Methods of muscle spasticity assessment in children with cerebral palsy: A scoping review. *Journal of Orthopaedic Surgery and Research*, *19*(1), 401. DOI: 10.1186/s13018-024-04894-7 PMID: 38992701

Novak, I., Mcintyre, S., Morgan, C., Campbell, L., Dark, L., Morton, N., Stumbles, E., Wilson, S. A., & Goldsmith, S. (2013). A systematic review of interventions for children with cerebral palsy: State of the evidence. *Developmental Medicine and Child Neurology*, *55*(10), 885–910. DOI: 10.1111/dmcn.12246 PMID: 23962350

Paul, S., Nahar, A., Bhagawati, M., & Kunwar, A. J. (2022). A review on recent advances of cerebral palsy. *Oxidative Medicine and Cellular Longevity*, *2022*(1), 2622310. DOI: 10.1155/2022/2622310 PMID: 35941906

Rathke, C. L., Pimentel, V. C. A., Alsina, P. J., do Espírito Santo, C. C., & Dantas, A. F. O. A. (2024). IoT-Based Wireless System for Gait Kinetics Monitoring in Multi-Device Therapeutic Interventions. *Sensors (Basel)*, *24*(17), 5799. DOI: 10.3390/s24175799 PMID: 39275710

Rozaire, J., Paquin, C., Henry, L., Agopyan, H., Bard-Pondarré, R., Naaim, A., Duprey, S., & Chaleat-Valayer, E. (2024). A systematic review of instrumented assessments for upper limb function in cerebral palsy: Current limitations and future directions. *Journal of Neuroengineering and Rehabilitation*, *21*(1), 56. DOI: 10.1186/s12984-024-01353-6 PMID: 38622731

Rozaire, J., Paquin, C., Henry, L., Agopyan, H., Bard-Pondarré, R., Naaim, A., Duprey, S., & Chaleat-Valayer, E. (2024). A systematic review of instrumented assessments for upper limb function in cerebral palsy: Current limitations and future directions. *Journal of Neuroengineering and Rehabilitation*, *21*(1), 56. DOI: 10.1186/s12984-024-01353-6 PMID: 38622731

Singh, D. N., Hashmi, M. F., & Sharma, S. K. (2020). Predictive analytics & modeling for modern health care system for cerebral palsy patients. *Multimedia Tools and Applications*, *79*(15), 10285–10307. DOI: 10.1007/s11042-019-07834-4

Skoutelis, V. C., Dimitriadis, Z., Kalamvoki, E., Vrettos, S., Kontogeorgakos, V., Dinopoulos, A., Papagelopoulos, P., & Kanellopoulos, A. (2022). Translation, reliability and validity of the Greek functional mobility scale (FMS) for children with cerebral palsy. *Disability and Rehabilitation*, *44*(8), 1436–1442. DOI: 10.1080/09638288.2020.1799439 PMID: 32744923

Thangam, S.. (2024). "Flex Sensor Data Analysis for Hand Rehabilitation using Wearable Glove." *2024 Third International Conference on Electrical, Electronics, Information and Communication Technologies (ICEEICT)*. IEEE.

Thangam, S., ... (2024). "IoT-Based Health Monitoring System for Forbidden Patients." *2024 10th International Conference on Advanced Computing and Communication Systems (ICACCS)*. Vol. 1. IEEE.

Virupaxappa, G., & Thangam, S. (2023). "Detection of Dystonia in Cerebral Palsy Using Dyskinesia Impairment Scale and Machine Learning," 2023 IEEE 3rd Mysore Sub Section International Conference (MysuruCon), HASSAN, India. DOI: 10.1109/MysuruCon59703.2023.10396938

von Elling-Tammen, L., Stark, C., Wloka, K. R., Alberg, E., Schoenau, E., & Duran, I. (2023). Predicting gross motor function in children and adolescents with cerebral palsy applying artificial intelligence using data on assistive devices. *Journal of Clinical Medicine*, *12*(6), 2228.

Wu, C. M., Chen, S. C., Chen, Y. J., & Efendi, A. (2024). A Personalized Contactless Emergency Aid System Designed for Individuals With Profound Physical Disabilities. *IEEE Access : Practical Innovations, Open Solutions*, *12*, 27115–27126.

Xiong, A., Wu, T., & Jia, J. (2024). Design of a Real-Time Monitoring System for Electroencephalogram and Electromyography Signals in Cerebral Palsy Rehabilitation via Wearable Devices. *Electronics (Basel)*, *13*(15), 2902. DOI: 10.3390/electronics13152902

Compilation of References

Aazam, M., Zeadally, S., & Harras, K. A. (2020). Health Fog for Smart Healthcare. IEEE Consumer Electronics Magazine, 9(2), 96-102. DOI: . Published by IEEE, Print ISSN: 2162-2248, Electronic ISSN: 2162-2256.DOI: 10.1109/MCE.2020.2968753

Abbady, H. E., Klinkenberg, E. T., de Moel, L., Nicolai, N., van der Stelt, M., Verhulst, A. C., Maal, T. J. J., & Brouwers, L. (2022). 3D-printed prostheses in developing countries: A systematic review. *Prosthetics and Orthotics International*, *46*(1), 19–30. DOI: 10.1097/PXR.0000000000000057 PMID: 34772868

Abbas, T., &Zlopasa, O. (2025). The Role of IoT and AI in Smart Prosthetics: Advancing Adaptive and Personalized Assistive Technologies.

Abbas, A., Aftab, M. J., & Naz, I. (2025). Experience of a University Teacher on the Self-Esteem of Visually Impaired Students. *Research Journal for Social Affairs*, *3*(2), 13–25. DOI: 10.71317/RJSA.003.02.0090

Abidi, M. H., Noor Siddiquee, A., Alkhalefah, H., & Srivastava, V. (2024). A comprehensive review of navigation systems for visually impaired individuals. *Heliyon*, *10*(11), e31825. DOI: 10.1016/j.heliyon.2024.e31825 PMID: 38841448

Abiraj, S., Janney, B., Prince, P. G. K., Sudhakar, T., & Jebaraj, E. (2024). AI-powered automated wheelchair with Lane detection. 2024 International Conference on Emerging Smart Computing and Informatics (ESCI), 1–5. DOI: 10.1109/ESCI59607.2024.10497306

Abraham, C. H., Ocansey, S., Boadi-Kusi, S. B., Faheem, F., Gyan, B. O., Nti, Y. A., Berchie, M., & Abu, E. K. (2023). Knowledge and practice of drivers on the provision of service to persons with visual disability: A survey of public transport drivers in a tertiary inclusion school in West Africa. *British Journal of Visual Impairment*, *41*(2), 414–424. DOI: 10.1177/02646196211044969

Abugabah, A., Nizamuddin, N., & Alzubi, A. A. (2020, September 4). Decentralized Telemedicine Framework for a Smart Healthcare Ecosystem. *IEEE Access : Practical Innovations, Open Solutions*, *8*, 166575–166588. DOI: 10.1109/ACCESS.2020.3021823

Abu-Jamie, T. N., & Abu-Naser, S. S. (2022). Classification of Sign-language Using VGG16. [IJAER]. *International Journal of Academic Engineering Research*, *6*(6), 36–46.

Abul Kalam Azad, T., Atkison, T., & Shahen Shah, A. F. M. 2024. A Review on Machine Learning in Intelligent Transportation Systems Applications. The Open Transportation Journal. [online] Available at: https://benthamopen.com/ABSTRACT/TOTJ-18-1

Accessibility Technology for blind & low vision people. (2025, January 30). Be My Eyes. https://www.bemyeyes.com/

Accessible pedestrian signals. (n.d.). Retrieved June 27, 2025, from https://www.okeenea.com/en/accessible-pedestrian-signal

AccessNow - pin-pointing accessibility worldwide. (2015, July 29). AccessNow. https://accessnow.com/

ADCET. (2025). *Deaf or hearing impaired.* Australian Disability Clearinghouse on Education and Training. https://www.adcet.edu.au/inclusive-teaching/specific-disabilities/deaf-hearing-impaired

Aderinto, N., Olatunji, G., Abdulbasit, M. O., Edun, M., Aboderin, G., & Egbunu, E. (2023). Exploring the efficacy of virtual reality-based rehabilitation in stroke: A narrative review of current evidence. *Annals of Medicine*, *55*(2), 2285907. DOI: 10.1080/07853890.2023.2285907 PMID: 38010358

Ahmad, I., Asghar, Z., Kumar, T., Li, G., Manzoor, A., Mikhaylov, K., Shah, S. A., Höyhtyä, M., Reponen, J., Huusko, J., & Harjula, E. (2022). Emerging technologies for next generation remote health care and assisted living. *IEEE Access : Practical Innovations, Open Solutions*, *10*, 56094–56132. DOI: 10.1109/ACCESS.2022.3177278

Ahmed, A., Kaiser, M. S., Rahman, M. S., Al Mamun, S., Rahman, M. M., & Mahmud, M. (2023, December). Internet of Educational Things (IoET): Enhancing Learning Experiences for People with Disabilities. In *International Conference on Trends in Electronics and Health Informatics* (pp. 729–754). Singapore: Springer Nature Singapore.

Ahmed, E., Islam, A., Sarker, F., Huda, M. N., & Abdullah-Al-Mamun, K. (2016). A road to independent living with smart homes for people with disabilities. In *2016 5th International conference on informatics, electronics and vision (ICIEV)* (pp. 472-477). IEEE. DOI: 10.1109/ICIEV.2016.7760048

Ahmed, H., & Malik, S. (2023). *Artificial intelligence (AI) in the digital healthcare and medical industry*. IGI Global.

Ainscow, M., Calderón-Almendros, I., Duk, C., & Viola, M. (2025). Using professional development to promote inclusive education in Latin America: Possibilities and challenges. *Professional Development in Education, 51*(1), 149–166. DOI: 10.1080/19415257.2024.2427285

Aira. (2025, February 14). Aira | Access Is a Human Right; Aira. https://aira.io/aira-app/

Akbari, A., Haghverd, F., & Behbahani, S. (2021). Robotic home-based rehabilitation systems design: From a literature review to a conceptual framework for community-based remote therapy during COVID-19 pandemic. *Frontiers in Robotics and AI, 8*, 612331. DOI: 10.3389/frobt.2021.612331 PMID: 34239898

Akhai, S. (2024). A Review on Optimizations in μ-EDM Machining of the Biomedical Material Ti6Al4V Using the Taguchi Method: Recent Advances Since 2020. *Latest Trends in Engineering and Technology*, 395-402.

Akhai, S. (2024). Smart Home Environment for Society: An Overview of IoT-Enabled Air Conditioners. In *Modelling of Virtual Worlds Using the Internet of Things* (Vol. 1, pp. 74-87). CRC Press.

Akhai, S. (2024). Towards Trustworthy and Reliable AI The Next Frontier. In *Explainable Artificial Intelligence (XAI) in Healthcare* (Vol. 1, pp. 119-129). CRC Press, Taylor & Francis Group.

Akhai, S. (2024a). Smart Home Environment for Society: An Overview of IoT-Enabled Air Conditioners. In Modelling of Virtual Worlds Using the Internet of Things (Vol. 1, pp. 74-87). CRC Press.

Akhai, S. (2024b). Towards Trustworthy and Reliable AI The Next Frontier. In Explainable Artificial Intelligence (XAI) in Healthcare (Vol. 1, pp. 119-129). CRC Press, Taylor & Francis Group.

Akhai, S., & Abbass, M. (2025). Air Conditioning for Healthier Living. In Managing the Health Risks of Climate Change (pp. 135–154). IGI Global Scientific Publishing. DOI: 10.4018/979-8-3693-4183-4.ch006

Akhai, S., & Khang, A. (2024). Innovations in Medical Manufacturing: A Review of 3D Printing, Robotics, and Internet of Things (IoT). In The Quantum Evolution (Vol. 1, pp. 226-241). CRC Press.

Akhai, S., & Kumar, V. (2024). Quantum resilience and distributed trust: The promise of blockchain and quantum computing in defense. In Sustainable Security Practices Using Blockchain, Quantum and Post-Quantum Technologies for Real Time Applications (pp. 125-153). Springer Nature Singapore.

Akhai, S., Abbass, M., Kaur, P., & Kaur, T. (2025). Digital Transformation Across Generations: Robotics and AI in Action. In *Impacts of Digital Technologies Across Generations* (pp. 23-40). IGI Global Scientific Publishing. DOI: 10.4018/979-8-3693-6366-9.ch002

Akhai, S. (2023). From Black Boxes to Transparent Machines: The Quest for Explainable AI. Social Science Research Network. DOI: 10.2139/ssrn.4390887

Akhai, S. (2023). Healthcare record management for healthcare 4.0 via blockchain: a review of current applications, opportunities, challenges, and future potential. In *Blockchain for Healthcare 4.0* (Vol. 1, pp. 211–223). CRC Press. DOI: 10.1201/9781003408246-11

Akhai, S. (2023). Navigating the Potential Applications and Challenges of Intelligent and Sustainable Manufacturing for a Greener Future. *Evergreen*, *10*(4), 2237–2243. DOI: 10.5109/7160899

Akhai, S. (2024). The Impact of Artificial Intelligence on Healthcare: Opportunities and Challenges. *Journal of Advanced Research in Medical Science & Technology*, *11*(1&2), 1–6. DOI: 10.24321/2394.6539.202401

Akhai, S., Singh, V. P., & John, S. (2016). Human performance in industrial design centers with small unit air conditioning systems. *Journal of Advanced Research in Production Industrial Engineering*, *3*(2), 5–11.

Akhai, S., Srivastava, P., Sharma, V., & Bhatia, A. (2021, August). Investigating weld strength of AA8011-6062 alloys joined via friction-stir welding using the RSM approach. *Journal of Physics: Conference Series*, *1950*(1), 012016. DOI: 10.1088/1742-6596/1950/1/012016

Akhai, S., & Wadhwa, A. S. (2024). Recent Advances in Bio-Tribology From Joint Lubrication to Medical Implants: A Review. *Journal of Materials*, *2*(2), 125–135.

Akhai, S., & Wadhwa, A. S. (2024). Wireless networking solutions for climate control and comfort in modern air conditioning systems. In *Intelligent Networks* (pp. 165–181). CRC Press. DOI: 10.1201/9781003541363-11

Al Khatib, I., Shamayleh, A., & Ndiaye, M. (2024, July). Healthcare and the internet of medical things: Applications, trends, key challenges, and proposed resolutions. *Informatics (MDPI), 11*(3), 47. DOI: 10.3390/informatics11030047

Alaftekin, M., Pacal, I., & Cicek, K. (2024). Real-time sign language recognition based on YOLO algorithm. *Neural Computing & Applications, 36*(14), 7609–7624. DOI: 10.1007/s00521-024-09503-6

Alahi, M. E. E., Sukkuea, A., Tina, F. W., Nag, A., Kurdthongmee, W., Suwannarat, K., & Mukhopadhyay, S. C. (2023). Integrating IoT-enabled technologies and artificial intelligence (AI) for smart city scenario: Recent advancements and future trends. *Sensors (Basel), 23*(11), 5206. DOI: 10.3390/s23115206 PMID: 37299934

Alam, E., Abu Sufian, P. D., & Leo, M. (2022). Vision-based human fall detection systems using deep learning: A review. *Computers in Biology and Medicine, 146*, 105626. DOI: 10.1016/j.compbiomed.2022.105626 PMID: 35680453

Alam, M., & Qureshi, N. (2023). *IoT in healthcare and telemedicine: Revolutionizing patient care*. IGI Global.

Alenezi, M., Wardat, S., & Akour, M. (2023). The need for integrating digital education in higher education: Challenges and opportunities. *Sustainability (Basel), 15*(6), 4782. DOI: 10.3390/su15064782

Alghabban, W. G., & Hendley, R. (2023). *Adaptive e-Learning and Dyslexia: An Empirical Evaluation and Recommendations for Future Work. Interacting with Computers*. OUCI., DOI: 10.1093/iwc/iwad036

Alharith, R., Ibrahim, A. O., Wahid, N., Ghazali, R., & Elsafi, A. (2024). Comparative Analysis of ResNet Models for Skin Cancer Diagnosis: Performance Evaluation and Insights. *Lecture Notes in Networks and Systems*, 370–378. DOI: 10.1007/978-3-031-66965-1_36

Al-Homoud, M. (2025). Aging in Place in Jordan: Assessing Home Modifications, Accessibility Barriers, and Cultural Constraints. *Buildings (Basel, Switzerland), 15*(17), 3125. DOI: 10.3390/buildings15173125

Aljebreen, M., Alamro, H., Al-Mutiri, F., Othman, K. M., Alsumayt, A., Alazwari, S., Hamza, M. A., & Mohammed, G. P. (2024). Enhancing traffic flow prediction in intelligent cyber-physical systems: A novel bi-LSTM-based approach with Kalman filter integration. *IEEE Transactions on Consumer Electronics, 70*(1), 1889–1902. DOI: 10.1109/TCE.2023.3335155

All_Aboard. (n.d.). "all_aboard" app effectively aids blind and visually impaired commuters in finding bus stops. Mass Eye and Ear. Retrieved June 27, 2025, from https://masseyeandear.org/news/press-releases/2024/01/all-aboard-app-effectively-aids-blind-and-visually-impaired-commuters

Almeida, D., Shmarko, K., & Lomas, E. (2022). The ethics of facial recognition technologies, surveillance, and accountability in an age of artificial intelligence: A comparative analysis of US, EU, and UK regulatory frameworks. *AI and Ethics*, *2*(3), 377–387. DOI: 10.1007/s43681-021-00077-w PMID: 34790955

Almufareh, A., Alabdulatif, A., Alyami, H., & Alzahrani, A. (2024). The role of smart learning platforms in promoting accessibility and inclusivity in higher education. *Education and Information Technologies*, *29*(2), 1573–1591. DOI: 10.1007/s10639-023-11986-2

Almufareh, M. F., Kausar, S., Humayun, M., & Tehsin, S. (2024). A conceptual model for inclusive technology: Advancing disability inclusion through artificial intelligence. *Journal of Disability Research*, *3*(1), 20230060. DOI: 10.57197/JDR-2023-0060

Almusaed, A., Almssad, A., Yitmen, I., & Homod, R. Z. (2023). Enhancing student engagement: Harnessing "AIED"'s power in hybrid education—A review analysis. *Education Sciences*, *13*(7), 632. DOI: 10.3390/educsci13070632

Al-Musawi, M. H., Turki, S. H., Al-Naymi, H. A. S., Al-salman, S. S., Boroujeni, V. V., Alizadeh, M., & Tavakoli, M. (2024). Localized delivery of healing stimulator medicines for enhanced wound treatment. *Journal of Drug Delivery Science and Technology*, *101*, 106212. DOI: 10.1016/j.jddst.2024.106212

Al-Remawi, M., & Aburub, F. (2024). "Clinical Applications of AI in Post-Cancer Rehabilitation," 2024 2nd International Conference on Cyber Resilience (ICCR), Dubai, United Arab EmiratesDOI: 10.1109/ICCR61006.2024.10533091

Alsharif, B., Alalwany, E., & Ilyas, M. (2024). Transfer learning with YOLOV8 for real-time recognition system of American Sign Language Alphabet. *Franklin Open*, *8*, 100165. DOI: 10.1016/j.fraope.2024.100165

Alsharif, B., Altaher, A. S., Altaher, A., Ilyas, M., & Alalwany, E. (2023). Deep Learning Technology to Recognize American Sign Language Alphabet. *Sensors (Basel)*, *23*(18), 7970. DOI: 10.3390/s23187970 PMID: 37766026

Alsolami, A. S. (2022). Teachers of special education and assistive technology: Teachers' perceptions of knowledge, competencies, and professional development. *SAGE Open*, *12*(1), 21582440221079900. DOI: 10.1177/21582440221079900

Alyami, S., Luqman, H., Al-Azani, S., Alowaifeer, M., Alharbi, Y., & Alonaizan, Y. (2025). *Isharah: A Large-Scale Multi-Scene Dataset for Continuous Sign Language Recognition* (No. arXiv:2506.03615). arXiv. https://doi.org//arXiv.2506.03615DOI: 10.48550

Alyami, S., Luqman, H., & Hammoudeh, M. (2024). Reviewing 25 years of continuous sign language recognition research: Advances, challenges, and prospects. *Information Processing & Management*, *61*(5), 103774. DOI: 10.1016/j.ipm.2024.103774

Aly, M., & Fathi, I. S. (2025). Recognizing American Sign Language gestures efficiently and accurately using a hybrid transformer model. *Scientific Reports*, *15*(1), 20253. DOI: 10.1038/s41598-025-06344-8 PMID: 40550837

American Academy of Dermatology Association. (2024). *Types of skin cancer*. Www.aad.org. https://www.aad.org/public/diseases/skin-cancer/types/common

Amin, M. S., Rizvi, S. T. H., & Hossain, M. (2022). A Comparative Review on Applications of Different Sensors for Sign Language Recognition. *Journal of Imaging*, *8*(4), 98. DOI: 10.3390/jimaging8040098

Analysis of the development and application status of smart zebra crossing. (2022, August 26). https://www.trafficsolution.cn/analysis-of-the-development-and-application-status-of-smart-zebra-crossing/

Anthony Jnr, B., Abbas Petersen, S., Helfert, M., Ahlers, D., & Krogstie, J. (2021). Modeling pervasive platforms and digital services for smart urban transformation using an enterprise architecture framework. *Information Technology & People*, *34*(4), 1285–1312. DOI: 10.1108/ITP-07-2020-0511

Anwar, A., Rehman, I. U., & Husamaldin, L. (2022, September). Smart education for people with disabilities (pwds): Conceptual framework for pwds emotions classification from student utterances (sus) during online learning. In 2022 IEEE International Smart Cities Conference (ISC2) (pp. 1-7). IEEE.

Arshi, O., Chaudhary, A., & Singh, R. (2023). "Navigating the Future of Healthcare: AI-Powered Solutions, Personalized Treatment Plans, and Emerging Trends in 2023," *2023 International Conference on Artificial Intelligence for Innovations in Healthcare Industries (ICAIIHI)*, Raipur, India. DOI: 10.1109/ICAIIHI57871.2023.10489554

Asha, V., Sumalatha, I., Mishra, A., Thethi, H. P., Kalra, R., & Almusawi, M. (2024, April). Utilizing artificial intelligence in telemedicine for efficient remote diagnosis and treatment plan. In 2024 IEEE 13th International Conference on Communication Systems and Network Technologies (CSNT) (pp. 1060-1065). IEEE.

Attar, R. W., Habes, M., Almusharraf, A., Alhazmi, A. H., & Attar, R. W. (2024). Exploring the impact of smart cities on improving the quality of life for people with disabilities in Saudi Arabia. *Frontiers in Built Environment, 10*, 1398425. DOI: 10.3389/fbuil.2024.1398425

Azad, A. K., Atkison, T., & Shah, A. F. M. (2024). A Review on Machine Learning in Intelligent Transportation Systems Applications. The Open Transportation Journal, 18(1).

Azevedo, G. A., Sampaio, R. R., Filho, A. S. N., Moret, M. A., & Murari, T. B. (2021). Sustainable urban mobility analysis for elderly and disabled people in São Paulo. *Scientific Reports, 11*(1), 1–10. DOI: 10.1038/s41598-020-80906-w PMID: 33436990

Aziz, R., Jawed, F., Khan, S. A., & Sundus, H. (2024). Wearable IoT Devices in Rehabilitation: Enabling Personalized Precision Medicine. In *Medical Robotics and AI-Assisted Diagnostics for a High-Tech Healthcare Industry* (pp. 281-308). IGI global.

Azzi, Z., Al Sayegh, H., Metwally, O., & Eissa, M. (2025). Review of Nondestructive Testing (NDT) Techniques for Timber Structures. *Infrastructures, 10*(2), 28. DOI: 10.3390/infrastructures10020028

Babatunde, A. O., Ogundijo, D. A., & Amusat, O. A.. (2024). Mobile health technologies in the prevention and management of hypertension: A scoping review. *Digital Health, 10*, 20552076241277172. Advance online publication. DOI: 10.1177/20552076241277172 PMID: 39221086

Bae, S. (2023). A study on the difficulty of communication through sign language in non-English-speaking countries. *Open Journal of Social Sciences, 11*(10), 494–506. DOI: 10.4236/jss.2023.1110028

Bagala, F., Becker, C., Cappello, A., Chiari, L., Aminian, K., Hausdorff, J. M., Zijlstra, W., & Klenk, J. (2012). Evaluation of accelerometer-based fall detection algorithms on real-world falls. *PLoS One*, *7*(5), e37062. DOI: 10.1371/journal.pone.0037062 PMID: 22615890

Bagher, M. M., Sajjadi, P., Wallgrün, J. O., La Femina, P. C., & Klippel, A. (2021). Move the object or move the user: The role of interaction techniques on embodied learning in VR. *Frontiers in Virtual Reality*, *2*, 695312. DOI: 10.3389/frvir.2021.695312

Baikuvekov, M., Tursynova, A., & Yespayev, G. (2024). "A Deep Learning for Cardiovascular Diseases Detection on Wearable Devices Data," in *Proc. IEEE 4th Int. Conf. Smart Inf. Syst. Technol. (SIST)*, Astana, Kazakhstan, May 2024, DOI: 10.1109/SIST61555.2024.10629525

Baker, M., & Winyard, S. (1998). *Lost vision: older visually impaired people in the UK*. Royal National Institute for the Blind.

Banerjee, K., Bali, V., Sharma, A., Aggarwal, D., Yadav, A. and Shukla, A., n.d. Traffic Accident Risk Prediction Using Machine Learning. IEEE.

Barbadekar, A., Ashtekar, V., & Chaudhari, A. (2023). Skin Cancer Classification and Detection Using VGG-19 and DesNet. *2023 International Conference on Computational Intelligence, Networks and Security (ICCINS)*, 1–6. DOI: 10.1109/ICCINS58907.2023.10449996

Bartolo, P. A., Borg, M., Callus, A. M., De Gaetano, A., Mangiafico, M., Mazzacano D'Amato, E., & Vincent, J. (2023). Aspirations and accommodations for students with disability to equitably access higher education: A systematic scoping review. [). Frontiers Media SA.]. *Frontiers in Education*, *8*, 1218120. DOI: 10.3389/feduc.2023.1218120

Bartusik-Aebisher, D., Rogóż, K., & Aebisher, D. (2025). Artificial Intelligence and ECG: A New Frontier in Cardiac Diagnostics and Prevention. *Biomedicines*, *13*(7), 1685. DOI: 10.3390/biomedicines13071685 PMID: 40722756

Bastola, A., Wang, H., Boroujeni, S. P. H., Brinkley, J., Moshayedi, A. J., & Razi, A. (2025). Driving toward inclusion: A systematic review of AI-powered accessibility enhancements for people with disability in autonomous vehicles. *IEEE Access : Practical Innovations, Open Solutions*, *13*, 61384–61415. DOI: 10.1109/ACCESS.2025.3555923

Batrakova, L., & Gredasova, V. (2016). Road Safety and Traffic Psychology. *Procedia Engineering*, *150*, 1876–1881.

Batura, O., Regeczi, D., Vassilev, A., Yagafarova, A., Bani, E., Bonneau, V., ... & DE STREEL, A. (2021). Artificial intelligence in road transport: annex to cost of non-Europe report.

Behera, A., & Behera, A. (2022). Shape-memory materials. *Advanced Materials: An Introduction to Modern Materials Science*, 1-42.

Bejani, M. M., & Ghatee, M. (2019). Convolutional neural network with adaptive regularization to classify driving styles on smartphones. *IEEE Transactions on Intelligent Transportation Systems*, *21*(2), 543–552. DOI: 10.1109/TITS.2019.2896672

Benouhiba, A., Holzer, S., Konstantinidi, S., Civet, Y., & Perriard, Y. (2025). The elastic frontier: Dielectric elastomer actuators in healthcare technology. *Smart Materials and Structures, 34*(3), 033001. DOI: 10.1088/1361-665X/adae6a

Berezi, I. U. (2025). Virtual Learning Environment: Redefining Higher Educational Delivery for Efficiency and Accessibility. *International Journal of Educational Management, Rivers State University., 1*(1), 451-467.

Berner, K., & Alves, A. N. (2023). A scoping review of the literature using speech recognition technologies by individuals with disabilities in multiple contexts. *Disability and Rehabilitation. Assistive Technology, 18*(7), 1139–1145. DOI: 10.1080/17483107.2021.1986583 PMID: 34670100

Beyene, W. M., Mekonnen, A. T., & Giannoumis, G. A. (2023). Inclusion, access, and accessibility of educational resources in higher education institutions: Exploring the Ethiopian context. *International Journal of Inclusive Education, 27*(1), 18–34. DOI: 10.1080/13603116.2020.1817580

Bezrukov, O. (2025, May 28). AI in transportation: Ethical balance between safety and privacy. Blog. https://tech-stack.com/blog/ai-in-transportation/

Bharadiya, J. P. (2023). Artificial intelligence in transportation systems a critical review. *American Journal of Computing and Engineering, 6*(1), 35–45. DOI: 10.47672/ajce.1487

Bhardwaj, A., Sharma, M., Kumar, S., Sharma, S., & Sharma, P. C. (2024). Transforming pediatric speech and language disorder diagnosis and therapy: The evolving role of artificial intelligence. *Health Sciences Review (Oxford, England), 100188*, 100188. Advance online publication. DOI: 10.1016/j.hsr.2024.100188

Bharti, I., Chauhan, K., & Aggarwal, P. (2024). Unveiling the future of ai in healthcare management: Analyzing trends of tomorrow rooted in the literature of yesterday. In *Healthcare Administration and Managerial Training in the 21st Century* (pp. 175–210). IGI Global.

Bhat, A., Rao, V. S., & Jayalakshmi, N. S. (2023). Review of the Evolution of Magnetorheological Fluid-Based Rehabilitative Devices: From the Perspective of Modeling, Sensors and Control Strategies. *IEEE Access : Practical Innovations, Open Solutions, 11*, 88759–88777. DOI: 10.1109/ACCESS.2023.3305674

Bhavnani, S. P., Parakh, K., Atreja, A., Druz, R., Graham, G. N., Hayek, S. S., Krumholz, H. M., Maddox, T. M., Majmudar, M. D., Rumsfeld, J. S., & Shah, B. R. (2017). 2017 Roadmap for Innovation—ACC Health Policy Statement on Healthcare Transformation in the Era of Digital Health, Big Data, and Precision Health: A Report of the American College of Cardiology Task Force on Health Policy Statements and Systems of Care. *Journal of the American College of Cardiology*, *70*(21), 2696–2718. DOI: 10.1016/j.jacc.2017.10.018 PMID: 29169478

Biased technology: The automated discrimination of facial recognition. (2024, February 29). ACLU of Minnesota. https://www.aclu-mn.org/en/news/biased-technology-automated-discrimination-facial-recognition

Bipin, P. B., & Abirami, S. (2023). *Smart Assistant for Visually Impaired People using Deep Learning Algorithms*. 2023 International Conference on Sustainable Computing and Smart Systems (ICSCSS). https://ieeexplore.ieee.org/document/10169851

Bizwire, K. (n.d.). Gwangju launches smart crosswalk system to assist elderly and mobility-impaired pedestrians. Be Korea-Savvy. Retrieved June 27, 2025, from http://koreabizwire.com/gwangju-launches-smart-crosswalk-system-to-assist-elderly-and-mobility-impaired-pedestrians/285633

Blackstone, S. W., Beukelman, D. R., & Yorkston, K. M. (2015). *Patient-provider communication: Roles for speech-language pathologists and other health care professionals*. Plural Publishing.

Blanck, P. (2023). On the importance of the Americans with Disabilities Act at 30. *Journal of Disability Policy Studies*, *34*(3), 176–198. DOI: 10.1177/10442073211036900 PMID: 39286446

Bocarejo, J. P., & Urrego, L. F. (2022). The impacts of formalization and integration of public transport in social equity: The case of Bogota. *Research in Transportation Business & Management*, *42*, 100560. DOI: 10.1016/j.rtbm.2020.100560

Bodemer, A. (2020). Skin-Cancer.pdf. https://www.va.gov/WHOLEHEALTHLIBRARY/docs/Skin-Cancer.pdf

Boldu, R., Matthies, D. J. C., Zhang, H., & Nanayakkara, S. (2020). AiSee. *Proceedings of the ACM on Interactive, Mobile, Wearable and Ubiquitous Technologies*, *4*(4), 1–25. DOI: 10.1145/3432196

Borthakur, P. P. (2025). The Role and Future Directions of 3D Printing in Custom Prosthetic Design. *Engineering Proceedings*, *81*(1), 10.

Boukerche, A., Tao, Y., & Sun, P. (2020). Artificial intelligence-based vehicular traffic flow prediction methods for supporting intelligent transportation systems. *Computer Networks*, *182*, 107484. DOI: 10.1016/j.comnet.2020.107484

Bragg, D., Koller, O., Bellard, M., Berke, L., Boudreault, P., Braffort, A., & Shillingsburg, T. (2021). Sign language recognition, generation, and translation: An interdisciplinary perspective. *Proceedings of the 21st International ACM SIGACCESS Conference on Computers and Accessibility*, 16-31.

Breaking barriers: Global accessibility in public transportation systems. (2025, June 9). KNOW-THE-ADA. https://know-the-ada.com/examining-accessibility-in-global-public-transportation-systems/

Bricout, J., Baker, P. M., Moon, N. W., & Sharma, B. (2021). Exploring the smart future of participation: Community, inclusivity, and people with disabilities. [IJEPR]. *International Journal of E-Planning Research*, *10*(2), 94–108. DOI: 10.4018/IJEPR.20210401.oa8

Brown, R. L., & Moloney, M. E. (2019). Intersectionality, work, and well-being: The effects of gender and disability. *Gender & Society*, *33*(1), 94–122. DOI: 10.1177/0891243218800636

Bruce, A., & Williams, L. A. (2025). Access and Citizenship for Those With Disabilities: Digitally Enabled Education and AI as a Bridge to Innovative Inclusion. In *Digital Citizenship and the Future of AI Engagement, Ethics, and Privacy* (pp. 31-78). IGI Global Scientific Publishing.

Building an accessible future for all: AI and the inclusion of Persons with Disabilities. (2024, December 2). United Nations Western Europe; United Nations. https://unric.org/en/building-an-accessible-future-for-all-ai-and-the-inclusion-of-persons-with-disabilities/

Bui, T., Liu, J., Cao, J., Wei, G., & Zeng, Q. (2024). Elderly fall detection in complex environment based on improved YOLOv5s and LSTM. *Applied Sciences (Basel, Switzerland)*, *14*(19), 9028. DOI: 10.3390/app14199028

Cacioppo, M., Loos, A., Lempereur, M., & Brochard, S. (2023). Bimanual movements in children with cerebral palsy: A systematic review of instrumented assessments. *Journal of Neuroengineering and Rehabilitation*, *20*(1), 26. DOI: 10.1186/s12984-023-01150-7 PMID: 36849971

Camedda, D., Banks, J., & Ringwood, B. (2024). Empowering Diversity: A Case Study on Inclusive Assessment and Universal Design for Learning in a Post-secondary Programme for Students with Intellectual Disabilities. *All Ireland Journal of Higher Education, 16*(2).

Campbell, P. (2024, July 1). Johns Hopkins researchers develop AI-enhanced navigation system for visually impaired. Johns Hopkins University Applied Physics Laboratory. https://www.jhuapl.edu/news/news-releases/240701-johns-hopkins-creates-navigation-system-for-the-visually-impaired

Carballo, R., Morgado, B., & Cortés-Vega, M. D. (2021). Transforming faculty conceptions of disability and inclusive education through a training programme. *International Journal of Inclusive Education, 25*(7), 843–859.Carballo, R., Morgado, B., & Cortés-Vega, M. D. (2021). Transforming faculty conceptions of disability and inclusive education through a training programme. *International Journal of Inclusive Education, 25*(7), 843–859. DOI: 10.1080/13603116.2019.1579874

Carter, D. L. H. D. (n.d.). Accessible Pedestrian Signals: A Guide to Best Practices. https://onlinepubs.trb.org/onlinepubs/nchrp/nchrp_w117a.pdf

Casey, H., Brady, N., & Guerin, S. (2013). 'Is seeing perceiving?'Exploring issues concerning access to public transport for people with sight loss. *British Journal of Visual Impairment, 31*(3), 217–227. DOI: 10.1177/0264619613495023

Casilari, E., & Oviedo-Jiménez, M. A. (2015). Automatic fall detection system based on the combined use of a smartphone and a smartwatch. *PLoS One, 10*(11), e0140929. DOI: 10.1371/journal.pone.0140929 PMID: 26560737

Cayamcela, M. E. M., & Lim, W. (2019). Fine-tuning a pre-trained convolutional neural network model to translate American sign language in real-time. *2019 International Conference on Computing, Networking and Communications (ICNC)*

Cerna, L., Mezzanotte, C., Rutigliano, A., Brussino, O., Santiago, P., Borgonovi, F., & Guthrie, C. (2021). Promoting inclusive education for diverse societies: A conceptual framework. *OECD Education Working Papers*, (260), 01–57.

Cerritelli, F., Chiera, M., Abbro, M., Megale, V., Esteves, J., Gallace, A., & Manzotti, A. (2021). The challenges and perspectives of the integration between virtual and augmented reality and manual therapies. *Frontiers in Neurology, 12*, 700211. DOI: 10.3389/fneur.2021.700211 PMID: 34276550

Chakraborty, M., Saha, S. and Sharmin, S., 2025. Quality-aware bus-driver scheduling for intelligent transportation system. Elsevier Transportation Research Part C: Emerging Technologies, [online] Available at: https://doi.org/DOI: 10.1016/j.trc.2024.104398

Chakraborty, C., Banerjee, A., Garg, L., & Rodrigues, J. J. P. C. (2020). *Internet of Medical Things for Smart Healthcare: COVID-19 Pandemic*. Published by Springer., DOI: 10.1007/978-981-15-8097-0

Chase, N., Maples, J., & Schipper, M. (2018, June). Autonomous vehicles: Uncertainties and energy implications. In *2018 EIA Energy Conference* (Vol. 5, p. 2018).

Chelli, A., & Pätzold, M. (2019). A machine learning approach for fall detection and daily living activity recognition. *IEEE Access : Practical Innovations, Open Solutions*, *7*, 38670–38687. DOI: 10.1109/ACCESS.2019.2906693

Chen, S. H., Lee, C. H., Jiang, B. C., & Sun, T. L. (2021). Using a Stacked Autoencoder for Mobility and Fall Risk Assessment via Time–Frequency Representations of the Timed Up and Go Test. *Frontiers in Physiology*, *12*, 668350. DOI: 10.3389/fphys.2021.668350 PMID: 34122139

Chen, T. L., Ciocarlie, M., Cousins, S., Grice, P. M., Hawkins, K., Hsiao, K., & Takayama, L. (2013). Robots for humanity: Using assistive robotics to empower people with disabilities. *IEEE Robotics & Automation Magazine*, *20*(1), 30–39. DOI: 10.1109/MRA.2012.2229950

Chen, X., & Wu, Y. (2023). *Artificial intelligence for medical signal processing*. IGI Global.

Chen, X., & Zhao, Y. (2023). *Harnessing AI for better health outcomes: Emerging trends*. IGI Global.

Chen, Y., Patel, R., & Lee, S. (2021). Building trust through inclusive design in assistive technologies. *International Journal of Inclusive Computing*, *12*(3), 150–165.

Chiramba, O., & Ndofirepi, E. S. (2023). Access and success in higher education: Disadvantaged students' lived experiences beyond funding hurdles at a Metropolitan South African university. *South African Journal of Higher Education*, *37*(6), 56–75. DOI: 10.20853/37-6-6021

Choi, G., & Seo, J. (2024). Accessibility, Usability, and Universal Design for Learning: Discussion of Three Key LX/UX Elements for Inclusive Learning Design. *TechTrends*, *68*(5), 936–945. DOI: 10.1007/s11528-024-00987-6

Chrysanthakopoulou, D. C., & Koutsojannis, C. (2025). Machine Learning Algorithms Introduce Evoked Potentials As Alternative Biomarkers for the Expanded Disability Status Scale Prognosis of Multiple Sclerosis Patients. *Cureus, 17*(3). Advance online publication. DOI: 10.7759/cureus.80335 PMID: 40206919

Cihan Camgoz, N., Koller, O., Hadfield, S., & Bowden, R. (2020). Sign Language Transformers: Joint End-to-End Sign Language Recognition and Translation. *2020 IEEE/CVF Conference on Computer Vision and Pattern Recognition (CVPR)*, 10020–10030. DOI: 10.1109/CVPR42600.2020.01004

Citaristi, I. (2022). International telecommunication union—itu. In *The Europa Directory of International Organizations 2022* (pp. 365–369). Routledge., https://www.taylorfrancis.com/chapters/edit/10.4324/9781003292548-75/international-telecommunication-union%E2%80%94itu-ileana-citaristi DOI: 10.4324/9781003292548-75

Clements, L. M., & Kockelman, K. M. (2017). Economic effects of automated vehicles. *Transportation Research Record: Journal of the Transportation Research Board, 2606*(1), 106–114. DOI: 10.3141/2606-14

Cleveland Clinic. (2021, November 19). *Skin Cancer Overview | Cleveland Clinic*. Cleveland Clinic. https://my.clevelandclinic.org/health/diseases/15818-skin-cancer

Coman, L. I., Ianculescu, M., Paraschiv, E. A., Alexandru, A., & Bădărău, I. A. (2024). Smart solutions for diet-related disease management: Connected care, remote health monitoring systems, and integrated insights for advanced evaluation. *Applied Sciences (Basel, Switzerland), 14*(6), 2351. DOI: 10.3390/app14062351

Conley, K., Foyer, A., Hara, P., Janik, T., Reichard, J., D'Souza, J., ... & Ababei, C. (2019). Vibration alert bracelet for notification of the visually and hearing impaired. Journal of Open Hardware.

Correia, C., Reis, R. L., Pashkuleva, I., & Alves, N. M. (2023). Adhesive and self-healing materials for central nervous system repair. *Biomaterials Advances, 151*, 213439. DOI: 10.1016/j.bioadv.2023.213439 PMID: 37146528

Craythorne, E., & Al-Niami, F. (2017). Skin cancer. *Medicine (Abingdon), 45*(7), 431–434. DOI: 10.1016/j.mpmed.2017.04.003

Creed, C., Al-Kalbani, M., Theil, A., Sarkar, S., & Williams, I. (2024). Inclusive AR/VR: Accessibility barriers for immersive technologies. *Universal Access in the Information Society, 23*(1), 59–73. DOI: 10.1007/s10209-023-00969-0

Crenshaw, K. (1989). Demarginalizing the intersection of race and sex: A black feminist critique of antidiscrimination doctrine, feminist theory and antiracist politics. *University of Chicago Legal Forum, 1989*(1), 139–167.

Cumming, T. M., & Rose, M. C. (2022). Exploring universal design for learning as an accessibility tool in higher education: A review of the current literature. *Australian Educational Researcher, 49*(5), 1025–1043. DOI: 10.1007/s13384-021-00471-7

Cusimano, G., Longo, A., Uffreduzzi, A., Bravi, M., & Taffoni, F. (2020). "Design and development of an instrumented glove for hand rehabilitation in children suffering from cerebral palsy: a digital manufacturing approach," 2020 IEEE International Workshop on Metrology for Industry 4.0 IoT, Roma, Italy, pp. 521-525 DOI: 10.1109/MetroInd4.0IoT48571.2020.9138274

D'Silva, J., & Kaur, M. (2020). Privacy concerns in smart home environments: A review. *Journal of Cybersecurity and Privacy, 2*(1), 1–18.

Dabla, P. K., Gruson, D., Gouget, B., Bernardini, S., & Homsak, E. (2021). Lessons learned from the COVID-19 pandemic: Emphasizing the emerging role and perspectives from artificial intelligence, mobile health, and digital laboratory medicine. *EJIFCC, 32*(2), 224. PMID: 34421492

Dabwan, B. A., Olayah, F. A., Halawani, H. T., Mashraqi, A. M., Abdelrahman, Y. A., & Shamsan, A. F. (2023). Classification of Sign language Using VGG16 and VGG19. 2023 7th International Symposium on Innovative Approaches in Smart Technologies (ISAS)

Dabwan, B. A., Jadhav, M. E., Gadkari, A. S., Ali, Y. A., Almula, S. M., Ismil, O. A., & Mohammad, A. A. (2024). Hand gesture classification for individuals with disabilities using the DenseNet121 model. *2024 International Conference on Advancements in Power, Communication and Intelligent Systems (APCI)*

Dahmani, M. G., Tarhouni, M., & Zidi, S. (2024). Vision Transformers (ViT) for Enhanced Skin Cancer Classification. *2024 IEEE International Conference on Artificial Intelligence & Green Energy (ICAIGE)*, 1–6. DOI: 10.1109/ICAIGE62696.2024.10776698

Dallaev, R. (2024). Advances in materials with self-healing properties: A brief review. *Materials (Basel), 17*(10), 2464. DOI: 10.3390/ma17102464 PMID: 38793530

Danemayer, J., Holloway, C., Cho, Y., Berthouze, N., Singh, A., Bhot, W., Dixon, O., Grobelnik, M., & Shawe-Taylor, J. (2023). Seeking information about assistive technology: Exploring current practices, challenges, and the need for smarter systems. *International Journal of Human-Computer Studies, 177*, 103078. DOI: 10.1016/j.ijhcs.2023.103078

Danley, K. (2024, October 25). Developments that will shape the future of smart wheelchairs. https://straitsresearch.com/article/key-advancements-in-smart-wheelchairs

Darcy, S., & Burke, P. F. (2018). On the road again: The barriers and benefits of automobility for people with disability. *Transportation Research Part A, Policy and Practice*, *107*, 229–245. DOI: 10.1016/j.tra.2017.11.002

Das, S., Mutsuddi, I., & Ray, N. (2025). Artificial Intelligence in Adaptive Education: A Transformative Approach. In *Advancing Adaptive Education: Technological Innovations for Disability Support* (pp. 21–50). IGI Global Scientific Publishing.

Dasgupta, R. (2024). *Application of artificial intelligence in healthcare sector*. IGI Global.

Das, K., Cockerell, C. J., Patil, A., Pietkiewicz, P., Giulini, M., Grabbe, S., & Goldust, M. (2021). Machine Learning and Its Application in Skin Cancer. *International Journal of Environmental Research and Public Health*, *18*(24), 13409. DOI: 10.3390/ijerph182413409 PMID: 34949015

Dayalan, K., Saman, D., Murugesan, H., & Prabhakaran, J. (2025). Sign language translation using random forest classifier. *AIP Conference Proceedings*.

Demir, A., Yilmaz, F., & Köse, O. (n.d.). *Early Detection of Skin Cancer Using Deep Learning Architectures: Resnet-101 and Inception-v3*. https://biyoklinikder.org/TIPTEKNO19_Bildiriler/095.pdf

Deng, Z., Liu, M., Li, L., Han, Q., & Min, W. (2025). VTAN: A Novel Video Transformer Attention-Based Network for Dynamic Sign Language Recognition. *Computers, Materials & Continua*, *82*(2), 2793–2812. DOI: 10.32604/cmc.2024.057456

Department of Transport. (2019). *Road Traffic Accident Reporting Guide*. Department for Transport.

Dereje, D., Lamba, D., Abessa, T. G., Kenea, C., Ramari, C., Osama, M., Kossi, O., Boma, P. M., Panda, J., Kushnir, A., Mourad, J., Mapinduzi, J., Fourtassi, M., Daniels, K., Deutsch, J., & Bonnechère, B. (2025). Unlocking the potential of serious games for rehabilitation in low and middle-income countries: Addressing potential and current limitations. *Frontiers in Digital Health*, *7*, 1505717. DOI: 10.3389/fdgth.2025.1505717 PMID: 39957725

Dev, P. S., Eljo, J. J. G., & Srinivasan, S. (2025). Navigating Mental Health Challenges in the Care of Elderly With Disabilities in Kerala: A Gerontological Social Work Perspective. In *Modern Digital Approaches to Care Technologies for Individuals With Disabilities* (pp. 33-56). IGI Global Scientific Publishing. DOI: DOI: 10.4018/979-8-3693-7560-0.ch003

Devi, V. A., Charulatha, T., & Dharishinie, P. (2023). A Survey on Sign Language Recognition and Training Module. ITM Web of Conferences

Dewang, Y., Sharma, V., Baliyan, V. K., Soundappan, T., & Singla, Y. K. (2025). Research Progress in Electroactive Polymers for Soft Robotics and Artificial Muscle Applications. *Polymers*, *17*(6), 746. DOI: 10.3390/polym17060746 PMID: 40292598

Dickerson, A. E., Molnar, L. J., Eby, D. W., Adler, G., Bedard, M., Berg-Weger, M., Classen, S., Foley, D., Horowitz, A., Kerschner, H., Page, O., Silverstein, N. M., Staplin, L., & Trujillo, L. (2007). Transportation and aging: A research agenda for advancing safe mobility. *The Gerontologist*, *47*(5), 578–590. DOI: 10.1093/geront/47.5.578 PMID: 17989400

Digital, A. C. L. (2024, January 4). IoT enabled elevator system – A big lift ahead in smart elevator technology. ACL Digital. https://www.acldigital.com/blogs/smart-elevator-technology

Digital, T. (n.d.). DIEZ and derq launch AI-powered smart pedestrian crossing system in DSO. Government of Dubai Media Office. Retrieved June 27, 2025, from https://mediaoffice.ae/en/news/2023/august/02-08/diez-and-derq-launch

Dildar, M., Akram, S., Irfan, M., Khan, H. U., Ramzan, M., Mahmood, A. R., Alsaiari, S. A., Saeed, A. H. M., Alraddadi, M. O., & Mahnashi, M. H. (2021). Skin Cancer Detection: A Review Using Deep Learning Techniques. *International Journal of Environmental Research and Public Health*, *18*(10), 5479. DOI: 10.3390/ijerph18105479 PMID: 34065430

Disability ethical AI. (2022, March 17). Disability Ethical AI. https://disabilityethicalai.org/

Disability, P. (2000). *Development: Issues Paper*. Dept. For International Development.

Dong, H., Lin, J., Tao, Y., Jia, Y., Sun, L., Li, W. J., & Sun, H. (2024). AI-enhanced biomedical micro/nanorobots in microfluidics. *Lab on a Chip*, *24*(5), 1419–1440. DOI: 10.1039/D3LC00909B PMID: 38174821

Dosovitskiy, A., Beyer, L., Kolesnikov, A., Weissenborn, D., Zhai, X., Unterthiner, T., Dehghani, M., Minderer, M., Heigold, G., Gelly, S., Uszkoreit, J., & Houlsby, N. (2021). *AN IMAGE IS WORTH 16X16 WORDS: TRANSFORMERS FOR IMAGE RECOGNITION AT SCALE*. https://arxiv.org/pdf/2010.11929

Dostalova, K., Tomasek, R., Kalova, M., Janura, M., Rosicky, J., Schnitzer, M., & Demel, J. (2022). Review of ankle rehabilitation devices for treatment of equinus contracture. *Expert Review of Medical Devices, 19*(9), 721–731. DOI: 10.1080/17434440.2022.2136029 PMID: 36225151

Douaidi, L., Senouci, S. M., El Korbi, I., & Harrou, F. 2023, June. Predicting electric vehicle charging stations occupancy: a federated deep learning framework. In *2023 IEEE 97th Vehicular Technology Conference (VTC2023-Spring)* (pp. 1-5). IEEE. DOI: 10.1109/VTC2023-Spring57618.2023.10199832

Dsane, D. N. A. A. B. (2024). Being understood: how to expand sign language access for the deaf community. Retrieved 19/08/2025 from https://blogs.worldbank.org/en/nasikiliza/how-to-expand-sign-language-access-for-the-deaf-community-

Eberle, U., Wenzig, J., & Mumm, N. (2022). Assessing the contribution of products to the United Nations' Sustainable Development Goals: A methodological proposal. *The International Journal of Life Cycle Assessment, 27*(7), 959–977. DOI: 10.1007/s11367-022-02063-8

Ed-dali, R. (2025). Bridging the gap: The role of assistive technologies in enhancing translation accessibility for visually impaired learners in Moroccan higher educational institutions. *Journal of Interdisciplinary Studies in Education, 14*(3), 121–148. DOI: 10.32674/991mea86

Edwards, M., Poed, S., Al-Nawab, H., & Penna, O. (2022). Academic accommodations for university students living with disability and the potential of universal design to address their needs. *Higher Education, 84*(4), 779–799. DOI: 10.1007/s10734-021-00800-w PMID: 35079174

Eisenberg, Y., Heider, A., Labbe, D., Gould, R., & Jones, R. (2024). Planning accessible cities: Lessons from high quality barrier removal plans. *Cities (London, England), 148*, 104837. DOI: 10.1016/j.cities.2024.104837

Ekpete, O. H. (2024). Assistive listening devices for individuals with hearing impairment. *Faculty of Natural and Applied Sciences Journal of Mathematics, and Science Education, 5*(2), 78-81. https://fnasjournals.com/index.php/FNAS-JMSE/article/view/390

Elbedoui, K., Mzoughi, H., & Slima, M. B. (2024). Deep Learning Approaches for Dermoscopic Image-Based Skin Cancer Diagnosis. *2024 IEEE 7th International Conference on Advanced Technologies, Signal and Image Processing (ATSIP)*, 1–7. DOI: 10.1109/ATSIP62566.2024.10638968

Elfakki, A. O., Sghaier, S., & Alotaibi, A. A. (2024). An Efficient System for Dyslexic Students Learning in A Virtual Environment. *Transylvanian Review, 32*(1). https://www.transylvanianreviewjournal.com/index.php/TR/article/view/1041 (transylvanianreviewjournal.com)

Elgohr, A., Elhadidy, M., El-Geneedy, M., Mohamed, S., & Mousa, M. (2025). Advancing Sign Language Recognition: A YOLO v.11-Based Deep Learning Framework for Alphabet and Transactional Hand Gesture Detection. *Proceedings of the AAAI Symposium Series, 6*, 209–217. DOI: 10.1609/aaaiss.v6i1.36055

Elkateb, S., Métwalli, A., Shendy, A., & Abu-Elanien, A. E. B. (2024). *Machine learning and IoT–based predictive maintenance approach for industrial applications*. Alexandria University, Arab Academy for Science, Technology and Maritime Transport. DOI: 10.1016/j.aej.2023.12.065

Ellis, K., Goggin, G., Haller, B. A., & Curtis, R. (Eds.). (2020). *The Routledge companion to disability and media* (p. 387). Routledge.

Elorduy, J. L., Pino, Y., & Gento, Á. M. (2025). Assessing public transport accessibility for people with physical disabilities in burgos, spain: A user-centered approach to inclusive urban mobility. *PLoS One*, *20*(4), e0322068. DOI: 10.1371/journal.pone.0322068 PMID: 40299992

El-Tanani, M., Satyam, S. M., Rabbani, S. A., El-Tanani, Y., Aljabali, A. A., Al Faouri, I., & Rehman, A. (2025). Revolutionizing Drug Delivery: The Impact of Advanced Materials Science and Technology on Precision Medicine. *Pharmaceutics*, *17*(3), 375. DOI: 10.3390/pharmaceutics17030375 PMID: 40143038

Enyan, M., Bing, Z., Amu-Darko, J. N. O., Issaka, E., Otoo, S. L., & Agyemang, M. F. (2025). Advances in smart materials soft actuators on mechanisms, fabrication, materials, and multifaceted applications: A review. *Journal of Thermoplastic Composite Materials*, *38*(1), 302–370. DOI: 10.1177/08927057241248028

Epp, S. (2024). Moving forward: Perspectives of adults with intellectual and developmental disabilities regarding the effectiveness of Individual Support Plans.

Erickson, G. 2025. Uncovering Responsible AI's Biggest Challenge: Privacy and Fairness. [online] Available at: https://www.nimblegravity.com/blog/responsible-ai-privacy-fairness

Fadhlillah, R., Susmartini, S., & Herdiman, L. (2020, February). Realtime health monitoring system design for children with cerebral palsy using internet of things. [). IOP Publishing.]. *Journal of Physics: Conference Series*, *1450*(1), 012119.

Fairchild, A., & Stuerzlinger, W. (2020). Designing smart home interfaces for visually impaired users. *Proceedings of the ACM on Interactive, Mobile, Wearable and Ubiquitous Technologies*, *4*(1), 1–22. PMID: 35846237

Fan, D., Yi, M., Kang, W., Wang, Y., & Lv, C. (n.d.). OPEN Continuous sign language. *Scientific Reports*.

Farham, B., & Baltazar, L. (2024). A review of smart materials in 4D printing for hygrothermal rehabilitation: Innovative insights for sustainable building stock management. *Sustainability (Basel)*, *16*(10), 4067. DOI: 10.3390/su16104067

Farina, D., Vujaklija, I., Brånemark, R., Bull, A. M., Dietl, H., Graimann, B., Hargrove, L. J., Hoffmann, K.-P., Huang, H., Ingvarsson, T., Janusson, H. B., Kristjánsson, K., Kuiken, T., Micera, S., Stieglitz, T., Sturma, A., Tyler, D., Weir, R. F., & Aszmann, O. C. (2023). Toward higher-performance bionic limbs for wider clinical use. *Nature Biomedical Engineering*, *7*(4), 473–485. DOI: 10.1038/s41551-021-00732-x PMID: 34059810

Features, C. (n.d.). Voice Systems Solutions. https://www.redbooks.ibm.com/redbooks/pdfs/sg246884.pdf

Fernandez, P., & Lopez, M. (2022). *Deep learning in medical imaging*. IGI Global.

Fernandez, P., & Lopez, M. (2023). *Deep learning based medical image analysis*. IGI Global.

Ficili, I., Giacobbe, M., Tricomi, G., & Puliafito, A. (2025). From Sensors to Data Intelligence: Leveraging IoT, Cloud, and Edge Computing with AI. *Sensors (Basel)*, *25*(6), 1763. DOI: 10.3390/s25061763 PMID: 40292910

Francisco-Martínez, C., Prado-Olivarez, J., Padilla-Medina, J. A., Díaz-Carmona, J., Pérez-Pinal, F. J., Barranco-Gutiérrez, A. I., & Martínez-Nolasco, J. J. (2021). Upper Limb Movement Measurement Systems for Cerebral Palsy: A Systematic Literature Review. *Sensors (Basel)*, *21*(23), 7884. DOI: 10.3390/s21237884 PMID: 34883885

Fuloria, N. K., Malviya, R., Verma, S., & Balusamy, B. (Eds.). (2023). *Big Data in Oncology: Impact, Challenges, and Risk Assessment*. CRC Press.

Fürst, E., & Vogelauer, C. (2013). Best and bad practices in public transport: approaches to a barrier-free design for the visually and hearing impaired. In *Proc. European Transport Conference 2013*.

Gafoor, A., & Amilan, S. (2024). Fintech adoption and financial well-being of persons with disabilities: The mediating role of financial access, financial knowledge and financial behaviour. *International Journal of Social Economics*, *51*(11), 1388–1401. DOI: 10.1108/IJSE-08-2023-0596

Gallagher, B. A., Hart, P. M., O'Brien, C., Stevenson, M. R., & Jackson, A. J. (2011). Mobility and access to transport issues as experienced by people with vision impairment living in urban and rural Ireland. *Disability and Rehabilitation*, *33*(12), 979–988. DOI: 10.3109/09638288.2010.516786 PMID: 20846055

Gallagher, K. A., Mills, J. L., Armstrong, D. G., Conte, M. S., Kirsner, R. S., Minc, S. D., Plutzky, J., Southerland, K. W., & Tomic-Canic, M. (2024). Current status and principles for the treatment and prevention of diabetic foot ulcers in the cardiovascular patient population: A scientific statement from the American Heart Association. *Circulation*, *149*(4), e232–e253. DOI: 10.1161/CIR.0000000000001192 PMID: 38095068

Gao, A., Murphy, R. R., Chen, W., Dagnino, G., Fischer, P., Gutierrez, M. G., Kundrat, D., Nelson, B. J., Shamsudhin, N., Su, H., Xia, J., Zemmar, A., Zhang, D., Wang, C., & Yang, G. Z. (2021). Progress in robotics for combating infectious diseases. *Science Robotics*, *6*(52), eabf1462. DOI: 10.1126/scirobotics.abf1462 PMID: 34043552

García-de-Villa, S., Ruiz, L. R., Neira, G. G. V., Álvarez, M. N., Huertas-Hoyas, E., Del-Ama, A. J., Rodriguez-Sanchez, M. C., Seco, F., & Jiménez, A. R. (2024). Validation of an IMU-based gait analysis method for assessment of fall risk against traditional methods. *IEEE Journal of Biomedical and Health Informatics*. PMID: 39074006

Garg, I., Verma, M., Kumar, H., Maurya, R., Negi, T., & Jain, P. (2025). Bioelectronic Therapeutics: A Revolutionary Medical Practice in Health Care. *Bioelectricity*, *7*(1), 2–28. DOI: 10.1089/bioe.2024.0039 PMID: 40342937

Garrad, T. A., & Nolan, H. (2023). Rethinking higher education unit design: Embedding universal design for learning in online studies. *Student Success*, *14*(1), 1–8.

Gaya-Morey, F. X., Manresa-Yee, C., & Buades-Rubio, J. M. (2024). Deep learning for computer vision based activity recognition and fall detection of the elderly: A systematic review. *Applied Intelligence*, *54*(19), 8982–9007. DOI: 10.1007/s10489-024-05645-1

GeeksforGeeks. 2025. CatBoost in Machine Learning. [online] Available at: https://www.geeksforgeeks.org/catboost-ml/

Gell, N. M., Rosenberg, D. E., Demiris, G., LaCroix, A. Z., & Patel, K. V. (2015). Patterns of technology use among older adults with and without disabilities. *The Gerontologist*, *55*(3), 412–421. DOI: 10.1093/geront/gnt166 PMID: 24379019

Gherman, B., Zima, I., Vaida, C., Tucan, P., Pisla, A., Birlescu, I., Machado, J., & Pisla, D. (2025). Robotic Systems for Hand Rehabilitation—Past, Present and Future. *Technologies*, *13*(1), 37. DOI: 10.3390/technologies13010037

Ghevondyan, M., Davtyan, M., & Aghayan, M. (2025). Dielectric elastomer actuators: Medical applications review. *Discover Materials*, *5*(1), 43. DOI: 10.1007/s43939-025-00225-7

Giansanti, D. (2025). Advancements in Ocular Neuro-Prosthetics: Bridging Neuroscience and Information and Communication Technology for Vision Restoration. *Biology (Basel)*, *14*(2), 134. DOI: 10.3390/biology14020134 PMID: 40001902

Giansanti, D., & Pirrera, A. (2025). Integrating AI and Assistive Technologies in Healthcare: Insights from a Narrative Review of Reviews. *Health Care*, *13*(5), 556. DOI: 10.3390/healthcare13050556 PMID: 40077118

Godfrey, A., Hetherington, V., Shum, H., Bonato, P., Lovell, N. H., & Stuart, S. (2018). From A to Z: Wearable technology explained. *Maturitas*, *113*, 40–47. DOI: 10.1016/j.maturitas.2018.04.012 PMID: 29903647

Golledge, R. G., Marston, J. R., & Costanzo, C. M. (1997). Attitudes of visually impaired persons toward the use of public transportation. *Journal of Visual Impairment & Blindness*, *91*(5), 446–459. DOI: 10.1177/0145482X9709100505

Gómez-García, C. A., Askar-Rodriguez, M., & Velasco-Medina, J. (2021, January). Platform for Healthcare Promotion and Cardiovascular Disease Prevention. *IEEE Journal of Biomedical and Health Informatics*, *25*(7), 2758–2767. DOI: 10.1109/JBHI.2021.3051967 PMID: 33449888

Gongor, F., & Tutsoy, O. (2025). On the Remarkable Advancement of Assistive Robotics in Human-Robot Interaction-Based Health-Care Applications: An Exploratory Overview of the Literature. *International Journal of Human-Computer Interaction*, *41*(2), 1502–1542. DOI: 10.1080/10447318.2024.2342101

Gonzalez-Vazquez, A., Garcia, L., Kilby, J., & McNair, P. (2023). Soft wearable rehabilitation robots with artificial muscles based on smart materials: A review. *Advanced Intelligent Systems*, *5*(4), 2200159. DOI: 10.1002/aisy.202200159

Gouda, W., Sama, N. U., Al-Waakid, G., Humayun, M., & Jhanjhi, N. Z. (2022). Detection of Skin Cancer Based on Skin Lesion Images Using Deep Learning. *Health Care*, *10*(7), 1183. DOI: 10.3390/healthcare10071183 PMID: 35885710

Gray, R., Indraratna, P., Lovell, N., & Ooi, S. (2022). *Digital health technology in the prevention of heart failure and coronary artery disease*. Cardiovascular Digital Health Journal, Elsevier. DOI: 10.1016/j.cvdhj.2022.09.002

Gray, M., & Cyan, L. (2022). Ethical guidelines for assistive smart technologies: Inclusion and accountability. *Ethics in Technology*, *5*(2), 89–107.

Greater Cambridge partnership. Smart pedestrian crossing trial. (2024, April 15). GOV.UK. https://www.gov.uk/algorithmic-transparency-records/greater-cambridge-partnership-smart-pedestrian-crossing-trial

Guerreiro, J., Sato, D., Asakawa, S., Dong, H., Kitani, K. M., & Asakawa, C. (2019). CaBot: Designing and evaluating an autonomous navigation robot for blind people. *Proceedings of the 21st International ACM SIGACCESS Conference on Computers and Accessibility*, 68–82. DOI: 10.1145/3308561.3353771

Gutiérrez, J., Rodríguez, V., & Martin, S. (2021). Comprehensive review of vision-based fall detection systems. *Sensors (Basel)*, *21*(3), 947. DOI: 10.3390/s21030947 PMID: 33535373

Habib, H., Jelani, S. A. K., & Najla, S. (2022). Revolutionising Inclusion: AI in Adaptive Learning for Students with Disabilities. *Multidisciplinary Science Journal*, *1*(01), 1–11.

Hakim, A., Huq, M. S., Shanta, S., & Ibrahim, B. S. K. K. (2017). Smartphone based data mining for fall detection: Analysis and design. *Procedia Computer Science*, *105*, 46–51. DOI: 10.1016/j.procs.2017.01.188

Hamidli, N. (2023). Introduction to UI/UX design: Key concepts and principles. *Preuzeto*, *28*(3), 2024.

Hamza, H. M., & Wali, A. (2023). Pakistan sign language recognition: Leveraging deep learning models with limited dataset. *Machine Vision and Applications*, *34*(5), 71. DOI: 10.1007/s00138-023-01429-8

Hanna, M., Pantanowitz, L., Jackson, B., Palmer, O., Visweswaran, S., Pantanowitz, J., & Rashidi, H. (2024). Ethical and Bias considerations in artificial intelligence (AI)/machine learning. *Modern Pathology*, •••, 100686. PMID: 39694331

Han, X., Guffanti, D., & Brunete, A. (2025). A Comprehensive Review of Vision-Based Sensor Systems for Human Gait Analysis. *Sensors (Basel)*, *25*(2), 498. DOI: 10.3390/s25020498 PMID: 39860869

Hariharan, U., Devarajan, D., Kumar, P. S., Rajkumar, K., Meena, M., & Akilan, T. (2025). Recognition of American sign language using modified deep residual CNN with modified canny edge segmentation. *Multimedia Tools and Applications*, *84*(31), 38093–38120. Advance online publication. DOI: 10.1007/s11042-025-20663-y

Harrou, F., Dairi, A., Taghezouit, B., & Sun, Y. (2019). An unsupervised monitoring procedure for detecting anomalies in photovoltaic systems using a one-class support vector machine. *Solar Energy*, *179*, 48–58. DOI: 10.1016/j.solener.2018.12.045

Harrou, F., Zerrouki, N., Sun, Y., & Houacine, A. (2017). Vision-based fall detection system for improving safety of elderly people. *IEEE Instrumentation & Measurement Magazine*, *20*(6), 49–55. DOI: 10.1109/MIM.2017.8121952

Harvey, A. R. (2008). *The functional mobility scale for children with cerebral palsy: reliability and validity*. University of Melbourne, School of Physiotherapy.

He, K., Zhang, X., Ren, S., & Sun, J. (2015). *Deep Residual Learning for Image Recognition*. https://arxiv.org/pdf/1512.03385

Hejazi, M., & Singh, Y. P. (2013). One-class support vector machines approach to anomaly detection. *Applied Artificial Intelligence*, *27*(5), 351–366. DOI: 10.1080/08839514.2013.785791

Hersh, M. A. (2016). Improving deafblind travelers' experiences: An international survey. *Journal of Travel Research*, *55*(3), 380–394. DOI: 10.1177/0047287514546225

Hilal, M., Khabbache, H., & Ali, D. A. (2024). Dropping out of school: A psychosocial approach. *Advances in Medicine, Psychology, and Public Health*, *1*(1), 26–36.

Hillman, M. R. (2006). *Assistive robotics*. Wiley Encyclopedia of Biomedical Engineering., DOI: 10.1002/9780471740360.ebs1029

Hosain, A. A., Santhalingam, P. S., Pathak, P., Košecká, J., & Rangwala, H. (2019). Sign Language Recognition Analysis using Multimodal Data. *2019 IEEE International Conference on Data Science and Advanced Analytics (DSAA)*, 203–210. DOI: 10.1109/DSAA.2019.00035

Hossain, M., Sadik, Kh., Rahman, Md. M., Ahmed, F., Hossain Bhuiyan, Md. N., & Khan, M. M. (2021, October 1). *Convolutional Neural Network Based Skin Cancer Detection (Malignant vs Benign)*. IEEE Xplore. DOI: 10.1109/IEMCON53756.2021.9623192

How generative AI boosts performance throughout our Group. (n.d.). SNCF Group. Retrieved June 27, 2025, from https://www.groupe-sncf.com/en/innovation/emerging-technologies/generative-ia

How stair lifts are adapting to smart home tech in 2025. (2025, May 8). Smart G Home. https://smartghome.com/smart-stair-lifts-in-2025/

Hsu, W. L., Liu, J. X., Yang, C. C., & Leu, J. S. (2023). A fall detection system based on FMCW radar range-Doppler image and bi-LSTM deep learning. *IEEE Sensors Journal, 23*(18), 22031–22039. DOI: 10.1109/JSEN.2023.3300994

Huang, C.-Y., Wu, C.-K., & Liu, P.-Y. (2022). Assistive technology in smart cities: A case of street crossing for the visually-impaired. *Technology in Society, 68*(101805), 101805. DOI: 10.1016/j.techsoc.2021.101805

Huang, X., Xue, Y., Ren, S., & Wang, F. (2023). Sensor-based wearable systems for monitoring human motion and posture: A review. *Sensors (Basel), 23*(22), 9047. DOI: 10.3390/s23229047 PMID: 38005436

Huarng, K. H. (2023). *Artificial intelligence in healthcare*. IGI Global.

Humphry, J., & Chesher, C. (2021). Preparing for smart voice assistants: Cultural histories and media innovations. *New Media & Society, 23*(7), 1971–1988. DOI: 10.1177/1461444820923679

Hussain, F., Hussain, F., Ehatisham-ul-Haq, M., & Azam, M. A. (2019). Activity-aware fall detection and recognition based on wearable sensors. *IEEE Sensors Journal, 19*(12), 4528–4536. DOI: 10.1109/JSEN.2019.2898891

Hussain, T., Ahmed, S., & Malik, A. (2023). *Design and development of AI-powered healthcare system*. IGI Global.

Hu, X., Yu, S., Zheng, J., Fang, Z., Zhao, Z., & Qu, X. (2025). A hybrid CNN-LSTM model for involuntary fall detection using wrist-worn sensors. *Advanced Engineering Informatics, 65*, 103178. DOI: 10.1016/j.aei.2025.103178

Iglesias-Pradas, S., Hernández-García, Á., Chaparro-Peláez, J., & Prieto, J. L. (2021). Emergency remote teaching and students' academic performance in higher education during the COVID-19 pandemic: A case study. *Computers in Human Behavior, 119*, 106713. DOI: 10.1016/j.chb.2021.106713 PMID: 34866769

Igual, R., Medrano, C., & Plaza, I. (2013). Challenges, issues and trends in fall detection systems. *Biomedical Engineering Online, 12*(1), 66. DOI: 10.1186/1475-925X-12-66 PMID: 23829390

Infrastructure Australia. 2018. Future Cities: Planning for our growing population. [online] Available at: https://www.infrastructureaustralia.gov.au/

Instituto Nacional de Estadística. (2023). Survey on Disability, Personal Autonomy and Dependency Situations [Online]. Retrieved June 10, 2025, from: https://www.ine.es/dyngs/INEbase/es/operacion.htm?c=Estadistica_C&cid=1254736176782&menu=resultados&idp=1254735573175#!tabs-1254736195764

Irigoyen, E., Larrea, M., & Graña, M. (2024). A Narrative Review of Haptic Technologies and Their Value for Training, Rehabilitation, and the Education of Persons with Special Needs. *Sensors (Basel)*, *24*(21), 6946. DOI: 10.3390/s24216946 PMID: 39517844

Ismail, M. I. M., & Mousa, M. A. (2025, August). Employing Computer Vision on a Smartphone to Help the Visually Impaired Cross the Road. In *Proceedings of the AAAI Symposium Series* (Vol. 6, No. 1, pp. 227-234). DOI: 10.1609/aaaiss.v6i1.36057

Iyer, A., & Umadevi, K. S. (2025). Design and analysis of TwinCardio framework to detect and monitor cardiovascular diseases using digital twin and deep neural network. *Scientific Reports*, *15*(1), 24376. DOI: 10.1038/s41598-025-08824-3 PMID: 40628887

Iyer, L. S. (2021). AI enabled applications towards intelligent transportation. *Transportation Engineering*, *5*, 100083. DOI: 10.1016/j.treng.2021.100083

Jalali, D. (2023, September 5). The ethics of artificial intelligence: Are AI voices legal? Voices. https://www.voices.com/blog/are-ai-voices-legal/

Jamieson, A. R., & Wijesundara, H. D. (2025). A review of adaptive equipment and technology for exercise and sports activities for people with disabilities. *Disability and Rehabilitation. Assistive Technology*, *20*(1), 33–45. DOI: 10.1080/17483107.2024.2372323 PMID: 38962933

Jamwal, R., Jarman, H. K., Roseingrave, E., Douglas, J., & Winkler, D. (2022). Smart home and communication technology for people with disability: A scoping review. *Disability and Rehabilitation. Assistive Technology*, *17*(6), 624–644. DOI: 10.1080/17483107.2020.1818138 PMID: 32924660

Jardinez, M. J., & Natividad, L. R. (2024). The Advantages and Challenges of Inclusive Education: Striving for Equity in the Classroom. *Shanlax International Journal of Education*, *12*(2), 57–65. DOI: 10.34293/education.v12i2.7182

Javaid, A., Zghyer, F., Kim, C., Spaulding, E. M., Isakadze, N., Ding, J., Kargillis, D., Gao, Y., Rahman, F., Brown, D. E., Saria, S., Martin, S. S., Kramer, C. M., Blumenthal, R. S., & Marvel, F. A. (2022). *Medicine 2032: The future of cardiovascular disease prevention with machine learning and digital health technology. American Journal of Preventive Cardiology, 12*, 100379. DOI: 10.1016/j.ajpc.2022.100379 PMID: 36090536

Javaid, S., Sajid, S., & Baloch, Y. K. (2025). UAlpha40: A comprehensive dataset of Urdu alphabet for Pakistan sign language. *Data in Brief, 59*, 111342. DOI: 10.1016/j.dib.2025.111342

Javed, A. R., Shahzad, F., Rehman, S., Zikria, Y. B., Razzak, I., Jalil, Z., & Xu, G. (2022). Future smart cities: Requirements, emerging technologies, applications, challenges, and future aspects. *Cities (London, England), 129*, 103794. DOI: 10.1016/j.cities.2022.103794

Jensen, M. T., Treskes, R. W., Caiani, E. G., Casado-Arroyo, R., Cowie, M. R., Dilaveris, P., & De Groot, N. (2021). ESC working group on e-cardiology position paper: Use of commercially available wearable technology for heart rate and activity tracking in primary and secondary cardiovascular prevention. *European Heart Journal. Digital Health, 2*(1), 49–59. DOI: 10.1093/ehjdh/ztab011 PMID: 36711174

Jiang, X., Ming, W. K., & You, J. H. S. (2019). *The Cost-Effectiveness of Digital Health Interventions on the Management of Cardiovascular Diseases: Systematic Review. Journal of Medical Internet Research, 21*(6), e13166. DOI: 10.2196/13166 PMID: 31210136

Jimbu, D., Cristea, A. E., Iliescu, D. M., Oprea, D., Iliescu, M. G., Caraban, B. M., & Bordei, P. (2024). 664 The importance of advanced technologies in functional rehabilitation of the hand. *Balneo and PRM Research Journal, 15*(1).

Jin, Z., Oresko, J., Huang, S., & Cheng, A. C. (2009, April). HeartToGo: a personalized medicine technology for cardiovascular disease prevention and detection. In *2009 IEEE/NIH Life Science Systems and Applications Workshop* (pp. 80-83). IEEE.

Jiralerspong, T., & Zhao, H. (2024). Soft Robotic Devices for Mechanotherapy of the Upper and Lower Extremities. *Advanced Materials Technologies*, •••, 2401530.

Jobin, A., & Levin, M. F. (2000). *Regulation of stretch reflex threshold in elbow flexors in children with cerebral palsy: a new measure of spasticity. Developmental Medicine &amp*. Child Neurology.

Jóhannsdóttir, L. G., Sigurðardóttir, S. G., Óskarsdóttir, M., & Islind, A. S. (2025). Digital nudging in digital health technologies: A systematic review. *Health and Technology*, *15*(6), 1037–1051. DOI: 10.1007/s12553-025-01000-7

Johnson, R., & Evans, T. (2023). *AI-enabled smart healthcare using biomedical signals*. IGI Global.

Joshi, V. D. (2024). *Artificial intelligence (AI) for healthcare: India retrospective*. IGI Global. DOI: 10.4018/979-8-3693-1934-5.ch003

Joy, J., Balakrishnan, K., & M, S. (2019). SiLearn: An intelligent sign vocabulary learning tool. *Journal of Enabling Technologies*, *13*(3), 173–187. DOI: 10.1108/JET-03-2019-0014

Jyothish, K. J., & Mishra, S. (2024). A survey on robotic prosthetics: Neuroprosthetics, soft actuators, and control strategies. *ACM Computing Surveys*, *56*(8), 1–44. DOI: 10.1145/3648355

Kablan, E. B., & Ayas, S. (2024). Skin lesion classification from dermoscopy images using ensemble learning of ConvNeXt models. *Signal, Image and Video Processing*, *18*(8-9), 6353–6361. Advance online publication. DOI: 10.1007/s11760-024-03321-y

Kanda, R., Akhai, S., & Bansal, R. (2013). Analysis of MOST technique for elimination of idle time by synchronization of different lines. *International Journal of Research in Advent Technology*, *1*(4), 151–158.

Kang, J., Patton, K., & Gardiner-Walsh, S. (2024). Success for all: Maximising digital accessibility in special education teacher preparation courses through universal design for learning. *Journal of Special Education Preparation*, *4*(3), 4–15. DOI: 10.33043/4a6kfo46

Kantaros, A., & Ganetsos, T. (2023). From static to dynamic: Smart materials pioneering additive manufacturing in regenerative medicine. *International Journal of Molecular Sciences*, *24*(21), 15748. DOI: 10.3390/ijms242115748 PMID: 37958733

Kantaros, A., Petrescu, F. I. T., Brachos, K., Ganetsos, T., & Petrescu, N. (2024). Leveraging 3D Printing for Resilient Disaster Management in Smart Cities. *Smart Cities*, *7*(6), 3705–3726. DOI: 10.3390/smartcities7060143

Kantaros, A., Petrescu, F. I. T., & Ganetsos, T. (2025). From Stents to Smart Implants Employing Biomimetic Materials: The Impact of 4D Printing on Modern Healthcare. *Biomimetics*, *10*(2), 125. DOI: 10.3390/biomimetics10020125 PMID: 39997148

Kaplan, A., Smith, J., & Lee, M. (2024). *Approaches to human-centered AI in healthcare*. IGI Global.

Karabulut, M. A., Shah, A. S., Ilhan, H., Pathan, A. S. K., & Atiquzzaman, M. (2023). Inspecting VANET with various critical aspects–a systematic review. *Ad Hoc Networks*, *150*, 103281. DOI: 10.1016/j.adhoc.2023.103281

Karim, M. R., Siddiqui, M. I. H., Assaifan, A. K., Aijaz, M. O., & Alnaser, I. A. (2024). Nanotechnology and Prosthetic Devices: Integrating Biomedicine and Materials Science for Enhanced Performance and Adaptability. *Journal of Disability Research*, *3*(3), 20240019. DOI: 10.57197/JDR-2024-0019

Karki, N., Anwar, A., Rehman, I. U., Husamaldin, L., & Saadati, P. (2023, September). Smart Attendance Monitoring System Using Face Recognition for People with Disabilities (PwDs). In 2023 IEEE International Smart Cities Conference (ISC2) (pp. 1-7). IEEE.

Katsivelis, N., Anastasiou, A., Petropoulou, O., Lambrou, G., Giokas, K., & Koutsouris, D. (2017). Applied technologies and Smart Home applications in the health sector. In *2017 IEEE 30th International Symposium on Computer-Based Medical Systems (CBMS)* (pp. 544-549). IEEE. DOI: 10.1109/CBMS.2017.48

Kaur, A. P., Nsugbe, E., Drahota, A., Oldfield, M., Mohagheghian, I., & Sporea, R. A. (2025). State-of-the-Art Fall Detection Techniques with Emphasis on Floor-Based Systems–A Review. *Biomedical Engineering Advances*, *9*, 100179. DOI: 10.1016/j.bea.2025.100179

Kaur, J., & Singh, D. (2023). *Smart healthcare*. IGI Global.

Khafar, N. H. B. A., Soomro, D. M., Rahman, R. A., Abdullah, M. N., Soho, I. A., & Rahimoon, A. A. (2019). Intelligent navigation system using ultrasonic sensor for visually impaired person (VIP). 2019 IEEE 6th International Conference on Engineering Technologies and Applied Sciences (ICETAS), 1–4. DOI: 10.1109/ICETAS48360.2019.9117297

Khalil, R. A., Safelnasr, Z., Yemane, N., Kedir, M., Shafiqurrahman, A., & Saeed, N. (2024). Advanced learning technologies for intelligent transportation systems: Prospects and challenges. *IEEE Open Journal of Vehicular Technology*, *5*, 397–427. DOI: 10.1109/OJVT.2024.3369691

Khang, A., & Akhai, S. (2024). Green intelligent and sustainable manufacturing: key advancements, benefits, challenges, and applications for transforming industry. *Machine Vision and Industrial Robotics in Manufacturing*, 405-417.

Khan, M. S., Yu, M., Feng, P., Wang, L., & Chambers, J. (2015). An unsupervised acoustic fall detection system using source separation for sound interference suppression. *Signal Processing*, *110*, 199–210. DOI: 10.1016/j.sigpro.2014.08.021

Khan, M., & Lee, J. (2023). *Machine learning solutions in smart healthcare*. IGI Global.

Khan, N. S., Abid, A., Abid, K., Farooq, U., Farooq, M. S., & Jameel, H. (n.d.). Speak Pakistan: Challenges in Developing Pakistan Sign Language using Information Technology. *South Asian Studies*.

Khan, S. S., & Hoey, J. (2017). Review of fall detection techniques: A data availability perspective. *Medical Engineering & Physics*, *39*, 12–22. DOI: 10.1016/j.medengphy.2016.10.014 PMID: 27889391

Khan, W. U., Shah, N., Muntean, G.-M., Farman, H., Nasralla, M. M., Ullah, S., & Shabir, M. (2021). A lightweight deep learning model for real-time human action recognition on resource-constrained devices. *Soft Computing*, *25*(24), 15371–15385.

Khasawneh, M. A. (2024). Accessibility matters: Investigating the usability of social media platforms for individuals with motor disabilities. *Studies in Media and Communication*, *12*(2), 1. DOI: 10.11114/smc.v12i2.6615

Khojasteh, S. B., Villar, J. R., Chira, C., González, V. M., & de la Cal, E. (2018). Improving Fall Detection Using an On-Wrist Wearable Accelerometer. *Sensors (Basel)*, *18*(5), 1350. DOI: 10.3390/s18051350 PMID: 29701721

Killari, V. (2022). MACHINE LEARNING ALGORITHMS FOR ASL IMAGE RECOGNITION WITH LENET5 FEATURE EXTRACTION. *international journal of advanced research in computer science*, *13*, 11–14. DOI: 10.26483/ijarcs.v13i3.6828

King, J. (n.d.). Privacy in an AI era: How do we protect our personal information? Retrieved June 26, 2025, from https://hai.stanford.edu/news/privacy-ai-era-how-do-we-protect-our-personal-information

King, M. R., & Colla, S. (2025). Muscle Rehabilitation Techniques and Prevention of Injury. *Veterinary Clinics: Equine Practice*.

Kiran, S., Khan, M. A., Javed, M. Y., Alhaisoni, M., Tariq, U., Nam, Y., Damaševičius, R., & Sharif, M. (2021). Multi-layered deep learning features fusion for human action recognition. *Computers, Materials & Continua*, *69*(3), 4061–4075. DOI: 10.32604/cmc.2021.017800

Kirillov, A., He, K., Girshick, R., Rother, C., & Dollár, P. (2019). Panoptic segmentation. In *Proceedings of the IEEE/CVF conference on computer vision and pattern recognition* (pp. 9404-9413).

Klingbeil, H., Baer, H. R., & Wilson, P. E. (2004). Aging with a disability. *Archives of Physical Medicine and Rehabilitation*, *85*, 68–73. DOI: 10.1016/j.apmr.2004.03.014 PMID: 15221734

Kocaaslan, R. (2024). The current state and future of robotic surgery in Urology: A Comprehensive Review. *Interdisciplinary Medicine. Health and Bioscience Researches*, *2024*, 77.

Koch, R. n.d. How AI in Traffic Management is Helping to Ease Traffic Congestion. [online] Available at: https://www.iotforall.com/how-ai-in-traffic-management-easing-congestion

Kolenik, T. (2022). Methods in digital mental health: smartphone-based assessment and intervention for stress, anxiety, and depression. In *Integrating Artificial Intelligence and IoT for Advanced Health Informatics: AI in the Healthcare Sector* (pp. 105–128). Springer International Publishing. DOI: 10.1007/978-3-030-91181-2_7

Kolluru, V., Mungara, S., & Chintakunta, A. N. (2018). Adaptive learning systems: Harnessing AI for customised educational experiences. *International Journal of Computer Science and Information Technologies*, *6*(3), 10–5121. DOI: 10.5121/ijcsity.2018.6302

Kothadiya, D., Bhatt, C., Sapariya, K., Patel, K., Gil-González, A.-B., & Corchado, J. M. (2022). Deepsign: Sign Language Detection and Recognition Using Deep Learning. *Electronics (Basel)*, *11*(11), 1780. DOI: 10.3390/electronics11111780

Krupp, M. M., Barlow, P. B., & Kyle, E. J. (2021). Developing a self-assessment tool for dental faculty to map professional growth. *Journal of Dental Education*, *85*(10), 1596–1605. DOI: 10.1002/jdd.12727 PMID: 34184247

Kulkarni, M. P. (n.d.). Innovations Challenges Managing Cab Aggregators.

Kulyk, O., & Gajos, K. Z. (2021). Enhancing accessibility and privacy in smart home devices for people with disabilities. *ACM Transactions on Accessible Computing*, *14*(4), 1–29.

Kumar, , HWadhwa, , A. SAkhai, , SKaushik, , A. (2024). Parametric analysis, modeling and optimization of the process parameters in electric discharge machining of aluminium metal matrix composite. *Engineering Research Express, 6*(2), 025542. DOI 10.1088/2631-8695/ad4ba9

Kumar, P., & Akhai, S. (2022). Effective energy management in smart buildings using VRV/VRF systems. In *Additive Manufacturing in Industry 4.0* (pp. 27-35). CRC Press. DOI: 10.1201/9781003360001-2

Kumar, A., & Das, S. (2023). *Machine learning for health informatics*. IGI Global.

Kumar, A., Kumar, M., Bhardwaj, V. P., Kumar, S., & Selvarajan, S. (2024). A novel skin cancer detection model using modified finch deep CNN classifier model. *Scientific Reports*, *14*(1), 11235. Advance online publication. DOI: 10.1038/s41598-024-60954-2 PMID: 38755202

Kumari, D., & Anand, R. S. (2023). Fusion of Attention-Based Convolution Neural Network and HOG Features for Static Sign Language Recognition. *Applied Sciences (Basel, Switzerland)*, *13*(21), 11993. DOI: 10.3390/app132111993

Kumar, K., & Ranjan, C. (2025). *Smart Materials: Electro-Rheological Fluids, Piezoelectric Smart Materials, and Shape Memory Alloys*. Walter de Gruyter GmbH & Co KG.

Kumar, S. A., Sasikala, S., & Arun, N. (2024). Enhancing the Communication of Speech-Impaired People Using Embedded Vision-based Gesture Recognition through Deep Learning. In *Exploration of Artificial Intelligence and Blockchain Technology in Smart and Secure Healthcare* (pp. 179–198). Bentham Science Publishers. DOI: 10.2174/9789815165432124070011

Kumar, S., Pandey, D., & Chandra, S. (2023). Revolutionizing biofeedback and beyond: a journey through the evolving landscape of biomechanics. *Biochemical and Cellular Archives*, *23*(S1), 23. DOI: 10.51470/BCA.2023.23.S1.1625

Kurni, M., & KG, S. (2024). IoT for Education. In *The Internet of Educational Things: Enhancing Students' Engagement and Learning Performance* (pp. 1-22). Cham: Springer Nature Switzerland.

Kurpad, N. B., Dhanyashree, S., Shivank, V., Surya Shobith, T. A. S., & Jinny, S. V. "AI-Infused Telemedicine for Rural Wellness: A Comprehensive Approach," 2024 5th International Conference on Innovative Trends in Information Technology (ICITIIT), Kottayam, India, 2024 DOI: 10.1109/ICITIIT61487.2024.10580661

Kwolek, B., & Kepski, M. (2014). Human fall detection on embedded platform using depth maps and wireless accelerometer. *Computer Methods and Programs in Biomedicine*, *117*(3), 489–501. DOI: 10.1016/j.cmpb.2014.09.005 PMID: 25308505

Kwolek, B., & Kepski, M. (2015). Improving fall detection by the use of depth sensor and accelerometer. *Neurocomputing*, *168*, 637–645. DOI: 10.1016/j.neucom.2015.05.061

Lakkaraju, H., Kamar, E., Caruana, R., & Horvitz, E. (2017). Identifying unknown unknowns in the open world: Representations and policies for guided exploration. Proceedings of the ... AAAI Conference on Artificial Intelligence. AAAI Conference on Artificial Intelligence, 31(1). DOI: 10.1609/aaai.v31i1.10821

Lamssaggad, A., Benamar, N., Hafid, A. S., & Msahli, M. (2021). A survey on the current security landscape of intelligent transportation systems. *IEEE Access : Practical Innovations, Open Solutions*, *9*, 9180–9208. DOI: 10.1109/ACCESS.2021.3050038

Lang, R., Kett, M., Groce, N., & Trani, J. F. (2011). Implementing the United Nations Convention on the rights of persons with disabilities: Principles, implications, practice and limitations. *Alter (Paris)*, *5*(3), 206–220. DOI: 10.1016/j.alter.2011.02.004

Lasker, J., & Bedrosian, J. (2001). Promoting acceptance of augmentative and alternative communication by adults with acquired communication disorders. *Augmentative and Alternative Communication*, *17*(3), 141–153. DOI: 10.1080/aac.17.3.141.153

Lazar, J., & Greenidge, K. D. (2020). Designing accessible voice interfaces for people with visual impairments. *Journal of Accessibility and Design for All*, *10*(1), 1–21.

Leal Filho, W., Tripathi, S. K., Andrade Guerra, J. B. S. O. D., Giné-Garriga, R., Orlovic Lovren, V., & Willats, J. (2019). Using the sustainable development goals towards a better understanding of sustainability challenges. *International Journal of Sustainable Development and World Ecology*, *26*(2), 179–190. DOI: 10.1080/13504509.2018.1505674

Lee, H., & Park, D. (2021). AI TTS smartphone app for communication of speech impaired people. Data Science and Digital Transformation in the Fourth Industrial Revolution, 219-229.

Lee, J. (2025). Smart Solutions for Student Well-being: AI-driven Mental Health Support in a Polytechnic. In *The Rise of Intelligent Machines* (pp. 211–242). Chapman and Hall/CRC.

Lee, R. J. T. (n.d.). Usability challenges assistive technologies: Bridging gap between innovation accessibility.

Lee, S., & Dey, A. K. (2020). Using smart glasses to assist visually impaired people in indoor navigation. *IEEE Pervasive Computing*, *19*(3), 54–63.

Levin, M. F., Piscitelli, D., & Khayat, J. (2024). Tonic stretch reflex threshold as a measure of disordered motor control and spasticity – A critical review. *Clinical Neurophysiology*, *165*, 138–150. DOI: 10.1016/j.clinph.2024.06.019

Li, X., & Dang, A. (2025). The disruptive effect of AI on urban planning. Nature Cities, 1-3.

Liang, F., Yang, X., Peng, W., Zhen, S., Cao, W., & Li, Q.. (2023). Applications of digital health approaches for cardiometabolic diseases prevention and management in the Western Pacific region. *The Lancet Regional Health. Western Pacific*, *43*, 100847. DOI: 10.1016/j.lanwpc.2023.100847 PMID: 38456090

Light, J., & McNaughton, D. (2022). Supporting the communication of people with complex communication needs: The role of augmentative and alternative communication. *Augmentative and Alternative Communication*, *38*(1), 1–13. DOI: 10.1080/07434618.2022.2025618 PMID: 35272537

Li, K. F. (2013). Smart home technology for telemedicine and emergency management. *Journal of Ambient Intelligence and Humanized Computing*, *4*(5), 535–546.

Lippi, L., Turco, A., Moalli, S., Gallo, M., Curci, C., Maconi, A., de Sire, A., & Invernizzi, M. (2023). Role of prehabilitation and rehabilitation on functional recovery and quality of life in thyroid cancer patients: A comprehensive review. *Cancers (Basel)*, *15*(18), 4502. DOI: 10.3390/cancers15184502 PMID: 37760472

Li, S., Fan, X., Zhang, Y., Trappe, W., Lindqvist, J., & Howard, R. E. (2017). Auto++ detecting cars using embedded microphones in real-time. *Proceedings of the ACM on Interactive, Mobile, Wearable and Ubiquitous Technologies*, *1*(3), 1–20. PMID: 30417164

Lise. (2023a, February 17). 7 good reasons to install audio beacons at public transport. Inclusive City Maker. https://www.inclusivecitymaker.com/install-audio-beacons-public-transport-network/

Lise. (2023b, March 10). Our audio beacons guide blind users at the Helsinki subway. Inclusive City Maker. https://www.inclusivecitymaker.com/audio-beacons-blind-visually-impaired-helsinki-subway/

Liu, T., Krentz, A. J., Huo, Z., & Ćurčin, V. (2025). Opportunities and Challenges of Cardiovascular Disease Risk Prediction for Primary Prevention Using Machine Learning and Electronic Health Records: A Systematic Review. *PMC*, PMID: 40351688.

Liu, Z., Mao, H., Wu, C.-Y., Feichtenhofer, C., Darrell, T., & Xie, S. (2022, March 2). *A convnet for the 2020s*. arXiv.org. https://arxiv.org/abs/2201.03545 DOI: 10.1109/CVPR52688.2022.01167

Liu, H., Hu, J., Zheng, Q., Feng, X., Zhan, F., Wang, X., Xu, G., & Hua, F. (2022). Piezo1 channels as force sensors in mechanical force-related chronic inflammation. *Frontiers in Immunology*, *13*, 816149. DOI: 10.3389/fimmu.2022.816149 PMID: 35154133

Liu, J., Li, X., Huang, S., Chao, R., Cao, Z., Wang, S., Wang, A., & Liu, L. (2023). A review of wearable sensors based fall-related recognition systems. *Engineering Applications of Artificial Intelligence*, *121*, 105993. DOI: 10.1016/j.engappai.2023.105993

Liu, L., Stroulia, E., Nikolaidis, I., Miguel-Cruz, A., & Rincon, A. R. (2016). Smart homes and home health monitoring technologies for older adults: A systematic review. *International Journal of Medical Informatics*, *91*, 44–59. DOI: 10.1016/j.ijmedinf.2016.04.007 PMID: 27185508

Liu, S., Qi, L., Qin, H., Shi, J., & Jia, J. (2018). *Path aggregation network for instance segmentation.* In *Proceedings of the IEEE conference on computer vision and pattern recognition* (pp. 8759–8768). DOI: 10.1109/CVPR.2018.00913

Liu, Y. H., Hung, P. C., Iqbal, F., & Fung, B. C. (2021). Automatic fall risk detection based on imbalanced data. *IEEE Access : Practical Innovations, Open Solutions*, *9*, 163594–163611. DOI: 10.1109/ACCESS.2021.3133297

Li, Y., Chen, M., Tang, Y., & Wu, Z. (2024). Impact of Road Environment and Driver Behaviour on Injury Severity. *Accident; Analysis and Prevention*, *188*, 107–118.

Li, Y., Liu, P., Fang, Y., Wu, X., Xie, Y., Xu, Z., Ren, H., & Jing, F. (2025). A Decade of Progress in Wearable Sensors for Fall Detection (2015–2024): A Network-Based Visualization Review. *Sensors (Basel)*, *25*(7), 2205. DOI: 10.3390/s25072205 PMID: 40218718

Li, Y., & Ma, X. (2020). Privacy-preserving techniques for smart home IoT devices: A survey. *IEEE Internet of Things Journal*, *7*(7), 5986–6003.

Loi, M., Christen, M., & Cioffi, F. (2022). Ethical challenges of AI in education: Equity, fairness, and data privacy. *Computers & Education*, *182*, 104483. DOI: 10.1016/j.compedu.2022.104483

Lokmic-Tomkins, Z., Bhandari, D., Bain, C., Borda, A., Kariotis, T. C., & Reser, D. (2023). Lessons learned from natural disasters around digital health technologies and delivering quality healthcare. *International Journal of Environmental Research and Public Health*, *20*(5), 4542. DOI: 10.3390/ijerph20054542 PMID: 36901559

Loshchilov, I., & Hutter, F. (n.d.). *DECOUPLED WEIGHT DECAY REGULARIZATION*. https://arxiv.org/pdf/1711.05101

Low, W. Y., Cao, M., De Vos, J., & Hickman, R. (2020). The journey experience of visually impaired people on public transport in London. *Transport Policy*, *97*, 137–148. DOI: 10.1016/j.tranpol.2020.07.018

Luan, T. H., Gao, L., Li, Z., Xiang, Y., Wei, G., & Sun, L. (2015). Fog computing: Focusing on mobile users at the edge. arXiv preprint arXiv:1502.01815.

Lu, C.-L., Liu, Z.-Y., Huang, J.-T., Huang, C.-I., Wang, B.-H., Chen, Y., Wu, N.-H., Wang, H.-C., Giarré, L., & Kuo, P.-Y. (2021). Assistive navigation using deep reinforcement learning guiding robot with UWB/voice beacons and semantic feedbacks for blind and visually impaired people. *Frontiers in Robotics and AI*, *8*, 654132. DOI: 10.3389/frobt.2021.654132 PMID: 34239900

Lum, K. Y., Goh, Y. H., & Lee, Y. B. (2020). American Sign Language Recognition Based on MobileNetV2. *Advances in Science, Technology and Engineering Systems Journal.*

Luo, J., Yan, Z., Guo, S., & Chen, W. (2021, May). Recent Advances in Atherosclerotic Disease Screening Using Pervasive Healthcare. *IEEE Reviews in Biomedical Engineering*, *15*, 293–308. DOI: 10.1109/RBME.2021.3081180 PMID: 34003754

Lynch, P., Singal, N., & Francis, G. A. (2024). Educational technology for learners with disabilities in primary school settings in low-and middle-income countries: A systematic literature review. *Educational Review*, *76*(2), 405–431. DOI: 10.1080/00131911.2022.2035685

Ma, D., Hirota, K., Dai, Y., & Jia, Z. (n.d.). *Dynamic Sign Language Recognition Based on Improved Residual-LSTM Network.*

MacLachlan, M., Banes, D., Bell, D., Borg, J., Donnelly, B., Fembek, M., Ghosh, R., Gowran, R. J., Hannay, E., Hiscock, D., Hoogerwerf, E.-J., Howe, T., Kohler, F., Layton, N., Long, S., Mannan, H., Mji, G., Odera Ongolo, T., Perry, K., & Hooks, H. (2018). Assistive technology policy: A position paper from the first global research, innovation, and education on assistive technology (GREAT) summit. *Disability and Rehabilitation. Assistive Technology*, *13*(5), 454–466. DOI: 10.1080/17483107.2018.1468496 PMID: 29790393

Mahmoud, M. M. E., Rodrigues, J. J. P. C., Ahmed, S. H., & Shah, S. C. (2018). Enabling Technologies on Cloud of Things for Smart Healthcare. IEEE Access, 6, 31950-31967. DOI: . Published by IEEE on June 8, 2018. Electronic ISSN: 2169-3536.DOI: 10.1109/ACCESS.2018.2845399

Mahmoudi-Dehaki, M., Nasr-Esfahani, N., & Vasan, S. (2025). The Transformative Role of Assistive Technology in Enhancing Quality of Life for Individuals With Disabilities. In *Assistive Technology Solutions for Aging Adults and Individuals With Disabilities* (pp. 45–72). IGI Global Scientific Publishing., DOI: 10.4018/979-8-3693-6308-9.ch003

Mahmud, T., Kayastha, R., Kisi, K., Ngu, A. H., & Alamgeer, S. (2025). Evaluating the Effectiveness of Plantar Pressure Sensors for Fall Detection in Sloped Surfaces. *Electronics (Basel)*, *14*(15), 3003. DOI: 10.3390/electronics14153003

Maithili, K., Ponmalar, A., Yamini, B., Karthikeyan, M., Anish, T. P., Maheswari, B., & Subramanian, R. S. (2024). Advances in AI and Machine Learning for Healthcare Informatics. In Machine Learning and Generative AI in Smart Healthcare (pp. 1-22). IGI Global.

Majumdar, S. R. (2017). The case of public involvement in transportation planning using social media. *Case Studies on Transport Policy*, *5*(1), 121–133. DOI: 10.1016/j.cstp.2016.11.002

Mala, S., Deep, U., Mala, E., & Akhai, S. (2025). Digital Health Technologies for Preventive Cardiology. In Impact of Digital Solutions for Improved Healthcare Delivery (pp. 379-400). IGI Global.

Mala, S., Deep, U., Mala, E., & Akhai, S. (2025). Digital Health Technologies for Preventive Cardiology. In *Impact of Digital Solutions for Improved Healthcare Delivery* (pp. 379–400). IGI Global.

Mane, V., Jadhav, M., & Kadam, I. "Human Disease Prediction Using Machine Learning," *2024 International Conference on Emerging Smart Computing and Informatics (ESCI)*, Pune, India, 2024, DOI: 10.1109/ESCI59607.2024.10497303

Mann, W. C. (2005). Aging, disability and independence: trends and perspectives. *Smart Technology for Aging, Disability, and Independence: The State of the Science*, 1-29. DOI: 10.1002/0471743941.ch1

Martínez-Villaseñor, L., Ponce, H., Brieva, J., Moya-Albor, E., Núñez-Martínez, J., & Peñafort-Asturiano, C. (2019). UP-fall detection dataset: A multimodal approach. *Sensors (Basel)*, *19*(9), 1988. DOI: 10.3390/s19091988 PMID: 31035377

Mathunjwa, B. M., Kor, R. Y. J., Ngarnkuekool, W., & Hsu, Y. L. (2025). A Comprehensive Review of Home Sleep Monitoring Technologies: Smartphone Apps, Smartwatches, and Smart Mattresses. *Sensors (Basel)*, *25*(6), 1771. DOI: 10.3390/s25061771 PMID: 40292882

Matin, B. K., Williamson, H. J., Karyani, A. K., Rezaei, S., Soofi, M., & Soltani, S. (2021). Barriers in access to healthcare for women with disabilities: A systematic review in qualitative studies. *BMC Women's Health*, *21*(1), 44. DOI: 10.1186/s12905-021-01189-5 PMID: 33516225

Matre, M. E., & Cameron, D. L. (2024). A scoping review on the use of speech-to-text technology for adolescents with learning difficulties in secondary education. *Disability and Rehabilitation. Assistive Technology*, *19*(3), 1103–1116. DOI: 10.1080/17483107.2022.2149865 PMID: 36427182

Mauldin, T. R., Canby, M. E., Metsis, V., Ngu, A. H., & Rivera, C. C. (2018). SmartFall: A smartwatch-based fall detection system using deep learning. *Sensors (Basel)*, *18*(10), 3363. DOI: 10.3390/s18103363 PMID: 30304768

Mavroudis, V., & Gritzalis, S. (2019). Security and privacy challenges in smart homes for vulnerable users. *Computers & Security*, *85*, 1–14.

Mavrou, K., Meletiou-Mavrotheris, M., Kärki, A., Sallinen, M., & Hoogerwerf, E. J. (2017). Opportunities and challenges related to ICT and ICT-AT use by people with disabilities: An explorative study into factors that impact on the digital divide. *Technology and Disability*, *29*(1-2), 63–75. DOI: 10.3233/TAD-170174

Ma, X., Shan, J., Ning, F., Li, W., & Li, H. (2023). EFFNet: A skin cancer classification model based on feature fusion and random forests. *PLoS One*, *18*(10), e0293266–e0293266. DOI: 10.1371/journal.pone.0293266 PMID: 37871038

Ma, X., Wang, Y., & Zhao, H. (2023). *Approaches and applications of deep learning in virtual medical care*. IGI Global.

Ma, Y., Xu, T., Han, S., & Kim, K. (2022). Ensemble Learning of Multiple Deep CNNs Using Accuracy-Based Weighted Voting for ASL Recognition. *Applied Sciences (Basel, Switzerland)*, *12*(22), 11766. DOI: 10.3390/app122211766

Ma, Y., Xu, T., & Kim, K. (2022). Two-Stream Mixed Convolutional Neural Network for American Sign Language Recognition. *Sensors (Basel)*, *22*(16), 5959. DOI: 10.3390/s22165959 PMID: 36015719

Mbua, E. M. (2023). Inclusive Education. *Principal Leadership*, *7*(1), 1–25.

McNaughton, D., Rackensperger, T., & McLemore, L. (2025). Supporting meaningful participation in society by adults with developmental disabilities who need and use AAC: Lived experiences, key research findings, and future directions. *Augmentative and Alternative Communication*, *41*(3), 1–14. DOI: 10.1080/07434618.2025.2504497 PMID: 40464637

Mehta, V., Dhall, A., Pal, S., & Khan, S. S. (2021, January). Motion and region aware adversarial learning for fall detection with thermal imaging. In *2020 25th international conference on pattern recognition (ICPR)* (pp. 6321-6328). IEEE. DOI: 10.1109/ICPR48806.2021.9412632

Mehta, S., & Gupta, L. (2023). *Applications of smart healthcare technologies*. IGI Global.

Messaoudi, M. D., Menelas, B.-A. J., & Mcheick, H. (2022). Review of navigation assistive tools and technologies for the visually impaired. *Sensors (Basel)*, *22*(20), 7888. DOI: 10.3390/s22207888 PMID: 36298237

Mhlongo, S., Mbatha, K., Ramatsetse, B., & Dlamini, R. (2023). Challenges, opportunities, and prospects of adopting and using smart digital technologies in learning environments: An iterative review. *Heliyon*, *9*(6), e16348. DOI: 10.1016/j.heliyon.2023.e16348 PMID: 37274691

Mian, S. M., Khan, M. S., Shawez, M., & Kaur, A. (2024). "Artificial Intelligence (AI), Machine Learning (ML) & Deep Learning (DL): A Comprehensive Overview on Techniques, Applications and Research Directions," 2024 2nd International Conference on Sustainable Computing and Smart Systems (ICSCSS), Coimbatore, India, DOI: 10.1109/ICSCSS60660.2024.10625198

Mikołajewska, E., Mikołajewski, D., Mikołajczyk, T., & Paczkowski, T. (2025). A Breakthrough in Producing Personalized Solutions for Rehabilitation and Physiotherapy Thanks to the Introduction of AI to Additive Manufacturing. *Applied Sciences (Basel, Switzerland)*, *15*(4), 2219. DOI: 10.3390/app15042219

Ministry of Transport (New Zealand). 2020. The Social Cost of Road Crashes and Injuries. [online] Available at: https://www.transport.govt.nz

Minuz, P., Albini, F. L., Imbalzano, E., Izzo, R., Masi, S., Pengo, M. F., Pucci, G., Scalise, F., Salvetti, M., Tocci, G., Cicero, A., Iaccarino, G., Savoia, C., Sechi, L., Parati, G., Borghi, C., Volpe, M., Ferri, C., Grassi, G., & Muiesan, M. L. (2023). Telemedicine and Digital Medicine in the Clinical Management of Hypertension and Hypertension-Related Cardiovascular Diseases: A Position Paper of the Italian Society of Arterial Hypertension (SIIA). *High Blood Pressure & Cardiovascular Prevention : the Official Journal of the Italian Society of Hypertension*, *30*(5), 387–399. DOI: 10.1007/s40292-023-00595-0 PMID: 37594686

Mirza, M. S., Munaf, S. M., Azim, F., Ali, S., & Khan, S. J. (2022). Vision-based Pakistani sign language recognition using bag-of-words and support vector machines. *Scientific Reports*, *12*(1), 21325. DOI: 10.1038/s41598-022-15864-6

Młodystach, Ł., Orczyk, M., & Tomaszewski, F. (2023). Evaluation of public transport in Poland form the perspective of the deaf and hard of hearing people towards the improvement of mobility. Archives of transport, 66(2), 61-76.

Moen, R. D., & Østensjø, S. (2023). Understanding the use and benefits of assistive devices among young children with cerebral palsy and their families in Norway: A cross-sectional population-based registry study. *Disability and Rehabilitation. Assistive Technology, 19*(4), 1454–1462. DOI: 10.1080/17483107.2023.2198563 PMID: 37026592

Mohamed, A., & Khan, F. (2023). *Artificial intelligence in the digital healthcare industry*. IGI Global.

Mohanty, C. T. (2003). *Feminism without borders: Decolonizing theory, practicing solidarity*. Duke University Press.

Monaco, R., Bergaentzlé, C., Vilaplana, J. A. L., Ackom, E., & Nielsen, P. S. (2024). Digitalisation of power distribution grids: Barrier analysis, ranking and policy recommendations. *Energy Policy, 188*, 114083. DOI: 10.1016/j.enpol.2024.114083

Monica, J. A., Malar, J. H., Arun, C., Sharmila, L., & Arif, M. (2025). Leveraging technology and universal design for inclusive and engaging learning in Indian higher education. In *Educational Philosophy and Sociological Foundation of Education* (pp. 177–212). IGI Global.

Monica, R., & Aleotti, J. (2023). Improving virtual reality navigation tasks using a haptic vest and upper body tracking. *Displays, 78*(102417), 102417. DOI: 10.1016/j.displa.2023.102417

Montanha, A., Oprescu, A. M., & Romero-Ternero, M. (2022). A context-aware artificial intelligence-based system to support street crossings for pedestrians with visual impairments. *Applied Artificial Intelligence, 36*(1), 2062818. Advance online publication. DOI: 10.1080/08839514.2022.2062818

Morris, J., & Zhang, L. (2023). *Role of AI and ML in clinical decision support*. IGI Global.

Mousa, M. A., Elgohr, A. T., & Khater, H. A. (2024). A novel hybrid deep neural network classifier for EEG emotional brain signals. *International Journal of Advanced Computer Science and Applications, 15*(6), 1045-1055. https://dx.doi.org/ DOI: 10.14569/IJACSA.2024.01506107

Mujeeb, A. A., Khan, A. H., Khalid, S., Mirza, M. S., & Khan, S. J. (2023). A Deep Learning Approach to Pakistani Sign Language Recognition. *2023 20th International Bhurban Conference on Applied Sciences and Technology (IBCAST)*, 255–260. DOI: 10.1109/IBCAST59916.2023.10712904

Mulfari, D., & Villari, M. (2024). A voice user interface on the edge for people with speech impairments. *Electronics (Basel), 13*(7), 1389. DOI: 10.3390/electronics13071389

Muñoz Ruiz, C. (2024). Shape Morphing Wearable For Regulating the Nervous System Through Breathing.

Naayini, P., Kumar, M. P., Bura, C., Jonnalagadda, A. K., & Kamatala, S. (2025). *AI-Powered Assistive Technologies for Visual Impairment.* ArXiv.org.

Naayini, P., Myakala, P. K., Bura, C., Jonnalagadda, A. K., & Kamatala, S. (2025). AI-powered assistive technologies for visual impairment. In arXiv [cs.HC]. arXiv. https://arxiv.org/abs/2503.15494

Nacheva, R., & Czaplewski, M. (2024). Artificial Intelligence In Helping People With Disabilities: Opportunities And Challenges. *HR and Technologies*, (1), 102–124.

Nahata, H., & Singh, S. P. (2020). Deep Learning Solutions for Skin Cancer Detection and Diagnosis. *Learning and Analytics in Intelligent Systems*, 159–182. DOI: 10.1007/978-3-030-40850-3_8

Naik, N. (2017, October). Choice of effective messaging protocols for IoT systems: MQTT, CoAP, AMQP and HTTP. In 2017 IEEE international systems engineering symposium (ISSE) (pp. 1-7). IEEE.

Nair, S., Liu, Y., & Zhao, W. (2023). Wearable technologies for chronic disease management in educational settings: Opportunities and challenges. *Frontiers in Digital Health*, *5*, 1178921. DOI: 10.3389/fdgth.2023.1178921

Nam, S. J., & Park, E. Y. (2017). The effects of the smart environment on the information divide experienced by people with disabilities. *Disability and Health Journal*, *10*(2), 257–263. DOI: 10.1016/j.dhjo.2016.11.001 PMID: 27899268

Naqvi, M., Syed Qasim Gilani, Syed, T., Marques, O., & Kim, H.-C. (2023). Skin Cancer Detection Using Deep Learning—A Review. *Skin Cancer Detection Using Deep Learning—a Review, 13*(11), 1911–1911. DOI: 10.3390/diagnostics13111911

Nascimento, L. M. S. D., Bonfati, L. V., Freitas, M. L. B., Mendes, J. J. A.Junior, Siqueira, H. V., & Stevan Jr, S. L. (2020). Sensors and systems for physical rehabilitation and health monitoring—A review. *Sensors (Basel)*, *20*(15), 4063. DOI: 10.3390/s20154063 PMID: 32707749

Nasra, P. (2024). Enhanced Melanoma Detection Using a Fine-Tuned EfficientNetV2-L Model on Dermoscopic Images. *2024 Second International Conference on Intelligent Cyber Physical Systems and Internet of Things (ICoICI)*, 1–7. DOI: 10.1109/ICoICI62503.2024.10696263

Nasr, M., Islam, M. M., Shehata, S., Karray, F., & Quintana, Y. (2021, October 8). Smart Healthcare in the Age of AI: Recent Advances, Challenges, and Future Prospects. *IEEE Access : Practical Innovations, Open Solutions*, *9*, 145248–145270. DOI: 10.1109/ACCESS.2021.3118960

Nasser, N., Ali, A., Karim, L., & Al-Helali, A. (2024). Enhancing mobility for the visually impaired with AI and IoT-enabled mobile applications. In ScienceOpen. DOI: 10.14293/PR2199.000775.v1

National Cancer Institute. (2018). *Melanoma of the Skin - Cancer Stat Facts*. SEER. https://seer.cancer.gov/statfacts/html/melan.html

National Disability Centre. (2024). Best practices for UX accessibility. National Disability Centre. https://nationaldisabilitycenter.org/resources/best-practice-ux-accessibility Orellana, A., Kanzki-Veloso, E., Arguello, G., & Wojnas, K. (2024). Students' Experiences When Using Real-Time Automated Captions and Subtitles in Live Online Presentations: A Phenomenological Study. *Qualitative Report, 29*(4).

National Safety Council. n.d. Night Driving Safety Facts. [online] Available at: https://www.nsc.org

Nazir, S., Nawaz, M., Adnan, A., Shahzad, S., & Asadi, S. (2019, September). Big Data Features, Applications, and Analytics in Cardiology—A Systematic Literature Review. *IEEE Access : Practical Innovations, Open Solutions*, *7*, 143742–143771. DOI: 10.1109/ACCESS.2019.2941898

Newaz, N. T., & Hanada, E. (2023). The methods of fall detection: A literature review. *Sensors (Basel)*, *23*(11), 5212. DOI: 10.3390/s23115212 PMID: 37299939

Nikitas, A., Michalakopoulou, K., Njoya, E. T., & Karampatzakis, D. (2020). Artificial intelligence, transport and the smart city: Definitions and dimensions of a new mobility era. *Sustainability (Basel)*, *12*(7), 2789. DOI: 10.3390/su12072789

Nisky, I., & Makin, T. R. (2024). A neurocognitive pathway for engineering artificial touch. *Science Advances, 10*(51), eadq6290. DOI: 10.1126/sciadv.adq6290 PMID: 39693427

Noh, B., Youm, C., Goh, E., Lee, M., Park, H., Jeon, H., & Kim, O. Y. (2021). XGBoost based machine learning approach to predict the risk of fall in older adults using gait outcomes. *Scientific Reports, 11*(1), 12183. DOI: 10.1038/s41598-021-91797-w PMID: 34108595

Nooruddin, S., Islam, M. M., Sharna, F. A., Alhetari, H., & Kabir, M. N. (2022). Sensor-based fall detection systems: A review. *Journal of Ambient Intelligence and Humanized Computing, 13*(5), 2735–2751. DOI: 10.1007/s12652-021-03248-z

Nourizadeh, M., Shadgan, B., Abbasidezfouli, S., Juricic, M., & Mulpuri, K. (2024). Methods of muscle spasticity assessment in children with cerebral palsy: A scoping review. *Journal of Orthopaedic Surgery and Research, 19*(1), 401. DOI: 10.1186/s13018-024-04894-7 PMID: 38992701

Novak, I., Mcintyre, S., Morgan, C., Campbell, L., Dark, L., Morton, N., Stumbles, E., Wilson, S. A., & Goldsmith, S. (2013). A systematic review of interventions for children with cerebral palsy: State of the evidence. *Developmental Medicine and Child Neurology, 55*(10), 885–910. DOI: 10.1111/dmcn.12246 PMID: 23962350

Ojasalo, J., Suomalainen, N., Seppälä, H., & Moonen, R. (2010). Better technologies and services for smart homes of disabled people: empirical findings from an explorative study among intellectually disabled. In *2010 2nd International Conference on Software Technology and Engineering* (Vol. 1, pp. V1-251). IEEE. DOI: 10.1109/ICSTE.2010.5608845

Okolo, G. I., Althobaiti, T., & Ramzan, N. (2024). Assistive Systems for Visually Impaired Persons: Challenges and Opportunities for Navigation Assistance. *Sensors (Basel), 24*(11), 3572. DOI: 10.3390/s24113572 PMID: 38894363

Oladele, D. A., Markus, E. D., & Abu-Mahfouz, A. M. (2021). Adaptability of assistive mobility devices and the role of the internet of medical things: Comprehensive review. *JMIR Rehabilitation and Assistive Technologies, 8*(4), e29610. DOI: 10.2196/29610 PMID: 34779786

Oladimeji, A., & Lee, S. (2021). Trust models for assistive smart systems: A systematic review. *Journal of Assistive Technologies, 15*(4), 263–279.

Oladimeji, D., Gupta, K., Kose, N. A., Gundogan, K., Ge, L., & Liang, F. (2023). Smart transportation: An overview of technologies and applications. *Sensors (Basel), 23*(8), 3880. DOI: 10.3390/s23083880 PMID: 37112221

Olayinka, O. H. (2021, 12(03), 711-726). Data driven customer segmentation and personalization strategies in modern business intelligence frameworks. World Journal of Advanced Research and Reviews, 12(03), 711–726. https://wjarr.com/content/data-driven-customer-segmentation-and-personalization-strategies-modern-business

Oliveira, R. B., Papa, J. P., Pereira, A. S., & Tavares, J. M. R. S. (2016). Computational methods for pigmented skin lesion classification in images: Review and future trends. *Neural Computing & Applications*, *29*(3), 613–636. DOI: 10.1007/s00521-016-2482-6

Ornaghi, H. L.Jr, Monticeli, F. M., & Agnol, L. D. (2023). A Review on Polymers for Biomedical Applications on Hard and Soft Tissues and Prosthetic Limbs. *Polymers*, *15*(19), 4034. DOI: 10.3390/polym15194034 PMID: 37836083

Oro, B. (2025). Perspective Chapter: Designing for Dignity–The Role of Esthetic Empathy in Assistive Technologies.

Oyedokun, T. T. (2025). Assistive technology and accessibility tools in enhancing adaptive education. In *Advancing adaptive education: Technological innovations for disability support* (pp. 125–162). IGI Global Scientific Publishing.

Özdemir, A. T., & Barshan, B. (2014). Detecting falls with wearable sensors using machine learning techniques. *Sensors (Basel)*, *14*(6), 10691–10708. DOI: 10.3390/s140610691 PMID: 24945676

Padhy, S., Tiwari, J., Rathore, S., & Kumar, N. (2019, December). Emergency signal classification for the hearing impaired using multi-channel convolutional neural network architecture. In *2019 IEEE Conference on Information and Communication Technology* (pp. 1-6). IEEE. DOI: 10.1109/CICT48419.2019.9066252

Pakistan Bureau of Statistics. (2021). *Population and housing census: Persons with disabilities*. Government of Pakistan. https://www.pbs.gov.pk/

Pan, T.-Y., Lo, L.-Y., Yeh, C.-W., Li, J.-W., Liu, H.-T., & Hu, M.-C. (2016). Real-time sign language recognition in complex background scene based on a hierarchical clustering classification method. 2016 IEEE second international conference on multimedia big data (BigMM)

Pan, M., Yuan, C., Liang, X., Dong, T., Liu, T., Zhang, J., Zou, J., Yang, H., & Bowen, C. (2022). Soft actuators and robotic devices for rehabilitation and assistance. *Advanced Intelligent Systems*, *4*(4), 2100140. DOI: 10.1002/aisy.202100140

Papageorgiou, G., Tsappi, E., & Wang, T. (2024). *Smart Urban Systems Planning for Active Mobility and Sustainability*. Elsevier Cities. [online], DOI: 10.1016/j.ifacol.2024.07.350

Papageorgiou, M., Diakaki, C., Dinopoulou, V., Kotsialos, A., & Wang, Y. (2003). Review of road traffic control strategies. *Proceedings of the IEEE*, *91*(12), 2043–2067. DOI: 10.1109/JPROC.2003.819610

Park, J., Bamford, J., Byun, H., & Chowdhury, S. (2017, November). Journey by visually impaired public transport users: Barriers and consequences. In Australasian Transport Research Forum (pp. 27-29).

Park, J., & Kim, S. (2023). AI-based privacy enhancement for assistive smart devices in home environments. *Sensors (Basel)*, *23*(4), 1789. PMID: 36850386

PARVEEN. N. (2022). Accessibility and disability for students with disabilities inside the higher education institutions. *National Institute of Educational Planning and Administration, New Delhi.*

Patel, N., & Gupta, L. (2024). *Deep learning frameworks in the healthcare industry.* IGI Global.

Patel, N., & Singh, R. (2023). *Emerging trends and future prospects of AI in healthcare.* IGI Global.

Patel, P., Pampaniya, S., Ghosh, A., Raj, R., Karuppaih, D., & Kandasamy, S. (2025). Enhancing Accessibility Through Machine Learning: A Review on Visual and Hearing Impairment Technologies. *IEEE Access : Practical Innovations, Open Solutions*, *13*, 33286–33307. DOI: 10.1109/ACCESS.2025.3539081

Patel, R., & Sharma, S. (2023). *AI in telehealth: Healthcare delivery transformation.* IGI Global.

Patel, S., Park, H., Bonato, P., Chan, L., & Rodgers, M. (2012). A review of wearable sensors and systems with application in rehabilitation. *Journal of Neuroengineering and Rehabilitation*, *9*(1), 1–17. DOI: 10.1186/1743-0003-9-21 PMID: 22520559

Pathak, K., Saikia, R., Das, A., Das, D., Islam, M. A., Pramanik, P., Parasar, A., Borthakur, P. P., Sarmah, P., Saikia, M., & Borthakur, B. (2023). 3D printing in biomedicine: Advancing personalized care through additive manufacturing. *Exploration of Medicine*, *4*(6), 1135–1167. DOI: 10.37349/emed.2023.00200

Patil, V., & Rao, S. (2023). *Application of machine learning and blockchain technology for smart healthcare applications.* IGI Global.

Patricks, V., Twiste, M., Granat, M., Curtin, S., & Worsley, P. (2025). Clinicians' Perspectives of Activity Monitoring Applications and Facilitators for Lower-Limb Prosthetic Service Provision. *Journal of Prosthetics and Orthotics*, *37*(1), 42–52. DOI: 10.1097/JPO.0000000000000518

Paul, S., Nahar, A., Bhagawati, M., & Kunwar, A. J. (2022). A review on recent advances of cerebral palsy. *Oxidative Medicine and Cellular Longevity, 2022*(1), 2622310. DOI: 10.1155/2022/2622310 PMID: 35941906

Paul, V. V., & Masood, J. A. I. S. (2024, July). Exploring Predictive Methods for Cardiovascular Disease: A Survey of Methods and Applications. *IEEE Access : Practical Innovations, Open Solutions, 12*, 101497–101505. DOI: 10.1109/ACCESS.2024.3430898

Pearson, S. R., & Shafik, M. (2024). Smart Cities enhancing the lives of people with disabilities. MATEC Web of Conferences, 401, 07004. DOI: 10.1051/matecconf/202440107004

Perlow, E. L., Wells, R. S., Hedayet, M., Xia, J., MacLean, H., Ding, E., & McCall, A. (2021). Hidden Inequality: Financial Aid Information Available to College Students with Disabilities Attending Public Four-Year Institutions. *Journal of Student Financial Aid, 50*(3), n3. DOI: 10.55504/0884-9153.1709

Pieri, K., & Cobb, S. V. G. (2019). Mobile app communication aid for Cypriot deaf people. *Journal of Enabling Technologies, 13*(2), 70–81. DOI: 10.1108/JET-12-2018-0058

Pierleoni, P., Belli, A., Palma, L., Pellegrini, M., Pernini, L., & Valenti, S. (2015). A high reliability wearable device for elderly fall detection. *IEEE Sensors Journal, 15*(8), 4544–4553. DOI: 10.1109/JSEN.2015.2423562

Pierzchlewicz, K., Kępa, I., Podogrodzki, J., &Kotulska, K. (2021). Spinal muscular atrophy: the use of functional motor scales in the era of disease-modifying treatment. *Child neurology open, 8*, 2329048X211008725.

Podder, K. K., Islam, M. R., Hossain, M. I., & Akhand, M. A. H. (2023). Signer-independent Arabic Sign Language recognition system using deep learning model. *Sensors (Basel), 23*(16), 7156. DOI: 10.3390/s23167156

Poli, M. (2021). COVID-19 effects in people's daily life, social media's role and the power of emotions and mind. In *Strategic Innovative Marketing and Tourism in the COVID-19 Era: 9th ICSIMAT Conference 2020* (pp. 141-151). Springer International Publishing. DOI: 10.1007/978-3-030-66154-0_16

Poli, M. (2021). Smart Technologies and the Case of People with Disabilities: A Preliminary Overview. *NiDS*, 217-222. DOI: 10.3233/FAIA210096

Popescu, M., Li, Y., Skubic, M., & Rantz, M. (2008, August). An acoustic fall detector system that uses sound height information to reduce the false alarm rate. In *2008 30th Annual International Conference of the IEEE Engineering in Medicine and Biology Society* (pp. 4628-4631). IEEE. DOI: 10.1109/IEMBS.2008.4650244

Pradhan, B., Das, S., Roy, D. S., Routray, S., Benedetto, F., & Jhaveri, R. H. (2023). An AI-Assisted Smart Healthcare System Using 5G Communication. *IEEE Access : Practical Innovations, Open Solutions*, *11*, 108339–108355. DOI: 10.1109/ACCESS.2023.3317174

Prasher, S., Nelson, L., & Gomathi, S. (2023). Resnet 50 Based Classification Model for Skin Cancer Detection Using Dermatoscopic Images. *2023 3rd Asian Conference on Innovation in Technology (ASIANCON)*, 1–5. DOI: 10.1109/ASIANCON58793.2023.10270158

Prokhorenkova, L., Gusev, G., Vorobev, A., Dorogush, A. V., & Gulin, A. 2018. CatBoost: Unbiased Boosting with CategoricalFeatures.InAdvancesinNeuralInformationProcessingSystems(NeurIPS). https://arxiv.org/abs/ 1810.11363

Providing accessible information onboard local bus and coach services. (n.d.). GOV. UK. Retrieved June 28, 2025, from https://www.gov.uk/government/publications/providing-accessible-information-onboard-local-bus-and-coach-services/providing-accessible-information-onboard-local-bus-and-coach-services

Puli, L., Layton, N., Bell, D., & Shahriar, A. Z. (2024). Financial inclusion for people with disability: A scoping review. *Global Health Action*, *17*(1), 2342634. DOI: 10.1080/16549716.2024.2342634 PMID: 38726584

Qasmi, F., & Fatima, S. K. (2024). Enhancing education and well-being through artificial intelligence: opportunities and challenges. In *International Conference on Breaking Barriers with Generative Intelligence* (pp. 154–164). Cham: Springer Nature Switzerland. DOI: 10.1007/978-3-031-65996-6_13

Qin, J., & Wang, M. (2025). Sign language recognition based on dual-channel star-attention convolutional neural network. *Scientific Reports*, *15*(1), 27685. DOI: 10.1038/s41598-025-13625-9

Rahman, M., Nobel, S. M. N., Meena, P. K., Meena, V. P., & Bahadur, J. (2025). Accelerated and Precise Skin Cancer Detection through an Enhanced Machine Learning Pipeline for Improved Diagnostic Accuracy. *Results in Engineering*, *25*, 104168–104168. DOI: 10.1016/j.rineng.2025.104168

Raj, C., Jain, C., & Arif, W. "HEMAN: Health monitoring and nous: An IoT based e-helathcare system for remote telemedicine",*International Conference on Wireless Communications, Signal Processing and Networking (WiSPNET)*,2017 DOI: 10.1109/WiSPNET.2017.8300134

Raj, C., & Kumar, A. (2023). *The essence of telemedicine in Health 4.0: A futuristic approach*. IGI Global.

Raj, O., & Bhatia, K. (2023). *Cutting-edge optimization stratagems assisting medical experts for complex mechanisms behind health and disease detection*. IGI Global.

Ramaiah, M. S., Nagarajan, S. K. S., Whig, P., & Dutta, P. K. (2025). AI-Powered Innovations Transforming Adaptive Education for Disability Support. In *Advancing Adaptive Education: Technological Innovations for Disability Support* (pp. 73–100). IGI Global Scientific Publishing.

Rao, E., & Nasir, M. A. R. B. (2024). *IMPACT OF AFFORDABILITY, ADAPTABILITY, AND AVAILABILITY IN ACHIEVING SUSTAINABILITY: A SYSTEM-DYNAMIC APPROACH* (Doctoral dissertation, College of Electrical & Mechanical Engineering (CEME), NUST).

Rao, K. (2021). Inclusive instructional design: Applying UDL to online learning. *The Journal of Applied Instructional Design, 10*(1), 1–10.

Rashed, A. N. Z., Yarrarapu, M., Prabu, R. T., Raj Antony, G. S., Edeswaran, L., Kumar, E. S., Aswitha, K., Snehith, N., & Ahammad, S. H. (2024). Connected smart elevator systems for smart power and time saving. *Scientific Reports*, *14*(1), 19330. DOI: 10.1038/s41598-024-69173-1 PMID: 39164299

Rassekh, E., & Snidaro, L. (2025). Survey on data fusion approaches for fall-detection. *Information Fusion*, *114*, 102696. DOI: 10.1016/j.inffus.2024.102696

Rastgoo, R., Kiani, K., & Escalera, S. (2021). Sign language recognition: A deep survey. *Expert Systems with Applications*, *164*, 113794. DOI: 10.1016/j.eswa.2020.113794

Rastogi, S., & Singh, J. (2023). Performance enhancement of vision based fall detection using ensemble of machine learning model. *Cluster Computing*, *26*(6), 4119–4132. DOI: 10.1007/s10586-022-03818-6

Rathi, N. D., & Deorankar, A. V. "Overview and an Approach to AI based Healthcare System by using NLP," *2023 Third International Conference on Advances in Electrical, Computing, Communication and Sustainable Technologies (ICAECT)*, Bhilai, India, 2023, DOI: 10.1109/ICAECT57570.2023.10117865

Rathke, C. L., Pimentel, V. C. A., Alsina, P. J., do Espírito Santo, C. C., & Dantas, A. F. O. A. (2024). IoT-Based Wireless System for Gait Kinetics Monitoring in Multi-Device Therapeutic Interventions. *Sensors (Basel), 24*(17), 5799. DOI: 10.3390/s24175799 PMID: 39275710

Reaber, G. (2024, May 2). From stations to exhibits: Enhancing public spaces with AI voice technology. https://www.respeecher.com/blog/enhancing-public-spaces-with-ai-voice-technology

Reddy, C. K., Kumar, C. P., Gowtham, A. R. P. S., Maharaju, R., & Valupadasu, R. (2024). Cloud-Based Skin Cancer Classification: Training and Deploying a Model on AWS. *Lecture Notes in Networks and Systems*, 423–434. DOI: 10.1007/978-981-99-9521-9_32

Reddy, M., & Rao, P. (2024). *Machine learning and generative AI in smart healthcare*. IGI Global.

Redmon, J., & Farhadi, A. (2018). YOLOv3: An incremental improvement. *arXiv preprint arXiv:1804.02767*. https://arxiv.org/abs/1804.02767

Rehman, T., & Malik, S. (2023). *Smart healthcare applications and services*. IGI Global.

Revolutionizing ride-hailing with AI-Powered Taxi App Development. (2024, December 18). Fullestop Blogs. https://www.fullestop.com/blog/ai-powered-taxi-app-development-revolutionizing-ride-hailing

Rezaei, N. (2025). *Promoting Activity in People with Dementia through Assistive Technologies: A Comprehensive Approach from Conceptual Design to System Development* (Doctoral dissertation, Technische Universität Wien).

Rice, P. (2024, September 11). Alexa integration, elevate your home with voice-controlled convenience: The PVE vacuum elevator. Anglian Lifts. https://anglian-lifts.co.uk/alexa-integration-pve-vacuum-lifts/

Rides for all with Lyft Up. (n.d.). Retrieved June 29, 2025, from https://www.lyft.com/lyftup/programs

Risser, R., Lexell, E. M., Bell, D., Iwarsson, S., & Ståhl, A. (2015). Use of local public transport among people with cognitive impairments–A literature review. *Transportation Research Part F: Traffic Psychology and Behaviour, 29*, 83–97. DOI: 10.1016/j.trf.2015.01.002

Rizzo, J. R., Beheshti, M., Hudson, T. E., Mongkolwat, P., Riewpaiboon, W., Seiple, W., Ogedegbe, O. G., & Vedanthan, R. (2023). The global crisis of visual impairment: An emerging global health priority requiring urgent action. *Disability and Rehabilitation. Assistive Technology, 18*(3), 240–245. DOI: 10.1080/17483107.2020.1854876 PMID: 33332166

Roboflow. (2023). *RF-DETR: A robust transformer for object detection* [GitHub repository]. GitHub. Retrieved March 5, 2025, from https://github.com/roboflow/rf-detr

Rode, P., & da Cruz, N. F. (2018). Governing urban accessibility: Moving beyond transport and mobility. *Applied Mobilities, 3*(1), 8–33. DOI: 10.1080/23800127.2018.1438149

Rominger, A., & Eiten, L. R. (2019). Hearing loss and hearing-related factors: Technology and environmental interventions. *Assistive Technologies and Environmental Interventions in Healthcare: An Integrated Approach*, 306-3Santoso, B. (2023). Inclusive digital financial services for persons with disabilities: Impact on economic empowerment and financial inclusion. *Indonesian Journal of Disability Studies, 10*(1), 105–124. DOI: 10.1002/9781394321759.ch18

Rony, M. K. K., Parvin, M. R., Wahiduzzaman, M., Akter, K., & Ullah, M. (2024). Challenges and advancements in the health-related quality of life of older people. *Advances in Public Health, 2024*(1), 8839631. DOI: 10.1155/2024/8839631

Rosli, H. F., Sabri, S. A., & Takril, N. F. (2024). Challenges and Solutions in Teaching and Learning for Students with Disabilities in Higher Education Institutions. *Journal of Quran Sunnah Education & Special Needs, 8*(2), 15–32. DOI: 10.33102/jqss.vol8no2.225

Roy, A., Karim, E., Bin Farukee, M., & Makedon, F. (2024, June). ChatGPT as an Assistive Technology: Enhancing Human-Computer Interaction for People with Speech Impairments. In *Proceedings of the 17th International Conference on PErvasive Technologies Related to Assistive Environments* (pp. 63-66). DOI: 10.1145/3652037.3663956

Rozaire, J., Paquin, C., Henry, L., Agopyan, H., Bard-Pondarré, R., Naaim, A., Duprey, S., & Chaleat-Valayer, E. (2024). A systematic review of instrumented assessments for upper limb function in cerebral palsy: Current limitations and future directions. *Journal of Neuroengineering and Rehabilitation, 21*(1), 56. DOI: 10.1186/s12984-024-01353-6 PMID: 38622731

S. Alsulamy. 2024. Predicting construction delay risks in Saudi Arabian projects: A comparative analysis of CatBoost, XGBoost, and LGBM. Automation in Construction 152 (2024), 105072. https://doi.org/. autcon.2024.105072.DOI: 10.1016/j

Sahoo, S., & Choudhury, B. (2023). AI advances in wheelchair navigation and control: A comprehensive review. *Journal of Process Management New Technologies, 11*(3-4), 115–132. DOI: 10.5937/jpmnt11-45181

Sajja, R., Sermet, Y., Cikmaz, M., Cwiertny, D., & Demir, I. (2024). Artificial intelligence-enabled intelligent assistant for personalised and adaptive learning in higher education. *Information (Basel), 15*(10), 596. DOI: 10.3390/info15100596

Saki, S., & Soori, M. (2025). Artificial intelligence, machine learning and deep learning in advanced transportation systems, A review. *Multimodal Transportation, 100242*(1), 100242. DOI: 10.1016/j.multra.2025.100242

Saldarriaga, A., Gutierrez-Velasquez, E. I., & Colorado, H. A. (2024). Soft hand exoskeletons for rehabilitation: Approaches to design, manufacturing methods, and future prospects. *Robotics (Basel, Switzerland), 13*(3), 50. DOI: 10.3390/robotics13030050

Sali, S., Chai, R., & Ganesan, B. (2025). Recent trends and digital technology applications in lower limb injury rehabilitation. In *Digital Technology in Public Health and Rehabilitation Care* (pp. 99–124). Academic Press. DOI: 10.1016/B978-0-443-22270-2.00007-1

Salmi, J., & D'Addio, A. (2021). Policies for achieving inclusion in higher education. *Policy Reviews in Higher Education, 5*(1), 47–72. DOI: 10.1080/23322969.2020.1835529

Samarpita, S., & Satpathy, R. N. "Applications of Machine Learning in Healthcare: An Overview," 2022 1st IEEE International Conference on Industrial Electronics: Developments & Applications (ICIDeA), Bhubaneswar, India, 2022, DOI: 10.1109/ICIDeA53933.2022.9970177

Samonte, M. J. C., Gazmin, R. A., Soriano, J. D. S., & Valencia, M. N. O. (2019, October). BridgeApp: An assistive mobile communication application for the deaf and mute. In *2019 International Conference on Information and Communication Technology Convergence (ICTC)* (pp. 1310-1315). IEEE. DOI: 10.1109/ICTC46691.2019.8939866

Santhiya, R. and GeethaPriya, C., 2021. Machine Learning Techniques for Intelligent Transportation Systems—An Overview. 2021 12th International Conference on Computing Communication and Networking Technologies (ICCCNT), pp.1–7. DOI: DOI: 10.1109/ICCCNT51525.2021.9579970

Sarker, A., Ul Islam, T., & Islam, M. R. (2025). A review on recent trends of bio-inspired soft robotics: Actuators, control methods, materials selection, sensors, challenges, and future prospects. *Advanced Intelligent Systems*, *7*(3), 2400414. DOI: 10.1002/aisy.202400414

Sarker, I. H. (2022). AI-based modelling: Techniques, applications and research issues towards automation, intelligent and smart systems. *SN Computer Science*, *3*(2), 158. DOI: 10.1007/s42979-022-01043-x PMID: 35194580

Sathe, N., Deodhe, V., Sharma, Y., & Shinde, A. "A Comprehensive Review of AI in Healthcare: Exploring Neural Networks in Medical Imaging, LLM-Based Interactive Response Systems, NLP-Based EHR Systems, Ethics, and Beyond," *2023 International Conference on Advanced Computing & Communication Technologies (ICACCTech)*, Banur, India, 2023, DOI: 10.1109/ICACCTech61146.2023.00108

Satyanarayanan, M. (2017). The emergence of edge computing. *Computer*, *50*(1), 30–39. DOI: 10.1109/MC.2017.9

Sayaf, A. M., Alamri, M. M., Alqahtani, M. A., & Alrahmi, W. M. (2022). Factors influencing university students' adoption of digital learning technology in teaching and learning. *Sustainability (Basel)*, *14*(1), 493. DOI: 10.3390/su14010493

Schlenger, J. 2024. Random Forest. 201–207. https://link.springer.com/chapter/10.1007/978-3-662-68313-2_24 C.M.C.Silva.2024.ADataScientist'sGuidetoBalancedAccuracy. https://blog.trainindata.com/a-data-scientists- guide-to-balanced-accuracy/

Schölkopf, B., Platt, J. C., Shawe-Taylor, J., Smola, A. J., & Williamson, R. C. (2001). Estimating the support of a high-dimensional distribution. *Neural Computation*, *13*(7), 1443–1471. DOI: 10.1162/089976601750264965 PMID: 11440593

Selvaraj, B., & Aruna, M. (2023). *A Review on Analyzing and Predicting the State of Cancer Disease using Machine Learning Algorithms*. DOI: 10.1109/ICIMIA60377.2023.10426268

Senbekov, M., Saliev, T., Bukeyeva, Z., Almabayeva, A., Zhanaliyeva, M., Aitenova, N., Toishibekov, Y., & Fakhradiyev, I. (2020). The Recent Progress and Applications of Digital Technologies in Healthcare: A Review. *Journal of Healthcare Engineering*, *2020*, 8830200. PMID: 33343657

Şengül, G., Karakaya, M., Misra, S., Abayomi-Alli, O. O., & Damaševičius, R. (2022). Deep learning based fall detection using smartwatches for healthcare applications. *Biomedical Signal Processing and Control, 71*, 103242. DOI: 10.1016/j.bspc.2021.103242

Shaheen, M. Y. (2021). Applications of artificial intelligence (AI) in healthcare: A review. *ScienceOpen Preprints, 1*(1). DOI: 10.14293/S2199-1006.1.SOR-.PPVRY8K.v1

Shah, F., Shah, M. S., Akram, W., Manzoor, A., Mahmoud, R. O., & Abdelminaam, D. S. (2021). Sign Language Recognition Using Multiple Kernel Learning: A Case Study of Pakistan Sign Language. *IEEE Access : Practical Innovations, Open Solutions, 9*, 67548–67558. DOI: 10.1109/ACCESS.2021.3077386

Shakespeare, T. (2017). *Disability: The basics*. Routledge. DOI: 10.4324/9781315624839

Shanmugam, P. S. T. (2025). 3D Printing in Prosthetic. *Compendium of 3D Bioprinting Technology*, 256.

Sharma, K., Verma, S., Sharma, S., & Jat, M. (2023). Neurorehabilitation Techniques. *Chief Editor Prof. Rajesh Kumar*, 41.

Sharma, A. (2024). Artificial intelligence in healthcare. In *Revolutionizing the healthcare sector with AI* (pp. 1–25). IGI Global. DOI: 10.4018/979-8-3693-3731-8.ch001

Sharma, B., Davies, J., Nicotra, E., Ji, A., Zhu, K., Phan, P. T., Nguyen, C. C., Hoang, T. T., Wan, J., Pruscino, P., Phan, H.-P., Lovell, N. H., & Do, T. N. (2025). A Soft Robotic Textile-Actuated Anthropomorphic Artificial Shoulder Mechanism. *Advanced Intelligent Systems, 7*(4), 2400807. DOI: 10.1002/aisy.202400807

Sheffield, Z., Paul, P., Krishnakumar, S., & Pan, D. (2025). Current Strategies and Future Directions of Wearable Biosensors for Measuring Stress Biochemical Markers for Neuropsychiatric Applications. *Advancement of Science, 12*(5), 2411339. DOI: 10.1002/advs.202411339 PMID: 39688117

Shinkansen, T. (n.d.). Retrieved June 27, 2025, from https://www.readspeaker.com/resources/tokaido-shinkansen/

Shirley, B., Thomas, J., & Roche, P. (2012, September). VoIPText: Voice chat for deaf and hard of hearing people. In 2012 IEEE Second International Conference on Consumer Electronics-Berlin (ICCE-Berlin) (pp. 19-23). IEEE.

Shrimal, H. (2024). *Integration of AI-powered vehicles with smart city infrastructure to transform the future of the automotive world* (No. 2024-28-0028). SAE Technical Paper

Shrivastava, R., & Pandey, M. (2021). Ensemble of multiple classifiers for accelerometer based human fall detection. In *Computer Networks and Inventive Communication Technologies: Proceedings of Third ICCNCT 2020* (pp. 865-874). Singapore: Springer Nature Singapore. DOI: 10.1007/978-981-15-9647-6_67

Shumba, A.-T., Montanaro, T., Sergi, I., Bramanti, A., Ciccarelli, M., Rispoli, A., Carrizzo, A., De Vittorio, M., & Patrono, L. (2023). Wearable Technologies and AI at the Far Edge for Chronic Heart Failure Prevention and Management: A Systematic Review and Prospects. *Sensors (Basel)*, *23*(15), 6896. Advance online publication. DOI: 10.3390/s23156896 PMID: 37571678

Singh, A. B., Khandelwal, C., &Dangayach, G. S. (2024). Revolutionizing healthcare materials: Innovations in processing, advancements, and challenges for enhanced medical device integration and performance. *Journal of Micromanufacturing*, 25165984241256234.

Singh, B., & Nayyar, A. (2024). Navigating deep learning models and health monitoring infrastructure financing in smart cities: Review from legal perceptions and future innovations. *Deep Learning in Engineering, Energy and Finance*, 80-114.

Singh, H. K., Yadav, A. K., & Claret, S. A. (2024, April). Voice Assistant for Hearing and Speech-Impaired Individuals Using Web framework. In 2024 2nd International Conference on Networking and Communications (ICNWC) (pp. 1-7). IEEE. DOI: 10.1109/ICNWC60771.2024.10537426

Singh, S., & Akhai, S. (2024, July). Electronics in precision control for mechanical engineering: A brief overview. In *AIP Conference Proceedings* (Vol. 3121, No. 1). AIP Publishing. DOI: 10.1063/5.0221464

Singh, S., & Akhai, S. (2025). Tracking Drug Authenticity and Expiry with Blockchain: A Comprehensive Overview. *Blockchain-Enabled Solutions for the Pharmaceutical Industry*, 175-188.

Singh, D. N., Hashmi, M. F., & Sharma, S. K. (2020). Predictive analytics & modeling for modern health care system for cerebral palsy patients. *Multimedia Tools and Applications*, *79*(15), 10285–10307. DOI: 10.1007/s11042-019-07834-4

Singh, S., & Sharma, R. (2023). *Telemedicine and AI redefining healthcare access and insurance*. IGI Global.

Singh, V. (2025). AI-Powered Assistive Technologies for People with Disabilities: Developing AI Solutions that Aid Individuals with Various Disabilities in Daily Tasks. *Journal of Engineering Research and Reports*, *27*(2), 292–309. DOI: 10.9734/jerr/2025/v27i21410

Singh, V., & Patel, N. (2023). *Telemedicine IoT networks and secure image transmission*. IGI Global.

Siviy, C., Baker, L. M., Quinlivan, B. T., Porciuncula, F., Swaminathan, K., Awad, L. N., & Walsh, C. J. (2023). Opportunities and challenges in the development of exoskeletons for locomotor assistance. *Nature Biomedical Engineering*, *7*(4), 456–472. DOI: 10.1038/s41551-022-00984-1 PMID: 36550303

Skoutelis, V. C., Dimitriadis, Z., Kalamvoki, E., Vrettos, S., Kontogeorgakos, V., Dinopoulos, A., Papagelopoulos, P., & Kanellopoulos, A. (2022). Translation, reliability and validity of the Greek functional mobility scale (FMS) for children with cerebral palsy. *Disability and Rehabilitation*, *44*(8), 1436–1442. DOI: 10.1080/09638288.2020.1799439 PMID: 32744923

Smart elevators for smart cities. (2019, October 27). Imdaad. https://www.imdaad.ae/case-studies/smart-elevators-for-smart-cities/

Smart Pedestrian Crossing – An EPS@ISEP 2020 Project. (n.d.). https://www.eps2020-wiki6.dee.isep.ipp.pt/lib/exe/fetch.php?media=smart_pedestrian_crossing_t6_eps_isep_2020.pdf

Smart ramp. (2022, March 15). DIGIFED. https://digifed.org/portfolio-item/smart-ramp/

Smart ramps to assist passengers with reduced mobility (PRM). (n.d.). Retrieved June 28, 2025, from https://danova-next-toolkit.com/smart-ramps-to-assist-passengers-with-reduced-mobility-prm/

Smita. (2025, June 16). AI in Transportation industry: Everything you need to know. ScalaCode. https://www.scalacode.com/guides/ai-in-transportation/

Smith, A., & Johnson, T. (2022). Accessibility and security considerations in smart home systems for visually impaired users. *Journal of Human-Computer Interaction*, *38*(5), 412–431.

Soar, J., & Croll, P. (2007). Assistive technologies for the frail elderly, chronic illness sufferers and people with disabilities-A case study of the development of a smart home. In *ACIS2007 Proceedings of the 18th Australasian Conference on Information Systems* (pp. 937–944). The University of Southern Queensland., https://eprints.qut.edu.au/14331/

Sood, S. K., Lamba, Y. S., & Singh, A. K. (2025). Exploring the Shift from 3D Printing to 4D Printing: A Review. *IEEE Sensors Journal*.

Soundscape, M. (2022, June 7). Microsoft Research. https://www.microsoft.com/en-us/research/product/soundscape/

Sozib, H. M.Hasan Mahmud Sozib. (2025). Wearable AI for Cardiovascular Health Monitoring: Enabling Early Detection and Prevention. *Journal of Computer Science and Technology Studies*, *7*(2), 30. DOI: 10.32996/jcsts.2025.7.2.30

Sridhar, A. R., Cheung, J. W., Lampert, R., Silva, J. N. A., Gopinathannair, R., Sotomonte, J. C., Tarakji, K., Fellman, M., Chrispin, J., Varma, N., Kabra, R., Mehta, N., Al-Khatib, S. M., Mayfield, J. J., Navara, R., Rajagopalan, B., Passman, R., Fleureau, Y., Shah, M. J., & Lakkireddy, D. (2024, October). State of the art of mobile health technologies use in clinical arrhythmia care. *Communications Medicine*, *4*(1), 218. Advance online publication. DOI: 10.1038/s43856-024-00618-4 PMID: 39472742

Srinivasan, S., & Rajavel, N. (2025). Technology Improves the Quality of Life for Elderly People. In *Perspectives on the Economics of Aging* (pp. 109-150). IGI Global Scientific Publishing.dooi: DOI: 10.2139/ssrn.5277229

Srinivasan, S., Rajavel, N., & Sanchez, N. K. (2025). The Impact of AI on Elderly Inmates in Central Prison. In *Exploration of AI in Contemporary Legal Systems* (pp. 281–314). IGI Global Scientific Publishing., DOI: 10.4018/979-8-3693-7205-0.ch013

Stefanov, D. H., Bien, Z., & Bang, W. C. (2004). The smart house for older persons and persons with physical disabilities: Structure, technology arrangements, and perspectives. *IEEE Transactions on Neural Systems and Rehabilitation Engineering*, *12*(2), 228–250. DOI: 10.1109/TNSRE.2004.828423 PMID: 15218937

Stremmel, C., & Breitschwerdt, R. (2023). Digital transformation in the diagnostics and therapy of cardiovascular diseases: Comprehensive literature review. *JMIR Cardio*, *7*, e44983. DOI: 10.2196/44983 PMID: 37647103

Subburam, R., Chandralekha, E., & Kandasamy, V. (2024). An elderly fall detection system using enhanced random forest in machine learning. *Engineering Proceedings*, *59*(1), 172.

Sucerquia, A., López, J. D., & Vargas-Bonilla, J. F. (2017). SisFall: A fall and movement dataset. *Sensors (Basel)*, *17*(1), 198. DOI: 10.3390/s17010198 PMID: 28117691

Suk, S., & Walter, A. (2018). Nighttime Visibility and Roadway Safety: A Literature Review. *Journal of Safety Research*, *67*, 1–7.

Sünderhauf, N., Brock, O., Scheirer, W., Hadsell, R., Fox, D., Leitner, J., Upcroft, B., Abbeel, P., Burgard, W., Milford, M., & Corke, P. (2018). The limits and potentials of deep learning for robotics. *The International Journal of Robotics Research, 37*(4-5), 405–420. DOI: 10.1177/0278364918770733

Sunu band. (2015). National Federation of the Blind. National Federation of the Blind Jernigan Institute Research Collaboration: Sunu Band. https://nfb.org/blog/national-federation-blind-jernigan-institute-research-collaboration-sunu-band

Svensson, I., Nordström, T., Lindeblad, E., Gustafson, S., Björn, M., Sand, C., & Nilsson, S. (2021). Effects of assistive technology for students with reading and writing disabilities. *Disability and Rehabilitation. Assistive Technology, 16*(2), 196–208. DOI: 10.1080/17483107.2019.1646821 PMID: 31418305

Swargiary, K. (2024). *Integrating IoT in Education:(Transforming Learning Through Smart Technologies)*. EdTech Research Association.

Szabó, P., Ara, J., Halmosi, B., Sik-Lanyi, C., & Guzsvinecz, T. (2023). Technologies designed to assist individuals with cognitive impairments. *Sustainability (Basel), 15*(18), 13490. DOI: 10.3390/su151813490

Szegedy, C., Vanhoucke, V., Ioffe, S., Shlens, J., & Wojna, Z. (2015, December 11). *Rethinking the inception architecture for computer vision*. arXiv.org. https://arxiv.org/abs/1512.00567

T. (2016). *TorchVision: PyTorch's Computer Vision library*. GitHub. https://github.com/pytorch/vision

T. R. Saravanan, S. Suvitha, D. Banavath, S. Gogula, J. Upadhyay, and M. Sudhakar, "Exploring AI and Machine Learning Integration in Medical Assistive Robotics: An Experimental Approach," in Fostering Cross-Industry Sustainability With Intelligent Technologies, 2024.

Tabucol, J., Kooiman, V. G., Leopaldi, M., Leijendekkers, R., Selleri, G., Mellini, M., Verdonschot, N., Oddsson, M., Carloni, R., Zucchelli, A., & Brugo, T. M. (2025). The MyFlex-ζ Foot: A Variable Stiffness ESR Ankle-Foot Prosthesis. *IEEE Transactions on Neural Systems and Rehabilitation Engineering, 33*, 653–663. DOI: 10.1109/TNSRE.2025.3534096 PMID: 40031158

Taimoor, N., & Rehman, S. (2021, December). Comprehensive Survey on Personalized Healthcare Services in Modern Healthcare Internet of Things. *IEEE Access : Practical Innovations, Open Solutions, 10*, 535–563. DOI: 10.1109/ACCESS.2021.3137364

Tajadod, F. (2021). *Voice command android-based smart home system for controlling door lock, lights, and home appliance for physically disabled people based on iot* (Doctoral dissertation, California State University San Marcos). https://scholarworks.calstate.edu/downloads/4m90f171q

Talk2lift brings the power of speech recognition on any elevator cabin, enabling passengers to voice-control. (2020, September 14). Talk2Lift; bmjwu. https://talk2lift.com/

Tamjeed, M., Tibdewal, V., Russell, M., McQuaid, M., Oh, T., & Shinohara, K. (2021). Understanding disability services toward improving graduate student support. In *Proceedings of the 23rd international ACM SIGACCESS conference on computers and accessibility* (pp. 1–14). DOI: 10.1145/3441852.3471231

Tan, M., & Le, Q. (2021). *EfficientNetV2: Smaller Models and Faster Training.* https://arxiv.org/pdf/2104.00298

Tan, M., Pang, R., & Le, Q. V. (2020). *EfficientDet: Scalable and Efficient Object Detection* (No. arXiv:1911.09070). arXiv. /arXiv.1911.09070DOI: 10.1109/CVPR42600.2020.01079

Tan, C. K., Lim, K. M., Chang, R. K. Y., Lee, C. P., & Alqahtani, A. (2023). HGR-ViT: Hand Gesture Recognition with Vision Transformer. *Sensors (Basel), 23*(12), 5555. DOI: 10.3390/s23125555 PMID: 37420722

Tan, C. K., Lim, K. M., Lee, C. P., Chang, R. K. Y., & Alqahtani, A. (2023). SDViT: Stacking of Distilled Vision Transformers for Hand Gesture Recognition. *Applied Sciences (Basel, Switzerland), 13*(22), 12204. DOI: 10.3390/app132212204

Tan, Q., Wu, C., Li, L., Shao, W., & Luo, M. (2022). Nanomaterial-Based Prosthetic Limbs for Disability Mobility Assistance: A Review of Recent Advances. *Journal of Nanomaterials, 2022*(1), 3425297. DOI: 10.1155/2022/3425297

Tanwar, P., Bansal, K., Sharma, A., & Dagar, N. "AI-Powered Chatbot for School Students to Address Healthcare FAQs Using Google Dialogflow," *2023 International Conference on Advances in Computation, Communication and Information Technology (ICAICCIT)*, Faridabad, India, 2023, pp. 45-50. DOI: 10.1109/ICAICCIT60255.2023.10465728

Tao, L., Volonakis, T., Tan, B., Jing, Y., Chetty, K., & Smith, M. (2018). Home activity monitoring using low resolution infrared sensor. *arXiv preprint arXiv:1811.05416.*

Taofik Ahmed Suleiman. (2023). *Abdulkareem Adinoyi," Telemedicine and Smart Healthcare—The Role of Artificial Intelligence, 5G, Cloud Services, and Other Enabling Technologies" in International Journal of Communications*. Network and System Science.

Taylor, D. L., Yeung, M., & Bashet, A. Z. (2021). Personalised and adaptive learning. *Innovative learning environments in STEM higher education: Opportunities, Challenges, and Looking Forward*, 17–34.

Techaraungrong, P., Suksakulchai, S., Kaewprapan, W., & Murphy, E. (2017). The design and testing of multimedia for teaching arithmetic to deaf learners. *Education and Information Technologies*, *22*(1), 215–237. DOI: 10.1007/s10639-015-9441-1

Text-to-speech voices designed for public transport. (n.d.). Acapela Group. https://www.acapela-group.com/tts-voices-for-transport/

Thacharodi, A., Singh, P., Meenatchi, R., Tawfeeq Ahmed, Z. H., Kumar, R. R., v, N., Kavish, S., Maqbool, M., & Hassan, S. (2024). Revolutionizing healthcare and medicine: The impact of modern technologies for a healthier future—A comprehensive review. *Health Care Science*, *3*(5), 329–349. DOI: 10.1002/hcs2.115 PMID: 39479277

Thakur, S., Kumar, A., Dijkstra, A., & Thakur, A. (2024). Occupational therapy-based rehabilitation of sciatic nerve pain. *Brain-X*, *2*(4), e70010. DOI: 10.1002/brx2.70010

Thangam, S., ... (2024). "IoT-Based Health Monitoring System for Forbidden Patients." *2024 10th International Conference on Advanced Computing and Communication Systems (ICACCS)*. Vol. 1. IEEE.

Thangam, S.. (2024). "Flex Sensor Data Analysis for Hand Rehabilitation using Wearable Glove." *2024 Third International Conference on Electrical, Electronics, Information and Communication Technologies (ICEEICT)*. IEEE.

Theodoridis, T., Solachidis, V., Vretos, N., & Daras, P. (2017, November). Human fall detection from acceleration measurements using a recurrent neural network. In *International conference on biomedical and health informatics* (pp. 145-149). Singapore: Springer Singapore.

Theodorikakos, S. (2023). *AR & VR application research for medical rehabilitation* (Master's thesis, Πανεπιστήμιο Πειραιώς).

Thomford, N. E., Bope, C. D., Agamah, F. E., Dzobo, K., Ateko, R. O., Chimusa, E., Mazandu, G. K., Ntumba, S. B., Dandara, C., & Wonkam, A. (2019). Implementing artificial intelligence and digital health in resource-limited settings? Top 10 lessons we learned in congenital heart defects and cardiology. *OMICS: A Journal of Integrative Biology*, *23*(11), 607–616. DOI: 10.1089/omi.2019.0142 PMID: 31592719

Tierney, C. (2024). Empowering Students through a Digital Badge in UDL. *All Ireland Journal of Higher Education, 16*(2).

TrainMate Robotic System Making Public Transportation. Public! (n.d.). Retrieved June 29, 2025, from https://onlinepubs.trb.org/onlinepubs/IDEA/FinalReports/Transit/Transit100.pdf

Tran, K. C., Gassi, M., Nehme, P., Rousseau, J., Nguyen, T. K., & Meunier, J. (2022, November). *Comparison of anomaly detection algorithms for near-fall detection with video surveillance. In 2022 E-Health and Bioengineering Conference (EHB) (pp. 01-04)*. IEEE.

TransPennine Express. (2024, Sep, 20). TransPennine Express tests UK-first AI speech-to-text announcements designed to improve journeys for hearing-impaired passengers [Press release]. Mediacentrefile. Retrieved June 28, 2025, from: https://mediacentre.tpexpress.co.uk/news/video-transpennine-express-tests-uk-first-ai-speech-to-text-announcements-designed-to-improve-journeys-for-hearing-impaired-passengers

Trewin, S., Basson, S., Muller, M., Branham, S., Treviranus, J., Gruen, D., Hebert, D., Lyckowski, N., & Manser, E. (2019). Considerations for AI fairness for people with disabilities. *AI Matters*, *5*(3), 40–63. DOI: 10.1145/3362077.3362086

Troussas, C., Krouska, A., & Sgouropoulou, C. (2020). Dynamic detection of learning modalities using fuzzy logic in students' interaction activities. In *Intelligent Tutoring Systems: 16th International Conference, ITS 2020, Athens, Greece, June 8–12, 2020, Proceedings 16* (pp. 205-213). Springer International Publishing. DOI: 10.1007/978-3-030-49663-0_24

Trovato, V., Sfameni, S., Rando, G., Rosace, G., Libertino, S., Ferri, A., & Plutino, M. R. (2022). A review of stimuli-responsive smart materials for wearable Technology in Healthcare: Retrospective, perspective, and prospective. *Molecules (Basel, Switzerland)*, *27*(17), 5709. DOI: 10.3390/molecules27175709 PMID: 36080476

Tschandl, P. (2018). The HAM10000 dataset, a large collection of multi-source dermatoscopic images of common pigmented skin lesions. *Harvard Dataverse*. https://doi.org/DOI: 10.7910/dvn/dbw86t

Tschandl, P., Rinner, C., Apalla, Z., Argenziano, G., Codella, N., Halpern, A., Janda, M., Lallas, A., Longo, C., Malvehy, J., Paoli, J., Puig, S., Rosendahl, C., Soyer, H. P., Zalaudek, I., & Kittler, H. (2020). Human–computer collaboration for skin cancer recognition. *Nature Medicine*, *26*(8), 1229–1234. DOI: 10.1038/s41591-020-0942-0 PMID: 32572267

Tyagi, S., Upadhyay, P., Fatima, H., Jain, S., & Sharma, A. K. (2023). *American Sign Language Detection using YOLOv5 and YOLOv8*. DOI: 10.21203/rs.3.rs-3126918/v1

Uber. (n.d.). Retrieved June 29, 2025, from https://www.uber.com/us/en/about/accessibility/

Ukasi, S., Pongampai, S., Panigrahi, B. K., Panda, S., Hajra, S., Kim, H. J., Vittayakorn, N., & Charoonsuk, T. (2024). Continuous tremor monitoring in Parkinson's disease: A wristwatch-inspired triboelectric sensor approach. *iScience*, *27*(12), 111480. DOI: 10.1016/j.isci.2024.111480 PMID: 39720518

Ullah, M., Hamayun, S., Wahab, A., Khan, S. U., Rehman, M. U., Haq, Z. U., Rehman, K. U., Ullah, A., Mehreen, A., Awan, U. A., Qayum, M., & Naeem, M. (2023). Smart technologies used as smart tools in the management of cardiovascular disease and their future perspective. *Current Problems in Cardiology*, *48*(11), 101922. DOI: 10.1016/j.cpcardiol.2023.101922 PMID: 37437703

Ultralytics. (2024). *YOLOv5 vs YOLOv8: Performance benchmarks*. Ultralytics Documentation. Retrieved March 5, 2025, from https://docs.ultralytics.com/compare/yolov5-vs-yolov8/#performance-benchmarks-yolov5-vs-yolov8

Ultralytics. (n.d.) *YOLOv5 architecture description*. https://docs.ultralytics.com/yolov5/tutorials/architecture_description/#1-model-structure

UNICEF report by Alessandaro Di Rosa and Megan T. Tucker (2022) https://www.unicef.org/media/131316/file/Accessible%20and%20inclusive%20digital%20solutions%20for%20girls%20with%20disabilities.pdf

United Nations. (n.d.). Transforming our world: The 2030 Agenda for Sustainable Development [Online]. Retrieved June 10, 2025, from: https://sdgs.un.org/2030agenda

Urrea, C., & Agramonte, R. (2023). Improving Exoskeleton Functionality: Design and Comparative Evaluation of Control Techniques for Pneumatic Artificial Muscle Actuators in Lower Limb Rehabilitation and Work Tasks. *Processes (Basel, Switzerland)*, *11*(12), 3278. DOI: 10.3390/pr11123278

Ushakov, D., Dudukalov, E., Shmatko, L., & Shatila, K. (2022). *Artificial Intelligence as a Factor of Public Transportation System Development*. Elsevier. [online], DOI: 10.1016/j.trpro.2022.06.276

Usmani, S., Saboor, A., Haris, M., Khan, M. A., & Park, H. (2021). Latest research trends in fall detection and prevention using machine learning: A systematic review. *Sensors (Basel)*, *21*(15), 5134. DOI: 10.3390/s21155134 PMID: 34372371

Vangelista, L., Zanella, A., & Zorzi, M. (2015). Long-range IoT technologies: The dawn of LoRa™. In Future Access Enablers for Ubiquitous and Intelligent Infrastructures: First International Conference, FABULOUS 2015, Ohrid, Republic of Macedonia, September 23-25, 2015. Revised Selected Papers 1 (pp. 51-58). Springer International Publishing.

Varaganti, P., & Seo, S. (2024). Recent advances in biomimetics for the development of bio-inspired prosthetic limbs. *Biomimetics*, *9*(5), 273. DOI: 10.3390/biomimetics9050273 PMID: 38786483

Velho, R., Holloway, C., Symonds, A., & Balmer, B. (2016). The effect of transport accessibility on the social inclusion of wheelchair users: A mixed method analysis. *Social Inclusion (Lisboa)*, *4*(3), 24–35. DOI: 10.17645/si.v4i3.484

Verma, R., Akhai, S., & Wadhwa, A. S. (2024). Use of smart materials in physiotherapy. In *Revolutionizing healthcare treatment with sensor technology* (pp. 300–319). IGI Global. DOI: 10.4018/979-8-3693-2762-3.ch019

Vervoort, D., Marvel, F. A., Isakadze, N., Kpodonu, J., & Martin, S. S. (2020). Digital cardiology: Opportunities for disease prevention. *Current Cardiovascular Risk Reports*, *14*(10). Advance online publication. DOI: 10.1007/s12170-020-00648-w

Vinayak Parkar, T., & Kamath, K. M. (2024). Next-gen healthcare: AI and IoT innovations and future trends. In *Intelligent systems and IoT applications* (pp. 150–173). IGI Global.

Virupaxappa, G., & Thangam, S. (2023). "Detection of Dystonia in Cerebral Palsy Using Dyskinesia Impairment Scale and Machine Learning," 2023 IEEE 3rd Mysore Sub Section International Conference (MysuruCon), HASSAN, India. DOI: 10.1109/MysuruCon59703.2023.10396938

Vishweshwar, S. M. (2023). Implications of Deepfake Technology on Individual Privacy and Security [St. Cloud State University]. https://repository.stcloudstate.edu/cgi/viewcontent.cgi?article=1199&context=msia_etds

Vocaturo, E., Zumpano, E., & Veltri, P. (2018). *Image pre-processing in computer vision systems for melanoma detection*. Bioinformatics and Biomedicine., DOI: 10.1109/BIBM.2018.8621507

Vojinovic, I., Panajotovic, T., Budimirovic, M., Jankovic, M., & Milic, D. (2024). User-centric Smart City Services for People with Disabilities and the Elderly: A UN SDG Framework Approach. *Economics, 18*(1), 20220103. https://www.degruyterbrill.com/document/doi/10.1515/econ-2022-0103/html

von Elling-Tammen, L., Stark, C., Wloka, K. R., Alberg, E., Schoenau, E., & Duran, I. (2023). Predicting gross motor function in children and adolescents with cerebral palsy applying artificial intelligence using data on assistive devices. *Journal of Clinical Medicine*, *12*(6), 2228.

Waidi, Y. O. (2025). Recent Advances in 4D-Printed Shape Memory Actuators. *Macromolecular Rapid Communications*, *46*(10), 2401141. DOI: 10.1002/marc.202401141 PMID: 40014667

Wang, H.-R., & Jing, Y.-H. "Research on the Application of Artificial Intelligence in the Development of Biomedicine and Oncology," *2023 International Conference on Intelligent Supercomputing and BioPharma (ISBP)*, Zhuhai, China, 2023 DOI: 10.1109/ISBP57705.2023.10061308

Wang, L., & Zhang, Y. (2024). Trust and privacy in IoT-enabled assistive technologies: A user-centered approach. *IEEE Transactions on Human-Machine Systems*, *54*(1), 45–56.

Wang, Q., Chen, Z., & Liu, S. (2022). *Advanced secure transmission of telemedicine-based bio-medical data using AI*. IGI Global.

Wang, S., Li, X., Liao, G., Liu, J., Liao, C., Liu, M., Liao, J., & Liu, L. (2024). A spatio-temporal graph neural network for fall prediction with inertial sensors. *Knowledge-Based Systems*, *293*, 111709. DOI: 10.1016/j.knosys.2024.111709

Wang, S., Xiao, J., Liu, Y., Zhang, S., & Yan, G. (2025). *Real-time detection of intelligent transportation system based on 3D point cloud*. Elsevier Expert Systems with Applications. [online], DOI: 10.1016/j.inffus.2025.103213

Wang, X., Ellul, J., & Azzopardi, G. (2020). Elderly fall detection systems: A literature survey. *Frontiers in Robotics and AI*, *7*, 71. DOI: 10.3389/frobt.2020.00071 PMID: 33501238

Wang, Y., Cui, Z., & Ke, R. (2023). *Machine learning for transportation research and applications*. Elsevier.

Wang, Z., Harrou, F., Sun, Y., & Genton, M. G. (2026). Exploring the magnitude-shape plot framework for anomaly detection in crowded video scenes. In *AI-Based Solutions for Engineering* (pp. 137–174). IGI Global Scientific Publishing.

Wanjiku Wang'ang'a, A. (2024). Social Economic Barriers to Information Communication Technology (ICT) Access for Persons with Disabilities in Africa: Literature Review. *East African Journal of Information Technology*, *7*(1), 318–327. DOI: 10.37284/eajit.7.1.2235

Warraich, H. J., Patrick-Lake, B., Saha, A., Rashid, L., Pai, V., Abbasi, A., Diamond, M. C., Tazbaz, T., & Califf, R. M. (2025). Digital health technologies for cardiometabolic disease and diabetes: A perspective from the U.S. Food and Drug Administration. *Journal of the American College of Cardiology*, *85*(5), 528–535. DOI: 10.1016/j.jacc.2024.10.075 PMID: 39641737

Warren, S., Craft, R. L., & Bosma, J. T. "Designing Smart Health Care Technology into the Home of the Future," presented at the United States, April 7, 1999. OSTI ID: 5696. DOI: 10.1109/IEMBS.1999.803832

Washburn, D., Sindhu, U., Balaouras, S., Dines, R. A., Hayes, N., & Nelson, L. E. (2009). Helping CIOs understand "smart city" initiatives. *Growth*, *17*(2), 1–17.

Wayfinder. (2024). https://paper.wayfinder.ai/wayfinder_paper_v1.pdf

WeWALK smart cane – smart cane for the visually impaired. (n.d.). Retrieved June 27, 2025, from https://wewalk.io/en/

WFD. (2025). *The Legal Recognition of National Sign Languages*. Retrieved 19/08/2025 from https://wfdeaf.org/the-legal-recognition-of-national-sign-languages

WHO. (2023a). *The critical role of accessibility in health information*. https://www.who.int/europe/news-room/feature-stories/item/the-critical-role-of-accessibility-in-health-information

WHO. (2023b). *Disability*. Retrieved 19/08/2025 from https://www.who.int/news-room/fact-sheets/detail/disability-and-health

WHO. (2025). *Deafness and hearing loss*. Retrieved 19/08/2025 from https://www.who.int/news-room/fact-sheets/detail/deafness-and-hearing-loss

WHO-UNICEF. (2022, May). Global report on assistive technology. https://www.unicef.org/reports/global-report-assistive-technology#:~:text=Highlights,replacements

Wicha, S., Sharp, B., Sureephong, P., Chakpitak, N., & Atkins, A. (2012). An animated dictionary for hearing-impaired students in Thailand. *Journal of Research in Special Educational Needs*, *12*(4), 234–244. DOI: 10.1111/j.1471-3802.2012.01239.x

Wightman, R. (2019). *PyTorch Image Models* [Review of *PyTorch Image Models*]. GitHub. https://github.com/huggingface/pytorch-image-models

Williamson, B., & Kizilcec, R. (2023). Data ethics in digital learning: Privacy, surveillance, and algorithmic accountability. *Learning, Media and Technology*, *48*(1), 1–18. DOI: 10.1080/17439884.2023.2167830

Willilams, J. D. (2023). Creating an Equitable Transit System for New York City. Metropolitan Transit Authority (MTA), New York City. https://advocate.nyc.gov/resources/reports/MTA-Accessibility-Report-PRINT-YR9jvk9Z6b9x.pdf

Willingham, T. B., Stowell, J., Collier, G., & Backus, D. (2024). Leveraging emerging technologies to expand accessibility and improve precision in rehabilitation and exercise for people with disabilities. *International Journal of Environmental Research and Public Health*, *21*(1), 79. DOI: 10.3390/ijerph21010079 PMID: 38248542

Wilson, D., & Baker, A. (2024). *Medical informatics: Concepts, methodologies, tools, and applications*. IGI Global.

World Cancer Research Fund. (2024, October 4). *Skin cancer statistics | world cancer research fund.* World Cancer Research Fund. https://www.wcrf.org/preventing-cancer/cancer-statistics/skin-cancer-statistics/

World Health Organization, & World Bank. (2011). World report on disability [Online]. Geneva: World Health Organization; 2011 Retrieved June 10, 2025. Available from: https://iris.who.int/handle/10665/44575

World Health Organization. (2019, October 8). *World report on vision*. Www.who.int. https://www.who.int/publications/i/item/9789241516570

World Health Organization. (2022). Global report on health equity for persons with disabilities [Online]. Retrieved June 10, 2025, from: https://www.who.int/publications/i/item/9789240063600

World Health Organization. (2022). *Global report on health equity for persons with disabilities*. World Health Organization. https://books.google.co.in/books?hl=en&lr=&id=mK2tEAAAQBAJ&oi=fnd&pg=PR3&dq=According+to+World+Health+Organization+(WHO)+16%25+of+the+world%E2%80%99s+population+(1+in+6+persons)+live+with+some+kind+of+disability,+out+of+them+approximately+200+million+face+considerable+difficulties+in+functioning.&ots=TN-gy_dDhd&sig=LoZ5EsaRiy-f-CECUZXK8NNCh9Q&redir_esc=y#v=onepage&q&f=false

World Health Organization. (2023, August 10). Blindness and vision impairment. https://www.who.int/news-room/fact-sheets/detail/blindness-and-visual-impairment

World Health Organization. (2023, August 10). *Blindness and vision impairment.* World Health Organization. https://www.who.int/news-room/fact-sheets/detail/blindness-and-visual-impairment

World Health Organization. 2017. Managing Speed. [online] Available at: https://www.who.int/publications-detail/9789241511712

World Health Organization. 2021. Global Status Report on Road Safety. [online] Available at: https://www.who.int/publications/i/item/9789241565685

Wu, C. H., Ho, J. M., & Lee, D. T. (2004). Travel-time prediction with support vector regression. *IEEE Transactions on Intelligent Transportation Systems*, *5*(4), 276–281. DOI: 10.1109/TITS.2004.837813

Wu, C. M., Chen, S. C., Chen, Y. J., & Efendi, A. (2024). A Personalized Contactless Emergency Aid System Designed for Individuals With Profound Physical Disabilities. *IEEE Access : Practical Innovations, Open Solutions*, *12*, 27115–27126.

Xiong, A., Wu, T., & Jia, J. (2024). Design of a Real-Time Monitoring System for Electroencephalogram and Electromyography Signals in Cerebral Palsy Rehabilitation via Wearable Devices. *Electronics (Basel)*, *13*(15), 2902. DOI: 10.3390/electronics13152902

Xue, X., Zeng, Y., Zhang, Y., Lee, S., & Yan, Z. (2021, July 26). A Study on an Application System for the Sustainable Development of Smart Healthcare in China. *IEEE Access : Practical Innovations, Open Solutions*, *9*, 111960–111974. DOI: 10.1109/ACCESS.2021.3099806

Xu, K., & Qin, S. (2023, May). An Interdisciplinary approach and advanced techniques for enhanced 3D-printed upper limb prosthetic socket design: A literature review. [). MDPI.]. *Actuators*, *12*(6), 223. DOI: 10.3390/act12060223

Xu, Y., Wang, Q., Lillie, J., Kamat, V., & Menassa, C. (2025). CoNav Chair: Design of a ROS-based smart wheelchair for shared control navigation in the built environment. In arXiv [cs.RO]. arXiv. https://arxiv.org/abs/2501.09680 DOI: 10.22260/ISARC2025/0046

Yadav, P., Udaya Kumar, D., & Karmakar, S. (2021). Inclusive design in higher educational institutes for people with disability. In *Design for Tomorrow—Volume 2: Proceedings of ICoRD 2021* (pp. 165-176). Springer Singapore. DOI: 10.1007/978-981-16-0119-4_14

Yamijala, S. M. S., Chodisetty, R. M., Chakravorty, C., & Sai, K. P. (2025). AI-Powered Learning Revolutionizing Smart Education With Personalized Learning Styles. In *Internet of Behaviour-Based Computational Intelligence for Smart Education Systems* (pp. 191–212). IGI Global.

Yang, H., Fang, H., Wang, C., Wang, Y., Qi, C., Zhang, Y., Zhou, Q., Huang, M., Wang, M., & Wu, M. (2024). 3D printing of customized functional devices for smart biomedical systems. *SmartMat*, *5*(5), e1244. DOI: 10.1002/smm2.1244

Yara Alkhalifah & Dimitrios Lytras, *Digital Twin in Cardiology*, 2025.

Yeung, A. W. K., Kulnik, S. T., Parvanov, E. D., Fassl, A., Eibensteiner, F., Völkl-Kernstock, S., Kletecka-Pulker, M., Crutzen, R., Gutenberg, J., Höppchen, I., Niebauer, J., Smeddinck, J. D., Willschke, H., & Atanasov, A. G. (2022). Research on digital technology use in cardiology: Bibliometric analysis. *Journal of Medical Internet Research*, *24*(5), e36086. DOI: 10.2196/36086 PMID: 35544307

Yeung, A. W. K., Litvinova, O., Bragazzi, N. L., Khader, Y., Rahman, M. M., Said, Z., Istepanian, R. S. H., Koulaouzidis, A., Aremu, A. O., Flanagan, J. M., Rabiee, N., Islam, S. M. S., Tewari, D., Venkatachalam, G., Orlando, G., Niebauer, J., Georgakilas, A. G., Saeb, M. R., Hrg, D., & Atanasov, A. G. (2024). *Digital health and mobile health: A bibliometric analysis of the 100 most cited papers and their contributing authors. Exploration of Digital Health Technologies*, *2*, 86–100. DOI: 10.37349/edht.2024.00013

Yihun, Y., & Delgado, P. (2025). Enhancing Personalized Rehabilitation: Integrating Assist-as-Needed System With Real-Time Feedback. *Journal of Engineering and Science in Medical Diagnostics and Therapy*, *8*(3), 031002. DOI: 10.1115/1.4066387

Yıldırım, M. Ş., Cavlak, M., Taştekin, B., Akçan, R., Tümer, A. R., & Balseven-Odabaşi, A. (2021). Road traffic injury-related disabilities in geriatric population. *Journal of Clinical Gerontology & Geriatrics*.

Yin, S., Yao, D. R., Song, Y., Heng, W., Ma, X., Han, H., & Gao, W. (2024). Wearable and Implantable Soft Robots. *Chemical Reviews*, *124*(20), 11585–11636. DOI: 10.1021/acs.chemrev.4c00513 PMID: 39392765

Yuan, T., da Rocha Neto, W. B., Rothenberg, C., Obraczka, K., Barakat, C., & Turletti, T. (2019). Harnessing machine learning for next-generation intelligent transportation systems: a survey. *Proceedings of the computational intelligence, communication systems and networks (CICSyN).*

Yu, X., Wang, C., Wu, W., & Xiong, S. (2025). A real-time skeleton-based fall detection algorithm based on temporal convolutional networks and transformer encoder. *Pervasive and Mobile Computing*, *107*, 102016. DOI: 10.1016/j.pmcj.2025.102016

Yu, X., Wan, J., An, G., Yin, X., & Xiong, S. (2024). A novel semi-supervised model for pre-impact fall detection with limited fall data. *Engineering Applications of Artificial Intelligence*, *132*, 108469. DOI: 10.1016/j.engappai.2024.108469

Zantalis, F., Koulouras, G., Karabetsos, S., & Kandris, D. (2019). A review of machine learning and IoT in smart transportation. *Future Internet*, *11*(4), 94. DOI: 10.3390/fi11040094

Zarei, M., Lee, G., Lee, S. G., & Cho, K. (2023). Advances in biodegradable electronic skin: Material progress and recent applications in sensing, robotics, and human–machine interfaces. *Advanced Materials*, *35*(4), 2203193. DOI: 10.1002/adma.202203193 PMID: 35737931

Zaugg, T. (2024). Future innovations for assistive technology and universal design for learning. *Assistive technology and universal design for learning: Toolkits for inclusive instruction*, 275–318.

Zawar, S., Udhani, R., & Sathe, S. (2024). Closing the Gap on Access to Assistive Technology. *Journal of Research in Medical and Interpathy Sciences*, *2*(1), 31–34.

Zaydi, M., Maleh, Y., & Khourdifi, Y. (2025). A new framework for agile cybersecurity risk management: Integrating continuous adaptation and real-time threat intelligence (ACSRM-ICTI). In *Agile Security in the Digital Era* (pp. 19-47). CRC Press.

Zemmouchi-Ghomari, L. (2025). Artificial intelligence in intelligent transportation systems. Journal of Intelligent Manufacturing and Special Equipment.

Zemmouchi-Ghomari, L. (2025). Artificial intelligence in intelligent transportation systems. *Journal of Intelligent Manufacturing and Special Equipment*, *6*(1), 26–42. DOI: 10.1108/JIMSE-11-2024-0035

Zerrouki, N., Harrou, F., Houacine, A., & Sun, Y. (2016, November). Fall detection using supervised machine learning algorithms: A comparative study. In *2016 8th international conference on modelling, identification and control (ICMIC)* (pp. 665-670). IEEE. DOI: 10.1109/ICMIC.2016.7804195

Zerrouki, N., Harrou, F., Sun, Y., Ait Djafer, A. Z., & Amrane, H. (2022, September). A survey on recent advances in fall detection systems using machine learning formalisms. In *2022 7th International Conference on Frontiers of Signal Processing (ICFSP)* (pp. 35-39). IEEE. DOI: 10.1109/ICFSP55781.2022.9924708

Zerrouki, N., Harrou, F., Sun, Y., & Houacine, A. (2016). A data-driven monitoring technique for enhanced fall events detection. *IFAC-PapersOnLine*, *49*(5), 333–338. DOI: 10.1016/j.ifacol.2016.07.135

Zerrouki, N., Harrou, F., Sun, Y., & Houacine, A. (2016). Accelerometer and camera-based strategy for improved human fall detection. *Journal of Medical Systems*, *40*(12), 284. DOI: 10.1007/s10916-016-0639-6 PMID: 27796842

Zerrouki, Y., Harrou, F., Zerrouki, N., Dairi, A., & Sun, Y. (2020). Desertification detection using an improved variational autoencoder-based approach through ETM-landsat satellite data. *IEEE Journal of Selected Topics in Applied Earth Observations and Remote Sensing*, *14*, 202–213. DOI: 10.1109/JSTARS.2020.3042760

Zhang, W. (2025). Enhancing Rehabilitation Assessment with Artificial Intelligence: A Comprehensive Investigation of Posture Quality Prediction Using Machine Learning. In *ITM Web of Conferences* (Vol. 70, p. 02025). EDP Sciences. DOI: 10.1051/itmconf/20257002025

Zhang, L., & Li, J. (2023). *Deep learning and sustainable telemedicine*. IGI Global.

Zhang, N., Cai, Y.-X., Wang, Y.-Y., Tian, Y.-T., Wang, X.-L., & Badami, B. (2019). Skin Cancer Diagnosis Based on Optimized Convolutional Neural Network. *Artificial Intelligence in Medicine*, *101756*. Advance online publication. DOI: 10.1016/j.artmed.2019.101756 PMID: 31980095

Zhang, R., Zhou, Y., Zhang, J., & Zhao, J. (2024). Cloud-integrated robotics: Transforming healthcare and rehabilitation for individuals with disabilities. *Proceedings of the Indian National Science Academy. Part A, Physical Sciences*, *90*(3), 752–763. DOI: 10.1007/s43538-024-00264-3

Zhang, X., Huang, X., Ding, Y., Long, L., Li, W., & Xu, X. (2024). Advancements in smart wearable mobility aids for visual impairments: A bibliometric narrative review. *Sensors (Basel)*, *24*(24), 7986. Advance online publication. DOI: 10.3390/s24247986 PMID: 39771730

Zhang, Y., & Jiang, X. (2024). Recent Advances on Deep Learning for Sign Language Recognition. *Computer Modeling in Engineering & Sciences*, *139*(3), 2399–2450. DOI: 10.32604/cmes.2023.045731

Zhang, Y.-T., Zheng, Y.-L., Lin, W.-H., Zhang, H.-Y., & Zhou, X.-L. (2013, February). Challenges and Opportunities in Cardiovascular Health Informatics. *IEEE Transactions on Biomedical Engineering*, *60*(3), 633–642. DOI: 10.1109/TBME.2013.2244892 PMID: 23380853

Zhang, Z., Wen, F., Sun, Z., Guo, X., He, T., & Lee, C. (2022). Artificial intelligence-enabled sensing technologies in the 5G/internet of things era: From virtual reality/augmented reality to the digital twin. *Advanced Intelligent Systems*, *4*(7), 2100228. DOI: 10.1002/aisy.202100228

Zhao, X., & Liu, H. (2021). Secure data sharing and privacy protection in smart healthcare and assistive devices. *IEEE Access : Practical Innovations, Open Solutions*, *9*, 123456–123468.

Zheng, Z., Wang, P., Liu, W., Li, J., Ye, R., & Ren, D. (2020). Distance-IoU loss: Faster and better learning for bounding box regression. *Proceedings of the AAAI Conference on Artificial Intelligence*, *34*(07), 12993–13000. DOI: 10.1609/aaai.v34i07.6999

Zhou, H., Hou, K.-M., Zuo, D., & Li, J. (2012). Intelligent urban public transportation for accessibility dedicated to people with disabilities. *Sensors (Basel)*, *12*(8), 10678–10692. DOI: 10.3390/s120810678 PMID: 23112622

Zhou, S., Loiacono, E. T., & Kordzadeh, N. (2024). Smart cities for people with disabilities: A systematic literature review and future research directions. *European Journal of Information Systems*, *33*(6), 845–862. DOI: 10.1080/0960085X.2023.2297974

Zhou, Y. (2024). User experience of lower extremity exoskeletons and its improvement methodologies: A narrative review. *Proceedings of the Institution of Mechanical Engineers. Part H, Journal of Engineering in Medicine*, *238*(11-12), 1052–1068. DOI: 10.1177/09544119241291194 PMID: 39552186

Zorec, K., Desmond, D., Boland, T., McNicholl, A., O'Connor, A., Stafford, G., & Gallagher, P. (2024). A whole-campus approach to technology and inclusion of students with disabilities in higher education in Ireland. *Disability & Society*, *39*(5), 1147–1172. DOI: 10.1080/09687599.2022.2114885

Zou, B., Li, J., He, S., & Zhang, Y. 2023. Weather Influence on Road Safety: A Data-Driven Analysis. Transportation Research Interdisciplinary Perspectives, 16, 100617. Data.gov. n.d. 1.08 Crash Data Report (Detail). https://catalog.data.gov/dataset/1-08-crash-data-report-detail- 498c3.

Zwack, C. C., Haghani, M., Hollings, M., Zhang, L., Gauci, S., Gallagher, R., & Redfern, J. (2023). *The evolution of digital health technologies in cardiovascular disease research.* npj. *Digital Medicine*, *6*(1), 1. DOI: 10.1038/s41746-022-00781-7 PMID: 36596833

About the Contributors

Ikram Ur Rehman is an Associate Professor of Computer Science and Programme Lead for Health Informatics (MSc) at the School of Computing and Engineering, University of West London, United Kingdom. He has been involved in numerous national and international mHealth projects in areas such as chronic disease management, social robotics, decision support systems, behavioural change management, telehealth, and telecare in developing countries. In addition, he has played a key role in eLearning projects, focusing on integrating new technologies like AI-driven adaptive learning, VR/AR for immersive experiences, and data analytics to personalise education, particularly for those with disabilities. His innovative efforts have enhanced the accessibility, interactivity, and effectiveness of educational programmes globally. Ikram has authored over 45 journal articles, peer-reviewed conference papers, and book chapters. He serves on editorial boards, review panels for numerous transactions and journals, and is a committee member for many international conferences. He has been an invited speaker at various industrial, scientific, and governmental events. In recognition of his academic achievements and contributions to teaching, he has received several accolades, including Academic of the Year (2021-2024), Innovation in Teaching and Learning Award (2022), and Teaching Excellence Award (2022). He is a Senior Fellow of the Higher Education Academy (SFHEA) and a member of IEEE, ACM, and IET. Furthermore, he is the Vice Chair of the IEEE Smart Cities Awards and Recognition Committee.

Moustafa M. Nasralla is the Head of the Department of Communications and Networks Engineering and an Associate Professor at Prince Sultan University, Riyadh, Saudi Arabia. He chairs the IEEE Smart Cities Awards and Recognition Committee and leads the Smart Systems Engineering Laboratory at Prince Sultan University, where he focuses on integrating advanced technologies into education and urban systems. Dr. Nasralla has secured national and international funding for projects, including Intelli-Student, an AI-powered smart education platform funded by the British Council, and 5G-Enabled Smart City Development in Saudi Arabia. Dr. Nasralla actively promotes the application of smart technologies in education and research. He is instrumental in advancing smart education through initiatives such as the 5G-Enabled Smart Cities Workshop at IEEE Smart Cities Conferences and the International Conference on Sustainability. His research interests include 6G, 5G, IoT, wireless sensor networks, machine learning, and multimedia communications, with applications in personalised learning environments and adaptive education systems. Dr. Nasralla has published over 80 high-impact articles and has received several distinguished reviewer awards. As a Fellow of the Higher Education Academy, he is dedicated to fostering innovation in education and integrating smart technologies to empower future generations.

Drishty Sobnath is an Assistant Professor in Computer Science. Prior to joining Heriot Watt, she was a Senior Lecturer at Solent University, Southampton, UK, as well as the Programme Leader of BSc (Hons) Computer Science, BSc (Hons) Software Engineering and MSc Computer Engineering. She was awarded her PhD in Software Engineering (mHealth) from Kingston University, London. Her work included implementation and testing of IoT solutions, wearables, and mobile application development to improve lifestyle of patients suffering from Chronic Obstructive Pulmonary Disease (COPD) in the UK and Netherlands. She teaches courses at both undergraduate and postgraduate levels in the fields of Data Science and Artificial Intelligence.

Muazzam Ali Khan Khattak is a Professor of AI and Computer Science and the Director of Science and Technology at Quaid-i-Azam University (QAU), Islamabad, Pakistan. Renowned for his commitment to advancing education, he is listed among the top 2% of scientists worldwide as recognized by Stanford University. Dr. Khattak's extensive experience in academia spans teaching, research, and academic administration. He has supervised over 100 undergraduate, master's, and PhD students and introduced advanced educational programs, including specializations in Artificial Intelligence and Data Science. His work emphasizes fostering equitable learning environments and using AI-driven technologies to support students and enhance teaching methodologies. A prolific researcher with over 200 publications, Dr. Khattak has secured national and international funding for projects integrating AI and IoT into education and society. He has also developed tools such as a Learning Management System (LMS) to facilitate online education for affiliated colleges and contributed to the establishment of new academic programs and departments. His leadership extends to organizing international conferences and workshops focused on health, education, sustainability, and smart technologies.

Sundus Ali is an Associate Professor in the Department of Telecommunications Engineering at the Department of Telecommunications Engineering, NED University of Engineering and Technology, Pakistan. With over 17 years of professional experience and a Senior Member of IEEE and IEEE ComSoc, she is an accomplished researcher, mentor, and academic leader with a strong record in wireless communication, Internet of Things (IoT), and analytical modeling. With a PhD in Electronic Engineering, Dr. Ali has led and co-led multiple nationally and internationally funded projects, including HEC NRPU, Sindh HEC, MoST Endowment Fund, and the British Council's PAK-UK Education Gateway. Her recent initiatives focus on proximity services, smart environment monitoring, and sustainable technology solutions for climate action. Dr. Ali has authored over 28 peer-reviewed journal papers and 12 conference publications, earning the NEDUET Best Researcher Award and NEDAASC Best Teacher Award. She also serves as Manager of the Business Incubation Center at NED University and Chairperson of the Academic Industry Council at National Incubation Center Karachi, where she drives university–industry collaboration, startup mentoring, and commercialization of research. Beyond academia, she is actively engaged in community and professional development, having organized and chaired several international conferences, delivered keynote talks, and facilitated capacity-building programs under Higher Education Commission, UNIDO, and FPCCI (Chambers of Commerce). With her blend of technical expertise, research excellence, and leadership in innovation ecosystems, Dr. Ali is committed to shaping the future of sustainable and inclusive technological development in Pakistan and beyond. She has supervised multiple postgraduate and doctoral theses, fostering a research culture that integrates innovation, sustainability, and societal relevance. Through her research, mentorship, and leadership in academic–industry ecosystems, Dr. Sundus Ali continues to play a transformative role in advancing Pakistan's technological capacity, particularly in IoT-driven environmental solutions, smart cities, and resilient communication systems. Her career reflects an enduring commitment to using science, innovation, and education as tools for sustainable development and positive societal change.

***

Mahapara Abbass is a distinguished academician and researcher in the Department of Civil Engineering at Maharishi Markandeshwar (Deemed to be University), renowned for her groundbreaking contributions to structural engineering and sustainable construction materials. With an impressive portfolio of publications in prestigious SCI and Scopus-indexed journals, including Multiscale Multidisciplinary Modeling, Experimentation and Design, and Lecture Notes in Civil Engineering, Dr. Abbass has also presented her work at esteemed conferences and authored/co-authored book chapters in critically acclaimed volumes, such as Advances in Geotechnics and Structural Engineering. Her expertise in geopolymer concrete, sustainable construction practices, and innovative materials has been recognized through publications in esteemed platforms like Elsevier, cementing her prominent role in advancing the frontiers of civil engineering.

Shalom Akhai has established himself as a prominent figure in the field of engineering, leveraging over 17 years of academic, research, and technical experience to make significant contributions. With a robust portfolio of over 50 publications in prestigious journals and conferences, Dr. Akhai demonstrates a commitment to advancing knowledge through scholarly work. Additionally, he has authored/co-authored several technical textbooks, further solidifying his expertise and dedication to education in the field. Beyond academia, Dr. Akhai's impact extends to real-world applications through the establishment of IGNIS Technical Solutions, a consultancy firm to translate his knowledge into real-world applications. His skills have resulted in the successful development of over 50 patents+, underscoring his innovative approach and influence in shaping the engineering landscape.

Meshall Alshalaan is pursuing a B.S in Computer Engineering at the University of California, San Diego and is a current member of the KAUST Gifted Student Program.

|Jaithun Shifaya B S - Contributing Author|Jaithun Shifaya is currently pursuing their Bachelor's degree in Information Technology at Velammal College of Engineering and Technology, Madurai. They are passionate about artificial intelligence, full-stack development, and academic research. They have presented a research paper on stock price prediction using machine learning at the Springer PEIS conference hosted by NIT Uttarakhand. They are also actively involved in developing AI-powered web applications that solve real-world problems.

Heba Elshimy is an academic and researcher in the field of Data and AI. Their research interests pertain to the application of deep learning in healthcare, especially in imaging diagnostics, decision support and explainability (xAI) of deep learning models in this domain.

Bulent Gursel Emiroğlu is working at Kırıkkale University. His research interest is Artificial Intelligence, Machine Learning, Deep Learning, Educational technology, Distance education.

Ghulam Fiza holds a Joint Master's degree in Telecommunication Engineering and Management from the University of Málaga, Spain, and Mehran University of

Engineering and Technology (MUET), Jamshoro. She is currently engaged in teaching and research in the Department of Telecommunications Engineering at NED University of Engineering and Technology, Karachi, Pakistan. Her experience includes academic and research roles at the University of Málaga, MUET, and University of Sindh. She has contributed to national projects under the HEC's National Centre of Robotics and Automation, focusing on intelligent monitoring systems for transportation infrastructure. Her research spans IoT, wireless sensor networks, machine and deep learning, 5G/6G technologies, image processing, and wireless body area networks. She is also active in international collaborations such as the PAK-UK Education Gateway Mobility Partnership.

Ananya Ganapathi is pursuing B.Tech at Amrita Vishwa Vidyapeetham,India

Fouzi Harrou received the M.Sc. degree in telecommunications and networking from the University of Paris VI, France, and the Ph.D. degree in systems optimization and security from the University of Technology of Troyes (UTT), France. He was an Assistant Professor with UTT for one year and with the Institute of Automotive and Transport Engineering, Nevers, France, for one year. He was also a Postdoctoral Research Associate with the Systems Modeling and Dependability Laboratory, UTT, for one year. He was a Research Scientist with the Chemical Engineering Department, Texas A&M University at Qatar, Doha, Qatar, for three years. He is actually a Senior Research Scientist with the Division of Computer, Electrical and Mathematical Sciences and Engineering, King Abdullah University of Science and Technology. His current research interests include statistical decision theory and its applications, fault detection and diagnosis, and deep learning. He is co-author of two books: "Statistical Process Monitoring Using Advanced Data-Driven and Deep Learning Approaches: Theory and Practical Applications" (Elsevier, 2020), and Advanced Road Traffic Modelling and Management Using Statistical and Deep Learning Methods, (Elsevier, 2021). He received two IEEE ECBIOS 2021 best paper awards and the Best Session Paper Award at the IEEE IPAS 2025 conference. Dr. Harrou is featured in Stanford University's list of the world's Top 2% scientists for 2020-2024.

Majida Kazmi has an extensive experience in the field of Artificial Intelligence and Embedded Computer Vision. Currently, she serves as an Associate Professor at NED University of Engineering and Technology, Karachi, Pakistan, and also holds key research positions, including Co-Principal Investigator at the Neurocomputation Lab under the National Centre of Artificial Intelligence, Head of the Embedded Systems and Computer Vision Lab and founding director of Asma M Hashmi STEM Centre. Her contributions to AI and technology have earned her multiple prestigious awards, including the National Engineering Excellence Gold Medal 2025, House of Habib, Ali Suleman Habib 2nd and 3rd Engineering Excellence Awards (2023, 2024), and the National Engineering Excellence Award 2024, FPCCI Talent of Pakistan 2024 underscoring her dedication to innovation and educational leadership.

Yogita Lamba is a final-year International Relations student at the IGNOU. She received a bachelor's degree in physics and computer science from Maitreyi College, University of Delhi and a master's degree in astrophysics from Amity University, Noida. Her current research focuses on the intersection of technology and society, with a particular interest in digitalization strategies for the vulnerable sections of the society. Through her work, Yogita aims to contribute to the development of inclusive technological solutions that address the unique challenges faced by older adults in a rapidly digitalizing world.

Nthabiseng Istorina Mahetlana is a Lecturer in the Department of Inclusive Education at the University of South Africa. She worked in the Department of Education for more than 15 years. Her specialization is in Inclusive Education. Her research interests are student support and reading difficulties. Dr Mahetlana is an active member of the scholarship projects that are engaged in the department.

Hira Mariam received the BE and M.Engg. in Telecommunication Engineering degrees in 2008 and 2011, and PhD in Electronic Engineering from NEDUET in 2021. She joined NEDUET in 2009, where she is involved in teaching undergraduate programme. She has an extensive teaching, research and administrative experience. Her research interests include 5G/6G communications, UAVs, deep learning and IoT networks.

Ajay Menon is a Computer Science graduate from Heriot-Watt University, Dubai (First-Class Honours). His research interests include machine learning, natural language processing, large language models, and intelligent systems, with academic and industry experience in developing AI-driven solutions.

Ratish Palanisamy holds a Bachelor's degree with First Class Honors in Computer Science from Heriot-Watt University. His work explores deep learning-based skin cancer detection systems to assist caregivers and dermatologists in monitoring visually impaired individuals, achieving high accuracy in lesion classification. His research interests include computer vision, AI/ML and NLP.

Sneha T Raghavan is pursuing her B.Tech CSE at Amrita Vishwa Vidyapeetham,India

Mehwish Raza received the Bachelor of Engineer- ing (B.E.) degree in Computer Engineering in 2012, and the Master of Engineering (M.E.) degree in Com- puter Architectures and System Designs in 2015, both from NED University of Engineering & Technology, Karachi, Pakistan. She is currently pursuing the Ph.D. in Computer Engineering, with a focus on the energy- efficient implementation of deep neural networks on FPGAs. She is serving as Lecturer in the Department of Computer and Information Systems Engineering at NED University of Engineering & Technology. Her research interests include approximate computing, edge computing, vision sensor nodes, and FPGA-based design solutions.

Thangam S. currently serves as an Assistant Professor (SG) at the Amrita School of Computing, Bengaluru.,Amrita Vishwa Vidyapeetham, India. Her area of interest in research includes Service Oriented Architecture, Networks, IoT, Artificial Intelligence, Data Structures and Cloud Computing. She completed her Ph. D. in Computer Science and Engineering from Anna University, Chennai. India. She has 26 years of teaching experience. She has published her research works in 25 international journals and conferences. She is a member of ISTE..

Deivanai Saravanan is pursuing her B.Tech CSE at Amrita Vishwa Vidyapeetham,India

Ajay K. Singh is working as an Associate Professor (Research) in the Department of Humanities and Social Science, Graphic Era (Deemed to be University) Dehradun. He has worked as Assistant Professor (Economics) in the School of Liberal Arts & Management, DIT University Dehradun for 6 years. He did Post-Doctorate Research with EDI of India, Ahmedabad, Gujarat (India). He received MPhil (Economics) from DAVV Indore (India), and PhD (Economics) from IIT Indore (India. He has published several research papers in the diversified area such as climate change, agricultural productivity, assessment of food security; estimation of GFSI, development of environmental sustainability index (ESI) and its association with socio-economic indicators; measurement and determinants of entrepreneurship ecosystem, and dimension of sustainable development and its interlinkages with economic development.

Ying Sun received the Ph.D. degree in statistics from Texas A&M, in 2011. She held a two-year postdoctoral research position at the Statistical and Applied Mathematical Sciences Institute and the University of Chicago. She was an Assistant Professor with Ohio State University for a year before joining KAUST, in 2014. At KAUST, she established and leads the Environmental Statistics research group, which works on developing statistical models and methods for complex data to address important environmental problems. She has made original contributions to environmental statistics, in particular in the areas of spatiotemporal statistics, functional data analysis, visualization, computational statistics, with an exceptionally broad array of applications. She received two prestigious awards: The Early Investigator Award in Environmental Statistics presented by the American Statistical Association and the Abdel El-Shaarawi Young Research Award from The International Environmetrics Society.

Srinivasan Vasan is an Assistant Professor in the Department of Humanities and Social Sciences at Graphic Era (Deemed to be University), with 14 years of teaching and field expertise. He has served in the Ministry of Health and Family Welfare, as a Guest Faculty, and as a Mobilization Training Specialist with the State Government. Recently, he contributed to a tuberculosis project funded by GFATM and USAID. He has published 60 papers, with 20 more under peer review in UGC-CARE and SCOPUS journals.

Fauzia Yasir received the B.E. and M.E. degrees in computer systems engineering from the NED University of Engineering and Technology, Karachi, Pakistan, in 2007 and 2014 respectively. Since 2013, she has been serving as Lecturer with the Department of Computer and Information Systems Engineering, NED University of Engineering and Technology.She is currently pursuing the Ph.D. degree and holds a key research position of Co-Principal Investigator of the Embedded Systems and Computer Vision Lab. Her research interests include digital systems design, digital image processing, natural language processing, language digitization and computer vision. She was a recipient of the House of Habib, Ali Suleman Habib Gold Medal and Engineering Excellence Award 2024.

Index

A

Accelerometer 123, 207, 208, 209, 210, 211, 212, 213, 214, 215, 216, 217, 218, 219, 220, 222, 223, 228, 230, 232, 234, 235, 448, 449, 450, 453, 454, 455, 457, 458, 461
Adaptive Prosthetics 396
AI 3, 5, 6, 8, 12, 16, 20, 34, 35, 42, 46, 47, 48, 49, 50, 53, 54, 56, 57, 61, 62, 63, 64, 66, 67, 69, 70, 71, 72, 73, 75, 76, 77, 78, 79, 80, 81, 82, 83, 84, 85, 86, 87, 88, 89, 90, 91, 92, 93, 94, 95, 96, 97, 98, 99, 100, 101, 102, 103, 104, 105, 106, 107, 108, 109, 110, 111, 112, 113, 114, 115, 116, 117, 119, 120, 121, 122, 123, 129, 133, 134, 135, 136, 137, 138, 139, 140, 141, 142, 143, 144, 145, 146, 147, 148, 149, 150, 151, 152, 153, 154, 155, 156, 157, 158, 159, 160, 161, 162, 163, 164, 165, 167, 169, 174, 177, 178, 179, 181, 185, 186, 194, 195, 196, 197, 198, 200, 225, 227, 235, 286, 309, 319, 320, 321, 322, 328, 340, 341, 347, 348, 349, 352, 353, 355, 357, 359, 360, 361, 363, 364, 366, 369, 370, 374, 375, 376, 378, 379, 380, 381, 382, 383, 384, 385, 386, 387, 388, 391, 396, 398, 400, 401, 402, 403, 436, 438, 439, 440
AI Integration 79, 359, 361, 381
Assistive Technology 3, 4, 11, 22, 36, 39, 40, 42, 68, 71, 72, 73, 150, 157, 162, 165, 273, 309, 386, 388, 390, 395, 441, 445, 463
Augmentation 146, 195, 207, 241, 246, 250, 252, 259, 261, 264, 265, 268, 271, 275, 284, 286, 287, 290, 291, 295, 296, 297, 299, 302, 303, 304, 305, 307, 308, 309, 397, 412, 416, 417, 435

C

Cerebral Palsy 128, 226, 358, 360, 366, 369, 370, 371, 382, 396, 443, 444, 446, 447, 448, 450, 452, 453, 458, 459, 462, 463, 464, 465
Cloud 20, 47, 79, 80, 82, 86, 88, 91, 113, 117, 130, 135, 136, 140, 144, 149, 164, 173, 199, 227, 321, 323, 324, 325, 328, 329, 330, 337, 341, 343, 345, 361, 368, 387, 395, 440, 444, 445, 448, 450, 451, 455, 457, 458, 459, 462
CNNs 82, 132, 133, 240, 241, 245, 247, 253, 254, 255, 259, 260, 261, 270, 274, 280, 282, 398, 404, 406, 407, 410, 411, 412
Computer Vision 119, 122, 133, 158, 166, 178, 230, 239, 241, 270, 273, 274, 277, 279, 280, 281, 309, 311, 312, 314, 322, 397, 398, 402, 403, 405, 406, 407, 408, 415, 440
ConvNeXt-T 411, 412

D

Deep Learning 77, 78, 79, 81, 82, 83, 86, 90, 100, 105, 110, 111, 113, 114, 118, 129, 132, 158, 162, 163, 166, 206, 207, 208, 209, 210, 212, 224, 228, 230, 231, 232, 233, 234, 239, 243, 244, 250, 269, 273, 274, 280, 282, 283, 284, 286, 297, 307, 308, 309, 311, 312, 313, 314, 393, 397, 398, 399, 402, 403, 404, 408, 412, 414, 415, 416, 418, 435, 437, 438, 439, 441
DenseNet 237, 254, 263, 265, 407, 408
Detection Stability 297
Digital Technology 1, 2, 8, 92, 118, 392
Disabilities 1, 2, 3, 4, 5, 6, 7, 8, 9, 10, 11, 12, 13, 14, 15, 16, 17, 18, 19, 20, 22, 23, 34, 35, 36, 38, 39, 40, 41, 42, 43, 44, 45, 46, 47, 48, 49, 50, 51, 52, 53, 54, 55, 56, 57, 58, 59, 60, 61, 62, 63, 65, 66, 67, 68, 69, 70, 71, 72, 73, 74, 79, 99, 100, 102, 103, 119, 124, 125, 129, 137, 145, 148, 149, 151, 155, 156, 160, 163, 164, 165, 166, 167,

168, 170, 173, 176, 177, 178, 180, 182, 185, 195, 196, 197, 200, 205, 206, 211, 225, 226, 227, 269, 273, 291, 308, 310, 312, 315, 316, 317, 318, 319, 320, 321, 323, 325, 327, 329, 331, 334, 336, 342, 350, 351, 352, 353, 354, 355, 357, 358, 359, 361, 364, 365, 369, 371, 372, 375, 376, 377, 379, 380, 381, 382, 385, 388, 395, 441, 444, 465
Disability Rehabilitation 357, 358, 359, 361, 363, 378, 379, 380, 381

E

EfficientNet 237, 250, 253, 263, 268, 409
EfficientNetV2-L 397, 410, 412, 415, 417, 418, 419, 421, 422, 423, 424, 427, 428, 431, 432, 434, 435, 439
Elbow Movement 453, 454, 458

F

Fall Detection 17, 19, 203, 204, 205, 206, 207, 208, 209, 210, 211, 212, 213, 215, 216, 217, 218, 219, 220, 222, 223, 224, 225, 226, 227, 228, 230, 231, 232, 233, 234, 235
Flex Sensors 444, 448, 452, 457, 458, 462

G

Generalization 192, 204, 207, 209, 212, 217, 229, 239, 241, 244, 250, 255, 259, 266, 268, 271, 274, 281, 282, 284, 286, 295, 297, 299, 301, 304, 417, 422, 435
Gesture Recognition 100, 158, 239, 255, 256, 257, 271, 283, 284, 297

H

Hand Gesture Recognition 257, 271
Healthcare Technology 85, 385
Higher Education 45, 46, 47, 48, 49, 50, 51, 54, 55, 58, 60, 61, 62, 63, 65, 66, 67, 68, 69, 70, 71, 72, 73, 74

I

Inclusive Innovation 382
Intelligent Transportation System 138, 166, 173, 182, 198, 199
Intelligent Transport System 200
Internet of Things 47, 79, 80, 85, 86, 93, 100, 117, 119, 135, 166, 319, 353, 354, 383, 384, 396, 439, 463

L

Lightweight Models 297

M

Malignant Lesion 430
MobileNetV2 237, 245, 246, 252, 254, 262, 263, 268, 270, 272
MQTT Protocol 447, 451, 462

N

Natural Language Processing 81, 97, 100, 119, 133, 166, 277, 281, 284, 402, 403, 411
Neurorehabilitation 367, 381, 392

P

Poor Vision 125

Q

Quality of Life 1, 2, 3, 4, 5, 6, 8, 9, 14, 16, 17, 18, 31, 33, 34, 35, 38, 40, 42, 45, 47, 99, 102, 204, 225, 226, 315, 316, 319, 322, 332, 351, 352, 359, 360, 363, 368, 371, 372, 390, 392, 398, 443, 444, 445, 453

R

Real-Time Monitoring 81, 87, 119, 204, 206, 227, 360, 366, 368, 381, 382, 445, 458, 465
Rehabilitation 39, 40, 41, 42, 60, 68, 71,

73, 82, 84, 88, 89, 91, 99, 102, 103, 110, 157, 233, 238, 357, 358, 359, 360, 361, 362, 363, 364, 365, 366, 367, 368, 369, 370, 376, 378, 379, 380, 381, 382, 383, 385, 386, 387, 388, 389, 390, 391, 392, 393, 394, 395, 396, 444, 445, 446, 447, 448, 452, 455, 458, 462, 463, 464, 465
ResNet 210, 237, 247, 250, 251, 252, 253, 254, 262, 263, 268, 272, 285, 408, 409, 411, 412, 415, 416, 417, 418, 421, 422, 423, 424, 426, 427, 428, 430, 431, 432, 434, 435, 437, 438, 439
Resnet-101 251, 254, 263, 408, 409, 412, 415, 416, 417, 418, 421, 422, 423, 424, 426, 427, 428, 430, 431, 432, 434, 435, 438
Risk Prediction 87, 89, 113, 181, 188, 192, 198, 210

S

Sign Language Recognition 269, 270, 273, 274, 275, 277, 282, 283, 290, 297, 308, 310, 311, 312, 313, 314
Skin Lesion 405, 406, 407, 409, 411, 412, 413, 415, 416, 434, 438, 439, 441
Smart Materials 319, 355, 357, 358, 359, 360, 361, 362, 363, 364, 365, 366, 367, 368, 377, 378, 379, 380, 381, 382, 385, 387, 388, 389, 390, 394, 396
Smart Systems 18, 73, 114, 315, 316, 317, 318, 319, 320, 322, 323, 325, 326, 327, 329, 330, 331, 332, 333, 335, 336, 342, 346, 347, 348, 349, 350, 351, 352, 355, 437
Smart Technology 2, 3, 4, 7, 17, 21, 40, 137, 323, 326, 350
Smartwatch 203, 204, 207, 208, 210, 211, 212, 213, 214, 215, 216, 218, 219, 220, 223, 224, 228, 230, 233, 321
Students With Disabilities 45, 46, 47, 48, 49, 50, 51, 52, 53, 54, 55, 56, 57, 58, 59, 60, 61, 62, 63, 65, 66, 69, 72, 74

T

Traffic Safety 133, 167, 175, 178, 181, 185, 190, 194
Transfer Learning 147, 210, 237, 239, 245, 252, 254, 255, 262, 263, 268, 272, 282, 310, 397, 408, 410, 412, 418, 423, 432, 442

V

VGG 237, 252, 263, 265, 407, 408, 437
Vision Transformers 237, 257, 263, 271, 406, 411, 437
ViT-B 411, 412, 416, 417, 418, 420, 421, 422, 423, 425, 426, 427, 428, 431, 432, 434, 435

W

Wearable 7, 17, 19, 55, 64, 71, 76, 85, 86, 87, 88, 89, 91, 92, 93, 94, 95, 99, 100, 110, 112, 116, 139, 140, 144, 159, 166, 174, 184, 204, 206, 209, 210, 213, 215, 224, 225, 228, 231, 232, 233, 279, 280, 281, 316, 320, 354, 359, 360, 361, 364, 367, 368, 373, 374, 375, 381, 382, 385, 388, 391, 393, 394, 395, 402, 437, 443, 444, 445, 448, 457, 458, 459, 462, 464, 465

Y

YOLOv5 274, 283, 286, 296, 297, 298, 299, 300, 302, 303, 305, 307, 308, 309, 313

www.ingramcontent.com/pod-product-compliance
Lightning Source LLC
LaVergne TN
LVHW081316300926
849161LV00008B/1780